BMA

The British
Medical Association

CONCISE GUIDE TO
MEDICINES
AND DRUGS

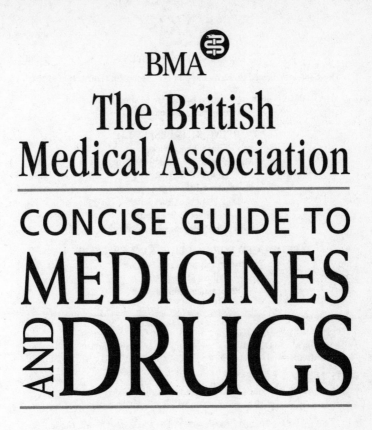

BMA
The British Medical Association

CONCISE GUIDE TO
MEDICINES
AND DRUGS

Chief Medical Editor

PROFESSOR JOHN A. HENRY MB FRCP

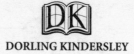

DORLING KINDERSLEY

This book is dedicated to the memory of Professor John Henry (1939–2007)

BMA Consulting Medical Editor Dr. Michael Peters MB BS
Contributor Ann Peters RGN

DORLING KINDERSLEY LTD
Editor Laura Nickoll
Managing Editor Adèle Hayward
Designer Vicky Read
Senior Art Editor Helen Spencer
DTP Designer Traci Salter
Art Director Peter Luff
Category Publisher Stephanie Jackson

PRODUCED FOR DORLING KINDERSLEY BY
Project Editor Teresa Pritlove
Editor Martyn Page
Proofreader Ann Baggaley

First UK Edition 2001
Second UK Edition 2005
Third UK Edition 2007, reprinted 2009 (with corrections)
The British Medical Association Concise Guide to Medicines and Drugs is based on
The British Medical Association New Guide to Medicines and Drugs (7th edition)
6 8 10 9 7 5

Published in the United Kingdom by Dorling Kindersley Limited
80 Strand, London WC2R 0RL, England

A CIP catalogue record for this book is available from the British Library
ISBN: 978-1-40532-640-7

Printed and bound in Great Britain by Clays Ltd. St Ives plc

see our complete catalogue at
www.dk.com

CONTENTS

INTRODUCTION

The British Medical Association Concise Guide to Medicines and Drugs provides clear information and practical advice on drugs and medicines that can be readily understood by a non-medical reader. The text reflects current medical knowledge and standard medical practice in this country. It is intended to complement and reinforce the advice of your doctor.

The book is divided into three parts. The first part covers the major groups of drugs. The second part gives detailed information about 260 individual drugs, arranged alphabetically. The third part consists of the drug finder and index.

PART 1: MAJOR DRUG GROUPS

This part of the book is subdivided into sections on each body system or major disease grouping. It contains descriptions of the principal drug groups and information on the uses, actions, effects, and risks associated with each. Common drugs in each group are listed to allow cross-reference to Part 2.

A–Z OF DRUGS

This part consists of profiles of 260 key drugs. Each profile gives detailed information and practical advice and is intended to provide reference and guidance for non-medical readers taking drug treatment. It is impossible, however, to take into account every variation in individual circumstances; readers should always follow a doctor's or pharmacist's instructions where they differ from the advice in this section.

The drugs have been selected to provide representative coverage of the principal classes of drugs in medical use today. For some disorders, a number of drugs are available and the most commonly used drugs have been chosen. Emphasis has also been placed on the drugs likely to be used in the home, although in a few cases drugs administered only in hospital have been included when the drug has been judged to be of sufficient general interest.

HOW TO UNDERSTAND THE PROFILES

For ease of reference, the information on each drug is arranged in a consistent format under standard headings.

Drug name Tells you the drug's generic name, brand names under which the drug is marketed, and combined preparations that contain the drug.

Quick reference Summarizes important facts regarding the drug.

General information Gives a brief summary of the drug's important characteristics.

Information for users Practical information on how and when to take the drug, the usual recommended dosage, how soon it takes effect, how long it is active, and advice on diet, storage, and missed doses.

Overdose action Indicates the symptoms that may occur if an overdose has been taken and tells you what immediate action is required.

Possible adverse effects Indicates adverse effects that may be experienced with the drug.

Interactions Tells you how the drug may interact with other drugs or substances taken at the same time.

Special precautions Describes circumstances in which the drug should be taken with special caution or in which it might not be suitable.

Prolonged use Tells you what effects the drug may have when taken long term and what monitoring may be advised.

PART 3: DRUG FINDER AND INDEX

The combined drug finder and index provides basic information on over 2,500 generic and brand-name drugs and drug groups and directs you to further information about them throughout the book.

PART 1

MAJOR DRUG GROUPS

Subdivided into sections dealing with each body system (such as heart and circulation) or major disease grouping (such as malignant and immune disease), this part of the book contains descriptions of the principal classes of drugs (such as corticosteroids), with information on the uses, actions, effects, and risks associated with each group of drugs. Individual drugs common to each group are listed to allow cross-reference to Part 2.

BRAIN AND NERVOUS SYSTEM

The human brain contains more than 100 billion nerve cells (neurons). These nerve cells receive electrochemical impulses from everywhere in the body. They interpret these impulses and send responsive signals back to various glands and muscles. The brain functions continuously as a switchboard for the human communications system. At the same time, it serves as the seat of emotions and mood, of memory, personality, and thought. Extending from the brain is an additional, large rod-shaped cluster of nerve cells that forms the spinal cord. Together, these two elements comprise the central nervous system.

Radiating from the central nervous system is the peripheral nervous system, which has three parts. One branches off the spinal cord and extends to skin and muscles throughout the body. Another, in the head, links the brain to the eyes, ears, nose, and taste buds. The third is a semi-independent network called the autonomic, or involuntary, nervous system. This is the part of the nervous system that controls unconscious body functions such as breathing, digestion, and glandular activity (see facing page).

Signals traverse the nervous system by electrical and chemical means. Electrical impulses carry signals from one end of a neuron to the other. To cross the gap between neurons, chemical neurotransmitters are released from one cell to bind on to the receptor sites of nearby cells. Excitatory transmitters stimulate action; inhibitory transmitters reduce it.

WHAT CAN GO WRONG

Disorders of the brain and nervous system may manifest as illnesses that show themselves as physical impairments, such as epilepsy or strokes, or mental and emotional impairments (for example, schizophrenia or depression).

Illnesses causing physical impairments can result from different types of disorder of the brain and nervous system. Death of nerve cells resulting from poor circulation can result in paralysis, while electrical disturbances of certain nerve cells cause the fits of epilepsy. Temporary changes in blood circulation within and around the brain are thought to

cause migraine. Parkinson's disease is caused by a lack of dopamine, a neurotransmitter that is produced by specialized brain cells.

The causes of disorders that trigger mental and emotional impairment are not known, but these illnesses are thought to result from the defective functioning of nerve cells and neurotransmitters. The nerve cells may be underactive, overactive, or poorly coordinated. Alternatively, mental and emotional impairment may be due to too much or too little neurotransmitter in one area of the brain.

WHY DRUGS ARE USED

By and large, the drugs described in this section do not eliminate nervous system disorders. Their function is to correct or modify the communication of the signals that traverse the nervous system. By doing so they can relieve symptoms or restore normal functioning and behaviour. In some cases, such as anxiety and insomnia, drugs are used to lower the level of activity in the brain. In other disorders (depression, for example) drugs are given to encourage the opposite effect, increasing the level of activity.

Drugs that act on the nervous system are also used for conditions that outwardly have nothing to do with nervous system disorders. Migraine headaches, for example, are often treated with drugs that cause the autonomic nervous system to send out signals constricting the dilated blood vessels that cause the migraine.

AUTONOMIC NERVOUS SYSTEM

The autonomic, or involuntary, nervous system governs the actions of the muscles of the organs and glands. Such vital functions as heart beat and digestion continue without conscious direction, whether we are awake or asleep.

The autonomic nervous system is divided into two parts: the sympathetic and parasympathetic nervous systems. The effects of one generally balance those of the other; the sympathetic has a mainly excitatory effect, while the parasympathetic, by contrast, has an opposite effect.

Although the functional pace of most organs results from the interplay between the two systems, the muscles in the blood vessel walls respond only to the signals of the sympathetic nervous system. Whether a vessel is dilated or constricted is determined by the relative stimulation of two sets of receptor sites: alpha sites and beta sites.

Blood vessels in the skin These are constricted by stimulation of alpha receptors by the sympathetic; the parasympathetic has no effect on them.

The heart The rate and strength of the heart are increased by the sympathetic and reduced by the parasympathetic.

The pupils These are dilated by the sympathetic and constricted by the parasympathetic.

The airways The bronchial muscles are relaxed and widened by the sympathetic and contracted and narrowed by the parasympathetic.

Intestines The activity of the intestinal wall muscles is reduced by the sympathetic and increased by the parasympathetic.

NEUROTRANSMITTERS

The sympathetic nervous system relies on epinephrine (adrenaline) and norepinephrine (noradrenaline), products of the adrenal glands, and neurons that act as both hormones and neurotransmitters. The parasympathetic nervous system depends on the neurotransmitter acetylcholine to transmit signals from cell to cell.

DRUGS THAT ACT ON THE SYMPATHETIC NERVOUS SYSTEM

The drugs that stimulate the sympathetic nervous system are called adrenergics (or sympathomimetics). They either promote the release of epinephrine (adrenaline) and norepinephrine (noradrenaline) or mimic their effects. Drugs that interfere with the action of the sympathetic nervous system are called sympatholytics. Alpha blockers act on alpha receptors; beta blockers act on beta receptors (see also Beta blockers, p.30).

DRUGS THAT ACT ON THE PARA-SYMPATHETIC NERVOUS SYSTEM

Drugs that stimulate the parasympathetic nervous system are called cholinergics (or para-

sympathomimetics); drugs that oppose its action are called anticholinergics. Many prescribed drugs have anticholinergic properties.

MAJOR DRUG GROUPS
◆ Analgesics
◆ Sleeping drugs
◆ Anti-anxiety drugs
◆ Antidepressant drugs
◆ Antipsychotic drugs
◆ Antimanic drugs
◆ Anticonvulsant drugs
◆ Drugs for parkinsonism
◆ Drugs for dementia
◆ Nervous system stimulants
◆ Drugs used for migraine
◆ Anti-emetics

Analgesics

Analgesics (painkillers) are drugs that relieve pain. Since pain is not a disease but a symptom, long-term relief depends on treatment of the underlying cause. For example, the pain of toothache can be relieved by drugs but can be cured only by appropriate dental treatment. If the underlying disorder, such as some rheumatic conditions, is irreversible, long-term analgesic treatment may be necessary.

Damage to body tissues as a result of disease or injury is detected by nerve endings that transmit signals to the brain. Interpretation of these sensations can be affected by a person's psychological state, so that pain is worsened by anxiety and fear, for example. Often a reassuring explanation of the cause of discomfort can make pain easier to bear and may even relieve it altogether. Anti-anxiety drugs (see p.13) are helpful when pain is accompanied by anxiety, and some of these drugs are also used to reduce painful muscle spasms. Some antidepressants (see p.14) act to block the transmission of impulses signalling pain and are particularly useful for nerve pains (neuralgia), which do not always respond to analgesics.

TYPES OF ANALGESIC

Analgesics are divided into the opioids (with similar properties to drugs derived from opium, such as morphine) and non-opioids. Non-opioids include all the other analgesics, including paracetamol, nefopam, and also non-steroidal anti-inflammatory drugs (NSAIDs), the most well known of which is aspirin. The non-opioids are all less powerful as painkillers than the opioids. Local anaesthetics (see facing page) are also used to relieve pain.

Opioid drugs and paracetamol act directly on the brain and spinal cord to alter the perception of pain. Opioids act like the endorphins, hormones naturally produced in the brain that stop the cell-to-cell transmission of pain sensation. NSAIDs prevent stimulation of the nerve endings at the site of the pain.

When pain is treated under medical supervision, it is common to start with paracetamol or an NSAID; if neither provides adequate pain relief, they may be combined. A mild opioid such as codeine may also be used. If the less powerful drugs are ineffective, a strong opioid such as morphine may be given. As there is now a wide variety of oral analgesic formulations, injections are seldom necessary to control even the most severe pain.

When using an over-the-counter preparation (for example, taking aspirin for a headache) you should seek medical advice if pain persists for longer than 48 hours, recurs, or is worse or different from previous pain.

NON-OPIOID ANALGESICS

Paracetamol This analgesic is believed to act by reducing the production of chemicals called prostaglandins in the brain. However, paracetamol does not affect prostaglandin production in the rest of the body, so it does not reduce inflammation, although it can reduce fever. Paracetamol can be used for everyday aches and pains, such as headaches, toothache, and joint pains. It is given as liquid to treat pain and reduce fever in children.

As well as being the most widely used analgesic, it is one of the safest when taken correctly. It does not usually irritate the stomach and allergic reactions are rare. However, an overdose can cause severe and possibly fatal liver or kidney damage. Its toxic potential may be increased in heavy drinkers.

Non-steroidal anti-inflammatory drugs (NSAIDs): aspirin Used for many years to relieve pain and reduce fever, aspirin also reduces inflammation by blocking the production of prostaglandins, which contribute to the swelling

and pain in inflamed tissue. Aspirin is useful for headaches, toothache, mild rheumatic pain, sore throat, and discomfort caused by feverish illnesses. Given regularly, it can also relieve the pain and inflammation of chronic rheumatoid arthritis (see Antirheumatic drugs, p.51).

Aspirin is found in combination with other substances in a variety of medicines (see Cold cures, p.28). It is also used in the treatment of some blood disorders, since aspirin helps to prevent abnormal clotting (see Drugs that affect blood clotting, p.38). For this reason, it is not suitable for people whose blood does not clot normally.

Aspirin in the form of soluble tablets, dissolved in water before being taken, is absorbed into the bloodstream more quickly, thereby relieving pain faster than tablets. Soluble aspirin is not less irritating to the stomach lining, however.

Aspirin is available in many forms, all of which have a similar effect, but because the amount of aspirin in a tablet of each type varies, it is important to read the packet for the correct dosage. It is not recommended for children aged under 16 years because its use has been linked to Reye's syndrome, a rare but potentially fatal liver and brain disorder.

Other non-steroidal anti-inflammatory drugs (NSAIDs) These drugs can relieve both pain and inflammation. NSAIDs are related to aspirin and also work by blocking the production of prostaglandins. They are most commonly used to treat muscle and joint pain and may also be prescribed for other types of pain including period pain. For further information on these drugs, see p.50.

COMBINED ANALGESICS

Mild opioids, such as codeine, are often found in combination preparations with non-opioids, such as paracetamol. The prefix "co-" is used to denote a drug combination. Although both opioids and paracetamol act centrally, these mixtures have the advantage of combining different mechanisms of action. Another advantage of combining analgesics is that the reductions in dose of the components may reduce the side effects of the preparation. Combinations can be helpful in reducing the number of tablets taken during long-term treatment.

OPIOID ANALGESICS

These drugs are related to opium, an extract of poppy seeds. They act directly on several sites in the central nervous system to block the transmission of pain signals. Because they act directly on the parts of the brain where pain is perceived, opioids are the strongest analgesics and are therefore used to treat the pain arising from surgery, serious injury, and cancer. These drugs are particularly valuable for relieving severe pain during terminal illnesses. In addition, their ability to produce a state of relaxation and euphoria is often of help in relieving the stress that accompanies severe pain.

Morphine is the best-known opioid analgesic. Others include diamorphine (heroin) and pethidine. The use of these powerful opioids is strictly controlled because the euphoria produced can lead to abuse and addiction. When these opioids are given under medical supervision to treat severe pain, the risk of addiction is negligible.

Opioid analgesics may prevent clear thought and cloud consciousness. Other possible adverse effects include nausea, vomiting, constipation, drowsiness, and depressed breathing. When they are taken in overdose, these drugs may induce a deep coma and lead to fatal breathing difficulties.

In addition to the powerful opioids, there are some less powerful drugs in this group that are used to relieve mild to moderate pain. They include dihydrocodeine and codeine. Their normally unwanted side effects of depressing respiration and causing constipation make them useful as cough suppressants (p.27) and as antidiarrhoeal drugs (p.44).

LOCAL ANAESTHETICS

These drugs are used to prevent pain, usually in minor surgical procedures (for example, dental treatment and stitching cuts). They can also be injected into the space around the spinal cord to numb the lower half of the body. This is called spinal or epidural anaesthesia and can be used for some major operations in people who are not fit for a general anaesthetic. Epidural anaesthesia is also used during childbirth.

Local anaesthetics block the passage of nerve impulses at the site of administration, deadening all feeling conveyed by the nerves with which they come into contact. They do not interfere with consciousness, however. Local anaesthetics are usually given by injection but can also be applied to the skin, mouth, and other areas lined with mucous membrane (such as the vagina), or the eye to relieve pain. Some local anaesthetics are formulated for injection together with epinephrine (adrenaline). Epinephrine constricts the blood vessels and prevents the local anaesthetic from being absorbed into the bloodstream. This action keeps the anaesthetic at the site, thus prolonging its effect.

Local anaesthetic creams are often used to numb the skin before injections in children and those people with a fear of needles.

COMMON DRUGS

Opioids Buprenorpine, Co-codamol, Codeine*, Co-dydramol, Diamorphine (heroin), Dihydrocodeine*, Dipipanone, Fentanyl, Meptazinol, Methadone*, Morphine*, Oxycodone, Pethidine, Tramadol*
NSAIDs (see p.50) Aspirin*, Diclofenac*, Etodolac, Fenbufen, Fenoprofen, Ibuprofen*, Indometacin, Ketoprofen*, Mefenamic acid*, Meloxicam*, Naproxen*, Piroxicam*
Other non-opioids Nefopam, Paracetamol*
Local anaesthetics Bupivacaine, Lidocaine
* See Part 2

Sleeping drugs

Difficulty in getting to sleep or staying asleep (insomnia) has many causes. Most people have sleepless nights from time to time, usually due to a temporary worry or discomfort from a minor illness. Persistent sleeplessness can be caused by psychological problems including anxiety or depression, or the pain and discomfort of a physical disorder.

WHY THEY ARE USED

For occasional sleeplessness, simple, common remedies to promote relaxation, such as taking a warm bath or a hot milk drink before bedtime, are usually the best treatment. Sleeping drugs (also known as hypnotics) are normally prescribed only when these self-help remedies have failed, and when lack of sleep is beginning to affect general health. They are used to re-establish the habit of sleeping, and should be used in the smallest dose and for the shortest possible time (not more than three weeks). It is best not to use sleeping tablets every night (see Risks and special precautions, right). Do not use alcohol to get to sleep as it can cause disturbed sleep and insomnia. Long-term treatment of sleeplessness depends on resolving the underlying cause.

TYPES OF SLEEPING DRUG

Benzodiazepines are the most commonly used class of sleeping drug because they have comparatively few adverse effects and are relatively safe in overdose. They are also used to treat anxiety (see p.13).

Barbiturates are now rarely used because of the risks of abuse, dependence, and toxicity in overdose. There is also a risk of prolonged sedation ("hangover").

Chloral derivatives effectively promote sleep but are little used now. If prescribed, triclofos causes fewer gastrointestinal side effects than chloral hydrate.

Other non-benzodiazepine sleeping drugs Zopiclone, zaleplon, and zolpidem are non-benzodiazepine sleeping drugs that work in a similar way to benzodiazepines. They are not intended for long-term use, and withdrawal symptoms have been reported.

Antihistamines are widely used to treat allergic symptoms (see p.58). Because they also cause drowsiness, they are sometimes used to promote sleep in children and the elderly.

Antidepressants may be used to promote sleep in depressed people (see p.14) and are effective in treating underlying depressive illness.

HOW THEY WORK

Most sleeping drugs promote sleep by depressing brain function. The drugs interfere with chemical activity in the brain and nervous system by reducing communication between nerve cells. This leads to reduced brain activity, allowing you to fall asleep more easily, but the nature of the sleep is affected by the drug. The main class of sleeping drugs, the benzodiazepines, is described on the facing page.

HOW THEY AFFECT YOU

A sleeping drug rapidly produces drowsiness and slowed reactions. Some people find that the drug makes them appear to be drunk, their speech slurred, especially if they delay going to bed after taking their dose. Most people find they usually fall asleep within one hour of taking the drug.

Because the sleep induced by drugs is not the same as normal sleep, many people find that they do not feel as well rested by it as by a night of natural sleep. This is the result of suppressed brain activity. Sleeping drugs also suppress the sleep during which dreams occur; both dream sleep and non-dream sleep are essential for a good night's sleep.

Some people experience a variety of "hangover" effects the following day. Some benzodiazepines may produce minor side effects, such as daytime drowsiness, dizziness, and unsteadiness, that can impair the ability to drive or operate machinery. Elderly people are likely to become confused and, for them, the selection of an appropriate drug is important.

RISKS AND SPECIAL PRECAUTIONS

Sleeping drugs become less effective after the first few nights and there may be a temptation to increase the dose. Apart from the antihistamines, most sleeping drugs can produce psychological and physical dependence when taken regularly for more than a few weeks, especially if they are taken in larger-than-normal doses.

When sleeping drugs are suddenly withdrawn, anxiety, convulsions, and hallucinations sometimes occur. Nightmares and vivid dreams may be a problem because the time spent in dream sleep increases. Sleeplessness will recur and may lead to a temptation to use sleeping drugs again. Anyone who wishes to stop taking sleeping drugs, particularly after prolonged use, should seek his or her doctor's advice to prevent these withdrawal symptoms from occurring.

COMMON DRUGS

Benzodiazepines Flurazepam, Loprazolam, Lormetazepam, Nitrazepam*, Temazepam*
Barbiturate Amobarbital
Other non-benzodiazepine sleeping drugs Clomethiazole, Promethazine*, Zaleplon, Zolpidem, Zopiclone*
* See Part 2

ANTI-ANXIETY DRUGS

Anti-anxiety drugs

A certain amount of stress can be beneficial, providing a stimulus to action. But too much will often result in anxiety, which might be described as fear or apprehension not caused by real danger.

Clinically, anxiety arises when the balance of certain chemicals in the brain is disturbed. The fearful feelings increase brain activity, stimulating the sympathetic nervous system (see Autonomic nervous system, p.8) and often triggering physical symptoms, for example, breathlessness, shaking, palpitations, digestive distress, and headaches.

WHY THEY ARE USED

Anti-anxiety drugs (also known as anxiolytics or minor tranquillizers) are prescribed for short-term relief of severe anxiety and nervousness caused by psychological problems. However, these drugs cannot resolve the causes. Tackling the underlying problem through counselling and perhaps psychotherapy offers the best hope of a long-term solution. Anti-anxiety drugs are also used in hospitals to calm and relax people undergoing uncomfortable medical procedures.

There are two main classes of drug for relieving anxiety: benzodiazepines and beta blockers. Benzodiazepines, which are the most widely used, are given as regular treatment for short periods to promote relaxation. Most benzodiazepines have a strong sedative effect, helping to relieve the insomnia that accompanies anxiety (see also Sleeping drugs, p.11).

Beta blockers are mainly used to reduce physical symptoms of anxiety, such as shaking and palpitations. These drugs are commonly prescribed for people who feel excessively anxious in certain situations, such as interviews or public appearances.

Many antidepressants, including SSRIs (see p.14), clomipramine, and venlafaxine, are proving useful in some anxiety disorders.

HOW THEY WORK

Benzodiazepines and related drugs depress activity in the part of the brain that controls emotion by promoting the action of the neurotransmitter gamma-aminobutyric acid (GABA), which binds to neurons, blocking transmission of electrical impulses and thereby reducing communication between brain cells. Benzodiazepines increase the inhibitory effect of GABA on brain cells, preventing the excessive brain activity that causes anxiety.

Buspirone is different from other anti-anxiety drugs; it binds mainly to serotonin (another neurotransmitter) receptors and does not cause drowsiness. Its effect is not felt for at least two weeks after treatment has begun.
Beta blockers block the action of a chemical transmitter called norepinephrine (noradrenaline) in the body, reducing the physical symptoms of anxiety. These symptoms are produced by an increase in the activity of the sympathetic nervous system. Sympathetic nerve endings release norepinephrine, which stimulates the heart, digestive system, and other organs. For more information on beta blockers, see p.30.

HOW THEY AFFECT YOU

Benzodiazepines and related drugs reduce feelings of restlessness and agitation, slow mental activity, and often produce drowsiness. They are said to reduce motivation and, if they are taken in large doses, may lead to apathy. They also have a relaxing effect on the muscles, and some benzodiazepines are used specifically for that purpose (see Muscle relaxants, p.54).

Minor adverse effects of these drugs include dizziness and forgetfulness. People who need to drive or operate potentially dangerous machinery should be aware that their reactions may be slowed. Because the brain soon becomes tolerant to and dependent on their effects, benzodiazepines are usually effective for only a few weeks at a time.

Beta blockers reduce the physical symptoms associated with anxiety, which may promote greater mental calmness. Because they do not cause drowsiness, they are safer for people who need to drive.

RISKS AND SPECIAL PRECAUTIONS

The benzodiazepines are safe for most people and are not likely to be fatal in overdose. The main risk is psychological and physical dependence, especially for regular users or

13

when larger-than-average doses have been used. For this reason, they are usually given for courses of two weeks or less. If they have been used for a longer period, they should be withdrawn gradually under medical supervision. If they are stopped suddenly, withdrawal symptoms, such as excessive anxiety, nightmares, and restlessness, may occur.

Benzodiazepines have been abused for their sedative effect, and are therefore prescribed with caution for people with a history of drug or alcohol abuse.

COMMON DRUGS

Benzodiazepines Alprazolam, Chlordiazepoxide, Diazepam/Lorazepam*, Oxazepam
Beta blockers Atenolol*, Bisoprolol*, Oxprenolol, Propranolol*
Other non-benzodiazepines Buspirone
* See Part 2

Antidepressant drugs

Occasional moods of discouragement or sadness are normal and usually pass quickly. However, more severe depression that is accompanied by despair, lethargy, loss of sex drive, and often poor appetite may call for medical attention. Such depression can arise from life stresses such as the death of someone close, an illness, or sometimes from no apparent cause.

There are three main types of drug for depression: tricyclic antidepressants (TCAs), selective serotonin re-uptake inhibitors (SSRIs), and monoamine oxidase inhibitors (MAOIs). Lithium, a metallic element, is used to treat manic depression (see Antimanic drugs, p.16). In some cases, it is used with an antidepressant for treating resistant depression. Several other antidepressants may be prescribed, including venlafaxine, mirtazepine, maprotiline, mianserin, and trazodone.

WHY THEY ARE USED

Minor depression does not usually require drug treatment; support and help in coming to terms with the cause is often all that is needed. Moderate or severe depression usually requires drug treatment, which is effective in most cases. Antidepressants may have

to be taken for many months. Treatment should not be stopped too soon because symptoms are likely to reappear. When treatment is stopped, the dose should be reduced gradually over several weeks because withdrawal symptoms may occur if the drugs are stopped suddenly.

TYPES OF ANTIDEPRESSANT

Treatment usually begins with either a TCA or an SSRI.
TCAs Some TCAs (such as amitriptyline) cause drowsiness, which is useful for sleep problems in depression. TCAs also cause anticholinergic effects (see Drugs that act on the parasympathetic nervous system, p.9), including blurred vision, dry mouth, and urinary difficulties.
SSRIs These drugs generally have fewer side effects than TCAs. The main unwanted effects are nausea and vomiting. Anxiety, headache, and restlessness may also occur at the beginning of treatment.
MAOIs These are especially effective in people who are anxious as well as depressed, or who suffer from phobias.
Lithium Salts of this metallic element are used to treat manic depression (see Antimanic drugs, p.16). They are sometimes used with an antidepressant drug for resistant depression.
Other antidepressants These drugs include venlafaxine, nefazodone, maprotiline, mianserin, and trazodone.

HOW THEY WORK

Normally, the brain cells release sufficient quantities of certain chemicals (known as neurotransmitters) in the brain to stimulate neighbouring cells. The neurotransmitters are constantly reabsorbed into the brain cells, where they are broken down by an enzyme called monoamine oxidase. Depression is thought to be caused by a reduction in the level of neurotransmitters being released. Antidepressants bring these levels back to normal.
TCAs and venlafaxine work by blocking the re-uptake of the neurotransmitters serotonin and norepinephrine (noradrenaline), thereby increasing the level of these neurotransmitters in the brain.
SSRIs act by blocking the re-uptake of only one neurotransmitter, serotonin.

MAOIs act by blocking the breakdown of neurotransmitters, mainly serotonin and norepinephrine (noradrenaline).

HOW THEY AFFECT YOU

The antidepressant effect of these drugs starts after 10 to 14 days of treatment, and it may be six to eight weeks before the full effect is seen. However, side effects may happen at once. Tolerance to these side effects usually occurs and treatment should be continued.

RISKS AND SPECIAL PRECAUTIONS

Overdose can be dangerous: tricyclic antidepressants can produce coma, fits, and disturbed heart rhythm, which may be fatal; monoamine oxidase inhibitors can also cause muscle spasms and even death. Both are prescribed with caution for people with heart problems or epilepsy.

When MAOIs are taken with certain drugs or foods rich in tyramine (for example, cheese, meat, yeast extracts, and red wine), they can produce a dramatic rise in blood pressure, with headache or vomiting. People taking MAOIs are given a card that lists prohibited drugs and foods. Because of this adverse interaction, MAOIs are used much less frequently today, and SSRIs or tricyclics are prescribed in preference to them. SSRIs are not generally prescribed to anyone under the age of 18, however.

COMMON DRUGS

Tricyclics Amitriptyline*, Amoxapine, Clomipramine*, Dosulepin*, Doxepin, Imipramine*, Lofepramine*, Nortriptyline, Trimipramine
SSRIs Citalopram/Escitalopram*, Fluoxetine*, Fluvoxamine, Paroxetine*, Sertraline*
MAOIs Isocarboxazid, Moclobemide, Phenelzine, Tranylcypromine
Other drugs Duloxetine, Flupentixol*, Maprotiline, Mianserin, Mirtazepine* Reboxetine, Trazodone, Tryptophan, Venlafaxine*
* See Part 2

Antipsychotic drugs

Psychosis is a term used to describe mental disorders that prevent the sufferer from thinking clearly, acting rationally, and recognizing reality. These disorders include schizophrenia and manic depression. Their precise causes are unknown, but several factors, including stress, heredity, and brain injury, may be involved. Temporary psychosis can also arise as a result of alcohol withdrawal or the abuse of mind-altering drugs. A variety of drugs is used to treat psychotic disorders (see Common drugs, p.16), and most have similar actions and effects. One exception is lithium, which is particularly useful for manic depression (see Antimanic drugs, p.16).

WHY THEY ARE USED

A person with a psychotic illness may recover spontaneously, so a drug will not always be prescribed. Long-term treatment is started only when normal life is seriously disrupted. Antipsychotic drugs (also called major tranquillizers or neuroleptics) do not cure the disorder, but they do help to control symptoms.

By controlling the symptoms of psychosis, antipsychotic drugs make it possible for most sufferers to live in the community and only be admitted to hospital for acute episodes.

The drug given to a particular individual depends on the nature of his or her illness and the expected adverse effects of that drug. Drugs differ in the amount of sedation produced; the need for sedation also influences the choice of drug.

Antipsychotics may also be given to calm or sedate a highly agitated or aggressive person, whatever the cause. Some antipsychotic drugs also have a powerful action against nausea and vomiting (see p.21), and are therefore sometimes used as premedication before a person has surgery.

HOW THEY WORK

It is thought that some forms of mental illness are caused by an increase in communication between brain cells due to overactivity of an excitatory chemical called dopamine. This may disturb normal thought processes and produce abnormal behaviour. Dopamine combines with receptors on the brain cells. Antipsychotic drugs reduce the transmission of nerve signals by binding to these receptors, thereby making the brain cells less sensitive to dopamine. Some new antipsychotic drugs, such as clozapine, risperidone, and sertindole, also bind to receptors for the chemical serotonin.

HOW THEY AFFECT YOU

Because antipsychotics depress the action of dopamine, they can disturb its balance with another chemical in the brain, acetylcholine. If an imbalance occurs, extrapyramidal side effects (EPSE) may appear. These include restlessness, disorders of movement, and parkinsonism (see Drugs for parkinsonism, p.18).

In these circumstances, a change to a different type of antipsychotic may be necessary. If this is not possible, an anticholinergic drug (see p.9) may be prescribed.

Antipsychotics may block the action of noradrenaline, another neurotransmitter in the brain. This lowers the blood pressure, especially when you stand up, causing dizziness. It may also prevent ejaculation.

RISKS AND SPECIAL PRECAUTIONS

It is important to continue taking these drugs even if all symptoms have gone, because the symptoms are controlled only by taking the prescribed dose.

Because antipsychotic drugs can have permanent as well as temporary side effects, the minimum necessary dosage is used. This minimum dose is found by starting with a low dose and increasing it until the symptoms are controlled. Sudden withdrawal after more than a few weeks can cause nausea, sweating, headache, and restlessness. Therefore, the dose is reduced gradually when treatment needs to be stopped.

The most serious long-term risk of antipsychotic treatment is a disorder known as tardive dyskinesia, which may develop after one to five years. This consists of repeated jerking movements of the mouth, tongue, and face, and sometimes of the hands and feet. The condition is less common with the newer antipsychotics (atypical antipsychotics) than the older drugs (typical antipsychotics).

HOW THEY ARE ADMINISTERED

Antipsychotics may be given by mouth as tablets, capsules, or syrup, or by injection. They can also be given in the form of a depot injection, which releases the drug slowly over several weeks. This is helpful for people who might forget to take their drugs or who might take an overdose.

COMMON DRUGS

Typical antipsychotics Benperidol, Chlorpromazine*, Flupentixol*, Fluphenazine, Haloperidol*, Levomepromazine, Pericyazine, Perphenazine, Pimozide, Pipotiazine, Prochlorperazine*, Promazine*, Sulpiride (see Amisulpride*), Trifluoperazine, Zuclopenthixol

Atypical antipsychotics Amisulpride*, Aripiprazole, Clozapine*, Olanzapine*, Quetiapine*, Risperidone*, Sertindole, Zotepine

Antimanic drugs Carbamazepine*, Lithium*

* See Part 2

Antimanic drugs

Changes in mood are normal, but when a person's mood swings become grossly exaggerated, with peaks of elation or mania alternating with troughs of depression, it becomes an illness known as manic depression. It is usually treated with salts of lithium (p.290), a drug that reduces the intensity of the mania, lifts the depression, and lessens the frequency of mood swings. Because it can take three weeks for lithium salts to work, an antipsychotic may be prescribed with lithium at first to give immediate relief of symptoms.

Lithium can be toxic if blood levels of the drug rise too high. Regular checks on the blood concentration of lithium should therefore be carried out during treatment. Symptoms of lithium poisoning include blurred vision, twitching, vomiting, and diarrhoea.

COMMON DRUGS

Carbamazepine*, Lithium*

* See Part 2

Anticonvulsant drugs

Electrical signals from nerve cells in the brain are normally finely coordinated to produce smooth movements of the arms and legs, but these signals can become irregular and chaotic, and trigger the disorderly muscular activity and mental changes that are characteristic of a seizure (also called a fit or convulsion). The most common cause of seizures is epilepsy, which occurs as a result of brain disease or injury. In epileptics, a fit may be triggered by an outside stimulus such as a flashing light. Seizures can also result from the toxic effects of certain drugs and, in young children, by a high temperature.

Anticonvulsant drugs are used both to reduce the risk of an epileptic seizure and to stop one that is in progress.

WHY THEY ARE USED

Isolated convulsions seldom require drug treatment, but anticonvulsant drugs are the usual treatment for controlling seizures caused by epilepsy. In most cases, they permit a person with epilepsy to lead a normal life.

Most people with epilepsy need to take anticonvulsants on a regular basis to prevent seizures. Usually a single drug is used, and treatment continues until there have been no attacks for at least two years.

If one drug is not effective, a different one will be tried. Occasionally, it is necessary to take a combination of drugs. Even when receiving treatment, a person can suffer seizures. Repeated seizures or status epilepticus can be halted by injection of diazepam or a similar drug.

The selection of anticonvulsant (antiepileptic) drug depends on the type of epilepsy, the age of the patient, and his or her particular response to individual drug treatment.

Generalized epilepsy In this form of epilepsy, there is widespread disturbance of electrical activity in the brain, and loss of consciousness occurs at the outset. In its simplest form, absence seizure, there is momentary loss of consciousness, during which the sufferer may stare into space. This form mainly affects children; convulsions do not occur.

Another form of generalized epilepsy causes a brief jerk of a limb (myoclonus).

The most severe type is a tonic-clonic (grand mal) seizure, which is characterized by loss of consciousness and convulsions that may last for a few minutes.

Sufferers may have one or more of these types of generalized epilepsy. Sodium valproate, lamotrigine, topiramate, levetiracetam, or the benzodiazepines are normally used for these types of epilepsy.

Partial (focal) epilepsy This type of epilepsy is caused by an electrical disturbance in only one part of the brain. The result is a disturbance of function, such as an abnormal sensation or movement of a limb, without loss of consciousness. Known as a simple partial seizure, this may precede a more serious attack associated with loss of consciousness (complex partial seizure), which may in turn progress to a generalized convulsive seizure.

Carbamazepine, lamotrigine, or phenytoin may be prescribed for this type of epilepsy.

Status epilepticus Repeated attacks without full recovery between, or a single attack lasting more than 10 minutes, occur in this form of epilepsy. Emergency treatment is required.

HOW THEY WORK

Brain cells bring about body movement by electrical activity that passes through the nerves to the muscles. In an epileptic seizure, uncontrolled electrical activity starts in one part of the brain and spreads to other parts, causing uncontrolled stimulation of brain cells. Most of the anticonvulsants have an inhibitory effect on brain cells and damp down electrical activity, preventing the excessive build-up that causes epileptic seizures.

HOW THEY AFFECT YOU

Ideally, the only effect an anticonvulsant should have is to reduce or prevent epileptic seizures. Unfortunately, no drug prevents seizures without potentially affecting normal brain function, often leading to poor memory, inability to concentrate, lack of coordination, and lethargy. It is important, therefore, to find a drug and dosage sufficient to prevent seizures without causing unacceptable side effects. The dose has to be carefully tailored to the individual. It is usual to start with a low dose of a selected drug and to increase it gradually until a balance is achieved between control of seizures and occurrence of side effects, many of which wear off after the first weeks of treatment.

Blood tests are used to monitor levels of some anticonvulsants in the body as an aid to dose adjustment.

RISKS AND SPECIAL PRECAUTIONS

Each anticonvulsant has its own specific adverse effects and risks; and some affect the liver's ability to break down other drugs and may influence the action of other drugs you are taking. Doctors try to prescribe the minimum number of anticonvulsants needed to control the seizures to reduce the risk of such interactions occurring.

Some anticonvulsants pose risks to a developing baby; if you are hoping to become pregnant, you should discuss the risks, and whether your medication should be changed, with your doctor. People taking anticonvulsants need to take them regularly as prescribed. If levels of anticonvulsant in the body fall suddenly, seizures are very likely to occur. The dose should not be reduced or treatment stopped, except on a doctor's advice. Certain driving restrictions may apply if you have had a seizure; you need to report this to the Driver and Vehicle Licensing Agency (DVLA).

If, for any reason, anticonvulsant drug treatment needs to be stopped, the dose should be reduced gradually. People on anticonvulsant therapy are advised to carry an identification tag giving full details of their condition and treatment.

COMMON DRUGS

Carbamazepine*, Clobazam, Clonazepam*, Diazepam*, Ethosuximide, Gabapentin*, Lamotrigine*, Levetiracetam, Lorazepam*, Oxcarbazepine, Phenobarbital*, Phenytoin*, Primidone, Sodium valproate*, Tiagabine, Topiramate, Vigabatrin

* See Part 2

Drugs for parkinsonism

Parkinsonism is a general term used to describe shaking of the head and limbs, muscular stiffness, an expressionless face, and inability to control or initiate movement. It is caused by an imbalance of chemicals in the brain; the effect of acetylcholine is increased by a reduction in the action of dopamine.

The most common cause of parkinsonism is Parkinson's disease, degeneration of the dopamine-producing cells in the brain. Other causes include the side effects of certain drugs, notably antipsychotics (see p.15), and narrowing of the blood vessels in the brain.

WHY THEY ARE USED

Drugs can relieve the symptoms of parkinsonism but, unfortunately, the degeneration of brain cells in Parkinson's disease cannot be halted, although drugs can minimize symptoms for many years.

HOW THEY WORK

Drugs to treat parkinsonism restore the balance between the chemicals dopamine and acetylcholine. They fall into two main groups: those that reduce the effect of acetylcholine (anticholinergic drugs) and those that boost the effect of dopamine.

Anticholinergics combine with receptors on brain cells, preventing acetylcholine from binding to them. This action reduces acetylcholine's relative overactivity and restores balance with dopamine.

Dopamine cannot pass from the blood to the brain, and therefore cannot be given to boost its levels in the brain. Levodopa (L-dopa), the chemical from which it is naturally produced in the brain, is combined with carbidopa (as co-careldopa) or benserazide (as co-beneldopa) to prevent it from being converted to dopamine before it reaches the brain. Amantadine (also used as an antiviral, see p.69) boosts dopamine levels in the brain by stimulating its release. Dopamine's action can also be boosted by other drugs, including bromocriptine, lisuride, pergolide, or apomorphine (injection only), which mimic the action of dopamine.

CHOICE OF DRUG

Anticholinergics are used to treat parkinsonism due to antipsychotic drugs, which have dopamine-blocking properties. They are not generally used to treat parkinsonism of unknown cause because they are less effective and may increase cognitive impairment. L-dopa is usually given when the disease impairs walking; its effectiveness usually wanes after two to five years, in which case other dopamine-boosting drugs may also be prescribed.

COMMON DRUGS

Dopamine-boosting drugs Amantadine*, Apomorphine, Bromocriptine*, Cabergoline, Entacapone, Levodopa* (as co-beneldopa/co-careldopa), Lisuride, Pergolide, Pramipexole, Ropinirole, Selegiline

Anticholinergic drugs Benzatropine, Orphenadrine*, Procyclidine*, Trihexyphenidyl/benzhexol
* See Part 2

COMMON DRUGS
Acetylcholinesterase inhibitors Donepezil*, Galantamine, Rivastigmine*
* See Part 2

Drugs for dementia

Dementia is a decline in mental function severe enough to affect normal social or occupational activities. It can be sudden and irreversible, due to a stroke or head injury for example. It can also develop gradually and may be a feature of disorders such as poor circulation in the brain, multiple sclerosis, and Alzheimer's disease. Much research is in progress on the cause of Alzheimer's disease, the single most common cause of dementia.

WHY THEY ARE USED
Drugs called acetylcholinesterase inhibitors have been found to improve the symptoms of dementia in Alzheimer's disease, although they do not prevent its long-term progression.

HOW THEY WORK
In healthy people, acetylcholinesterase (an enzyme in the brain) breaks down the neurotransmitter acetylcholine, balancing its levels and limiting its effects. In Alzheimer's disease, there is a deficiency of acetylcholine. Acetylcholinesterase inhibitors block the action of the enzyme acetylcholinesterase, raising brain levels of acetylcholine, thus increasing alertness and slowing the rate of deterioration.

HOW THEY AFFECT YOU
Following assessment by a specialist of mental function, drug treatment is started at a low dose and increased gradually to minimize side effects. Any improvements should begin to appear in about three weeks. Assessment is repeated at six-monthly intervals to decide whether or not the treatment is having any benefit.

RISKS AND SPECIAL PRECAUTIONS
It is important to continue taking these drugs if they prove effective because there is a gradual loss of improvement after treatment is stopped. Side effects include urinary difficulties, nausea, vomiting, and diarrhoea. These drugs may increase the risk of convulsions in some people.

Nervous system stimulants

A person's state of mental alertness varies throughout the day and is under the control of chemicals in the brain, some of which are depressant, causing drowsiness, and others that are stimulant, heightening awareness.

It is thought that an increase in the activity of the depressant chemicals may be responsible for a condition called narcolepsy, which is a tendency to fall asleep during the day for no obvious reason. In this case, the nervous system stimulants are administered to increase wakefulness. These drugs include the amphetamines (usually dexamfetamine), the related drug methylphenidate, and modafinil. Amphetamines are used less often these days because of the risk of dependence. A common home remedy for increasing alertness is caffeine, a mild stimulant that is present in coffee, tea, and cola. Respiratory stimulants related to caffeine are used to improve breathing.

WHY THEY ARE USED
In adults who suffer from narcolepsy, some of these drugs prevent excessive drowsiness during the day. Stimulants do not cure narcolepsy and, since the disorder usually lasts throughout the sufferer's lifetime, may have to be taken indefinitely. Methylphenidate or dexamfetamine are sometimes given to children suffering from attention deficit hyperactivity disorder (ADHD). Stimulants were once used as part of the treatment for obesity because reduced appetite is a side effect of amphetamines but they are no longer thought appropriate for weight reduction. Diet is now the main treatment, together with orlistat or sibutramine if necessary.

Caffeine is added to some analgesics to counteract the effects of caffeine withdrawal, which can cause headaches, but no clear medical justification exists for this.

Respiratory stimulants such as theophylline, aminophylline, and doxapram are related to caffeine and are used to improve breathing. They act on the respiratory centre, the part of the brain that controls breathing. They are sometimes used in hospitals to help people who have difficulty in breathing, mainly very young babies and adults with severe chest infections.

Apart from their use in narcolepsy, nervous system stimulants are not useful in the long term because the brain soon develops tolerance to them.

HOW THEY WORK
The level of wakefulness is controlled by a part of the brain stem called the reticular activating system (RAS). Activity in this area depends on the balance between chemicals, some of which are excitatory (including norepinephrine (noradrenaline), and some inhibitory, such as gamma aminobutyric acid (GABA). Stimulants promote release of noradrenaline increasing activity in the RAS and other parts of the brain, so raising alertness.

HOW THEY AFFECT YOU
In adults, the central nervous system stimulants taken in the prescribed dose for narcolepsy increase wakefulness, thereby allowing normal concentration and thought processes to occur. They may also reduce appetite and cause tremors. In hyperactive children, they reduce the general level of activity to a more normal level and increase the attention span.

RISKS AND SPECIAL PRECAUTIONS
Some people, especially the elderly or those with previous psychiatric problems, are particularly sensitive to stimulants and may experience adverse effects, even when the drugs are given in comparatively low doses. They need to be used with caution in children because they can retard growth if taken for prolonged periods. An excess of these drugs given to a child may depress the nervous system, producing drowsiness or even loss of consciousness. Palpitations may also occur.

These drugs reduce the level of natural stimulants in the brain, so after regular use for a few weeks a person may become physically dependent on them for normal func-

tion. If they are abruptly withdrawn, the excess of natural inhibitory chemicals in the brain depresses central nervous system activity, producing withdrawal symptoms. These may include lethargy, depression, increased appetite, and difficulty in staying awake.

Stimulants can produce overactivity in the brain if used inappropriately or in excess, resulting in extreme restlessness, sleeplessness, nervousness, or anxiety. They also stimulate the sympathetic branch of the autonomic nervous system (see p.8), causing shaking, sweating, and palpitations. More serious risks of exceeding the prescribed dose are fits and a major disturbance in mental functioning that may result in delusions and hallucinations. Because these drugs have been abused, amphetamines and methylphenidate are classified as controlled drugs.

COMMON DRUGS
Respiratory stimulants Doxapram, Theophylline/aminophylline*
Other drugs Atomoxetine, Caffeine, Dexamfetamine, Methylphenidate, Modafinil, Sibutramine*
* See Part 2

Drugs used for migraine

Migraine is a term applied to recurrent severe headaches affecting only one side of the head and caused by changes in the blood vessels around the brain and scalp. They may be accompanied by nausea and vomiting and preceded by warning signs, usually an impression of flashing lights or numbness and tingling in the arms. Occasionally, speech may be impaired, or the attack may be disabling. The cause of migraine is unknown, but an attack may be triggered by a blow to the head, physical exertion, certain foods and drugs, or emotional factors such as excitement, tension, or shock. A family history of migraine also increases the chance of an individual suffering from it.

WHY THEY ARE USED
Drugs are used either to relieve symptoms or to prevent attacks. Different drugs are used in each approach, but none cures the underlying disorder. However, a susceptibility to migraine headaches can clear up spontaneously

and, if you are taking drugs regularly, your doctor may recommend that you stop them after a few months to see if this has happened.

In most people, migraine headaches can be relieved by a mild analgesic (painkiller), such as paracetamol or a non-steroidal anti-inflammatory drug (NSAID), or a stronger one like codeine (see Analgesics, p.9). If nausea and vomiting accompany the migraine, tablets may not be absorbed sufficiently from the gut. Absorption can be increased if they are taken as soluble tablets in water or with an anti-emetic (see below, right).

Some drugs used to relieve attacks can be given by injection, inhaler, nasal spray, or suppository. Preparations that contain caffeine should be avoided since headaches may be caused by excessive use or on stopping treatment. $5HT_1$ agonist drugs (such as sumatriptan) are used if analgesics are not effective. Ergotamine is used less often now.

The factors that trigger an individual's attacks should be identified and avoided. Anti-anxiety drugs are not usually prescribed if stress is a precipitating factor because of the potential for dependence. If the attacks occur more often than once a month and significantly disrupt daily life, drugs to prevent migraine may be taken every day. Drugs used to prevent migraine are beta blockers (see p.30), such as metoprolol or propranolol, and pizotifen (an antihistamine and serotonin blocker). Other drugs that have been used include nifedipine, amitriptyline (an antidepressant, see p.14), verapamil, and cyproheptadine.

HOW THEY WORK

A migraine begins when blood vessels surrounding the brain constrict, producing the typical migraine warning signs. The constriction is thought to be due to certain chemicals found in food or produced by the body. The neurotransmitter serotonin causes large blood vessels in the brain to constrict. Pizotifen and propranolol block the effect of chemicals on blood vessels, thereby preventing attacks.

The next stage of a migraine attack occurs when blood vessels in the scalp and around the eyes dilate (widen). As a result, chemicals called prostaglandins are released, producing pain. Aspirin and paracetamol relieve this pain by blocking prostaglandins. Codeine acts directly on the brain, altering pain perception (see Analgesics, p.9). Ergotamine and $5HT_1$ agonists relieve pain by narrowing dilated blood vessels in the scalp.

HOW THEY AFFECT YOU

Each drug has its own adverse effects. $5HT_1$ agonists may cause chest tightness and drowsiness. Ergotamine may cause drowsiness, tingling sensations in the skin, cramps, and weakness in the legs, and vomiting may be made worse. Pizotifen may cause drowsiness and weight gain. For effects of propranolol, see p.359, and for analgesics, see p.9.

RISKS AND SPECIAL PRECAUTIONS

$5HT_1$ agonists should not usually be used by people with high blood pressure, angina, or coronary heart disease. Ergotamine can damage blood vessels by prolonged overconstriction, so it should be used with caution by those with poor circulation. Excessive use can lead to dependence and many adverse effects, including headache. You should not take more than your doctor advises in any one week.

HOW THEY ARE ADMINISTERED

These drugs are usually taken by mouth as tablets or capsules. Sumatriptan can also be taken as an injection or a nasal spray. Ergotamine can be taken as suppositories, or as tablets that dissolve under the tongue.

COMMON DRUGS

Drugs to prevent migraine Amitriptyline*, Cyproheptadine, Nifedipine*, Pizotifen*, Propranolol*, Sodium valproate*, Verapamil*

$5HT_1$ agonists Almotriptan, Eletriptan, Frovatriptan, Naratriptan, Rizatriptan, Sumatriptan*, Zolmitriptan
Other drugs to relieve migraine Codeine*, Ergotamine*, NSAIDs (see p.50), Paracetamol*, Tolfenamic acid
* See Part 2

Anti-emetics

Drugs used to treat or prevent vomiting or the feeling of sickness (nausea) are known as anti-emetics. Vomiting is a reflex action for getting rid of harmful substances, but it may also be a symptom of disease. Vomiting and nausea are often caused by a digestive tract infection, travel sickness, pregnancy, or vertigo (a balance disorder involving the inner ear). They can also occur as a side effect of some drugs, especially those used for cancer, radiation therapy, or general anaesthesia.

Commonly used anti-emetics include metoclopramide, domperidone, haloperidol, cyclizine, ondansetron, granisetron, prochlorperazine, promethazine, and cinnarizine. The phenothiazine and butyrophenone drug groups are also used as antihistamines (see p.58) and to treat some types of mental illness (see Antipsychotic drugs, p.15).

WHY THEY ARE USED

Doctors usually diagnose the cause of vomiting before prescribing an anti-emetic because the vomiting may be caused by an infection of the digestive tract or some other condition of the abdomen that might require treatment such as surgery. Treating only the vomiting and nausea might delay diagnosis, correct treatment, and recovery.

Anti-emetics may be taken to prevent travel sickness (using one of the antihistamines), vomiting resulting from anticancer (see p.96) and other drug treatments (metoclopramide, haloperidol, domperidone, ondansetron, and prochlorperazine, for example).

Vertigo is a spinning sensation in the head often accompanied by nausea and vomiting. It is usually caused by a disease affecting the organ of balance in the inner ear. Anti-emetics are prescribed to relieve the symptoms.

Ménière's disease is a disorder in which excess fluid builds up in the inner ear, causing vertigo, noises in the ear, and gradual deafness. It is usually treated with cinnarizine, betahistine, prochlorperazine, or an anti-anxiety drug (see p.13). A diuretic (see p.32) may also be given to reduce the excess fluid in the ear.

Anti-emetics are also used to help the nausea that occurs in vertigo and are occasionally used to relieve cases of severe vomiting during pregnancy. You should not take an anti-emetic during pregnancy except on medical advice. No anti-emetic drug should be taken for longer than a couple of days without consulting your doctor.

HOW THEY WORK

Nausea and vomiting occur when the vomiting centre in the brain is stimulated by signals from three places in the body: the digestive tract, the part of the inner ear controlling balance, and the brain itself via thoughts and emotions and via its chemoreceptor trigger zone, which responds to harmful substances in the blood. Anti-emetic drugs may act at one or more of these places. Some help the stomach to empty its contents into the intestine. A combination may be used that works at different sites and has an additive effect.

HOW THEY AFFECT YOU

As well as treating vomiting and nausea, many anti-emetic drugs may make you feel drowsy. However, for preventing travel sickness on long journeys, a sedating antihistamine may be an advantage.

Some anti-emetics (in particular, phenothiazines and antihistamines) can block the parasympathetic nervous system (see Autonomic nervous system, p.8), causing dry mouth, blurred vision, or difficulty in passing urine. Phenothiazines may also lower blood pressure, leading to dizziness or fainting.

RISKS AND SPECIAL PRECAUTIONS

Because some antihistamines can make you drowsy, it may be advisable not to drive while taking them. Phenothiazines, butyrophenones, and metoclopramide can produce uncontrolled movements of the face and tongue, so they are used with caution in people with parkinsonism.

COMMON DRUGS

Antihistamines Cinnarizine*, Cyclizine, Meclozine, Promethazine*

Phenothiazines Chlorpromazine*, Levomepromazine, Perphenazine, Prochlorperazine*, Trifluoperazine

5HT₃ antagonists Granisetron, Ondansetron*, Tropisetron

Butyrophenones Haloperidol*

Other drugs Betahistine*, Dexamethasone*, Domperidone*, Hyoscine hydrobromide*, Metoclopramide*, Nabilone

* **See Part 2**

RESPIRATORY SYSTEM

The respiratory system consists of the lungs and the air passages, such as the trachea (windpipe) and bronchi, by which air reaches them. Through the process of inhaling and exhaling air (breathing) the body obtains the oxygen necessary for survival, and to expel carbon dioxide, which is the waste product of the basic human biological process.

Air enters the trachea, which branches into two main bronchi, one for each lung. Within the lungs, the air passes into bronchioles, smaller tubes whose muscular walls may contract or dilate in response to drugs and nerve signals. The bronchioles open out into tiny, blood-vessel lined air sacs (alveoli), which allow oxygen to pass into the bloodstream and carbon dioxide to pass from the bloodstream for expiration.

WHAT CAN GO WRONG

Difficulty in breathing may be due to narrowing of the air passages, from spasm, as in asthma and bronchitis, or from swelling of the linings of the air passages, as in bronchiolitis and bronchitis. Breathing difficulties may also be due to an infection of the lung tissue, as in pneumonia and bronchitis, or to damage to the small air sacs (alveoli) from emphysema or from inhaled dusts or moulds, which cause pneumoconiosis and farmer's lung. Smoking and air pollution can affect the respiratory system in many ways, leading to diseases such as lung cancer and bronchitis.

Sometimes difficulty in breathing may be due to congestion of the lungs from heart disease, to an inhaled object such as a peanut, or to infection or inflammation of the throat. Symptoms of breathing difficulties often include a cough and a tight feeling in the chest.

WHY DRUGS ARE USED

Drugs with a variety of actions are used to clear the air passages, soothe inflammation, and reduce the production of mucus. Some can be bought without a prescription as single- or combined-ingredient preparations, often with an analgesic (see p.9).

Decongestants (see p.27) reduce swelling inside the nose, thereby making it possible to breathe more freely. If the cause of the congestion is an allergic response, an antihistamine (see p.58) is often recommended to relieve symptoms or prevent attacks. Bacterial infections of the respiratory tract are usually treated with antibiotics (see p.62), although most respiratory tract infections are viral.

Bronchodilators (see below) are drugs that widen the bronchi. They are used to prevent and relieve asthma attacks. Corticosteroids (see p.80) reduce inflammation in the swollen inner layers of the airways. They are used to prevent asthma attacks. Other drugs, such as sodium cromoglicate, may be used for treating allergies and preventing asthma attacks but are not effective once an asthma attack has begun.

A variety of drugs are used to relieve a cough, depending on the type of cough involved. Some drugs make it easier to eliminate phlegm; others suppress the cough by inhibiting the cough reflex.

MAJOR DRUG GROUPS

◆ Bronchodilators
◆ Drugs for asthma
◆ Decongestants
◆ Drugs to treat coughs
◆ See also sections on Allergy (p.58) and Infections (p.61)

Bronchodilators

Air entering the lungs passes through narrow tubes called bronchioles. In asthma and bronchitis the bronchioles become narrower, either as a result of contraction of the muscles in their walls, or as a result of mucus congestion. This narrowing of the bronchioles obstructs the flow of air into and out of the lungs and causes breathlessness.

Bronchodilators are prescribed to widen the bronchioles and improve breathing. There are three main groups of bronchodilator: sympathomimetics, anticholinergics, and xanthine drugs, which are related to caffeine. They are all used for relief of symptoms, and do not affect the underlying disease process. Anticholinergics are thought to be more effective in, and are used particularly for, bronchitis. In asthma, they are less effective, and are usually prescribed as additional therapy when control with other drugs is inadequate. Sympathomimetics are the first choice drugs in the management of asthma, and are frequently used in bronchitis. Xanthines have been used for many years, both for asthma and bronchitis. They usually need precise adjustment of dosage to be effective while avoiding side effects. This makes them more difficult to use, and they are reserved for people whose condition cannot be controlled by other bronchodilators alone.

WHY THEY ARE USED

Bronchodilators help to dilate the bronchioles of people suffering from asthma and bronchitis. However, they are of little benefit to those suffering from severe chronic bronchitis.

Bronchodilators are usually taken when they are needed in order to relieve an attack of breathlessness that is in progress. Some people find it helpful to take an extra dose of their bronchodilator immediately before undertaking any activity that is likely to provoke an attack of breathlessness. A patient who requires treatment with a sympathomimetic inhaler more than once daily should see his or her doctor about preventative treatment with an inhaled corticosteroid. Sympathomimetic drugs are mainly used for the rapid relief of breathlessness; anticholinergic and xanthine drugs are used both for acute attacks and long term.

HOW THEY WORK

Bronchodilator drugs act by relaxing the muscles surrounding the bronchioles. Sympathomimetic and anticholinergic drugs achieve this by interfering with nerve signals passed to the muscles through the autonomic nervous system (see p.8). Xanthine drugs are thought to relax the muscle in the bronchioles by a direct effect on the muscle fibres, but their precise action is not known.

Bronchodilator drugs usually improve breathing within a few minutes of administration. Corticosteroids usually start to increase the sufferer's capacity for exercise within a few days, and most people find that the frequency of their attacks of breathlessness is reduced.

Because sympathomimetic drugs stimulate a branch of the autonomic nervous system that controls the heart rate, they may sometimes cause palpitations and trembling. Typical side effects of anticholinergic drugs include dry mouth, blurred vision, and difficulty in passing urine. Xanthine drugs may cause headaches and nausea.

RISKS AND SPECIAL PRECAUTIONS

Since most bronchodilators are not taken by mouth, but inhaled, they do not commonly cause serious side effects. However, because of their possible effect on heart rate, xanthine and sympathomimetic drugs need to be prescribed with caution to people with heart problems, high blood pressure, or an overactive thyroid gland. Smoking tobacco and drinking alcohol increase excretion of xanthines from the body, reducing their effects. Stopping smoking after being stabilized on a xanthine may result in a rise in blood concentration, and an increased risk of side effects. It is advisable to stop smoking before starting treatment. The anticholinergic drugs may not be suitable for people with urinary retention or those who have a tendency to glaucoma.

COMMON DRUGS

Sympathomimetics Bambuterol, Ephedrine*, Epinephrine*, Formoterol, Fenoterol, Salbutamol*, Salmeterol*, Terbutaline*
Anticholinergics Ipratropium bromide*, Tiotropium*
Xanthines Theophylline/aminophylline*
* See Part 2

Drugs for asthma

Asthma is a chronic lung disease that is characterized by episodes in which the bronchioles constrict due to oversensitivity. The attacks are usually, but not always, reversible; asthma is also known as reversible airways obstruction. About 5 per cent of adults and 10 per cent of children have the disease. Sometimes the inflammation causing the constriction is due to an identifiable allergen in the atmosphere, such as house dust mites, but often there is no obvious trigger. Breathlessness is the main symptom, and wheezing, coughing, and chest tightness are common. Asthma sufferers often have attacks during the night and wake up with breathing difficulty. The illness varies in severity, and it can be life threatening.

There are a number of drugs that are used in the control of asthma. Where drugs are needed only to control an occasional attack, a sympathomimetic bronchodilator will probably be used in the form of an inhaler. When the patient needs continuous preventative treatment there are a number of choices: often an inhaled corticosteroid may be used (with a sympathomimetic inhaler if attacks persist). More severe cases may require higher-dose corticosteroids or the addition of a long-acting sympathomimetic bronchodilator. If this is not adequate, the addition of an anticholinergic drug, or theophylline, or these in combination with others already tried, may be needed. There are also leukotriene antagonists (see p.60), which may be used alone or with corticosteroids; they are less effective in severe cases when patients are taking high doses of other drugs. Some people who suffer from very severe asthma may need such large doses of corticosteroids that tablets have to be taken. Antihistamines have been prescribed for asthma in the past but this has not proved to be a successful treatment.

WHY THEY ARE USED

In asthma, the airways (bronchioles) constrict, which makes it difficult to get air into or out of the lungs. Bronchodilators (sympathomimetics, anticholinergics, and theophylline) (see p.23) relax the constricted muscles around the bronchioles. Short-acting sympathomimetics act almost immediately when inhaled and are used to provide relief of symptoms during an attack, and in more severe cases the long-acting sympathomimetics may be used to help with continuous protective cover. Anticholinergic drugs do not act as rapidly as the sympathomimetics. They are used for continuous prevention. Theophylline/amino-

phylline must be given by mouth or injection; the tablets are used for regular continuous dosing, and the injection is used in hospital to gain control of severe asthma. Drugs that are not bronchodilators, such as corticosteroids and leukotriene receptor antagonists, are not useful for dealing with an acute attack of asthma, but they are effective for long-term protection.

Antihistamines have been tried in the treatment of asthma but, although they are useful for other allergic conditions, they are not very effective in asthma.

HOW THEY WORK

Inhaling a drug directly into the lungs is the best way of obtaining benefit without experiencing excessive side effects. A selection of devices for delivering the drug into the airways is described below.

Inhalers or puffers release a small dose when they are pressed, but require some skill to use effectively. A large hollow plastic "spacer" can help you to inhale your drug more easily. Cartridges deliver larger amounts of drug than inhalers and are easier to use because the drug is taken in as you breathe normally.

In severe attacks, nebulizers pump compressed air through a solution of drug to produce a fine mist that is inhaled through a face mask. Nebulizers deliver large doses of the drug to the lungs, rapidly relieving breathing difficulty.

Bronchodilators act by relaxing the muscles surrounding the bronchioles. Corticosteroids are used for their anti-inflammatory properties. By suppressing airway inflammation they reduce swelling (oedema) inside the bronchioles, complementing relaxation of the walls by the bronchodilators in opening up the tubes. Reducing the inflammation also has the effect of reducing the amount of mucus produced, and this again helps to clear the airways. Corticosteroids usually start to increase the sufferer's capacity for exercise within a few days, and most people find that the frequency of their attacks of breathlessness is greatly reduced.

Leukotrienes, which used to be called "slow reacting substances", occur naturally in the body. They are chemically related to the prostaglandins, but are much more potent in producing an inflammatory reaction; they are also much more potent than histamine at causing bronchoconstriction. Leukotrienes seem to play an important part in asthma. Drugs have been developed that block their receptors (leukotriene receptor antagonists) and therefore reduce the inflammation and bronchoconstriction of asthma. Cromoglicate and nedocromil act by stabilizing mast cells in the lungs, preventing them from releasing histamine, leukotrienes, and other inflammation-causing chemicals.

RISKS AND SPECIAL PRECAUTIONS

The drugs taken by inhalation act locally and are used in much lower doses than would be needed as tablets. They do not commonly cause serious side effects, but the dry powder inhalations can cause a reflex bronchospasm as the powder hits the lining of the airways; this can be avoided by first using a short-acting sympathomimetic. Inhaled corticosteroids may encourage fungal growth in the mouth and throat (thrush). This can be minimized by using a spacer and by rinsing your mouth out and gargling after each inhalation. High doses of inhaled steroids may suppress adrenal gland function, reduce bone density, and increase the risk of glaucoma. Sympathomimetics and theophylline by mouth may affect heart rate, and should be prescribed with caution to people with heart problems, high blood pressure, or an overactive thyroid gland. The effects of theophylline may last longer if you have a viral infection, heart failure, or liver cirrhosis. The drugs also interact with many other drugs. Anticholinergics must be used with caution in patients who have prostate problems or urinary retention. Leukotriene receptor antagonists may produce a syndrome with several potentially serious effects including worsening lung function and heart complications.

COMMON DRUGS

Sympathomimetics Bambuterol, Ephedrine*, Epinephrine*, Fenoterol, Formoterol, Salbutamol*, Salmeterol*, Terbutaline*

Anticholinergics Ipratropium bromide*, Tiotropium*

Leukotriene antagonists Montelukast*, Zafirlukast

Corticosteroids Beclometasone*, Budesonide*, Ciclesonide, Fluticasone*, Prednisolone*

Xanthines Theophylline/aminophylline*

Other drugs Nedocromil, Sodium cromoglicate*

* See Part 2

Decongestants

The usual cause of a blocked nose is swelling of the delicate mucous membrane that lines the nasal passages and excessive production of mucus as a result of inflammation. This may be caused by an infection (for example, a common cold) or it may be caused by an allergy (for example, to pollen – a condition known as allergic rhinitis or hay fever). Congestion can also occur in the sinuses (the air spaces in the skull), resulting in sinusitis. Decongestants are drugs that reduce swelling of the mucous membrane and suppress the production of mucus, helping to clear blocked nasal passages and sinuses. Antihistamines (see p.58) counter the allergic response in allergy related conditions. If the symptoms are persistent, either topical corticosteroids (see p.120) or sodium cromoglicate (p.386) may be preferred.

WHY THEY ARE USED

Most common colds and blocked noses do not need to be treated with decongestants. Simple home remedies such as steam inhalation, possibly with the addition of an aromatic oil such as menthol or eucalyptus, are often effective. Decongestants are used when such measures are ineffective or when there is a particular risk from untreated congestion (for example, in people who suffer from recurrent middle-ear or sinus infections).

Decongestants are available in the form of drops or sprays applied directly into the nose (topical decongestants), or they can be taken by mouth. Small quantities of decongestant drugs are added to many over-the-counter cold remedies (see Cold cures, p.28).

HOW THEY WORK

When the mucous membrane lining the nose is irritated by infection or allergy, the blood vessels supplying the membrane become enlarged. This leads to fluid accumulation in the surrounding tissue and encourages the production of larger-than-normal amounts of mucus.

Most decongestants belong to the sympathomimetic group of drugs that stimulate the sympathetic branch of the autonomic nervous system (see p.8). One effect of this action is to constrict the blood vessels, thereby reducing swelling of the lining of the nose and sinuses.

HOW THEY AFFECT YOU

When applied topically in the form of drops or sprays, these drugs start to relieve congestion within a few minutes. Decongestants by mouth take a little longer to act, but their effect may also last longer. Used in moderation, topical decongestants have few adverse effects, because they are not absorbed by the body in large amounts.

Used for too long or in excess, topical decongestants can, after giving initial relief, do more harm than good, causing a "rebound congestion". This effect is a sudden increase in congestion due to widening of the blood vessels in the nasal lining because the blood vessels are no longer constricted by the decongestant. Rebound congestion can be prevented by taking the minimum effective dose and by using decongestant preparations only when absolutely necessary. Decongestants taken by mouth do not cause rebound congestion but are more likely to cause other side effects.

COMMON DRUGS

Used topically Ephedrine*, Ipratropium*, Oxymetazoline, Phenylephrine, Xylometazoline
Taken by mouth Ephedrine*, Phenylephrine, Pseudoephedrine
* See Part 2

Drugs to treat coughs

Coughing is a natural response to irritation of the lungs and air passages, designed to expel harmful substances from the respiratory tract. Common causes of coughing include infection of the respiratory tract (for example, bronchitis or pneumonia), inflammation of the airways caused by asthma, or exposure to certain irritant substances such as smoke or chemical fumes. Depending on their cause, coughs may be productive – that is, phlegm-producing – or they may be dry.

In most cases, coughing is a helpful reaction that assists the body in ridding itself of excess phlegm and substances that irritate the respiratory system; suppressing the cough may actually delay recovery. However, repeated bouts of coughing can be distressing, and may increase irritation of the air passages. In such cases, medication to ease the cough may be recommended.

There are two main groups of cough remedies, according to whether the cough is productive or dry.

PRODUCTIVE COUGHS

Mucolytics and expectorants are sometimes recommended for productive coughs when simple home remedies such as steam inhalation have failed to "loosen" the cough and make it easier to cough up phlegm. Mucolytics alter the consistency of the phlegm, making it less sticky and easier to cough up. These are often given by inhalation. However, there is little evidence that they are effective. Dornase alfa may be given to people who suffer from cystic fibrosis; the drug, given by inhalation via a nebulizer, is an enzyme that improves lung function by thinning the mucus. Expectorant drugs are taken by mouth to loosen a cough. There is some evidence that guaifenesin is effective but, overall, evidence of benefit is poor. Expectorants are included in many over-the-counter cough remedies.

DRY COUGHS

In dry coughs, no advantage is gained from promoting the expulsion of phlegm. Drugs used for dry coughs are given to suppress the coughing mechanism by calming the part of the brain that governs the coughing reflex. Antihistamines are often given for mild coughs, particularly in children. A demulcent, such as a simple linctus, can be used to soothe a dry, irritating cough. For persistent coughs, mild opioid drugs such as codeine may be prescribed (see also Analgesics, p.9). All cough suppressants have a generally sedating effect on the brain and nervous system and commonly cause drowsiness and other side effects.

SELECTING A COUGH MEDICATION

There is a bewildering variety of over-the-counter medications available for the treatment of coughs. Most preparations consist of a syrupy base to which active ingredients and flavourings are added. Many contain a number of different active ingredients, sometimes with contradictory effects: it is not uncommon to find an expectorant (for a productive cough) and a decongestant included in the same preparation.

It is important to select the correct type of medication for your cough to avoid the risk that you may make your condition worse. For example, using a cough suppressant for a productive cough may prevent you from getting rid of excess infected phlegm and may delay recovery. It is best to choose a preparation with a single active ingredient that is appropriate for your type of cough. Diabetics may need to select a sugar-free product. If you are in any doubt about which product to choose, ask your doctor or pharmacist for advice. Since there is a danger that use of over-the-counter cough remedies to alleviate symptoms may delay the diagnosis of a more serious underlying disorder, it is important to seek medical advice for any cough that persists for longer than a few days or if a cough is accompanied by additional symptoms such as fever or blood in the phlegm.

COLD CURES

Many preparations are available over the counter to treat different symptoms of the common cold. The main ingredient in most of these preparations is a mild analgesic, such as aspirin or paracetamol, accompanied by a decongestant (see p.26), an antihistamine (see p.58), and sometimes caffeine. In some cases, the dose of each added ingredient is too low to provide any benefit. There is no evidence to suggest that vitamin C (see p.90) speeds recovery. However, zinc supplements (see p.93) may be effective in shortening the duration of a cold.

While some people find these drugs help to relieve symptoms, over-the-counter cold cures do not alter the course of the illness. Most doctors recommend using a product with a single analgesic as the best way of alleviating symptoms. Other decongestants or antihistamines may be taken if needed. These medicines are not harmless, and care should be taken to avoid overdose if different brands are used.

COMMON DRUGS

Expectorants Ammonium chloride, Guaifenesin
Mucolytics Carbocysteine, Dornase alfa, Mecysteine
Steam inhalation Eucalyptus, Menthol
Opioid cough suppressants Codeine*, Dextromethorphan, Methadone*, Pholcodine
Non-opioid cough suppressants Antihistamines (see p.27)
* **See Part 2**

HEART AND CIRCULATION

The blood transports oxygen, nutrients, and heat, contains chemical messages in the form of drugs and hormones, and carries away waste products for excretion by the kidneys. Blood is pumped by the heart to and from the lungs, and then in a separate circuit to the rest of the body, including the brain, digestive organs, muscles, kidneys, and skin.

The heart is a pump with four chambers – two atria and two ventricles. The atrium and ventricle on the left side pump oxygenated blood to the body, while those on the right pump deoxygenated blood to the lungs. Backflow of blood is stopped by one-way valves at the chamber exits. Arteries carry blood away from the heart. Their muscle walls are elastic, contracting and dilating in response to nerve signals. Veins carry blood back to the heart. Their walls are thinner and less elastic than those of arteries.

WHAT CAN GO WRONG

The efficiency of the circulation may be impaired by weakening of the pumping action of the heart (heart failure) or by irregularity of the heart rate (arrhythmia). In addition, the blood vessels may be narrowed and clogged by fatty deposits (atherosclerosis). This may reduce blood supply to the brain, the extremities (peripheral vascular disease), or the heart muscle (coronary heart disease), causing angina. These last disorders can be complicated by the formation of clots that may block a blood vessel. A clot in the arteries supplying the heart muscle is known as coronary thrombosis; a clot in an artery inside the brain is the most frequent cause of stroke.

One common circulatory disorder is abnormally high blood pressure (hypertension), in which the pressure of circulating blood on the vessel walls is increased for reasons not yet fully understood. One factor may be loss of elasticity of the vessel walls (arteriosclerosis). Several other conditions, such as migraine and Raynaud's disease, are caused by temporary alterations to blood vessel size.

WHY DRUGS ARE USED

Because people suffering from heart disease often have more than one problem, several drugs may be prescribed at once. Many act directly on the heart to alter the rate and rhythm of the heart beat. These are known as anti-arrhythmics and include beta blockers and digoxin.

Other drugs affect the diameter of the blood vessels, either by dilating them (vasodilators) to improve blood flow and reduce blood pressure, or by constricting them (vasoconstrictors).

Drugs may also reduce blood volume and fat levels, and alter clotting ability. Diuretics (used in the treatment of hypertension and heart failure) increase the body's excretion of water. Lipid-lowering drugs reduce blood cholesterol levels, thereby minimizing the risk of atherosclerosis. Drugs to reduce blood clotting are administered if there is a risk of abnormal blood clots forming in the heart, veins, or arteries. Drugs that increase clotting are given when the body's natural clotting mechanism is defective.

MAJOR DRUG GROUPS

◆ Digitalis drugs
◆ Beta blockers
◆ Vasodilators
◆ Diuretics
◆ Anti-arrhythmics
◆ Anti-angina drugs
◆ Antihypertensive drugs
◆ Lipid-lowering drugs
◆ Drugs that affect blood clotting

Digitalis drugs

Digitalis is the collective term for the naturally occurring substances (also called cardiac glycosides) that are found in the leaves of plants of the foxglove family and used to treat certain heart disorders. The principal drugs in this group are digoxin and digitoxin. Digoxin is more commonly used because it is shorter acting and dosage is easier to adjust (see also Risks and special precautions, p.30).

WHY THEY ARE USED

Digitalis drugs do not cure heart disease but improve the heart's pumping action and thereby relieve many of the symptoms that result from poor heart function. They are useful for treating conditions in which the heart beats irregularly or too rapidly (notably in atrial fibrillation, see Anti-arrhythmics, p.33), when it pumps too weakly (in congestive heart failure), or when the heart muscle is damaged and weakened following a heart attack.

Digitalis drugs can be used for a short period when the heart is working poorly, but in many cases they have to be taken indefinitely. Their effect does not diminish with time. In heart failure, digitalis drugs are often given together with a diuretic drug (see p.32).

HOW THEY WORK

The normal heart beat results from electrical impulses generated in nerve tissue within the heart. These cause the heart muscle to contract and pump blood. By reducing the flow of electrical impulses in the heart, digitalis makes the heart beat more slowly.

The force with which the heart muscle contracts depends on chemical changes in the heart muscle. By promoting these chemical changes, digitalis increases the force of muscle contraction each time the heart is stimulated. This compensates for the loss of power that occurs when some of the muscle is damaged following a heart attack. The stronger heart beat increases blood flow to the kidneys. This increases urine production and helps to remove the excess fluid that often accumulates as a result of heart failure.

HOW THEY AFFECT YOU

Digitalis relieves the symptoms of heart failure – fatigue, breathlessness, and swelling of the legs – and increases your capacity for exercise. The frequency with which you need to pass urine is also increased initially.

RISKS AND SPECIAL PRECAUTIONS

Digitalis drugs can be toxic; if blood levels rise too high, symptoms of digitalis poisoning (including nausea, appetite loss, vomiting, diarrhoea, confusion, and visual disturbance) may occur. It is important to report such symptoms to your doctor promptly.

Digoxin is normally removed from the body by the kidneys; if kidney function is impaired, the drug is more likely to accumulate in the body and cause toxic effects. Digitoxin, which is broken down in the liver, is sometimes preferred in such cases. Digitoxin can accumulate after repeated dosage if liver function is severely impaired.

Both digoxin and digitoxin are more toxic when blood potassium levels are low. Potassium deficiency is commonly due to diuretics, so that people taking these with digitalis drugs need to have the effects of both drugs and blood potassium levels carefully monitored. Potassium supplements may be required.

COMMON DRUGS

Digitoxin, Digoxin*
* See Part 2

Beta blockers

Beta blockers are drugs that interrupt the transmission of stimuli through beta receptors. Since the actions that they block originate in the adrenal glands (and elsewhere) they are also sometimes called beta adrenergic blocking agents. There are two types of beta receptor in the body: beta 1 and beta 2. Beta 1 receptors are located mainly in the heart muscle; beta 2 receptors in the airways and blood vessels. Cardioselective drugs act mainly on beta 1 receptors: non-cardioselective drugs on both types. Used mainly in heart disorders, these drugs are occasionally prescribed for other conditions.

WHY THEY ARE USED

Beta blockers are used for treating angina (see p.35) and irregular heart rhythms (see p.34). They may also be used for treating hypertension (see p.36) but are not usually used to initiate treatment. They are sometimes given after a heart attack to reduce the likelihood of abnormal heart rhythms or further damage to the heart muscle. They are also prescribed to improve heart function in heart muscle disorders, known as cardiomyopathies.

Beta blockers may also be given to prevent migraine headaches (see p.20), or to reduce the physical symptoms of anxiety (see p.13).

These drugs may be given to control symptoms of an overactive thyroid gland. A beta blocker is sometimes given in the form of eye drops in glaucoma (see p.114) to lower the fluid pressure inside the eye.

HOW THEY WORK

By occupying the beta receptors, in different parts of the body, beta blockers nullify the stimulating action of norepinephrine (noradrenaline), the main "fight or flight" hormone. As a result, they reduce the force and speed of the heart beat and prevent the dilation of the blood vessels surrounding the brain and leading to the extremities.

Heart Slowing of the heart rate and reduction of the force of the heart beat reduces the workload of the heart, helping to prevent angina and abnormal heart rhythms. This action may worsen heart failure, however.

Lungs Constriction of the airways may provoke breathlessness in asthmatic people or those with chronic bronchitis.

Brain Dilation of the blood vessels that surround the brain is inhibited, thereby preventing migraine.

Blood vessels Constriction of the blood vessels may cause coldness of the hands and feet.

Blood pressure The pressure is lowered due to reduction in the rate and force at which the heart pumps blood around the body.

Eye Beta blocker eye drops reduce fluid production, lowering pressure inside the eye.

Muscles Muscle tremor caused by anxiety or overactivity of the thyroid gland is reduced.

HOW THEY AFFECT YOU

Beta blockers are taken to treat angina. They reduce the frequency and severity of attacks. As part of the treatment for hypertension, beta blockers help to lower blood pressure and thus reduce the risks that are associated with this condition. Beta blockers help to prevent severe attacks of arrhythmia, in which the heart beat is wild and uncontrolled.

Because beta blockers affect many parts of the body, they often produce minor side effects. By reducing the heart rate and air flow to the lungs, they may reduce the capacity for strenuous exercise, although this is unlikely to be noticed by somebody whose physical activity was previously limited by heart problems. Many people experience cold hands and feet while taking these drugs as a result of the reduction in the blood supply to the limbs. Reduced circulation can also lead to temporary impotence during treatment.

RISKS AND SPECIAL PRECAUTIONS

The main risk of beta blockers is that of provoking breathing difficulties as a result of their blocking effect on beta receptors in the lungs. Cardioselective beta blockers, which act principally on the heart, are thought less likely than non-cardioselective ones to cause such problems. But all beta blockers are prescribed with caution for people who have asthma, bronchitis, or other forms of respiratory disease.

Beta blockers are not commonly prescribed to people who have poor circulation in the limbs because they reduce blood flow and may aggravate such conditions. They may be of some benefit in heart failure, but treatment is usually initiated by specialists. People with diabetes who need to take beta blockers should be aware that they may notice a change in the warning signs of low blood sugar; in particular, they may find that symptoms such as palpitations and tremor are suppressed.

Beta blockers should not be stopped suddenly after prolonged use; this may provoke a sudden and severe recurrence of symptoms of the original disorder, even a heart attack. The blood pressure may also rise markedly. When treatment with beta blockers needs to be stopped, it should be withdrawn gradually under medical supervision.

COMMON DRUGS

Cardioselective Acebutolol*, Atenolol*, Betaxolol, Bisoprolol*, Celiprolol, Esmolol, Metoprolol*, Nebivolol
Non-cardioselective Carvedilol, Labetalol, Nadolol, Oxprenolol, Pindolol, Propranolol*, Sotalol*, Timolol*
* See Part 2

Vasodilators

Vasodilators are drugs that widen blood vessels. Their most obvious use is to reverse narrowing of the blood vessels when this leads to reduced blood flow and, consequently, a lower oxygen supply to parts of the body. This problem occurs in angina, when narrowing of the coronary arteries reduces blood supply to the heart muscle. Vasodilators are often used to treat high blood pressure (hypertension).

WHY THEY ARE USED

Vasodilators improve blood flow and thus the oxygen supply to areas of the body where they are most needed. In angina, dilation of blood vessels throughout the body reduces the force with which the heart needs to pump and thereby eases its workload (see also Antiangina drugs, p.35). This may also be helpful in treating congestive heart failure when other treatments are not effective.

Because blood pressure is partly dependent on the diameter of blood vessels, vasodilators are often helpful for hypertension (see p.36).

In peripheral vascular disease, narrowed blood vessels in the legs cannot supply sufficient blood to the extremities, often leading to pain in the legs during exercise. Unfortunately, because the vessels are narrowed by atherosclerosis, vasodilators have little effect.

Vasodilators have also been used to treat senile dementia, in the hope of increasing oxygen supply to the brain. The benefits of this have not yet been proved.

HOW THEY WORK

Vasodilators widen the blood vessels by relaxing the muscles surrounding them, either by affecting the action of the muscles directly (nitrates, hydralazine, and calcium channel blockers), or by interfering with the nerve signals that govern contraction of the blood vessels (alpha blockers). ACE (angiotensin-converting enzyme) inhibitors block the activity of an enzyme in the blood that is responsible for producing angiotensin II, a powerful vasoconstrictor. Angiotensin II blockers prevent angiotensin II from constricting the blood vessels by blocking its receptors within the vessels.

HOW THEY AFFECT YOU

As well as relieving the symptoms of the disorders for which they are taken, vasodilators can have many minor side effects related to their action on the circulation. Flushing and headaches are common at the start of treatment. Dizziness and fainting may also occur due to lowered blood pressure. Dilation of the blood vessels can also cause fluid build-up, leading to swelling, particularly of the ankles.

RISKS AND SPECIAL PRECAUTIONS

The major risk is of blood pressure falling too low; vasodilators are used with caution in people with unstable blood pressure. It is also advisable to sit or lie down after taking the first dose of a vasodilator.

COMMON DRUGS

ACE inhibitors Captopril*, Cilazapril, Enalapril*, Fosinopril, Lisinopril*, Perindopril, Quinapril, Ramipril*, Trandolapril

Angiotensin II blockers Candesartan*, Irbesartan*, Losartan*, Telmisartan, Valsartan*

Alpha blockers Doxazosin*, Indoramin, Prazosin, Terazosin

Potassium channel activators Nicorandil*

Nitrates Glyceryl trinitrate*, Isosorbide dinitrate/mononitrate*

Calcium channel blockers Amlodipine*, Diltiazem*, Felodipine*, Lacidipine, Lercanidipine, Nicardipine, Nifedipine*, Nisoldipine, Verapamil*

Other drugs Hydralazine, Minoxidil*

Peripheral vasodilators Cilastazol, Naftidrofuryl*, Pentoxifylline

* See Part 2

Diuretics

Diuretic drugs help to turn excess body water into urine. As the urine is expelled, two disorders are relieved: the tissues become less water-swollen (oedema) and the heart action improves because it has to pump a smaller volume of blood. There are several classes of diuretic, each of which has different uses, modes of action, and effects (see Types of diuretic, facing page). But all diuretics act on the kidneys, the organs that govern the water content of the body.

WHY THEY ARE USED

Diuretics are most commonly used in the treatment of high blood pressure (hypertension). By removing a larger amount of water than usual from the bloodstream, the kidneys reduce the total volume of blood circulating. This drop in volume causes a reduction of the pressure within the blood vessels (see Antihypertensive drugs, p.36).

Diuretics are also widely used to treat heart failure in which the heart's pumping mechanism has become weak. In the treatment of this disorder, they remove fluid that has accumulated in the tissues and lungs. The resulting drop in blood volume reduces the work of the heart.

Other conditions for which diuretics are often prescribed include nephrotic syndrome (a kidney disorder that causes oedema), liver cirrhosis (in which fluid may accumulate in the abdominal cavity), and premenstrual syndrome (when hormonal activity can lead to fluid retention and bloating).

Less commonly, diuretics are used to treat glaucoma (see p.114) and Ménière's disease (see Anti-emetics, p.21).

TYPES OF DIURETIC

Thiazides The most commonly prescribed diuretics, thiazides are often given with potassium supplements, or in conjunction with a potassium-sparing diuretic (see below), because they may lead to potassium deficiency.

Loop diuretics These fast-acting, powerful drugs increase urine output for a few hours and are therefore sometimes used in emergencies. They can cause excessive potassium loss, which may need to be prevented as for thiazides. Large doses given into a vein may disturb hearing.

Potassium-sparing diuretics These mild diuretics are usually used in conjunction with a thiazide or a loop diuretic to prevent excessive loss of potassium.

Osmotic diuretics Prescribed only rarely, osmotics are used to maintain the urine flow through the kidneys after surgery or injury, and to reduce pressure rapidly in the brain or eye.

Acetazolamide This mild diuretic is used mainly to treat glaucoma (see p.114).

HOW THEY WORK

The kidneys' normal filtration process takes water, salts (mainly potassium and sodium), and waste products out of the bloodstream. Most of the salts and water are returned to the bloodstream, but some are expelled from the body together with the waste products in the urine. Diuretics interfere with this filtration process by reducing the amounts of sodium and water taken back into the bloodstream, thus increasing the volume of urine produced. Modifying the filtration process in this way means that the water content of the blood is reduced; less water in the blood causes excess water present in the tissues to be drawn out and eliminated in urine.

HOW THEY AFFECT YOU

All diuretics increase the frequency with which you need to pass urine. This is most noticeable at the start of treatment. People who have suffered from oedema may notice that swelling – particularly of the ankles – is reduced, and those with heart failure may find that breathlessness is relieved.

RISKS AND SPECIAL PRECAUTIONS

Diuretics can cause blood chemical imbalances, of which a fall in potassium levels (hypokalaemia) is the most common. Hypokalaemia can cause confusion, weakness, and trigger abnormal heart rhythms (especially in people taking digitalis drugs). Potassium supplements or a potassium-sparing diuretic usually corrects the imbalance. A diet that is rich in potassium (containing plenty of fresh fruits and vegetables) may be helpful.

Some diuretics may raise blood levels of uric acid, increasing the risk of gout. They may also raise blood sugar levels, causing problems for diabetics.

COMMON DRUGS

Loop diuretics Bumetanide*, Furosemide/frusemide*, Torasemide

Potassium-sparing diuretics Amiloride*, Eplerenone, Spironolactone*, Triamterene*

Thiazides Bendroflumethiazide*, Chlortalidone, Cyclopenthiazide, Hydrochlorothiazide*, Hydroflumethiazide, Indapamide*, Metolazone, Xipamide

* See Part 2

Anti-arrhythmics

The heart contains two upper and two lower chambers, which are known as the atria and ventricles (see p.29). The pumping actions of these two sets of chambers are normally co-ordinated by electrical impulses that originate in the heart's pacemaker and then travel along conducting pathways so that the heart beats with a regular rhythm. If this coordination breaks down, the heart will beat abnormally, either irregularly or faster or slower than usual. The general term for abnormal heart rhythm is arrhythmia.

Arrhythmias may occur as a result of a birth defect, coronary heart disease, or other less common heart disorders. A variety of more general conditions, including overactivity of the thyroid gland, and certain drugs, such as caffeine and anticholinergic drugs, can also disturb heart rhythm.

Arrhythmias can be divided into two groups: tachycardias (such as atrial fibrillation), in which the heart rate is faster than normal; and bradycardias (such as heart block), in which the rate is slower.

Atrial fibrillation In this common type of arrhythmia, the atria contract irregularly at such a high rate that the ventricles cannot keep pace. The condition is treated with digoxin, verapamil, amiodarone, or a beta blocker.

Ventricular tachycardia This condition arises from abnormal electrical activity in the ventricles that causes the ventricles to contract rapidly. Regular treatment with quinidine, disopyramide, or procainamide is usually given. Amiodarone may be used if these drugs are not effective.

Supraventricular tachycardia This condition occurs when extra electrical impulses arise in the pacemaker or atria, stimulating the ventricles into contracting rapidly. Attacks may disappear on their own without treatment, but drugs such as adenosine, digoxin, verapamil, or propranolol may be given.

Heart block When impulses are not conducted from the atria to the ventricles, the ventricles start to beat at a slower rate. Some cases of heart block do not require treatment. For more severe heart block accompanied by dizziness and fainting, the fitting of an artificial pacemaker is usually necessary.

A wide range of drugs is used to regulate heart rhythm, including beta blockers, digitalis drugs, and calcium channel blockers. Other drugs used are disopyramide, lidocaine, procainamide, and quinidine.

WHY THEY ARE USED

Minor disturbances of heart rhythm are common and do not usually require drug treatment. However, if the heart's pumping action is seriously affected, the circulation of blood throughout the body may become inefficient, and drug treatment may be necessary.

Drugs may be taken to treat individual attacks of arrhythmia, or they may be taken on a regular basis to prevent or control abnormal heart rhythms. The particular drug prescribed depends on the type of arrhythmia to be treated, but because people differ in their response, it may be necessary to try several in order to find the most effective one. When the arrhythmia is sudden and severe, it may be necessary to inject a drug immediately to restore normal heart function.

HOW THEY WORK

The heart's pumping action is governed by electrical impulses under the control of the sympathetic nervous system (see Autonomic nervous system, p.8). These signals pass through the heart muscle, causing the two pairs of chambers – the atria and ventricles – to contract in turn.

All anti-arrhythmic drugs alter the conduction of electrical signals in the heart. However, each drug or drug group has a different effect on the sequence of events controlling the pumping action. Some block the transmission of signals to the heart (beta blockers); some affect the way in which signals are conducted within the heart (digitalis drugs); others affect the response of the heart muscle to the signals received (calcium channel blockers, disopyramide, procainamide, and quinidine).

HOW THEY AFFECT YOU

These drugs usually prevent symptoms of arrhythmia and may restore a regular heart rhythm. Although they do not prevent all arrhythmias, they usually reduce the frequency and severity of any symptoms.

Unfortunately, as well as suppressing arrhythmias, many of these drugs tend to depress normal heart function, and may produce dizziness on standing up, or increased breathlessness on exertion. Mild nausea and visual disturbances are also fairly frequent. Verapamil can cause constipation, especially when it is prescribed in high doses. Disopyramide may interfere with the parasympathetic nervous system (see Autonomic nervous system, p.8), resulting in a number of anticholinergic effects.

RISKS AND SPECIAL PRECAUTIONS

These drugs, under certain circumstances, may further disrupt heart rhythm, and therefore they are used only when the likely benefit outweighs the risks.

Quinidine can be toxic if an overdose is taken, resulting in a syndrome called cinchonism, which includes disturbed hearing, giddiness, and impaired vision (even blindness). Because some people are particularly sensitive to this drug, a test dose is usually given before regular treatment is started.

Amiodarone may accumulate in the tissues over time, and may lead to light-sensitive rashes, changes in thyroid function, and lung problems.

COMMON DRUGS

Beta blockers (see also p.30), Sotalol*
Calcium channel blockers Felodipine* Verapamil*
Digitalis drugs (see also p.29), Digitoxin, Digoxin*
Other drugs Adenosine, Amiodarone*, Bretylium, Disopyramide, Flecainide, Lidocaine, Mexiletine, Moracizine, Procainamide, Propafenone, Quinidine
* See Part 2

Anti-angina drugs

Angina is chest pain produced when insufficient oxygen reaches the heart muscle. This is usually caused by a narrowing of the blood vessels (coronary arteries) that carry blood and oxygen to the heart muscle. In the most common type of angina (classic angina), pain usually occurs during physical exertion or emotional stress. In variant angina, pain may also occur at rest. In classic angina, the narrowing of the coronary arteries results from deposits of fat, known as atheroma, on the walls of the arteries. In the variant type, however, angina is caused by contraction (spasm) of the muscle fibres in the artery walls.

Atheroma deposits build up more rapidly in the arteries of smokers and people who eat a high-fat diet. This is why, as a basic component of angina treatment, doctors recommend that smoking should be given up and the diet changed. Overweight people are also advised to lose weight in order to reduce the demands placed on the heart. While such changes in lifestyle often produce an improvement in symptoms, drug treatment to relieve angina is also frequently necessary.

The drugs used to treat angina include beta blockers, nitrates, calcium channel blockers, and potassium channel openers.

WHY THEY ARE USED

Frequent episodes of angina can be disabling and, if left untreated, can lead to an increased risk of a heart attack. Drugs can both relieve angina attacks and reduce their frequency. People who suffer only occasional episodes are usually prescribed a rapid-acting drug to take at the first signs of an attack, or before an activity that is known to bring on an attack. Glyceryl trinitrate, a rapid-acting nitrate drug, is usually prescribed for this purpose.

If attacks become more frequent or more severe, regular preventative treatment may be advised. Beta blockers, long-acting nitrates, and calcium channel blockers are used as regular medication to prevent attacks. The introduction of adhesive patches to administer nitrates through the patient's skin has extended the duration of action of glyceryl trinitrate, making treatment easier.

Drugs can often control angina for many years, but they cannot cure the disorder. When severe angina cannot be controlled by drugs, then surgery to increase the blood flow to the heart may be recommended.

HOW THEY WORK

Nitrates and calcium channel blockers dilate blood vessels by relaxing the muscle layer in the blood vessel walls (see also Vasodilators, p.31). Blood is more easily pumped through the dilated vessels, reducing the strain on the heart.

Beta blockers reduce heart muscle stimulation during exercise or stress by interrupting signal transmission in the heart. Decreased heart muscle stimulation means that less oxygen is required, reducing the risk of angina attacks. For further information on beta blockers, see p.30.

HOW THEY AFFECT YOU

Treatment with one or more of these medicines usually effectively controls angina. Drugs to prevent attacks allow sufferers to undertake more strenuous activities without provoking pain, and if an attack does occur, nitrates usually provide effective relief.

These drugs do not usually cause serious adverse effects but can produce a variety of minor symptoms. By dilating blood vessels throughout the body, nitrates and calcium channel blockers can cause dizziness (especially on standing) and may cause fainting. Other possible side effects are headaches at the start of treatment, flushing of the skin (especially of the face), and ankle swelling. Beta blockers often cause cold hands and feet, and sometimes they may produce tiredness and a feeling of heaviness in the legs.

COMMON DRUGS

Calcium channel blockers Amlodipine*, Diltiazem*, Felodipine*, Nicardipine, Nifedipine*, Nisoldipine, Verapamil*
Beta blockers (see p.30)
Nitrates Glyceryl trinitrate*, Isosorbide dinitrate/mononitrate*
Potassium channel opener Nicorandil*
Other drugs Aspirin*, Heparin/low molecular weight heparins (Enoxaparin, Dalteparin)*, Ivabradine, Simvastatin*
* See Part 2

Antihypertensive drugs

Blood pressure is the force exerted by the blood against the artery walls. Two measurements are taken: one indicates force while the heart's ventricles are contracting (systolic pressure). This reading is a higher figure than the other one, which measures the blood pressure during ventricle relaxation (diastolic pressure). Blood pressure varies among individuals and normally increases with age. If a person's blood pressure is higher than normal on at least three separate occasions, a doctor may diagnose the condition as hypertension.

Blood pressure may be elevated as a result of an underlying disorder, which the doctor will try to identify. Usually, however, it is not possible to determine a cause. This condition is referred to as essential hypertension.

Although hypertension does not usually cause any symptoms, severely raised blood pressure may produce headaches, palpitations, and general feelings of ill-health. It is important to reduce high blood pressure because it can have serious consequences, including stroke, heart attack, heart failure, and kidney damage. Certain groups are particularly at risk from high blood pressure. These risk groups include diabetics, smokers, people with pre-existing heart damage, and those whose blood contains a high level of fat. High blood pressure is more common among black people than among whites, and in countries, such as Japan, where the diet is high in salt.

A small reduction in blood pressure may be brought about by reducing weight, exercising regularly, and avoiding an excessive amount of salt in the diet. However, for more severely raised blood pressure, one or more antihypertensive drugs may be prescribed. Several classes of drug have antihypertensive properties, including the centrally acting antihypertensives, diuretics (p.32), beta blockers (p.30), calcium channel blockers (p.34), ACE (angiotensin-converting enzyme) inhibitors (see Vasodilators, p.31), and alpha blockers.

WHY THEY ARE USED

Antihypertensive drugs are prescribed when diet, exercise, and other simple remedies have not brought about an adequate reduction in blood pressure, and your doctor sees a risk of serious consequences if the condition is not treated. These drugs do not cure hypertension and may have to be taken indefinitely. However, it is sometimes possible to taper off drug treatment when blood pressure has been reduced to a normal level for a year or more.

HOW THEY WORK

Blood pressure depends not only on the force with which the heart pumps blood, but also on the diameter of blood vessels and volume of blood in circulation: blood pressure is increased either if the vessels are narrow or the volume of blood is high. Antihypertensives lower blood pressure either by dilating the blood vessels or by reducing blood volume. Each type of antihypertensive acts in a different way to lower blood pressure.

Centrally acting drugs act on the mechanism in the brain that controls the diameter of the blood vessels.

Beta blockers reduce the force of the heart beat.

Diuretics act on the kidneys to reduce blood volume.

ACE inhibitors act on enzymes in the blood to dilate blood vessels.

Vasodilators and calcium channel blockers act on the arterial wall muscles to prevent constriction.

Alpha blockers block nerve signals that trigger constriction of blood vessels.

CHOICE OF DRUG

Drug treatment depends on the severity of the hypertension. At the beginning of treatment for mild or moderately high blood pressure, a single drug is used. A thiazide diuretic is often chosen for initial treatment, but it is also increasingly common to use a calcium channel blocker or an ACE inhibitor. If a single drug does not reduce the blood pressure sufficiently, a combination of these drugs may be used. Some people who have moderate hypertension require an additional drug, in which case an alpha blocker or beta blocker may also be prescribed.

Severe hypertension is usually controlled with a combination of several drugs, which may need to be given in high doses. Your doctor may need to try a number of drugs before finding a combination that controls blood pressure without unacceptable side effects.

HOW THEY AFFECT YOU

Treatment with antihypertensive drugs relieves symptoms such as headache and palpitations. However, since most people with hypertension have few, if any, symptoms, side effects may be more noticeable than any immediate beneficial effect. Some antihypertensive drugs may cause dizziness and fainting at the start of treatment because they can sometimes cause an excessive fall in blood pressure. It may take a while for your doctor to determine a dosage that avoids such effects. For detailed information on the adverse effects of drugs that are used to treat hypertension, consult the individual drug profiles in Part 2.

RISKS AND SPECIAL PRECAUTIONS

Because your doctor needs to know exactly how treatment with a particular drug affects your hypertension – the benefits as well as the side effects – it is important for you to keep using the antihypertensive medication as prescribed, even though you may feel that the problem is under control. Sudden withdrawal of some of these drugs may cause a potentially dangerous rebound increase in blood pressure. The dose needs to be reduced gradually under medical supervision.

COMMON DRUGS

ACE inhibitors (see p.31)
Angiotensin II blocker Candesartan*
Beta blockers (see p.30)
Calcium channel blockers Amlodipine*, Diltiazem*, Felodipine*, Isradipine, Lacidipine, Lercanidipine, Nicardipine, Nifedipine*, Nisoldipine, Verapamil*
Centrally acting antihypertensives Clonidine, Methyldopa, Moxonidine*
Diuretics (see p.32)
Alpha blockers Doxazosin*, Indoramin, Prazosin, Terazosin
Vasodilators (see p.31)
* See Part 2

Lipid-lowering drugs

The blood contains several types of fats, or lipids. They are necessary for normal body function but can be damaging in excess, particularly saturated fats such as cholesterol. The main risk is atherosclerosis, in which fatty deposits (atheroma) build up in the arteries, restricting and disrupting blood flow. This can increase the likelihood of abnormal blood clots forming, leading to potentially fatal disorders such as stroke and heart attack.

For most people, reducing their fat intake reduces the risk of atherosclerosis; but for those with an inherited tendency to high blood levels of fat (hyperlipidaemia), lipid-lowering drugs may also be recommended.

WHY THEY ARE USED

Lipid-lowering drugs are generally used only when dietary measures have failed to control hyperlipidaemia. They may be prescribed at an earlier stage to people at increased risk of atherosclerosis – such as diabetics and those already suffering from circulatory disorders. The drugs may help the body to remove existing atheroma in the blood vessels and prevent accumulation of new deposits. Low-dose simvastatin is available over the counter to help lower cholesterol levels in certain people.

For maximum benefit, lipid-lowering drugs are used in conjunction with a low-fat diet and a reduction in other risk factors such as obesity and smoking. The choice of drug depends on the type of lipid causing problems, so a full medical history, examination, and laboratory analysis of blood samples are needed before drug treatment is prescribed.

HOW THEY WORK

Cholesterol and triglycerides are two of the major fats in the blood. One or both may be raised, influencing the choice of lipid-lowering drug. Bile salts contain a large amount of cholesterol and are normally released into the bowel to aid digestion before being reabsorbed into the blood. Drugs that bind to bile salts reduce cholesterol levels by blocking their reabsorption, allowing them to be lost from the body.

Other drugs act on the liver. Fibrates and nicotinic acid and its derivatives can reduce the level of both cholesterol and triglycerides in the blood. Fish oil preparations reduce blood triglycerides. Statins lower blood cholesterol. It is now believed that low-grade inflammation is one of the causes of atheroma, and statins have an anti-inflammatory action, which may partly explain their effectiveness.

Lipid-lowering drugs do not correct the underlying cause of raised levels of fat in the blood, so it is usually necessary to continue with diet and drug treatment indefinitely. Stopping treatment usually leads to a return of high blood lipid levels.

HOW THEY AFFECT YOU

Because hyperlipidaemia and atherosclerosis are usually without symptoms, you are unlikely to notice any short-term benefits from these drugs. Rather, the aim of treatment is to reduce long-term complications. There may be minor side effects from some of these drugs.

The statin drugs appear to be well tolerated and are widely used to lower cholesterol levels when diet alone is not effective.

RISKS AND SPECIAL PRECAUTIONS

Drugs that bind to bile salts can limit absorption of some fat-soluble vitamins, and vitamin supplements may therefore be needed. The fibrates can increase susceptibility to gallstones and occasionally upset the balance of fats in the blood. Statins are used with caution in people with reduced kidney or liver function, and monitoring of blood samples is often advised. You should consult your doctor or pharmacist before taking simvastatin.

COMMON DRUGS

Statins Atorvastatin*, Fluvastatin, Pravastatin*, Rosuvastatin*, Simvastatin*

Drugs that bind to bile salts Colestipol, Colestyramine*, Ezetimibe*, Ispaghula

Fibrates Bezafibrate*, Ciprofibrate, Fenofibrate, Gemfibrozil

Other drugs acting on the liver Omega-3 acid ethyl esters, Omega-3 marine triglycerides

Nicotinic acid and derivatives Acipimox, Nicotinic acid

* See Part 2

Drugs that affect blood clotting

When bleeding occurs as a result of injury or surgery, the body normally acts swiftly to stem the flow by sealing the breaks in the blood vessels. This occurs in two stages – first when cells called platelets accumulate as a plug at the opening in the blood vessel wall, and then when these platelets produce chemicals that activate clotting factors in the blood to form a protein called fibrin. Vitamin K plays an important role in this process. An enzyme in the blood called plasmin ensures that clots are broken down when the injury has been repaired.

Some disorders interfere with this process, either preventing clot formation or creating clots uncontrollably. If the blood does not clot, there is a danger of excessive blood loss. Inappropriate development of clots may block the supply of blood to a vital organ.

DRUGS USED TO PROMOTE BLOOD CLOTTING

Fibrin formation depends on the presence in the blood of several clotting-factor proteins. When Factor VIII is absent or at low levels, an inherited disease called haemophilia exists; the symptoms almost always appear only in males. Factor IX deficiency causes another bleeding condition called Christmas disease, named after the person in whom it was first identified. Lack of these clotting factors can lead to uncontrolled bleeding or excessive bruising following even minor injuries.

Regular drug treatment for haemophilia is not normally required. However, if severe bleeding or bruising occurs, a concentrated form of the missing factor, extracted from normal blood, may be injected in order to promote clotting and thereby halt bleeding. Injections may need to be repeated for several days after injury.

It is sometimes useful to promote blood clotting in non-haemophiliacs when bleeding is difficult to stop (for example, following surgery). In such cases, blood clots are sometimes stabilized by reducing the action of plasmin with an antifibrinolytic (or haemostatic) drug like tranexamic acid; this is also occasionally given to haemophiliacs before minor surgery such as tooth extraction.

A tendency to bleed may also occur with deficiency of vitamin K, which is required for the production of several blood clotting factors. It is absorbed from the intestine in fats, but some diseases of the small intestine or pancreas cause fat to be poorly absorbed. As a result, the level of vitamin K in the circulation is low, causing impaired blood clotting. A similar problem sometimes occurs in newborn babies due to absence of vitamin K. Injections of phytomenadione, a vitamin K preparation, are used to restore levels to normal.

DRUGS USED TO PREVENT ABNORMAL BLOOD CLOTTING

Blood clots normally form only as a response to injury. In some people, however, there is a tendency for clots to form in the blood vessels without apparent cause. Disturbed blood flow occurring as a result of the presence of fatty deposits – atheroma – inside the blood vessels increases the risk of the formation of this type of abnormal clot (or thrombus). In addition, a portion of a blood clot (known as an embolus) formed in response to injury or surgery may sometimes break off and be removed in the bloodstream. The likelihood of this happening is increased by long periods of little or no activity. When an abnormal clot forms, there is a risk that it may become lodged in a blood vessel, thereby blocking the blood supply to a vital organ such as the brain or heart.

Three main types of drugs are used to prevent and disperse clots: antiplatelet drugs, anticoagulants, and thrombolytics.

ANTIPLATELET DRUGS

Taken regularly by people with a tendency to form clots in the fast-flowing blood of the heart and arteries, these drugs are also given to prevent clots from forming after heart surgery. They reduce the tendency of platelets to stick together when blood flow is disrupted.

The most widely used antiplatelet drug is aspirin (see also Analgesics, p.9), which has an antiplatelet action even when given in much lower doses than would be necessary to reduce pain. In these low doses adverse effects that may occur when aspirin is given in pain-relieving doses are unlikely. Other antiplatelet drugs are clopidogrel and dipyridamole.

ANTICOAGULANTS

Anticoagulants help to maintain normal blood flow in people at risk from clot formation. They can either prevent the formation of blood clots in the veins or stabilize an existing clot so that it does not break away and become a circulation-stopping embolism. All anticoagulants reduce the activity of certain blood clotting factors, but each drug's mode of action differs. These medicines do not dissolve clots that have already formed, however: these are treated with thrombolytic drugs (see right).

Anticoagulants fall into two groups: those that are given by intravenous injection and act immediately, and those that are given by mouth and take effect after a few days.

INJECTED ANTICOAGULANTS

Heparin is the most widely used drug of this type and it is used mainly in hospital during or after surgery. It is also given during kidney dialysis to prevent clots from forming in the dialysis equipment. Because heparin cannot be taken by mouth, it is less suitable for long-term treatment in the home.

A number of synthetic injected anticoagulants have recently been developed. Some act for a longer time than heparin, and others are alternatives for people who react adversely to heparin.

ORAL ANTICOAGULANTS

Warfarin is the most widely used of the oral anticoagulants. These drugs are mainly prescribed to prevent the formation of clots in veins and in the chambers of the heart (they are less likely to prevent clot formation in arteries). Oral anticoagulants may be given following injury or surgery (in particular, heart valve replacement) when there is a high risk of embolism. They are also given long term as preventative treatment to people at risk of strokes. A common problem with these drugs is that overdosage may lead to bleeding from the nose or gums, or in the urinary tract. For this reason, the dosage needs to be carefully calculated; regular blood tests are performed to ensure that the clotting mechanism is correctly adjusted.

The action of oral anticoagulants may be affected by many other drugs, and it may therefore be necessary to alter the dosage of anticoagulant when other drugs also need to be given. People prescribed oral anticoagulants should carry a warning list of drugs that they should not be given. In particular, no anticoagulant should be taken together with aspirin except on the direction of a doctor.

THROMBOLYTICS

Also known as fibrinolytics, these drugs are used to dissolve clots that have already formed. They are usually given in hospital intravenously to clear a blocked blood vessel (in coronary thrombosis, for example). The sooner they are given after the start of symptoms, the more likely they are to reduce the size and severity of a heart attack. Thrombolytic drugs may be given either intravenously or directly into the blocked blood vessel. The main thrombolytics are streptokinase and alteplase, which act by increasing the blood level of plasmin, the enzyme that breaks down fibrin. When given promptly, alteplase appears to be tolerated better than streptokinase.

The most common problems with use of these drugs are increased susceptibility to bleeding and bruising, and allergic reactions to streptokinase, such as rashes, breathing difficulty, or general discomfort. Once streptokinase has been given, patients are given a card indicating this, because further treatment with the same drug may be less effective.

COMMON DRUGS

Blood clotting factors Factor VIIa, Factor VIII, Factor IX, Fresh frozen plasma

Antifibrinolytic or haemostatic drugs Aprotinin, Etamsylate, Tranexamic acid

Vitamin K Phytomenadione

Antiplatelet drugs Abciximab, Aspirin*, Clopidogrel*, Dipyridamole*, Eptifibatide, Tirofiban

Injected anticoagulants Danaparoid, Desirudin, Epoprostenol, Fondaparinux, Heparin*, Lepirudin

Thrombolytic drugs Alteplase, Reteplase, Streptokinase*, Tenecteplase*

Oral anticoagulants Acenocoumarol/nicoumalone, Warfarin*

Heparin/low molecular weight heparins (Dalteparin, Enoxaparin, Tinzaparin)*

* See Part 2

GASTROINTESTINAL TRACT

The gastrointestinal tract, also known as the digestive or alimentary tract, is the pathway through which food passes as it is processed to enable the nutrients it contains to be absorbed for use by the body. It consists of the mouth, oesophagus, stomach, duodenum, small intestine, large intestine (including the colon and rectum), and anus. In addition, a number of other organs are involved in the digestion of food: the salivary glands in the mouth, the liver, pancreas, and gallbladder. These organs, together with the gastrointestinal tract, form the digestive system.

The digestive system breaks down the large, complex chemicals – proteins, carbohydrates, and fats – present in the food we eat into simpler molecules that can be used by the body (see also Nutrition, p.90).

The stomach holds food and passes it into the intestine. The lining of the stomach releases gastric juice that partly digests food. The stomach wall continuously produces thick mucus that forms a protective coating.

The duodenum is the tube that connects the stomach to the intestine. Its lining may be damaged by excess acid from the stomach.

The pancreas produces enzymes that digest proteins, fats, and carbohydrates into simpler substances; pancreatic juices neutralize the acidity of the food passing from the stomach.

The gallbladder stores bile, which is produced by the liver, and releases it into the duodenum. Bile assists the digestion of fats by reducing them to smaller units that are more easily acted upon by digestive enzymes.

The small intestine is a long tube in which food is broken down by digestive juices from the gallbladder and pancreas. The mucous lining of the small intestine consists of tiny, finger-like projections called villi that provide a large surface area through which the products of digestion are absorbed into the bloodstream.

The large intestine receives both undigested food and indigestible material from the small intestine. Water and mineral salts pass through the lining into the bloodstream.

When a sufficient mass of undigested material, together with some of the body's waste products, has accumulated, it is expelled from the body as faeces.

MOVEMENT OF FOOD THROUGH THE GASTROINTESTINAL TRACT

Food is propelled through the gastrointestinal tract by rhythmic waves of muscular contraction called peristalsis.

Muscle contraction in the gastrointestinal tract is controlled by the autonomic nervous system (p.8) and is therefore easily disrupted by drugs that either stimulate or inhibit the activity of the autonomic nervous system. Excessive peristaltic action may cause diarrhoea, and constipation may result from slowed peristalsis.

WHAT CAN GO WRONG

Inflammation of the lining of the stomach or intestine (gastroenteritis) is usually the result of an infection or parasitic infestation. Damage may also occur through the inappropriate production of digestive juices, leading to minor complaints like acidity and major disorders like peptic ulcers. The lining of the intestine can be damaged by abnormal functioning of the immune system (inflammatory bowel disease). The rectum and anus can become painful and irritated by damage to the lining, tears in the skin at the opening of the anus (anal fissure), or enlarged veins (haemorrhoids).

Constipation, diarrhoea, and irritable bowel syndrome are the most frequently experienced gastrointestinal complaints, and they usually occur when something disrupts the normal muscle contractions that propel food residue through the bowel.

WHY DRUGS ARE USED

Many drugs for gastrointestinal disorders are taken by mouth and act directly on the digestive tract without first entering the bloodstream. Such drugs include certain antibiotics and other drugs used to treat infestations. Some antacids for peptic ulcers and excess stomach acidity, and the bulk-forming agents for constipation and diarrhoea, also pass through the system unabsorbed.

However, for many disorders, drugs with a systemic effect are required, including anti-ulcer drugs, opioid antidiarrhoeal drugs, and some of the drugs for inflammatory bowel disease.

MAJOR DRUG GROUPS

◆ Antacids
◆ Anti-ulcer drugs
◆ Antidiarrhoeal drugs
◆ Drugs for irritable bowel syndrome
◆ Laxatives
◆ Drugs for inflammatory bowel disease
◆ Drugs for rectal and anal disorders
◆ Drug treatment for gallstones
◆ Drug treatment for pancreatic disorders

Antacids

Digestive juices in the stomach contain acid and enzymes that break down food before it passes into the intestine. The wall of the stomach is normally protected from the action of digestive acid by a layer of mucus that is constantly secreted by the stomach lining. Problems arise when the stomach lining is damaged or too much acid is produced and eats away at the mucous layer.

Excess acid that leads to discomfort, commonly referred to as indigestion, may result from anxiety, overeating or eating certain foods, coffee, alcohol, or smoking. Some drugs, notably aspirin and non-steroidal anti-inflammatory drugs, can irritate the stomach lining and even cause ulcers to develop.

Antacids are used to neutralize acid and thus relieve pain. They are simple chemical compounds that are mildly alkaline and some also act as chemical buffers. Their chalky taste is often disguised with flavourings.

WHY THEY ARE USED

Antacids may be needed when simple remedies (such as a change in diet or a glass of milk) fail to relieve indigestion. They are especially useful after a meal to neutralize the acid surge that sometimes occurs after a meal.

Doctors prescribe these drugs in order to relieve dyspepsia (pain in the chest or upper abdomen caused by or aggravated by acid) in disorders such as inflammation or ulceration of the oesophagus, stomach lining, and duo-

denum. Antacids usually relieve pain resulting from ulcers in the oesophagus, stomach, or duodenum within a few minutes. Regular treatment with antacids reduces the acidity of the stomach, thereby encouraging the healing of any ulcers that may have formed.

TYPES OF ANTACID

Aluminium compounds These drugs have a prolonged action and are widely used, especially for the treatment of indigestion and dyspepsia. They may cause constipation, but this is often countered by combining this type of antacid with one containing magnesium. Aluminium compounds can interfere with the absorption of phosphate from the diet, causing muscle weakness and bone damage if taken in high doses over a long period.

Magnesium compounds Like the aluminium compounds, these have a prolonged action. In large doses magnesium compounds can cause diarrhoea, and in people who have impaired kidney function, a high blood magnesium level may build up, causing weakness, lethargy, and drowsiness.

Sodium bicarbonate This antacid, the only sodium compound used as an antacid, acts quickly, but its effect soon passes. It reacts with stomach acids to produce gas, which may cause bloating and belching. Sodium bicarbonate is not advised for people with heart or kidney disease, because the excess sodium can lead to accumulation of water (oedema) in the legs and lungs and may raise blood pressure.

Combined preparations Antacids may be combined with other substances called alginates and antifoaming agents. Alginates are intended to float on the contents of the stomach and produce a neutralizing layer to subdue acid that can otherwise rise into the oesophagus, causing heartburn.

Antifoaming agents (usually dimeticone) are used to relieve flatulence. In some preparations, a local anaesthetic is combined with the antacid to relieve discomfort in oesophagitis. The value of these additives is dubious.

HOW THEY WORK

By neutralizing stomach acid, antacids prevent inflammation, relieve pain, and allow the mucous layer and lining to mend. When used in the treatment of ulcers, they prevent acid from attacking damaged stomach lining and so allow the ulcer to heal.

HOW THEY AFFECT YOU

If antacids are taken according to the instructions, they are usually effective in relieving abdominal discomfort caused by acid. The speed of action, dependent on the ability to neutralize acid, varies. Their duration of action also varies; the short-acting drugs may have to be taken quite frequently.

Although most antacids have few serious side effects when used only occasionally, some may cause diarrhoea, and others may cause constipation (see Types of antacid, facing page).

RISKS AND SPECIAL PRECAUTIONS

Antacids should not be taken to prevent abdominal pain on a regular basis except under medical supervision, as they may suppress the symptoms of stomach cancer. Your doctor is likely to want to arrange tests such as endoscopy or barium X-rays before prescribing long-term treatment.

Antacids can interfere with the absorption of other drugs. Therefore, if you are taking a prescription medicine, you should check with your doctor or pharmacist before taking an antacid.

COMMON DRUGS

Antacids Aluminium hydroxide*, Calcium carbonate, Hydrotalcite, Magnesium carbonate, Magnesium hydroxide*, Magnesium trisilicate, Sodium bicarbonate
Antifoaming agents Dimeticone, Simeticone
Other drugs Alginates*
* See Part 2

Anti-ulcer drugs

Normally, the linings of the oesophagus, stomach, and duodenum are protected from the irritant action of stomach acids or bile by a thin covering layer of mucus. If this is damaged, or if large amounts of stomach acid are formed, the underlying tissue may become eroded, causing a peptic ulcer (break in the gut lining). An ulcer often leads to abdominal pain, vomiting, and changes in

appetite. The most common type of ulcer occurs just beyond the stomach, in the duodenum. The exact cause of peptic ulcers is not understood, but a number of risk factors have been identified, including heavy smoking, the regular use of aspirin or similar drugs, and family history. An organism found in almost all patients who have peptic ulcers, *Helicobacter pylori*, is believed to be the main causative agent.

The symptoms caused by ulcers may be relieved by an antacid (see facing page), but healing is slow. The usual treatment is with an anti-ulcer drug, such as an H_2 blocker, a proton pump inhibitor, bismuth, or sucralfate, combined with antibiotics to eradicate the *Helicobacter pylori* infection which seems to cause many ulcers.

WHY THEY ARE USED

Anti-ulcer drugs are used to relieve symptoms and heal the ulcer. Untreated ulcers may erode blood vessel walls or perforate the stomach or duodenum.

Eradication of *Helicobacter pylori* by a proton pump inhibitor, or by rantidine bismuth citrate combined with two antibiotics (known as "triple therapy"), may provide a cure in one to two weeks. Surgery is reserved for complications such as obstruction, perforation, haemorrhage, and when there is a possibility of cancer.

HOW THEY WORK

Drugs protect ulcers from the action of stomach acid, allowing the tissue to heal. H_2 blockers, misoprostol, and proton pump inhibitors reduce the amount of acid released; bismuth and sucralfate form a protective coating over the ulcer. Bismuth also has an antibacterial effect. It is combined with an H_2 blocker in ranitidine bismuth citrate.

HOW THEY AFFECT YOU

These drugs begin to reduce pain in a few hours and usually allow the ulcer to heal in four to eight weeks. They produce few side effects, although H_2 blockers can cause confusion in the elderly. Bismuth may blacken the faeces and sucralfate may cause constipation; misoprostol, diarrhoea; and proton pump inhibitors, either constipation or diarrhoea. Triple therapy is given for one or two weeks. If *Helicobacter pylori* is eradicated, maintenance therapy should not be necessary. Sucralfate is usually prescribed for up to 12 weeks, and bismuth and misoprostol for four to eight weeks. Because they may mask symptoms of stomach cancer, H_2 blockers and proton pump inhibitors are normally prescribed only when tests have ruled out this disorder.

COMMON DRUGS

Proton pump inhibitors Esomeprazole, Lansoprazole*, Omeprazole*, Pantoprazole, Rabeprazole*

H_2 blockers Cimetidine*, Famotidine, Nizatidine, Ranitidine*

Other drugs Antacids (see p.42), Antibiotics (see p.62), Carbenoxolone, Misoprostol*, Ranitidine bismuth citrate, Sucralfate*, Tripotassium dicitratobismuthate (bismuth chelate)

* See Part 2

Antidiarrhoeal drugs

Diarrhoea is an increase in the fluidity and frequency of bowel movements. In some cases diarrhoea protects the body from harmful substances in the intestine by hastening their removal. The most common causes of diarrhoea are viral infection, food poisoning, and parasites. But it also occurs as a symptom of other illnesses. It can be a side effect of some drugs and may follow radiation therapy for cancer. Diarrhoea may also be caused by anxiety.

An attack of diarrhoea usually clears up quickly without medical attention. The best treatment is to abstain from food and to drink plenty of clear fluids. Rehydration solutions containing sugar as well as potassium and sodium salts are widely recommended for preventing dehydration and chemical imbalances, particularly in children. You should consult your doctor if the condition does not improve within 48 hours; the diarrhoea contains blood; severe abdominal pain and vomiting are present; you have just returned from a foreign country; or the diarrhoea occurs in a small child or an elderly person.

Severe diarrhoea can impair absorption of drugs, and anyone taking a prescribed drug should seek advice from a doctor or pharmacist. Women taking oral contraceptives may require additional contraceptives (see p.105).

The main types of drugs used to relieve nonspecific diarrhoea are opioids, and bulk-forming and adsorbent agents. Antispasmodic drugs may also be used to relieve accompanying pain (see Drugs for irritable bowel syndrome, facing page).

WHY THEY ARE USED

An antidiarrhoeal drug may be prescribed to provide relief when simple remedies are not effective, and once it is certain the diarrhoea is neither infectious nor toxic.

Opioids are the most effective anti-diarrhoeals. They are used when the diarrhoea is severe and debilitating. Bulking and adsorbent agents have a milder effect and are often used when it is necessary to regulate bowel action over a prolonged period (for example, in people with colostomies or ileostomies).

HOW THEY WORK

Opioids decrease the muscles' propulsive activity so that faecal matter passes more slowly through the bowel.

Bulk-forming agents and adsorbents absorb water and irritants in the bowel, resulting in larger, firmer stools at less frequent intervals.

HOW THEY AFFECT YOU

Drugs that are used to treat diarrhoea reduce the urge to move the bowels. Opioids and antispasmodics may relieve abdominal pain. All antidiarrhoeals may cause constipation if used in excess.

RISKS AND SPECIAL PRECAUTIONS

Used in relatively low doses for a limited period of time, the opioid drugs are unlikely to produce adverse effects. However, these drugs are not recommended for acute diarrhoea in children and should be used with caution when diarrhoea is caused by an infection, since they may slow the elimination of microorganisms from the intestine. All antidiarrhoeals should be taken with plenty of water. It is important not to take a bulk-forming agent together with an opioid or antispasmodic drug, because a bulky mass could form and obstruct the bowel.

COMMON DRUGS

Antispasmodics Alverine, Atropine*, Dicycloverine (dicyclomine)*, Hyoscine*, Mebeverine*, Peppermint oil, Propantheline

Opioids Codeine*, Co-phenotrope*, Loperamide*, Morphine/diamorphine*

Antibacterials Ciprofloxacin*

Bulk-forming agents and adsorbents Ispaghula Kaolin, Methylcellulose*, Sterculia

Other drugs Aluminium hydroxide*, Colestyramine*

* See Part 2

Drugs for irritable bowel syndrome

Irritable bowel syndrome is a common, often stress-related, condition in which the waves of muscular contraction that normally move the bowel contents smoothly through the intestines become strong and irregular. This disruption often causes pain, and may be associated with diarrhoea or constipation.

Symptoms are often relieved by adjusting the amount of fibre in the diet, but medication may also be needed. Bulk-forming agents may be given to regulate consistency of the bowel contents. If pain is severe, an antispasmodic drug may be given. These drugs are anticholinergics (see Drugs that act on the parasympathetic nervous system, p.9), which reduce the transmission of nerve signals to the bowel wall. Tricyclic antidepressants are sometimes used because their anticholinergic action has a calming effect on the bowel.

COMMON DRUGS

Antispasmodics Atropine*, Dicycloverine*, Hyoscine*, Mebeverine*

Opioids Loperamide*

Other drugs Peppermint oil

* See Part 2

Laxatives

When your bowels do not move as frequently as usual and the faeces are hard and difficult to pass, you are suffering from constipation. The most common cause is lack of sufficient fibre in your diet; fibre supplies the bulk that makes the faeces soft and easy to pass. The simplest remedy is more fluid and a diet that contains plenty of foods that are high in fibre, but laxative drugs may also be used.

Ignoring the urge to defecate can also cause constipation, because the faeces become dry, hard to pass, and too small to stimulate the muscles that propel them through the intestine.

Certain drugs may be constipating: for example, opioid analgesics, tricyclic antidepressants, and antacids containing aluminium. Some diseases, such as hypothyroidism (an underactive thyroid gland) and scleroderma (a rare disorder of connective tissue characterized by the hardening of the skin), can also lead to constipation.

The onset of constipation in a middle-aged or elderly person may be an early symptom of bowel cancer. Consult your doctor about any persistent change in bowel habit.

TYPES OF LAXATIVE

Bulk-forming agents These are relatively slow-acting but are less likely than other laxatives to interfere with normal bowel action. If the constipation is accompanied by abdominal pain, take them only after consulting your doctor because there is a risk of intestinal obstruction.

Stimulant (contact) laxatives These laxatives are for occasional use when other treatments have failed or when rapid onset of action is needed. They should not normally be used for longer than a week at a time, because they can cause abdominal cramps and diarrhoea.

Softening agents These treatments are often used when hard faeces cause pain as the bowels are opened – especially after surgery, when straining must be avoided, or if you have haemorrhoids (see p.47). Liquid paraffin was once used to relieve faecal impaction (blockage of the bowel by faeces) but, because of its side effects, it has largely been replaced by docusate sodium.

Osmotic laxatives Preparations that contain magnesium carbonate or citrate may be used to evacuate the bowel before surgery or investigative procedures. They are not normally used for the long-term relief of constipation, however, because they can cause chemical imbalances in the blood.

Lactulose is an alternative to bulk-forming laxatives for long-term treatment of chronic constipation. It may cause stomach cramps and flatulence but is usually well tolerated.

WHY THEY ARE USED

Since prolonged use is harmful, laxatives should be used for very short periods only. They may prevent pain and straining in people with either hernias or haemorrhoids (see facing page). Doctors may prescribe them for the same reason after abdominal surgery or childbirth. Laxatives are also used to clear the bowel before investigative procedures such as colonoscopy. They may be prescribed for elderly or bedridden patients because lack of exercise can often lead to constipation.

HOW THEY WORK

Laxatives act on the large intestine by increasing the speed with which faecal matter passes through the bowel, or increasing its bulk and/or water content. Stimulants cause the bowel muscles to contract, increasing the speed at which faecal matter goes through the intestine. Bulk-forming laxatives absorb water in the bowel, thereby increasing the volume of faeces, making them softer and easier to pass. Lactulose also causes fluid to accumulate in the intestine. Osmotic laxatives act by keeping water in the bowel, and thereby make the bowel movements softer. This also increases the bulk of the faeces and enables them to be passed more easily. Lubricant liquid paraffin preparations make bowel movements softer and easier to pass without increasing their bulk. Prolonged use can interfere with the absorption of some essential vitamins.

RISKS AND SPECIAL PRECAUTIONS

Laxatives can cause diarrhoea if taken in overdose, and constipation if overused. The most serious risk of prolonged use of most laxatives is developing dependence on the laxative for normal bowel action. Use of a laxative should therefore be discontinued as soon as normal bowel movements have been re-established. Children should not be given laxatives except in special circumstances on the advice of a doctor.

COMMON DRUGS

Stimulant laxatives Bisacodyl, Dantron, Docusate, Glycerol, Senna, Sodium picosulfate
Bulk-forming agents Bran, Ispaghula, Methylcellulose*, Sterculia
Softening agents Arachis oil, Liquid paraffin
Osmotic laxatives Lactulose*, Macrogols, Magnesium citrate, Magnesium hydroxide*, Magnesium sulphate, Sodium acid phosphate
* **See Part 2**

Drugs for inflammatory bowel disease

Inflammatory bowel disease is the term used for disorders in which inflammation of the intestinal wall causes recurrent attacks of abdominal pain, general feelings of ill-health, and frequently diarrhoea, with blood and mucus present in the faeces. Loss of appetite and poor absorption of food may often result in weight loss.

There are two main types of inflammatory bowel disease: Crohn's disease and ulcerative colitis. In Crohn's disease (also called regional enteritis), any part of the digestive tract may become inflamed, although the small intestine is the most commonly affected site. In ulcerative colitis, it is the large intestine (colon) that becomes inflamed and ulcerated, often producing bloodstained diarrhoea.

The exact cause of these disorders is not known, although stress-related, dietary, infectious, and genetic factors may all be important.

Establishing a proper diet and a less stressful lifestyle may help to alleviate these conditions. Bed rest during attacks is also advisable. However, these simple measures alone do not usually relieve or prevent attacks, and drug treatment is often necessary.

Three types of drug are used to treat inflammatory bowel disease: corticosteroids (see p.80), immunosuppressants (see p.99), and aminosalicylate anti-inflammatory drugs such as sulfasalazine. Nutritional supplements (used especially for Crohn's disease) and antidiarrhoeal drugs (see p.44) may also be used. Surgery to remove damaged areas of the intestine may be needed in severe cases.

Newer drugs are currently being developed. Infliximab (see p.268) offers hope of controlling Crohn's disease.

WHY THEY ARE USED

Drugs cannot cure inflammatory bowel disease, but treatment is needed, not only to control symptoms, but also to prevent complications, especially severe anaemia and perforation of the intestinal wall. Aminosalicylates are used to treat acute attacks of ulcerative colitis and Crohn's disease, and they may be continued as maintenance therapy. People who have severe bowel inflammation are usually prescribed a course of corticosteroids, particularly during a sudden flare-up. Once the disease is under control, an immunosuppressant drug may be prescribed to prevent a relapse.

HOW THEY WORK

Corticosteroids and sulfasalazine damp down the inflammatory process, allowing the damaged tissue to recover. They act in different ways to prevent migration of white blood cells into the bowel wall, which may be responsible in part for the inflammation of the bowel.

HOW THEY AFFECT YOU

Taken to treat attacks, these drugs relieve symptoms within a few days, and general health improves gradually over a period of a few weeks. Aminosalicylates usually provide long-term relief from the symptoms of inflammatory bowel disease.

Treatment with an immunosuppressant drug may take several months before the condition improves; and regular blood tests to monitor possible drug side effects are often required.

RISKS AND SPECIAL PRECAUTIONS

Immunosuppressant and corticosteroid drugs can cause serious adverse effects and are prescribed only when potential benefits outweigh the risks involved.

The side effects of corticosteroids can be reduced by the use of budesonide in a topical preparation (enema) that releases the drug at the site of inflammation.

It is important to continue taking these drugs as instructed because stopping them

abruptly may cause a sudden flare-up of the disorder. Doctors usually supervise a gradual reduction in dosage when such drugs are stopped, even when they are given as a short course for an attack. Antidiarrhoeal drugs should not be taken on a routine basis because they may mask signs of deterioration or cause sudden bowel dilation or rupture.

HOW THEY ARE ADMINISTERED

Antidiarrhoeals are usually taken in the form of tablets, although mild ulcerative colitis in the last part of the large intestine may be treated with suppositories or an enema containing a corticosteroid or aminosalicylate.

COMMON DRUGS

Corticosteroids Budesonide*, Hydrocortisone*, Prednisolone*
Immunosuppressants Azathioprine*, Mercaptopurine*, Methotrexate*
Aminosalicylates Balsalazide, Mesalazine*, Olsalazine, Sulfasalazine*
Other drugs Colestyramine*, Infliximab*, Metronidazole*
* See Part 2

Drugs for rectal and anal disorders

The most common disorder of the rectum (the last part of the large intestine) and anus (the opening from the rectum) is haemorrhoids, commonly known as piles. They occur when haemorrhoidal veins become swollen or irritated, often due to prolonged local pressure such as that caused by a pregnancy or a job requiring long hours of sitting. Haemorrhoids may cause irritation and pain, especially on defecation, and are aggravated by constipation and straining during defecation. In some cases haemorrhoids may bleed, and occasionally clots form in the swollen veins, leading to severe pain, a condition called thrombosed haemorrhoids.

Other common disorders include anal fissure (painful cracks in the anus) and pruritus ani (itching around the anus). Anal disorders of all kinds occur less frequently in people who have soft, bulky stools.

A number of both over-the-counter and prescription-only preparations are available for the relief of such disorders.

WHY THEY ARE USED

Preparations for relief of haemorrhoids and anal discomfort fall into three main groups: creams or suppositories that act locally to relieve inflammation and irritation; glyceryl trinitrate ointment, which reduces pain by relieving anal pressure and increasing blood flow; and measures that relieve constipation, which contributes to the formation of, and discomfort from, haemorrhoids and anal fissure.

Locally acting treatments often contain a soothing agent with antiseptic, astringent, or vasoconstrictor properties. Such ingredients include zinc oxide, bismuth, hamamelis (witch hazel), and Peru balsam. Some of these also include a mild local anaesthetic (see p.11) such as lidocaine. In some cases a doctor may prescribe an ointment containing a corticosteroid to relieve inflammation around the anus (see Topical corticosteroids, p.120).

People who suffer from haemorrhoids or anal fissure are generally advised to include in their diets plenty of fluids and fibre-rich foods, such as fresh fruits, vegetables, and whole grain products, both to prevent constipation and to ease defecation. A mild bulk-forming or softening laxative (see p.45) may also be prescribed.

Neither of these treatments can shrink large haemorrhoids, although they may provide relief while anal fissures heal naturally. Severe, persistently painful haemorrhoids that continue to be troublesome in spite of these measures may need to be removed surgically or, more commonly, by banding. This is a procedure in which a small rubber band is applied tightly to a haemorrhoid, thereby blocking off its blood supply; the haemorrhoid will eventually wither away.

HOW THEY AFFECT YOU

The treatments described above usually relieve discomfort, especially during defecation. Most people experience no adverse effects, although preparations containing local anaesthetics may cause irritation or even a rash in the anal area. It is rare for ingredients in locally acting preparations to be absorbed into the body in sufficient quantities to cause generalized side effects.

The main risk is that self-treatment of haemorrhoids may delay diagnosis of bowel cancer. It is therefore always wise to consult your doctor if symptoms of haemorrhoids are present, especially if you have noticed bleeding from the rectum or a change in bowel habits.

COMMON DRUGS

Soothing and astringent agents Aluminium acetate, Bismuth, Peru balsam, Zinc oxide
Topical corticosteroids Hydrocortisone*
Local anaesthetics (see p.11)
Laxatives (see p.45)
Other drugs Glyceryl trinitrate*
* **See Part 2**

Drug treatment for gallstones

The formation of gallstones is the most common disorder of the gallbladder, which is the storage and concentrating unit for bile, a digestive juice produced by the liver. During digestion, bile passes from the gallbladder via the bile duct into the small intestine, where it assists in the digestion of fats. Bile is composed of several ingredients, including bile acids, bile salts, and bile pigments. It also has a significant amount of cholesterol, which is dissolved in bile acid. If the amount of cholesterol in the bile increases, or if the amount of bile acid is reduced, a proportion of the cholesterol cannot remain dissolved, and under certain circumstances this excess accumulates in the gallbladder as gallstones.

Gallstones may be present in the gall bladder for years without causing symptoms. However, if they become lodged in the bile duct they cause pain and block the flow of bile. If the bile accumulates in the blood, it may cause an attack of jaundice, or the gallbladder may become infected and inflamed.

Drug treatment with ursodeoxycholic acid is only effective against stones made principally of cholesterol (some contain other substances), and even these take many months to dissolve. Therefore, surgery and ultrasound have become widely used, as techniques have improved. Surgery and ultrasound treatments are always used to remove stones blocking the bile duct.

WHY THEY ARE USED
Even if you have not experienced any symptoms, once gallstones have been diagnosed your doctor may advise treatment because of the risk of blockage of the bile duct. Drug treatment is usually preferred to surgery for small cholesterol stones or when there is a possibility that surgery may be risky.

HOW THEY WORK
Ursodeoxycholic acid is a substance that is naturally present in bile. It acts on chemical processes in the liver to regulate the amount of cholesterol in the blood by controlling the amount that passes into the bile. Once the cholesterol level in the bile is reduced, the bile acids are able to start dissolving the stones in the gallbladder. To achieve maximum effect, ursodeoxycholic acid treatment usually needs to be accompanied by adherence to a low-cholesterol, high-fibre diet.

HOW THEY AFFECT YOU
Drug treatment may often take years to dissolve gallstones completely. You will not, therefore, feel any immediate benefit from the drug, but you may have some minor side effects, the most usual of which is diarrhoea. If this occurs, your doctor may adjust the dosage. The effect of drug treatment on the gallstones is usually monitored at regular intervals by means of ultrasound or X-ray examinations.

Even after successful treatment with drugs, gallstones often recur when the drug is stopped. In some cases drug treatment and dietary restrictions may be continued even after the gallstones have dissolved, to prevent a recurrence.

Although the drug reduces cholesterol in the gallbladder, it increases the level of cholesterol in the blood because it reduces its excretion in the bile. Doctors therefore prescribe it with caution to people who have atherosclerosis (fatty deposits in the blood vessels). The drug is not usually given to people who have liver disorders because it can interfere with normal liver function. Surgical or ultrasound treatment is used for those with liver problems.

COMMON DRUGS
Pancreatic enzymes Amylase, Lipase, Pancreatin, Protease
Drugs for gallstones Ursodeoxycholic acid
Other drugs Colestyramine*
* See Part 2

Drug treatment for pancreatic disorders

The pancreas releases certain enzymes into the small intestine that are necessary for digestion of a range of foods. If the release of pancreatic enzymes is impaired (by chronic pancreatitis or cystic fibrosis, for example), enzyme replacement therapy may be necessary. Replacement of enzymes does not cure the underlying disorder, but it restores normal digestion. Pancreatic enzymes should be taken just before or with meals, and usually take effect immediately. Your doctor will probably advise you to eat a diet that is high in protein and carbohydrates and low in fat.

Pancreatin, the generic name for those preparations containing pancreatic enzymes, is extracted from pig pancreas. Treatment must be continued indefinitely as long as the pancreatic disorder persists.

MUSCLES, BONES, AND JOINTS

The basic architecture of the human body comprises 206 bones, over 600 muscles, and a complex assortment of other tissues that enable the body to move efficiently.

Bones support the body, provide protection for organs, and enable movement.

Tendons attach the muscles that control body movement to the bones.

Muscles work bones that act as levers: when the muscle contracts, movement occurs at the joint.

Ligaments are bands of tough fibrous tissue that hold joints together.

Cartilage covers each bone end, reducing friction between the ends of two bones.

WHAT CAN GO WRONG

Although tough, these structures often suffer damage. Muscles, tendons, and ligaments can be strained or torn by violent movement, which may cause inflammation, making the affected tissue swollen and painful. Joints, especially those that bear the body's weight – hips, knees, ankles, and vertebrae – are prone to wear and tear. The cartilage covering the bone ends may tear, causing pain and inflammation. Joint damage also occurs in rheumatoid arthritis, which is thought to be a form of autoimmune disorder. Gout, in which uric acid crystals form in some joints, may also cause inflammation, a condition known as gouty arthritis.

Another problem affecting the muscles and joints includes nerve injury or degeneration, which alters nerve control over muscle contraction. Myasthenia gravis, in which transmission of signals between nerves and muscles is reduced, affects muscle control as a result. Bones may also be weakened by vitamin, mineral, or hormone deficiencies.

WHY DRUGS ARE USED

A simple analgesic drug or one that has an anti-inflammatory effect will provide pain relief in most of the conditions described above. For severe inflammation, a doctor may inject a drug with a more powerful anti-inflammatory effect, such as a corticosteroid, into the affected site. In cases of severe progressive rheumatoid arthritis, antirheumatic drugs may halt the disease's progression and relieve symptoms.

Drugs that help to eliminate excess uric acid from the body are often prescribed to treat gout. Muscle relaxants that inhibit transmission of nerve signals to the muscles are used to treat muscle spasm. Drugs that increase nervous stimulation of the muscle are prescribed for myasthenia gravis. Bone disorders in which the mineral content of the bone is reduced are treated with supplements of minerals, vitamins, and hormones.

MAJOR DRUG GROUPS

◆ Non-steroidal anti-inflammatory drugs
◆ Antirheumatic drugs
◆ Corticosteroids for rheumatic disorders
◆ Drugs for gout
◆ Muscle relaxants
◆ Drugs used for myasthenia gravis
◆ Drugs for bone disorders

Non-steroidal anti-inflammatory drugs

Drugs in this group, often referred to as NSAIDs, are used to relieve the pain, stiffness, and inflammation of painful conditions affecting the muscles, bones, and joints. NSAIDs are called "non-steroidal" to distinguish them from corticosteroid drugs (see p.80), which also damp down inflammation.

WHY THEY ARE USED

NSAIDs are widely prescribed for the treatment of osteoarthritis, rheumatoid arthritis, and other rheumatic conditions. They reduce pain and inflammation in the joints, but they do not alter the progress of these diseases.

The response to the various drugs in this group varies between individuals. It is sometimes necessary to try several different NSAIDs before finding the one that best suits a particular individual.

Because NSAIDs do not change the progress of a disease, additional treatment is often necessary, particularly for rheumatoid arthritis (see p.52).

NSAIDs are also commonly prescribed to relieve back pain, headaches, gout (see p.53), menstrual pain (see p.104), mild pain following surgery, and pain from soft tissue injuries, such as sprains and strains (see also Analgesics, p.9).

HOW THEY WORK

Prostaglandins are chemicals released by the body at the site of injury. They are responsible for producing inflammation and pain following tissue damage. NSAIDs block an enzyme, cyclo-oxygenase (COX) which is involved in the production of prostaglandins, and thus reduce pain and inflammation (see Analgesics, p.9).

HOW THEY AFFECT YOU

NSAIDs are rapidly absorbed from the digestive system and most start to relieve pain within an hour. When used regularly they reduce pain, inflammation, and stiffness and may restore or improve the function of a damaged or painful joint.

Most NSAIDs are short acting and need to be taken a few times a day for optimal pain relief. Some need to be taken only twice daily. Others, such as piroxicam, are very slowly eliminated from the body and are effective when taken once a day.

RISKS AND SPECIAL PRECAUTIONS

Most NSAIDs carry a low risk of serious adverse effects although nausea, indigestion, and altered bowel action are common. However, the main risk from NSAIDs is that, occasionally, they can cause bleeding in the stomach or duodenum. Therefore, the lowest effective dose is given for the shortest duration. NSAIDs should be avoided altogether by people who have suffered from peptic ulcers.

Most NSAIDs are not recommended during pregnancy or for breast-feeding mothers. Caution is also advised for people with kidney or liver abnormalities or heart disease, or those people with a history of hypersensitivity to other drugs.

NSAIDs may impair blood clotting and are, therefore, prescribed with caution to people with bleeding disorders or who are taking drugs that reduce blood clotting.

MISOPROSTOL

An NSAID may cause bleeding when its anti-prostaglandin action occurs where it is not wanted, such as in the digestive tract. To protect against this side effect, a prostaglandin-like drug called misoprostol is sometimes prescribed with the NSAID. Preparations are available that incorporate both misoprostol and an NSAID. Misoprostol is also used to help heal peptic ulcers (see p.43).

COX-2 INHIBITORS

NSAIDs block two types of COX, COX-1 and COX-2, at different sites in the body; blocking COX-1 leads to the upper gastrointestinal tract irritation of NSAIDs, while blocking COX-2 leads to the anti-inflammatory effect. COX-2 inhibitors block COX-2 but not COX-1. COX-2 inhibitors are not prescribed to anyone who has had a heart attack or stroke, because they are thought slightly to increase the risk of recurrence, nor are they prescribed to people with peripheral artery disease (poor circulation). They are prescribed with caution to anyone at risk of any of these conditions.

COMMON DRUGS

Aceclofenac, Acemetacin, Aspirin*, Diclofenac*, Diflunisal, Felbinac, Fenbufen, Fenoprofen, Flurbiprofen, Ibuprofen*, Indometacin, Ketoprofen*, Mefenamic acid*, Meloxicam*, Nabumetone, Naproxen*, Piroxicam*, Sulindac, Tenoxicam, Tiaprofenic acid

COX-2 inhibitors Celecoxib*, Etodolac, Etoricoxib, Lumiracoxib

* See Part 2

Antirheumatic drugs

These drugs are used in the treatment of various rheumatic disorders, the most crippling and deforming being rheumatoid arthritis, an autoimmune disease in which the body's mechanism for fighting infection contributes to the damage of its own joint tissue. There is pain, stiffness, and swelling of the joints that, over many months, can lead to deformity. Flare-ups of rheumatoid arthritis also cause a general feeling of being unwell, fatigue, and loss of appetite.

Treatments for rheumatoid arthritis include drugs, rest, physiotherapy, changes in diet, and immobilization of joints. The disorder cannot yet be cured, but in many cases it does not progress to permanent disability. It also sometimes subsides spontaneously for prolonged periods.

WHY THEY ARE USED

The aim of drug treatment is to relieve the symptoms of pain and stiffness, maintain mobility, and prevent deformity. Drugs for rheumatoid arthritis fall into two main categories: those that alleviate symptoms, and those that modify, halt, or slow the underlying disease process. Drugs in the first category include aspirin (p.146) and other NSAIDs (see Non-steroidal anti-inflammatory drugs, p.50). These drugs are usually prescribed as a first treatment.

Drugs in the second category are known collectively as disease-modifying antirheumatic drugs (DMARDs). They may be given if the rheumatoid arthritis is severe or if initial drug treatment has proved to be ineffective. DMARDs may prevent further joint damage and disability, but they are not prescribed routinely because the disease may stop spontaneously and because they have potentially severe adverse effects (see Some types of disease-modifying antirheumatic drug, below, for further information on individual drugs).

Corticosteroids (see p.80) are sometimes used in the treatment of rheumatoid arthritis, but are used only for limited periods because they depress the immune system, increasing susceptibility to infection.

SOME TYPES OF DISEASE-MODIFYING ANTIRHEUMATIC DRUG

Chloroquine Originally developed to treat malaria (see p.75), chloroquine and related drugs are less effective than penicillamine or gold. Prolonged use may cause eye damage, but only if too high a dose is used.

Immunosuppressants These are prescribed if other drugs do not provide relief and if the rheumatoid arthritis is severe and disabling.

Regular observation and blood tests must be carried out because immunosuppressants can cause severe complications.

Sulfasalazine Used mainly for ulcerative colitis (p.46), sulfasalazine was originally introduced to treat rheumatoid arthritis and is effective in some cases.

Gold-based drugs These are effective and may be given orally or by injection for many years. Side effects can include a rash and digestive disturbances. Gold may sometimes damage the kidneys, which recover once treatment is stopped; regular urine tests are usually carried out, however. Gold can also suppress blood cell production in bone marrow. Therefore, periodic blood tests are also carried out.

Monoclonal antibodies such as infliximab (see p.268) target a particular body protein that is responsible for rheumatoid arthritis. Monoclonal antibodies often cause allergy-type reactions, especially at the start of treatment. Infections, particularly of the upper respiratory and urinary tracts, are common.

HOW THEY WORK

It is not known precisely how most DMARDs stop or slow the disease process. Some may reduce the body's immune response, which is thought to be partly responsible for the disease (see also Immunosuppressant drugs, p.99). Monoclonal antibodies such as infliximab (see p.268) combine with a body protein called "tumour necrosis factor alpha" (TNF), which is overactive in rheumatoid arthritis. By reducing the level of TNF activity, they can improve the arthritis. When effective, DMARDs prevent damage to the cartilage and bone, thereby reducing progressive deformity and disability. The effectiveness of each drug varies depending on individual response.

HOW THEY AFFECT YOU

DMARDs are generally slow acting; it may be four to six months before benefit is noticed. So, treatment with aspirin or other NSAIDs is usually continued until remission occurs. Prolonged treatment with DMARDs can markedly improve symptoms. Arthritic pain is relieved, joint mobility increased, and general symptoms of ill health fade. Side effects (which vary between individual drugs) may be noticed before beneficial effects, so patience is required. Regular monitoring of the kidneys, liver, and bone marrow are needed. Severe adverse effects may require treatment to be abandoned.

COMMON DRUGS

Immunosuppressants Azathioprine*, Ciclosporin*, Cyclophosphamide*, Leflunomide, Methotrexate*
NSAIDs (see p.50)
DMARDs Auranofin, Chloroquine*, Hydroxychloroquine, Infliximab*, Penicillamine, Sodium aurothiomalate, Sulfasalazine*
* See Part 2

Corticosteroids for rheumatic disorders

The adrenal glands, which lie on the top of the kidneys, produce a number of important hormones. Among these are the corticosteroids, so named because they are made in the outer part (cortex) of the glands. The corticosteroids play an important role, influencing the immune system and regulating the carbohydrate and mineral metabolism of the body. A number of drugs that mimic the natural corticosteroids have been developed.

These drugs have many uses and are discussed in detail under Corticosteroids (see p.80). This section concentrates on those corticosteroids injected into an affected site to treat joint disorders.

WHY THEY ARE USED

Corticosteroids given by injection are particularly useful for treating joint disorders – most notably rheumatoid arthritis and osteoarthritis – when one or only a few joints are involved, and when pain and inflammation have not been relieved by other drugs. In such cases, it is possible to relieve symptoms by injecting each of the affected joints individually. Corticosteroids may also be injected to relieve pain and inflammation caused by strained or contracted muscles, ligaments, and/or tendons – for example, in frozen shoulder or tennis elbow. They may also be given for bursitis, tendinitis, or swelling that is compressing a nerve. Cortico-steroid injections are sometimes used in order to relieve pain and stiffness sufficiently to permit physiotherapy.

HOW THEY WORK

Corticosteroid drugs have two important actions that are believed to account for their effectiveness. They block the production of prostaglandins – chemicals responsible for triggering inflammation and pain – and depress the accumulation and activity of the white blood cells that cause the inflammation. An injection concentrates the corticosteroids, and their effects, at the site of the problem, thus giving the maximum benefit where it is most needed.

HOW THEY AFFECT YOU

Corticosteroids usually produce dramatic relief from symptoms when the drug is injected into a joint. Often a single injection is sufficient to relieve pain and swelling, and to improve mobility. When used to treat muscle or tendon pain, they may not always be effective because it is difficult to position the needle so that the drug reaches the right spot. In some cases, repeated injections are necessary.

Because these drugs are concentrated in the affected area, rather than being dispersed in significant amounts in the body, the generalized adverse effects that sometimes occur when corticosteroids are taken by mouth are unlikely. Minor side effects, such as loss of skin pigment at the injection site, are uncommon. Occasionally, a temporary increase in pain (steroid flare) may occur. In such cases, rest, local application of ice, and analgesic medication may relieve the condition. Sterile injection technique is critically important.

COMMON DRUGS

Dexamethasone*, Hydrocortisone*, Methylprednisolone, Prednisolone*, Triamcinolone
* See Part 2

Drugs for gout

Gout is a disorder that arises when the blood contains increased levels of uric acid, which is a by-product of normal body metabolism.

When its concentration in the blood is excessive, uric acid crystals may form in various parts of the body, especially in the joints of the foot (most often the big toe), the knee, and the hand, causing intense pain and inflammation known as gouty arthritis. Crystals may form as white masses, known as tophi, in soft tissue, and in the kidneys as stones. Attacks of gouty arthritis can recur, and may lead to damaged joints and deformity. Kidney stones can cause kidney damage.

An excess of uric acid can be caused either by increased production or by decreased elimination by the kidneys, which remove it from the body. The disorder tends to run in families and is far more common in men than women. The risk of attack is increased by high alcohol intake, the consumption of certain foods (red meat, sardines, anchovies, yeast extract, and offal such as liver, brains, and sweetbreads), and obesity. An attack may be triggered by drugs such as thiazide diuretics (see p.32) or anticancer drugs (see p.96), or excessive drinking. Changes in diet and a reduction in the consumption of alcohol may be an important part of treatment.

Drugs used to treat acute attacks of gouty arthritis include NSAIDs (see Non-steroidal anti-inflammatory drugs, p.50), and colchicine. Other drugs, which lower the blood level of uric acid, are used for the long-term prevention of gout. These include uricosuric drugs (such as sulfinpyrazone) and allopurinol, the drug of choice. Aspirin is not prescribed for pain relief because it slows excretion of uric acid.

WHY THEY ARE USED

Drugs may be prescribed either to treat an attack of gout or to prevent recurrent attacks that could lead to deformity of affected joints and kidney damage. The NSAIDs and colchicine are both used to treat an attack of gout and should be taken as soon as an attack begins. Because colchicine is relatively specific in relieving the pain and inflammation arising from gout, doctors sometimes administer it in order to confirm their diagnosis of the condition before prescribing an NSAID.

If symptoms recur, your doctor may advise long-term treatment with either allopurinol or a uricosuric drug. One of these drugs must usually be taken indefinitely. Since they can trigger attacks of gout at the beginning of treatment, colchicine is sometimes given with these drugs for a few months.

HOW THEY WORK

Allopurinol reduces the level of uric acid in the blood by interfering with the activity of xanthine oxidase, an enzyme that is involved in the production of uric acid in the body. Sulfinpyrazone increases the rate at which uric acid is excreted by the kidneys. The process by which colchicine reduces inflammation and relieves pain is not understood. The actions of NSAIDs are described on p.51.

HOW THEY AFFECT YOU

Drugs used in the long-term treatment of gout are usually successful in preventing attacks and joint deformity. However, response may be slow. Colchicine can disturb the digestive system, causing diarrhoea, in which case treatment is stopped.

RISKS AND SPECIAL PRECAUTIONS

Since they increase the output of uric acid through the kidneys, uricosuric drugs can cause uric acid crystals to form in the kidneys. They are not, therefore, usually prescribed for those people who already have kidney problems. In such cases, allopurinol may be preferred. It is always important to drink plenty of fluids while taking drugs for gout in order to prevent kidney crystals from forming. Regular blood tests to monitor levels of uric acid in the blood may be required.

COMMON DRUGS

Drugs to treat attacks Colchicine*, NSAIDs (but not aspirin, see p.50)
Drugs to treat high uric acid caused by cytotoxic drugs Rasburicase
Drugs to prevent attacks Allopurinol*, Sulfinpyrazone
* **See Part 2**

Muscle relaxants

Several drugs are available to treat muscle spasm – the involuntary, painful contraction of a muscle or a group of muscles that can stiffen an arm or leg or make it almost impossible to straighten your back. There are various causes. It can follow an injury, or come on without warning. It may also be brought on by a disorder like osteoarthritis, the pain in the affected joint triggering abnormal tension in a nearby muscle.

Spasticity is another form of muscle tightness seen in some neurological disorders, such as multiple sclerosis, stroke, or cerebral palsy. Spasticity can sometimes be helped by physiotherapy, but in severe cases drugs may be used to relieve symptoms.

WHY THEY ARE USED

Muscle spasm resulting from direct injury is usually treated with a non-steroidal anti-inflammatory drug (see p.50) or an analgesic. However, if the spasm is severe, a muscle relaxant may also be tried for a short period.

In spasticity, the person's legs may become so stiff and uncontrollable that walking unaided is impossible. In such cases, a drug may be used to relax the muscles. Relaxation of the muscles often permits physiotherapy to be given for longer-term relief from spasms.

The muscle relaxant, botulinum toxin, may be injected locally to relieve muscle spasm in small groups of accessible muscles, such as those around the eye or in the neck.

HOW THEY WORK

Muscle-relaxant drugs work in one of several ways. The centrally acting drugs damp down the passage of the nerve signals from the brain and spinal cord that cause muscles to contract, thus reducing excessive stimulation of muscles as well as unwanted muscular contraction. Tizanidine stimulates the alpha receptors in the blood vessels. Dantrolene reduces the sensitivity of the muscles to nerve signals. When injected locally, botulinum toxin prevents transmission of impulses between nerves and muscles.

HOW THEY AFFECT YOU

Drugs taken regularly for a spastic disorder of the central nervous system usually reduce stiffness and improve mobility. They may restore the use of the arms and legs when this has been impaired by muscle spasm.

Unfortunately, most centrally acting drugs can have a generally depressant effect on nervous activity and produce drowsiness, particularly at the beginning of treatment. Too high a dosage can excessively reduce the muscles' ability to contract and can therefore cause weakness. For this reason, the dosage needs to be carefully adjusted to find a level that controls symptoms but which, at the same time, maintains sufficient muscle strength.

RISKS AND SPECIAL PRECAUTIONS

The main long-term risk associated with centrally acting muscle relaxants is that the body becomes dependent. If the drugs are withdrawn suddenly, the stiffness may become worse than before drug treatment.

Rarely, dantrolene can cause serious liver damage. Anyone who is taking this drug should have his or her blood tested regularly to assess liver function.

Unless used very cautiously, botulinum toxin can paralyse unaffected muscles, and might interfere with functions such as speech and swallowing.

COMMON DRUGS

Centrally acting drugs Baclofen*, Diazepam*, Orphenadrine*
Other drugs Botulinum toxin*, Dantrolene, Tizanidine
* See Part 2

Drugs used for myasthenia gravis

Myasthenia gravis is a disorder that occurs when the immune system (see p.95) becomes defective and produces antibodies that disrupt the signals being transmitted between the nervous system and muscles that are under voluntary control. As a result, the body's muscular response is progressively weakened. The first muscles to be affected are those controlling the eyes, eyelids, face, pharynx, and larynx, with muscles in the arms and legs becoming involved as the disease progresses. Myasthenia gravis is often linked to a disorder of the thymus gland, which is the source of the destructive antibodies concerned.

Various methods can be used in the treatment of myasthenia gravis, including removal of the thymus gland (called a thymectomy) or temporarily clearing the blood of antibodies (a procedure known as plasmapheresis, or plasma exchange). Drugs that improve muscle function, principally neostigmine and pyridostigmine, may be prescribed. They may be used alone or together with other drugs that depress the immune system – usually azathioprine (see Immunosuppressant drugs, p.99) or corticosteroids (see p.80). Intravenous immunoglobulins may also be used in severe cases where there are breathing and swallowing problems.

WHY THEY ARE USED

Drugs that improve the muscle response to nerve impulses have several uses. One such drug, edrophonium, acts very quickly and, once administered, brings about a dramatic improvement in the symptoms. This effect is used to confirm the diagnosis of myasthenia gravis. However, because of its short duration of action, edrophonium is not used for long-term treatment. Pyridostigmine and neostigmine are preferred for long-term treatment, especially when removal of the thymus gland is not feasible or does not provide adequate relief. These drugs may be given following surgery to counteract the effects of a muscle-relaxant drug given prior to certain surgical procedures.

HOW THEY WORK

Normal muscle action occurs when a nerve impulse triggers a nerve ending to release a neurotransmitter, which combines with a specialized receptor on the muscle cells and causes the muscles to contract. In myasthenia gravis, the body's immune system destroys many of these receptors, so that the muscle is less responsive to nervous stimulation. Drugs used to treat the disorder increase the amount of neurotransmitter at the nerve ending by blocking the action of an enzyme that normally breaks it down. Increased levels of the neurotransmitter permit the remaining receptors to function more efficiently.

HOW THEY AFFECT YOU

These drugs usually restore the muscle function to a normal or near-normal level, particularly when the disease takes a mild form. Unfortunately, the drugs can produce unwanted muscular activity by enhancing the transmission of nerve impulses elsewhere in the body.

Common side effects include vomiting, nausea, diarrhoea, and muscle cramps in the arms, legs, and abdomen.

RISKS AND SPECIAL PRECAUTIONS

Muscle weakness can suddenly worsen even when it is being treated with drugs. Should this occur, it is important not to take larger doses of the drug to try to relieve the symptoms, because excessive drug levels can interfere with the transmission of nerve impulses to muscles, causing further weakness. Administration of other drugs, including some antibiotics, can also markedly increase the symptoms of myasthenia gravis. If your symptoms suddenly worsen, consult your doctor.

COMMON DRUGS

Azathioprine*, Corticosteroids (see p.80), Distigmine, Edrophonium, Neostigmine, Pyridostigmine*
* **See Part 2**

Drugs for bone disorders

Bone is a living structure. Its hard, mineral quality is created by the action of the bone cells. These cells continuously deposit and remove phosphorus and calcium, which are stored in a honeycombed protein framework called the matrix. Because the rates of deposit and removal (the bone metabolism) are about equal in adults, the bone mass remains fairly constant.

Removal and renewal is regulated by hormones and influenced by a number of factors, notably the level of calcium in the blood, which depends on the intake of calcium and vitamin D from the diet, the actions of various hormones, plus everyday movement and weight-bearing stress. When normal bone metabolism is altered, various bone disorders result.

OSTEOPOROSIS

In osteoporosis, the strength and density of bone are reduced. Such wasting occurs when the rate of removal of mineralized bone exceeds the rate of deposit. In most people, bone density decreases very gradually from the age of 30. But bone loss can dramatically increase when a person is immobilized for a period, and this is an important cause of osteoporosis in elderly people. Hormone deficiency is another important cause, commonly occurring in women with lowered oestrogen levels after the menopause or removal of the ovaries. Osteoporosis also occurs in disorders in which there is excess production of adrenal or thyroid hormones. Osteoporosis can result from long-term treatment with corticosteroid drugs.

People with osteoporosis often have no symptoms, but, if the vertebrae become so weakened that they are unable to bear the body's weight, they may collapse spontaneously or after a minor accident. Subsequently, the individual suffers from back pain, reduced height, and a round-shouldered appearance. Osteoporosis also makes a fracture of an arm, leg, or hip more likely.

Most doctors emphasize the need to prevent the disorder by an adequate intake of protein and calcium and by regular exercise throughout adult life. Oestrogen supplements, however, are no longer usually recommended to prevent osteoporosis.

The condition of bones damaged by osteoporosis cannot usually be improved, but drug treatment can help to prevent further deterioration and help fractures to heal. For people whose diet is deficient in calcium or vitamin D, supplements may be prescribed. However, these are of limited value and are often less useful than drugs that inhibit removal of calcium from the bones. In the past, the hormone calcitonin was used, but it has now been largely superseded by drugs such as etidronate and alendronate. These drugs, known as bisphosphonates, bind very tightly to bone matrix, preventing its removal by bone cells.

OSTEOMALACIA AND RICKETS

In osteomalacia (called rickets when it affects children), a lack of vitamin D leads to loss of calcium, resulting in softening of the bones. There is pain and tenderness and a risk of fracture and bone deformity. In children, growth is retarded.

Osteomalacia is most commonly caused by a lack of vitamin D. This can result from an inadequate diet, inability to absorb the vitamin, or insufficient exposure of the skin to sunlight (the action of the sun on the skin produces vitamin D inside the body). Individuals who are at special risk include those whose absorption of vitamin D is impaired by an intestinal disorder, like Crohn's disease or coeliac disease. People with dark skins living in Northern Europe are also susceptible. Chronic kidney disease is an important cause of rickets in children and of osteomalacia in adults, since healthy kidneys play an essential role in the body's metabolism of vitamin D.

Long-term relief depends on treating the underlying disorder where possible. In rare cases, treatment may be lifelong.

VITAMIN D

A number of substances that are related to vitamin D may be used in the treatment of bone disorders. These drugs include alfacalcidol, calcitriol, and ergocalciferol. The substance that is prescribed depends on the underlying problem.

COMMON DRUGS

Alendronic acid*, Alfacalcidol, Calcitonin, Calcitriol, Calcium carbonate, Ergocalciferol, Etidronate*, Fluoride, Pamidronate, Risedronate*, Salcatonin (calcitonin (salmon)), Strontium, Teriparatide, Vitamin D*

* **See Part 2**

ALLERGY

Allergy, a hypersensitivity to certain substances, is a reaction of the body's immune system. Through a variety of mechanisms (see Malignant and immune disease, p.95), the immune system protects the body by eliminating unrecognized foreign substances, such as microorganisms (bacteria or viruses).

One way in which the immune system acts is through the production of antibodies. When the body encounters a particular foreign substance (or allergen) for the first time, one type of white blood cell, the lymphocyte, produces antibodies that attach themselves to another type of white blood cell, the mast cell. If the same substance is encountered again, the allergen binds to the antibodies on the mast cells, causing the release of chemicals known as mediators.

The most important mediator is histamine. Its release can produce a rash, swelling, narrowing of the airways, and a drop in blood pressure. Although these effects are important in protecting the body against infection, they may also be triggered inappropriately in an allergic reaction.

WHAT CAN GO WRONG

One of the most common allergic disorders, hay fever, is caused by an allergic reaction to inhaled grass pollen leading to allergic rhinitis – swelling and irritation of the nasal passages and watering of the nose and eyes. Other substances, such as house-dust mites, animal fur, and feathers, may cause a similar reaction in susceptible people.

Asthma, another allergic disorder, may result from the action of leukotrienes rather than histamine. Other allergic conditions include urticaria (hives) or other rashes (sometimes in response to a drug), some forms of eczema and dermatitis, and allergic alveolitis (farmer's lung). Anaphylaxis is a serious systemic allergic reaction that occurs when an allergen reaches the bloodstream (see also Epinephrine, p.231).

WHY DRUGS ARE USED

Antihistamines and drugs that inhibit mast cell activity are used to prevent and treat allergic reactions. Other drugs minimize symptoms, and include decongestants (see p.26) to clear the nose in allergic rhinitis, bronchodilators (see p.23) to widen the airways of those with asthma, and corticosteroids applied to skin affected by eczema (see p.125).

MAJOR DRUG GROUPS

◆ Antihistamines
◆ Leukotriene antagonists
◆ Corticosteroids (see p.80)

Antihistamines

Antihistamines are the most widely used drugs in the treatment of allergic reactions of all kinds. They can be subdivided according to their chemical structure, each subgroup having slightly different actions and characteristics (see table, p.60). Their main action is to counter the effects of histamine, one of the chemicals released in the body when there is an allergic reaction (see left).

Histamine is also involved in other body functions, including blood vessel dilation and constriction, contraction of muscles in the respiratory and gastrointestinal tracts, and the release of digestive juices in the stomach. The antihistamine drugs described here are also known as H_1 blockers because they block the action of histamine only on certain receptors, known as H_1 receptors. Another group of antihistamines, known as H_2 blockers, is used in the treatment of peptic ulcers (see Anti-ulcer drugs, p.43).

Some antihistamines have a significant anticholinergic action. This is used to advantage in a variety of conditions, but it also accounts for certain undesired side effects.

WHY THEY ARE USED

Antihistamines relieve allergy-related symptoms when it is not possible to prevent exposure to the substance that has provoked the reaction. They are most commonly used in the prevention of allergic rhinitis (hay fever), the inflammation of the nose and upper airways that results from an allergic reaction to a substance such as pollen, house dust, or animal fur. Antihistamines are more effective when taken before the start of an attack. If they are taken only after an attack has begun, beneficial effects may be delayed.

Antihistamines are not usually effective in asthma caused by similar allergens because the symptoms of this allergic disorder are not solely caused by the action of histamine, but are likely to be the result of more complex mechanisms. Antihistamines are usually the first drugs to be tried in the treatment of allergic disorders but alternatives can be prescribed (see Other allergy treatments, p.60).

Antihistamines are also prescribed for the itching, swelling, and redness of allergic reactions involving the skin (such as urticaria (hives) and dermatitis. Irritation from chickenpox may be reduced by these drugs. Allergic reactions to insect stings may also be reduced by antihistamines. In such cases the drug may be taken by mouth or applied topically. Applied as drops, antihistamines can reduce inflammation and irritation of the eyes and eyelids in allergic conjunctivitis.

Antihistamines are often included as an ingredient in cough and cold preparations (see p.28), when the anticholinergic effect of drying mucus secretions and their sedative effect on the coughing mechanism may be helpful.

Because most antihistamines have a depressant effect on the brain, they are sometimes used to promote sleep, especially when discomfort from itching is disturbing sleep (see also Sleeping drugs, p.11). The depressant effect of antihistamines on the brain also extends to the centres that control nausea and vomiting. Antihistamines are therefore often effective for preventing and controlling these symptoms (see Anti-emetics, p.21).

Occasionally, antihistamines are used to treat fever, rash, and breathing difficulties that may occur in adverse reactions to blood transfusions and allergic reactions to drugs. Promethazine and alimemazine are also used as premedication to provide sedation and to dry secretions during surgery, particularly in children.

HOW THEY WORK

Antihistamines block the action of histamine on H_1 receptors. These are found in various body tissues, particularly the small blood vessels in the skin, nose, and eyes. This helps prevent the dilation of the vessels, thus reducing the redness, watering, and swelling. In addition, the anticholinergic action of these drugs contributes to this effect by reducing the secretions from tear glands and nasal passages. Antihistamine drugs pass from the blood into the brain. In the brain, the blocking action of the antihistamines on histamine activity may produce general sedation and depression of various brain functions, including the vomiting and coughing mechanisms.

HOW THEY AFFECT YOU

Antihistamines frequently cause a degree of drowsiness and may affect coordination, leading to clumsiness. Some newer drugs have little or no sedative effect (see table, p.60).

Anticholinergic side effects, including dry mouth, blurred vision, and difficulty passing urine, are common. Most side effects diminish with continued use and can often be helped by an adjustment in dosage or a change to a different drug.

RISKS AND SPECIAL PRECAUTIONS

It is advisable not to drive or operate machinery while taking antihistamines, particularly those more likely to cause drowsiness (see table, p.60). Antihistamines can also increase the sedative effects of alcohol, sleeping drugs, opioid analgesics, and anti-anxiety drugs.

In high doses, or in children, some antihistamines can cause excitement, agitation, and even, in extreme cases, hallucinations and convulsions. Abnormal heart rhythms have occurred after high doses with some antihistamines or when drugs that interact with them, such as antifungals and antibiotics, have been taken at the same time. Heart rhythm problems may also affect people with liver disease, electrolyte disturbances, or abnormal heart activity. A person who has these conditions, or who has glaucoma or prostate trouble, should seek medical advice before taking antihistamines because their various drug actions may make such conditions worse.

COMMON DRUGS

Non-sedating Acrivastine, Cetirizine*, Fexofenadine, Levocetirizine, Loratadine/Desloratadine*, Mizolastine

Sedating Alimemazine, Chlorphenamine*, Cinnarizine*, Clemastine, Hydroxyzine, Promethazine*
* See Part 2

OTHER ALLERGY TREATMENTS

Sodium cromoglicate This drug (see p.386) prevents the release of histamine from mast cells (see p.58) in response to exposure to an allergen, thereby preventing the physical symptoms of allergies. Sodium cromoglicate is commonly given by inhaler for the prevention of allergy-induced rhinitis (hay fever) or asthma attacks and by drops for the treatment of allergic eye disorders.

Leukotriene antagonists Like histamine, leukotrienes are substances that occur naturally in the body and seem to play an important part in asthma. Drugs such as montelukast (see p.321) and zafirlukast (leukotriene antagonists) have been developed to prevent asthma attacks from occurring. They are not bronchodilators, however, and will not relieve an existing attack (see Drugs for asthma, p.24).

Corticosteroids These drugs for allergic rhinitis and asthma are usually given by inhaler, providing a high dose to the affected area.

The dose of the drug to the rest of the body is very low, reducing the risk of long-term adverse effects.

Desensitization This may be tried in conditions such as allergic rhinitis due to pollen sensitivity and insect venom hypersensitivity, when avoidance, antihistamines, and other treatments have not been effective and tests have shown one or two specific allergens to be responsible. Desensitization often provides incomplete relief and can be time-consuming.

Treatment involves a series of injections containing increasing doses of an extract of the allergen. It is not understood how this prevents allergic reactions, but controlled exposure may trigger the immune system into producing increasing levels of antibodies so that the body no longer responds dramatically when the allergen is encountered naturally.

Desensitization must be carried out under medical supervision because it can provoke a severe allergic response. Therefore, it is important that you remain near emergency medical facilities for at least one hour after each injection.

COMPARISON OF ANTIHISTAMINES

The table below indicates the main uses of some common antihistamines and lists their relative strength of anticholinergic action, sedative effects, and duration of action.

KEY
● Drug used ■ Strong ◪ Medium □ Minimal
▲ Long (over 12 hours) ◮ Medium (6–12 hours)
△ Short (4–6 hours)

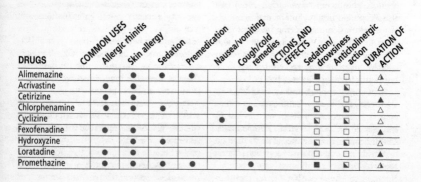

DRUGS	COMMON USES Allergic rhinitis	Skin allergy	Sedation	Premedication	Nausea/vomiting	Cough/cold remedies	ACTIONS AND EFFECTS Sedation/drowsiness	Anticholinergic action	DURATION OF ACTION
Alimemazine		●	●	●			■	□	△
Acrivastine	●	●					□	◪	△
Cetirizine	●	●					□	□	▲
Chlorphenamine	●	●	●			●	◪	◪	△
Cyclizine					●		◪	◪	△
Fexofenadine	●	●					□	□	▲
Hydroxyzine		●	●				◪	◪	△
Loratadine	●	●					□	□	▲
Promethazine	●	●	●	●		●	■	◪	△

INFECTIONS AND INFESTATIONS

The human body provides a suitable environment for the growth of many types of microorganism, including bacteria, viruses, fungi, yeasts, and protozoa. It may also become the host for animal parasites such as insects, worms, and flukes.

Microorganisms (microbes) exist all around us and can be transmitted from person to person in many ways: direct contact, inhalation of infected air, and consumption of contaminated food or water. Not all microorganisms cause disease; many types of bacteria exist on the skin surface or in the bowel without causing ill effects, while others cannot live either in or on the body.

Normally, the immune system protects the body from infection. Invading microbes are killed before they can multiply in sufficient numbers to cause serious disease. (See also Malignant and immune disease, p.95.)

TYPES OF INFECTING ORGANISM

A typical bacterium consists of a single cell with a protective wall. Some bacteria are aerobic (requiring oxygen) and are therefore more likely to infect surface areas such as the skin or respiratory tract. Others are anaerobic and multiply in oxygen-free surroundings such as the bowel or deep wounds. Bacteria can cause symptoms of disease in two principal ways: by releasing toxins that harm body cells and by provoking an inflammatory response in the infected tissues.

Viruses are smaller than bacteria and consist simply of a core of genetic material surrounded by a protein coat. A virus can multiply only in a living cell, by using the host tissue's replicating material.

Protozoa are single-celled parasites and are slightly bigger than bacteria. Many protozoa live in the human intestine and are harmless. However, other types cause malaria, sleeping sickness, and dysentery.

INFESTATIONS

Invasion by parasites that live on the body (such as lice) or in the body (such as tapeworms) is known as infestation. Since the body lacks strong natural defences against infestation, antiparasitic treatment is necessary. Infestation is often associated with tropical climates and poor standards of hygiene.

WHAT CAN GO WRONG

Infectious diseases occur when the body is invaded by microbes. This may be caused by the body having little or no natural immunity to the invading organism, or the number of invading microbes being too great for the body's immune system to overcome. Serious infections can occur when the immune system does not function properly or when a disease weakens or destroys the immune system, as occurs in AIDS (acquired immune deficiency syndrome).

Infections (such as childhood infectious diseases or those with flu-like symptoms) can cause generalized illness or they may affect a specific part of the body (as in wound infections). Some parts are more susceptible to infection than others – respiratory tract infections are relatively common, whereas bone and muscle infections are rare.

Some symptoms are the result of damage to body tissues by the infection, or by toxins released by the microbes. In other cases, the symptoms result from the body's defence mechanisms.

Most bacterial and viral infections cause fever. Bacterial infections may also result in inflammation and pus in the affected area.

WHY DRUGS ARE USED

Treatment of an infection is necessary only when the type or severity of symptoms shows that the immune system has not overcome the infection.

Bacterial infection can be treated with antibiotic or antibacterial drugs. Some of these drugs kill the infecting bacteria, whereas others merely prevent them from multiplying.

Unnecessary use of antibiotics may result in the development of resistant bacteria.

Some antibiotics can be used to treat a broad range of infections, while others are effective against a particular type of bacterium or in a certain part of the body. Antibiotics are most commonly given by mouth, or by injection in severe infections, but they may be applied topically for a local action.

Antiviral drugs are used for severe viral infections that threaten body organs or survival. Antivirals may be used in topical preparations, given by mouth, or administered by injection, usually in hospital.

Other drugs used to fight infection include antiprotozoal drugs for protozoal infections such as malaria; antifungal drugs for infection by fungi and yeasts, including *Candida* (thrush); and anthelmintics to eradicate worm and fluke infestations. Infestation by skin parasites is usually treated with the topical application of insecticides (see p.122).

MAJOR DRUG GROUPS

◆ Antibiotics
◆ Drugs for meningitis
◆ Antibacterial drugs
◆ Drug treatment for Hansen's disease
◆ Antituberculous drugs
◆ Antiviral drugs
◆ Vaccines and immunization
◆ Antiprotozoal drugs
◆ Antimalarial drugs
◆ Antifungal drugs
◆ Anthelmintic drugs

Antibiotics

One in six prescriptions that British doctors write every year is for antibiotics. These drugs are usually safe and effective in the treatment of bacterial disorders ranging from minor infections, like conjunctivitis, to life-threatening diseases like pneumonia, meningitis, and septicaemia. They are similar in function to the antibacterial drugs (see p.66), but the early antibiotics all had a natural origin in moulds and fungi, although most are now synthesized.

Since 1941, when the first antibiotic, penicillin, was introduced, many different classes have been developed. Each one has a different chemical composition and is effective against a particular range of bacteria. None is effective against viral infections (see Antiviral drugs, p.69).

Some of the antibiotics have a broad spectrum of activity against a wide variety of bacteria. Others are used in the treatment of infection by only a few specific organisms. For a description of each common class of antibiotic, see Classes of antibiotic p.64.

WHY THEY ARE USED

We are surrounded by bacteria – in the air we breathe, on the mucous membranes of our mouth and nose, on our skin, and in our intestines – but we are protected, most of the time, by our immunological defences. When these break down, or when bacteria already present migrate to a vulnerable new site, or when harmful bacteria not usually present invade the body, infectious disease sets in.

The bacteria multiply uncontrollably, destroying tissue, releasing toxins, and, in some cases, threatening to spread via the bloodstream to such vital organs as the heart, brain, lungs, and kidneys. The symptoms of infectious disease vary widely, depending on the site of infection and type of bacteria.

Confronted with a sick person and suspecting a bacterial infection, the doctor identifies the organism causing the disease before prescribing any drug. However, tests to analyse blood, sputum, urine, stool, or pus usually take 24 hours or more. In the meantime, especially if the person is in discomfort or pain, the doctor usually makes a preliminary drug choice, based on an educated guess as to the causative organism. In starting this "empirical treatment", as it is called, the doctor is guided by the site of the infection, the nature and severity of the symptoms, the likely source of infection, and the prevalence of any similar illnesses in the community at that time.

In such circumstances, pending laboratory identification of the trouble-making bacteria, the doctor may initially prescribe a broad-spectrum antibiotic, which is effective against a wide variety of bacteria. As soon as tests provide more exact information, the doctor may switch the person to the recommended antibiotic treatment for the identified bacteria. In some cases, more than one antibiotic is prescribed, to be sure of eliminating all strains of bacteria.

In most cases, antibiotics can be given by mouth. However, in serious infections when

USES OF ANTIBIOTICS

The table below shows common drugs in each class of antibiotic used to treat infections in different parts of the body. (It is not intended as a guide to prescribing.) For comparison, some antibacterial drugs (p.66) are included under "sulphonamides" and "Other drugs".

ANTIBIOTIC	Ear, nose, throat, and mouth	Respiratory tract	Skin and soft tissue	Gastrointestinal tract	Eye	Kidney and urinary tract	Brain and nervous system	Heart and blood	Bones and joints	Genital tract
Penicillins										
Amoxicillin	●	●	●			●		●	●	
Ampicillin	●	●	●			●	●	●		
Benzylpenicillin	●	●	●				●	●		●
Co-amoxiclav	●	●	●			●				
Flucloxacillin	●		●					●	●	
Phenoxymethylpenicillin	●	●	●							
Cephalosporins										
Cefaclor	●	●				●				
Cefalexin		●	●			●				
Cefotaxime		●		●			●	●		
Macrolides										
Azithromycin	●	●	●							●
Clarithromycin	●	●	●	●						
Erythromycin	●	●	●	●	●				●	●
Tetracyclines										
Doxycycline	●	●	●			●				●
Oxytetracycline	●	●	●							
Tetracycline	●	●	●		●	●				●
Aminoglycosides										
Amikacin		●	●	●		●	●		●	
Gentamicin		●	●	●	●	●	●	●	●	
Neomycin			●	●						
Netilmicin		●	●	●		●	●		●	
Streptomycin		●						●		
Tobramycin		●	●	●		●	●		●	
Sulphonamides										
Co-trimoxazole		●				●				
Other drugs										
Chloramphenicol	●				●		●			
Ciprofloxacin		●		●		●				●
Clindamycin		●	●	●					●	
Colistin		●								
Dapsone			●							
Fusidic acid			●		●			●	●	
Levofloxacin	●	●	●			●				
Linezolid		●	●							
Metronidazole	●		●	●				●	●	●
Nalidixic acid						●				
Nitrofurantoin						●				
Teicoplanin			●					●	●	
Trimethoprim		●	●			●				
Vancomycin			●					●	●	

high blood levels of the drug are needed rapidly, or when a type of antibiotic is needed that cannot be given by mouth, the drug may be given by injection. Antibiotics are also included in topical preparations for localized skin, eye, and ear infections (see also Anti-infective skin preparations, p.120, and Drugs for ear disorders, p.117).

HOW THEY WORK

Depending on the type of drug and the dosage, antibiotics are either bactericidal, killing organisms directly, or bacteriostatic, halting the multiplication of bacteria and enabling the body's natural defences to overcome the remaining infection.

Penicillins and cephalosporins are bactericidal, destroying bacteria by preventing them from making normal cell walls; most other antibiotics act inside the bacteria by interfering with the chemical activities essential to their life cycle.

CLASSES OF ANTIBIOTIC

Penicillins The first antibiotic drugs to be developed, penicillins are still widely used to treat many common infections. Some are not effective when they are taken by mouth and therefore have to be given by injection in hospital. Unfortunately, certain strains of bacteria are resistant to penicillin treatment, and other drugs may have to be substituted.

Cephalosporins These broad-spectrum antibiotics, similar to the penicillins, are often used when penicillin treatment has proved ineffective. Some can be given by mouth, but others are given only by injection. About 10 per cent of people who are allergic to penicillins are also allergic to cephalosporins. Some cephalosporins can occasionally damage the kidneys, particularly if used with aminoglycosides.

Macrolides Erythromycin is the most common drug in this group. It is a broad-spectrum antibiotic that is often prescribed as an alternative to penicillins or cephalosporins. Erythromycin is also effective against certain diseases, such as Legionnaires' disease (a rare type of pneumonia), that cannot be treated with other antibiotics. The main risk with erythromycin is that it can occasionally impair liver function.

Tetracyclines These have a broader spectrum of activity than other classes of antibiotic. However, increasing bacterial resistance (see Antibiotic resistance, facing page) has limited their use, but they are still widely prescribed. As well as being used for the treatment of infections, tetracyclines are also used in the long-term treatment of acne, although this application is probably not related to their antibacterial action. A major drawback to the use of tetracycline antibiotics in pregnant women and young children is that they are deposited in developing bones and teeth.

With the exception of doxycycline, drugs from this group are poorly absorbed through the intestines, and when given by mouth they have to be administered in high doses in order to reach effective levels in the blood. Such high doses increase the likelihood of diarrhoea as a side effect. The absorption of tetracyclines can be further reduced by interaction with calcium and other minerals. Drugs from this group should not therefore be taken with iron tablets or milk products.

Aminoglycosides These potent drugs are effective against a wide range of bacteria. They are not as widely used as some other antibiotics, however, since they have to be given by injection and have potentially serious side effects. Their use is therefore limited to hospital treatment of serious infections. They are often given with other antibiotics. Possible adverse effects include a severe skin rash and damage to the kidneys and nerves in the ear.

Lincosamides The lincosamide clindamycin is not commonly used because it is more likely than other antibiotics to cause serious disruption of bacterial activity in the bowel. It is reserved mainly for treating bone, joint, abdominal, and pelvic infections that do not respond well to other antibiotics. It is also used topically for acne and vaginal infections.

Quinolones These drugs, often called antibacterials, are derived from chemicals rather than living organisms. Quinolones have a wide spectrum of activity. They are used in the treatment of urinary infections and are widely effective in acute diarrhoeal diseases, including that caused by salmonella, as well as in the treatment of enteric fever.

The absorption of quinolones is reduced by antacids containing magnesium and aluminium. Quinolones are generally well tolerated but can, rarely, cause convulsions in some people. These drugs are less frequently used in children because there is a theoretical risk of damage to the developing joints.

HOW THEY AFFECT YOU

Antibiotics stop most common types of infection within days. Because they do not relieve symptoms directly, your doctor may advise additional medication, such as analgesics (see p.9), to relieve pain and fever until the antibiotics take effect.

It is important to complete the course of medication as prescribed by your doctor, even if all your symptoms have disappeared. Failure to do this can lead to a resurgence of the infection in an antibiotic-resistant form (see Antibiotic resistance, below).

Most antibiotics used in the home do not cause any adverse effects if taken in the recommended dosage. In people who do experience adverse effects, nausea and diarrhoea are among the more common ones (see also individual drug profiles in Part 2). Some people may be hypersensitive to certain types of antibiotic, which can result in a variety of serious adverse effects.

ANTIBIOTIC RESISTANCE

The increasing use of antibiotics in the treatment of infection has led certain types of bacteria to become resistant to the effects of particular antibiotics. This resistance to the drug usually occurs when bacteria develop mechanisms of growth and reproduction that are not disrupted by the effects of the antibiotics. In other cases, bacteria produce enzymes that neutralize the antibiotics.

Antibiotic resistance may develop in a person during prolonged treatment when a drug has failed to eliminate the infection quickly. The resistant strain of bacteria is able to multiply, thereby prolonging the illness. It may also infect other people and result in the spread of resistant infection.

One particularly important example of a resistant strain of bacteria is methicillin-resistant staphylococcus aureus (MRSA), which resists most antibiotics but can be treated with other drugs such as teicoplanin and vancomycin.

Doctors try to prevent the development of antibiotic resistance by selecting the drug that is most likely to eliminate the bacteria present in each individual case as quickly and as thoroughly as possible. Failure to complete a course of antibiotics that has been prescribed by your doctor increases the likelihood that the infection will recur in a resistant form.

RISKS AND SPECIAL PRECAUTIONS

Most antibiotics used for short periods outside a hospital setting are safe for most people. The most common risk, particularly with cephalosporins and penicillins, is a severe allergic reaction to the drug that can cause rashes and sometimes swelling of the face and throat. If this happens, the drug should be stopped and immediate medical advice sought. If you have had a previous allergic reaction to an antibiotic, all other drugs in that class and related classes should be avoided. It is therefore important to inform your doctor if you have previously suffered an adverse reaction to treatment with an antibiotic (with the exception of minor bowel disturbances).

Another risk of antibiotic treatment, especially if it is prolonged, is that the balance among microorganisms normally inhabiting the body may be disturbed. In particular, antibiotics may destroy the bacteria that normally limit the growth of Candida, a yeast that is often present in the body in small amounts. This can lead to overgrowth of Candida (thrush) in the mouth, vagina, or bowel, and an antifungal drug (p.76) may be needed.

A rarer, but more serious, result of disruption of normal bacterial activity in the body is a disorder known as pseudomembranous colitis, in which bacteria resistant to the antibiotic multiply in the bowel, causing violent, bloody diarrhoea. This potentially fatal disorder can occur with any antibiotic, but is most common with the lincosamides.

COMMON DRUGS

Aminoglycosides Amikacin, Gentamicin*, Neomycin, Netilmicin, Streptomycin, Tobramycin
Cephalosporins Cefaclor, Cefadroxil, Cefalexin*, Cefixime, Cefpodoxime, Ceftazidime

Tetracyclines Doxycycline*, Oxytetracycline, Tetracycline*
Macrolides Azithromycin, Clarithromycin*, Erythromycin*
Penicillins Amoxicillin/co-amoxiclav*, Azlocillin, Benzylpenicillin, Co-fluampicil, Flucloxacillin, Phenoxymethyl-penicillin*, Piperacillin/tazobactam
Lincosamides Clindamycin
Other drugs Aztreonam, Chloramphenicol*, Ciprofloxacin*, Colistin, Fusidic acid, Imipenem, Levofloxacin*, Linezolid, Metronidazole*, Rifampicin*, Teicoplanin, Trimethoprim*, Vancomycin
* See Part 2

Drugs for meningitis

Meningitis is inflammation of the meninges (the membranes surrounding the brain and spinal cord), and it can be caused by both bacteria and viruses. Bacterial meningitis can kill previously well individuals in a matter of hours.

If bacterial meningitis is suspected, intramuscular or intravenous antibiotics will be needed immediately, and admission to hospital is arranged.

In cases of bacterial meningitis caused by *Haemophilus influenzae* or *Neisseria meningitidis*, people who have been in contact with an infected person are advised to have a preventative course of antibiotics, usually rifampicin (see p.371) or ciprofloxacin (see p.185).

Antibacterial drugs

This broad classification of drugs comprises agents that are similar to antibiotics (p.62) in function but dissimilar in origin. The original antibiotics were derived from living organisms such as moulds and fungi. Antibacterials were developed from chemicals. The sulphonamides were the first drugs to be given for the treatment of bacterial infections, and they provided the mainstay of the treatment of infection before penicillin (the first antibiotic) became generally available. Increasing bacterial resistance and the development of antibiotics that are more effective and less toxic have reduced the use of sulphonamides.

WHY THEY ARE USED
Sulphonamides are less commonly used these days, and co-trimoxazole is reserved for rare cases of pneumonia in immunocompromised patients.

Trimethoprim is used for chest and urinary tract infections. The drug used to be combined with sulfamethoxazole as co-trimoxazole, but because of the side effects of sulfamethoxazole, trimethoprim on its own is usually preferred now.

Antibacterials for tuberculosis are discussed on p.67. Others, sometimes classified as antimicrobials, include metronidazole, which is used for a variety of genital infections and some serious infections of the abdomen, pelvic region, heart, and central nervous system. Other antibacterials are used to treat urinary infections. These include nitrofurantoin and quinolones (see Classes of antibiotic, p.64) such as nalidixic acid, which can be used to cure or prevent recurrent infections. The quinolones are effective against a broad spectrum of bacteria. More potent relatives of nalidixic acid include norfloxacin, which is used to treat urinary tract infections, and ciprofloxacin, levofloxacin, and ofloxacin. These are all also used to treat many serious bacterial infections.

HOW THEY WORK
Most antibacterials function by preventing growth and multiplication of bacteria. For example, folic acid, a chemical necessary for the growth of bacteria, is produced within bacterial cells by an enzyme that acts on a chemical called para-aminobenzoic acid. Sulphonamides interfere with the release of the enzyme. This prevents folic acid from being formed. The bacterium is therefore unable to function properly and dies.

HOW THEY AFFECT YOU
Antibacterials usually take several days to eliminate bacteria. During this time your doctor may recommend additional medication to alleviate pain and fever. Possible side effects of sulphonamides include loss of appetite, nausea, a rash, and drowsiness.

RISKS AND SPECIAL PRECAUTIONS
Like antibiotics, most antibacterials can cause allergic reactions in susceptible people.

Possible symptoms that should always be brought to your doctor's attention include rashes and fever. If such symptoms occur, a change to another drug is likely to be necessary. Treatment with sulphonamides carries a number of serious but uncommon risks. Some drugs in this group can cause crystals to form in the kidneys, a risk that can be reduced by drinking adequate amounts of fluid during prolonged treatment. Because sulphonamides may also occasionally damage the liver, they are not usually prescribed for people with impaired liver function. These drugs are also less frequently used in children because there is a theoretical risk of damage to the developing joints.

COMMON DRUGS

Quinolones Ciprofloxacin*, Levofloxacin*, Moxifloxacin, Nalidixic acid, Norfloxacin, Ofloxacin
Sulphonamides Co-trimoxazole*, Sulfadiazine
Other drugs Clofazimine, Dapsone, Daptomycin, Linezolid, Metronidazole*, Nitrofurantoin, Tinidazole, Trimethoprim*
* See Part 2

Drug treatment for Hansen's disease

Hansen's disease, more commonly known as leprosy, is a bacterial infection caused by *Mycobacterium leprae*. It is rare in the United Kingdom but relatively common in parts of Africa, Asia, and Latin America.

Hansen's disease progresses slowly, first affecting the peripheral nerves and causing loss of sensation in the hands and feet. This leads to frequent unnoticed injuries and consequent scarring. Later, the nerves of the face may also be affected.

Treatment involves the use of three drugs together to prevent resistance from developing. Usually, dapsone, rifampicin, and clofazimine will be given for at least two years. If one of these drugs cannot be used, a second-line drug (ofloxacin, minocycline, or clarithromycin) might be substituted. Complications during treatment may require use of prednisolone, aspirin, chloroquine, or even thalidomide.

Antituberculous drugs

Tuberculosis is an infectious bacterial disease acquired, often in childhood, by inhaling the tuberculosis bacilli that are present in the spray of a sneeze or cough from an actively infected person. It may also, rarely, be acquired from infected unpasteurized cow's milk. The disease usually starts in a lung and takes one of two forms: primary or reactivated infection.

In 90 to 95 per cent of those with a primary infection, the body's immune system suppresses the infection but does not kill the bacilli. They remain alive but dormant and may cause the reactivated form of the disease. After they are reactivated, the tuberculosis bacilli may spread via the lymphatic system and bloodstream throughout the body.

The first symptoms of primary infection may include a cough, fever, tiredness, night sweats, and weight loss. Tuberculosis is confirmed through clinical investigations, which may include a chest X-ray, isolation of the bacilli from the person's sputum, and a positive reaction (localized inflammation) to the Mantoux test, an injection of tuberculin (a protein extracted from tuberculosis bacilli) into the skin.

The gradual emergence in adults of the destructive and progressive form of tuberculosis is caused by the reactivated infection. It occurs in 5 to 10 per cent of those who have had a previous primary infection. Another form, reinfection tuberculosis, occurs when someone with the dormant, primary form is reinfected. This type of tuberculosis is clinically identical to the reactivated form. Reactivation is more likely in people whose immune system is suppressed, such as the elderly, those taking corticosteroids or other immunosuppressants, and those with AIDS. Reactivation tuberculosis may be difficult to identify because the symptoms may start in any part of the body seeded with the bacilli. It is most often first seen in the upper lobes of the lung, and is frequently diagnosed after a chest X-ray. The early symptoms may be identical to those of primary infection: a cough, tiredness, night sweats, fever, and weight loss.

If it is left untreated, tuberculosis continues to destroy tissue, spreading throughout the body and eventually causing death. It was one of the most common causes of death in the United Kingdom until the 1940s, but the disease is now on the increase again worldwide. Vulnerable groups are the homeless and people who have suppressed immune systems.

WHY THEY ARE USED

A person diagnosed as having tuberculosis is likely to be treated with three or four antituberculous drugs. This helps to overcome the risk of drug-resistant strains of the bacilli emerging (see Antibiotic resistance, p.65).

The standard drug combination for the treatment of tuberculosis consists of rifampicin, isoniazid, and pyrazinamide. In areas where there is high prevalence of drug-resistant tuberculosis, or a large number of organisms is present, ethambutol may be added. However, other drugs may be substituted if the initial treatment fails or drug sensitivity tests indicate that the bacilli are resistant to these drugs.

The standard duration of treatment for a newly diagnosed tuberculosis infection is a six-month regimen as follows: isoniazid, rifampicin, pyrazinamide, and ethambutol daily for two months, followed by isoniazid and rifampicin daily for four months. The duration of treatment can be extended from nine months to up to two years in people at particular risk, such as those with a suppressed immune system or those in whom tuberculosis has infected the central nervous system.

Corticosteroids may be added to the treatment, if the patient does not have a suppressed immune system, to reduce the amount of tissue damage.

Both the number of drugs required and the long duration of treatment may make treatment difficult, particularly for those who are homeless. To help with this problem, supervised administration of treatment is available when required, both in the community and in hospital.

Tuberculosis in patients with HIV infection or AIDS is treated with the standard antituberculous drug regimen; but lifelong preventative treatment with isoniazid may be necessary.

HOW THEY WORK

Antituberculous drugs act in the same way as antibiotics, either by killing bacilli or preventing them from multiplying. (See also Antibiotics, p.62).

HOW THEY AFFECT YOU

The drugs start to combat the disease within days, but benefits are not usually noticeable for a few weeks. As the infection is eradicated, the body repairs the damage caused by the disease. Symptoms gradually subside, and appetite and general health improve.

RISKS AND SPECIAL PRECAUTIONS

Antituberculous drugs may cause nausea, vomiting, and abdominal pain and occasionally lead to serious allergic reactions. When this happens, another drug is substituted.

Rifampicin and isoniazid may affect liver function; isoniazid may adversely affect the nerves as well. Ethambutol can cause changes in colour vision. Dosage is carefully monitored, especially in children, the elderly, and those with reduced kidney function.

TUBERCULOSIS PREVENTION

A vaccine prepared from an artificially weakened strain of cattle tuberculosis bacteria can provide immunity from tuberculosis by provoking the development of natural resistance to the disease (see Vaccines and immunization, p.70). The BCG vaccine is a form of tuberculosis bacillus that provokes the body's immune response but does not cause the illness because it does not invade tissues. The vaccine is given to people who are at risk of tuberculosis and for whom a skin test is negative. Babies born to immigrants in this category are immunized, without having a skin test, within a few weeks of birth.

The vaccine is usually injected into the upper arm. A small pustule usually appears 6 to 12 weeks later, by which time the person can be considered immune.

COMMON DRUGS

Amikacin, Capreomycin, Ciprofloxacin*, Clarithromycin*, Cycloserine, Ethambutol*, Isoniazid*, Protionamide, Pyrazinamide, Rifabutin, Rifampicin*, Streptomycin

* See Part 2

Antiviral drugs

Viruses are simpler and smaller organisms than bacteria and are less able to sustain themselves. These organisms can survive and multiply only by penetrating body cells. Because viruses perform few functions independently, medicines that disrupt or halt their life cycle without harming human cells have been difficult to develop.

There are many different types of virus; and viral infections cause illnesses with various symptoms and degrees of severity. Common viral illnesses include the cold, influenza and flu-like illnesses, cold sores, and childhood diseases such as chickenpox, mumps, and measles. Throat infections, pneumonia, acute bronchitis, gastroenteritis, and meningitis are often, but not always, due to a virus.

Fortunately, the body's natural defences are usually strong enough to overcome infections such as these, with drugs given to ease pain and lower fever. However, the more serious viral diseases, such as pneumonia and meningitis, need close medical supervision.

Another difficulty with viral infections is the speed with which the virus multiplies. By the time symptoms appear, the viruses are so numerous that antiviral drugs have little effect. Antiviral agents must be given early in the course of a viral infection. They may also be used prophylactically (as a preventative). Some viral infections can be prevented by vaccination (see p.70).

WHY THEY ARE USED

Antiviral drugs are helpful in the treatment of various conditions caused by the herpes virus: cold sores, encephalitis, genital herpes, chickenpox, and shingles.

Aciclovir and penciclovir are applied topically to treat outbreaks of cold sores, herpes eye infections, and genital herpes. They can reduce the severity and duration of an outbreak, but they do not eliminate the infection permanently. Aciclovir, famciclovir, and valaciclovir are given by mouth or, under exceptional circumstances, by injection, to prevent chickenpox or severe, recurrent attacks of herpes virus infections in those people who are already weakened by other conditions.

Influenza may sometimes be prevented by oseltamivir or treated with zanamivir. Oseltamivir may also be used to treat the symptoms of influenza in at-risk people, such as those over 65 or people with respiratory diseases such as COPD (chronic obstructive pulmonary disease) or asthma, cardiovascular disease, kidney disease, immunosuppression, or diabetes mellitus.

The interferons are proteins produced by the body and involved in the immune response and cell function. Interferon alpha and beta are effective in reducing the activity of hepatitis B and hepatitis C. Lamivudine is also used to treat hepatitis B, and ribavirin is used for hepatitis C.

Ganciclovir is sometimes used for cytomegalovirus (CMV). Respiratory syncytial virus (RSV) has been treated with ribavirin, and prevented by palivizumab. Drug treatment for AIDS is discussed on p.100.

HOW THEY WORK

Some antivirals act by altering the "building blocks" for the cells' genetic material (DNA), so that the virus cannot multiply. Others stop viruses multiplying by blocking enzyme activity within the host cell. Halting multiplication prevents the virus from spreading to uninfected cells and improves symptoms rapidly. However, in herpes infections, it does not eradicate the virus from the body. Infection may therefore flare up on another occasion.

HOW THEY AFFECT YOU

Topical antiviral drugs usually start to act immediately. Providing that the treatment is applied early enough, an outbreak of herpes can be cut short. Symptoms usually clear up within two to four days. Antiviral ointments may cause irritation and redness. Antivirals given by mouth or injection can occasionally cause nausea and dizziness.

RISKS AND SPECIAL PRECAUTIONS

Because some of these drugs may affect the kidneys adversely, they are prescribed with caution to people with reduced kidney function. Some antivirals can adversely affect the activity of normal body cells, particularly those in the bone marrow. Idoxuridine is therefore available only for topical use.

COMMON DRUGS

Aciclovir*, Amantadine, Cidofovir, Famciclovir, Fomivirsen, Foscarnet, Ganciclovir, Inosine pranobex, Oseltamivir*, Palivizumab, Penciclovir, Ribavirin, Valaciclovir, Valganciclovir, Zanamivir, Zidovudine/Lamivudine*

* See Part 2

See also Drugs for HIV, p.100

Vaccines and immunization

Many infectious diseases, including most of the common viral infections, occur only once during a person's lifetime. The reason is that the antibodies produced in response to the disease remain afterwards, prepared to repel any future invasion as soon as the first infectious germs appear. The duration of such immunity varies, but it can last a lifetime.

Protection against many infections can now be provided artificially by the use of vaccines derived from altered forms of the infecting organism. These vaccines stimulate the immune system in the same way as a genuine infection, and provide lasting, active immunity. Because each type of microbe stimulates the production of a specific antibody, a different vaccine must be given for each disease.

Another type of immunization, called passive immunization, relies on giving antibodies (see Immunoglobulins, p.72).

WHY THEY ARE USED

Some infectious diseases cannot be treated effectively or are potentially so serious that prevention is the best treatment. Routine immunization not only protects the individual but may gradually eradicate the disease completely, as is the case with smallpox.

Newborn babies receive antibodies for many diseases from their mothers, but this protection lasts only for about three months. Most children from 2 months to 15 years are vaccinated against common childhood infectious diseases. Additionally, travellers to many countries, especially the tropics, are advised to be vaccinated against diseases common in those areas. Rabies, yellow fever, and hepatitis B vaccines may be required for remote areas.

Effective lifelong immunization can sometimes be achieved by a single dose of the vaccine. However, in many cases, reinforcing doses, commonly called booster shots, are needed later to maintain reliable immunity.

Vaccines do not provide immediate protection against infection, and it may be up to four weeks before full immunity is able to develop. When immediate protection from infectious disease is needed (for example, following exposure to infection) it may be necessary to establish passive immunity with immunoglobulins (see p.72).

HOW THEY WORK

Vaccines provoke the immune system into creating antibodies that help the body to resist specific infectious diseases. Many vaccines (known as live vaccines) are made from artificially weakened forms of the disease-causing germ; but even these are effective in stimulating sufficient growth of antibodies. Other vaccines rely either on inactive (or killed) disease-causing germs, or inactive derivatives of them, but their effect on the immune system remains the same. Effective antibodies are created, thereby establishing active immunity.

HOW THEY AFFECT YOU

The degree of protection varies among different vaccines. Some provide reliable lifelong immunity; others may not give full protection against a disease, or the effects may last for as little as six months. Influenza vaccines usually protect only against the variety of virus causing the latest outbreak of flu. New varieties appear during most years.

Any vaccine may cause side effects but they are usually mild and soon disappear. The most common reactions are a red, slightly raised, tender area at the site of injection, and a slight fever or a flu-like illness lasting for one or two days.

RISKS AND SPECIAL PRECAUTIONS

Serious reactions are rare and, for most children, the risk is far outweighed by the protection given. A family or personal history of seizures is not necessarily a contraindication to immunization; but sometimes immunization may be delayed if the condition is unstable. Children with any infection more

COMMON VACCINATIONS

INFECTION	HOW GIVEN	AGE GIVEN
Diphtheria/tetanus/pertussis/polio/ *Haemophilus influenzae* type b (Hib) (DTaP/IPV/Hib)	1 injection	2 months.
Pneumococcal infection (PCV – pneumococcal conjugate vaccine)	1 injection	
Diphtheria/tetanus/pertussis/polio/Hib (DTaP/IPV/Hib)	1 injection	3 months.
Meningitis C (Meningococcal group C) (MenC)	1 injection	
Diphtheria/tetanus/pertussis/polio/Hib (DTaP/IPV/Hib)	1 injection	4 months.
Meningitis C (MenC)	1 injection	
Pneumococcal infection (PCV)	1 injection	
Hib/meningitis C (Hib/MenC)	1 injection	Around 12 months.
Measles/mumps/rubella (MMR)	1 injection	Around 13 months.
Pneumococcal infection (PCV)	1 injection	
Diphtheria/tetanus/pertussis/polio (DTaP/IPV or dTaP/IPV)	1 injection	3–5 years.
Measles/mumps/rubella (MMR)	1 injection	
Diphtheria/tetanus/polio (Td/IPV)	1 injection	13–18 years.
Tuberculosis	1 injection	Infants and children in areas of UK with high incidence, or whose parents or grandparents are from a high-risk area; at-risk workers (e.g. healthcare or hostel staff).
Hepatitis A	1 injection	Single dose for people of any age who are at risk. Booster 6 –12 months after initial shot. Boosters may be given every 10–20 years if needed.
Hepatitis B	1 injection	3 inoculations at any age, with the second and third shots 1 and 6 months after the first. Booster after 5 years if needed.
Typhoid	1 injection	Single dose for people of any age who are at risk.
Influenza	1 injection	Given routinely from the age of 65. Also given to people of any age who are at risk of serious illness or death if they develop influenza.
Pneumococcal disease	1 injection	Single dose given routinely from the age of 65. Also given to people of any age who are at risk.

severe than a common cold will not be given any routine vaccination until they have recovered.

Live vaccines should not be given during pregnancy, because they may affect a developing baby, nor should they be given to people whose immune systems are weakened by disease or drug treatment. Those taking high doses of corticosteroids (p.80) are advised to delay vaccination until the end of drug treatment.

The risk of high fever following the DTaP/IPV/Hib (combined diphtheria, tetanus, acellular pertussis, inactivated polio, and *Haemophilus influenzae* type b) vaccine can be reduced by giving paracetamol at the time of the vaccination. The pertussis vaccine may rarely cause a mild fit, which is brief, usually associated with fever, and stops without treatment. Children who have experienced such fits recover completely without neurological or developmental problems.

IMMUNOGLOBULINS

Antibodies, which can result from exposure to snake and insect venom as well as infectious disease, are found in the serum of the blood (the part remaining after the red cells and clotting agents are removed). The concentrated serum of people who have survived diseases or poisonous bites is called immunoglobulin. Given by injection, it creates passive immunity. Immunoglobulin from blood donated by a wide cross-section of donors is likely to contain antibodies to most common diseases. Specific immunoglobulins against rare diseases or toxins are derived from the blood of selected donors who are likely to have high levels of antibodies to that disease. These are called hyperimmunoglobulins. Some immunoglobulins are extracted from horse blood following repeated doses of the toxin.

Because immunoglobulins do not stimulate the body to produce its own antibodies, their effect is not long-lasting and diminishes progressively over three or four weeks. Continued protection requires repeated injections of immunoglobulins.

Adverse effects from immunoglobulins are uncommon. Some people are sensitive to horse globulins, and approximately a week after the injection they may experience a reaction known as serum sickness, in which they have fever, a rash, joint swelling, and pain. Serum sickness usually ends in a few days but should be reported to your doctor before any further immunization.

TRAVEL VACCINATIONS

These are not normally needed for travel to Western Europe, North America, Australia, or New Zealand (but you should make sure that your tetanus and polio boosters are up to date). Consult your doctor if you are visiting other destinations. Check that children travelling with you have had all the routine childhood vaccinations and any that are necessary for the areas you will be travelling in.

If you are visiting an area where there is yellow fever, an International Certificate of Vaccination will be needed. You may also need this certificate in the future. Many countries that you might want to visit require an International Certificate of Vaccination if you have already been to a country where yellow fever is present.

You are at risk of other infectious diseases in many parts of the world, and appropriate vaccinations are a wise precaution. For example, a zone called the "Meningitis Belt" runs in a wide band across Africa from the Sahara down to Kenya. Anyone intending to visit this zone should have meningococcal vaccine A, C, W135, and Y. Visitors to Saudi Arabia at certain times of the year may also be required to have had the meningitis group A, C, W135, and Y vaccine.

You may need extra vaccinations if you are backpacking or planning a lengthy stay. For example, hepatitis A vaccine would be sensible for anyone travelling to a developing country, but a long-stay traveller should consider having hepatitis B and BCG (tuberculosis) as well. Rabies vaccination is recommended to anyone travelling into remote areas.

All immunization should be completed well before departure as the vaccinations do not give instant protection (BCG needs 3 months), and some (for example, typhoid) need more than one dose to be effective.

The Department of Health publishes a booklet called *Health Advice for Travellers Anywhere in the World*. This booklet gives information on the requirements for vaccination and is available from some travel agents and post offices.

TRAVEL IMMUNIZATION

The immunizations you will need before you travel depend on the part of the world you intend to visit, but some diseases can be contracted almost anywhere. Make sure that you are immunized against diphtheria, tetanus, and polio and have had boosters if necessary. Ask your doctor or pharmacist for up-to-date information on vaccination for specific areas.

DISEASE	NUMBER OF DOSES	WHEN EFFECTIVE	PERIOD OF PROTECTION	WHO SHOULD BE IMMUNIZED
Hepatitis A	2 injections 6–12 months apart	2–4 weeks after 1st dose	10 years	Frequent travellers to the Mediterranean or developing countries
Hepatitis B	3 injections, 1 month between 1st and 2nd doses, 5 months between 2nd and 3rd doses	Immediately after 2nd dose	3–5 years	People travelling to countries in which hepatitis B is prevalent; those who might need medical or dental treatment while travelling in a developing country; and people likely to have unprotected sex.
Japanese B encephalitis	3 injections, 1 week between 1st and 2nd doses and 3 weeks between 2nd and 3rd doses	10–14 days after last dose	About 1 year	People staying for an extended period in rural areas of the Indian subcontinent, China, Southeast Asia, and the Far East.
Meningitis A, C, W135, and Y	1 injection	2–3 weeks	5 years	People travelling to sub-Saharan Africa. Immunization certificate needed if travelling to Saudi Arabia for the Hajj and Umrah pilgrimages.
Rabies	3 injections. 1 week between 1st and 2nd doses, 3 weeks between 2nd and 3rd doses	Immediately after 3rd dose	2–3 years	People travelling to areas where rabies is endemic and who are at high risk (such as veterinary surgeons, people working with animals, and those travelling into remote country)
Typhoid	1 injection	2 weeks after last injection	3 years	People travelling to areas with poor sanitation and those at high risk, such as laboratory workers.
Yellow fever	1 injection	After 10 days	10 years	People travelling to parts of South America and sub-Saharan Africa.
Cholera	2 oral doses, one week apart	After 1 week	2 years	People travelling to areas where cholera is endemic or epidemic. Vaccination does not provide complete protection; travellers should pay scrupulous attention to food, water, and personal hygiene.

Antiprotozoal drugs

Protozoa are single-celled organisms that are present in soil and water. They may be transmitted to or between humans via contaminated food or water, sexual contact, or insect bites. There are many types of protozoal infection, each of which causes a different disease, depending on the organism involved. Trichomoniasis, toxoplasmosis, cryptosporidium, giardiasis, and pneumocystis pneumonia are probably the most common protozoal infections seen in the United Kingdom. The rarer infections are usually contracted as a result of exposure to infection in another part of the world.

Many types of protozoa infect the bowel, causing diarrhoea and generalized symptoms of ill-health. Others may infect the genital tract or skin. Some protozoa may penetrate vital organs such as the lungs, brain, and liver. Prompt diagnosis and treatment are important in order to limit the spread of the infection within the body and, in some cases, prevent it from spreading to other people. Increased attention to hygiene is an important factor in controlling the spread of the disease.

A variety of medicines is used in the treatment of these diseases. Some, such as metronidazole and tetracycline, are also commonly used for their antibacterial action. Others, such as pentamidine, are rarely used except in treating specific protozoal infections.

HOW THEY AFFECT YOU

Protozoa are often difficult to eradicate from the body. Drug treatment may therefore need to be continued for several months in order to eliminate the infecting organisms completely and thus prevent recurrence of the disease. In addition, unpleasant side effects such as nausea, diarrhoea, and abdominal cramps are often unavoidable because of the limited choice of drugs and the need to maintain dosage levels that will effectively cure the disease. For detailed information on the risks and adverse effects of individual antiprotozoal drugs, consult the appropriate drug profile in Part 2.

TYPES OF PROTOZOAL DISEASE

Amoebiasis *(Entamoeba histolytica)*, or amoebic dysentery, is an infection of the bowel (and sometimes the liver and other organs) usually transmitted in contaminated food or water. Its major symptom is violent, sometimes bloody, diarrhoea. Treatment is with diloxanide, metronidazole, or tinidazole.

Balantidiasis *(Balantidium coli)* is an infection of the bowel, specifically the colon, that is usually transmitted through contact with infected pigs. Possible symptoms include diarrhoea and abdominal pain. Treatment of the infection is with tetracycline, metronidazole, or diodohydroxyquinoline.

Cryptosporidiosis *(Cryptosporidium)* affects the bowel (and occasionally the respiratory tract and bile ducts). Cryptosporidiosis is spread through contaminated food or water or by contact with animals or other humans. Symptoms include diarrhoea and abdominal pain. There are no specific drugs to treat it, but paromomycin, azithromycin, or eflornithine may be effective.

Giardiasis *(Giardia lamblia)*, or lambliasis, affects the bowel and is usually transmitted in contaminated food or water; but it may also be spread by some types of sexual contact. Its major symptoms are generalized ill-health, diarrhoea, flatulence, and abdominal pain. Treatment is with mepacrine, metronidazole, or tinidazole.

Leishmaniasis *(Leishmania)* is a mainly tropical and subtropical disease caused by organisms spread through sandfly bites. It affects the mucous membranes of the mouth, nose, and throat and may, in its severe form, invade organs such as the liver. Treatment is with paromomycin, sodium stibogluconate, pentamidine, or amphotericin.

Pneumocystis pneumonia *(Pneumocystis jiroveci)* is a potentially fatal lung infection usually affecting only people with reduced resistance to infection, such as those who are HIV positive. Symptoms include fever, cough, breathlessness, and chest pain. Treatment is with drugs such as atovaquone, co-trimoxazole, pentamidine, and dapsone with trimethoprim.

Toxoplasmosis *(Toxoplasma gondii)* is usually spread via cat faeces or by eating undercooked meat. Although usually symptomless, toxoplasmosis may cause generalized ill-health, mild fever, and eye inflammation. Treatment is necessary only if the eyes are involved or the patient is immunosuppressed (such as in HIV). It may also pass from mother to baby during pregnancy, leading to severe disease in the fetus. Treatment usually consists of pyrimethamine with sulfadiazine, azithromycin, clarithromycin, or clindamycin, or, during pregnancy, spiramycin.

Trichomoniasis *(Trichomonas vaginalis)* most often affects the vagina, causing irritation and an offensive discharge. In men, it may occur in the urethra. It is usually sexually transmitted. Treatment is with metronidazole or tinidazole.

Trypanosomiasis *(Trypanosoma)*, or African trypanosomiasis (sleeping sickness), is spread by the tsetse fly and causes fever, swollen glands, and drowsiness. South American trypanosomiasis (Chagas' disease) is spread by assassin bugs and causes inflammation, enlargement of internal organs, and infection of the brain. Sleeping sickness is treated with pentamidine, suramin, eflornithine, or melarsoprol. Chagas' disease is treated with primaquine or nifurtimox.

Antimalarial drugs

Malaria is one of the main killing diseases in the tropics. It is most likely to affect people who live in or travel to such places.

The disease is caused by protozoa (see p.73) whose life cycle is far from simple. The malaria parasite, which is called *Plasmodium*, lives in and depends on the female *Anopheles* mosquito during one part of its life cycle. It lives in and depends on human beings during other parts of its life cycle.

Transferred to humans in the saliva of the female mosquito as she penetrates ("bites") the skin, the malaria parasite enters the bloodstream and settles in the liver, where it multiplies asexually.

Following its stay in the liver, the parasite (or plasmodium) enters another phase of its life cycle, circulating in the bloodstream, penetrating and destroying red blood cells, and reproducing again. If the plasmodia then transfer back to a female *Anopheles* mosquito via another "bite", they breed sexually, and are again ready to start a human infection.

Following the emergence of plasmodia from the liver, the symptoms of malaria occur: episodes of high fever and profuse sweating alternate with equally agonizing episodes of shivering and chills. One of the four strains of malaria (*Plasmodium falciparum*) can produce a single severe attack that can be fatal unless treated. The others cause recurrent attacks, sometimes extending over many years.

A number of drugs are available for prevention of malaria; the choice depends on the region in which the disease can be contracted and the resistance to the commonly used drugs. In most areas, *Plasmodium falciparum* is resistant to chloroquine (see Choice of drug, below). In all regions, four drugs are commonly used for treating malaria: quinine, mefloquine, Malarone (a brand-name drug containing the antimalarials proguanil with atovaquone), and Riamet (a brand-name drug containing the antimalarials artemether with lumefantrine).

CHOICE OF DRUG

The following list is for guidance only. Because prevalent strains of malaria change very rapidly, and the risk may vary in different areas and/or countries, you must always seek specific medical advice before travelling. The parts of the world in which malaria is prevalent, and travel to which may make antimalarial drug treatment advisable, can be divided into six zones. Due to drug resistance, specific antimalarials are recommended for each zone. They may include:

Zone 1 North Africa, the Middle East, and Central Asia Chloroquine, proguanil, and doxycycline.

Zone 2 Sub-Saharan Africa Mefloquine, doxycycline, and Malarone.

Zone 3 South Asia Chloroquine, proguanil, mefloquine, doxycycline, and Malarone.

Zone 4 Southeast Asia Chloroquine, proguanil, mefloquine, Malarone, and doxycycline.

Zone 5 Oceania Doxycycline, mefloquine, and Malarone.

Zone 6 Central and South America and the Caribbean Chloroquine, proguanil, mefloquine, doxycycline, and Malarone.

WHY THEY ARE USED

The medical response to malaria takes three forms: prevention, treatment of attacks, and the complete eradication of the plasmodia (radical cure).

For someone planning a trip to an area where malaria is prevalent, drugs are given that destroy the parasites as they enter the liver. This preventative treatment needs to start up to three weeks before departure and continue for 1–4 weeks after returning (the exact timings depend on the drugs taken).

Drugs such as mefloquine, Riamet, and Fansidar (a brand-name drug containing the antimalarials pyrimethamine and sulfadoxine) can produce a radical cure but chloroquine does not. After chloroquine treatment of non-falciparum malaria, a 14- to 21-day course of primaquine is administered. The drug is highly effective in destroying plasmodia in the liver but is weak against plasmodia in the blood. Primaquine is recommended only after a person leaves the malarial area because of the high risk of reinfection.

HOW THEY WORK

Taken to prevent the disease, the drugs kill the plasmodia in the liver, preventing them from multiplying. Once plasmodia have multiplied, the same drugs may be used in higher doses to kill plasmodia that re-enter the bloodstream. If these drugs are not effective, primaquine may be used to destroy any plasmodia that are still present in the liver.

HOW THEY AFFECT YOU

The low doses of antimalarial drugs taken for prevention rarely produce noticeable effects. Drugs taken for an attack usually begin to relieve symptoms within a few hours. Most of them can cause nausea, vomiting, and diarrhoea. Quinine can cause disturbances in vision and hearing. Mefloquine can cause sleep disturbance, dizziness, and difficulties in coordination.

RISKS AND SPECIAL PRECAUTIONS

When drugs are given to prevent or cure malaria, the full course of treatment must be taken. No drugs give long-term protection; a new course of treatment is needed for each journey.

Most of these drugs do not produce severe adverse effects, but primaquine can cause the blood disorder haemolytic anaemia, particularly in people with glucose-6-phosphate dehydrogenase (G6PD) deficiency. Blood tests are taken before treatment to identify susceptible individuals. Mefloquine is not prescribed for those who have had psychological disorders or convulsions.

OTHER PROTECTIVE MEASURES

Because *Plasmodium* strains continually develop resistance to the available drugs, prevention using drugs is not absolutely reliable.

Protection from mosquito bites is of the highest priority. Such protection includes the use of insect repellents and mosquito nets impregnated with permethrin insecticide, as well as covering any exposed skin after dark.

COMMON DRUGS

Drugs for prevention Chloroquine*, Doxycycline*, Mefloquine*, Proguanil*, Proguanil with atovaquone (Malarone)*

Drugs for treatment Artemether with lumefantrine (Riamet), Chloroquine*, Mefloquine*, Primaquine, Proguanil with atovaquone (Malarone)*, Pyrimethamine with sulfadoxine (Fansidar)*, Quinine*

* See Part 2

Antifungal drugs

We are continually exposed to fungi – in the air we breathe, the food we eat, and the water we drink. Fortunately, most of them cannot live in the body, and few are harmful. But some can grow in the mouth, skin, hair, or nails, causing irritating or unsightly changes, and a few can cause serious and possibly fatal disease. The most common fungal infections are caused by the tinea group. These include tinea pedis (athlete's foot), tinea cruris (jock itch), tinea corporis (ringworm), and tinea capitis (scalp ringworm). Caused by a variety of organisms, they are spread by direct or indirect contact with infected humans or animals. Infection is encouraged by warm, moist conditions.

Problems may also result from the proliferation of a fungus normally present in the body; the most common example is excessive growth of *Candida*, a yeast that causes thrush infection of the mouth, vagina, and bowel. It can also infect other organs if it spreads through the body via the bloodstream. Overgrowth of *Candida* may occur in people taking antibiotics (p.62) or oral contraceptives (p.105), in pregnant women, or in those with diabetes or immune system disorders such as HIV.

Superficial fungal infections (those that attack only the outer layer of the skin and mucous membranes) are relatively common and, although irritating, do not usually present a threat to general health. Internal fungal infections (for example, of the lungs, heart, or other organs) are very rare, but may be serious and prolonged.

Because antibiotics and other antibacterial drugs have no effect on fungi and yeasts, a different type of drug is needed. Drugs for fungal infections are either applied topically to treat minor infections of the skin, nails, and mucous membranes or given by mouth or injection to eliminate serious fungal infections of the internal organs and nails.

WHY THEY ARE USED

Drug treatment is necessary for most fungal infections since they rarely improve alone. Measures such as careful washing and drying of the affected areas may help, but they are not a substitute for antifungal drugs. The use of over-the-counter preparations to increase the acidity of the vagina is not usually effective except when accompanied by drug treatment.

Fungal infections of the skin and scalp are usually treated with a cream or shampoo. Drugs for vaginal thrush are most commonly applied in the form of vaginal pessaries or cream applied with a special applicator. For very severe or persistent vaginal infections, a short course of fluconazole or itraconazole

may be given by mouth. Mouth infections are usually eliminated by lozenges dissolved in the mouth or an antifungal solution or gel applied to the affected areas. For severe or persistent nail infections, either griseofulvin or terbinafine are given by mouth until the infected nails have grown out.

In the rare cases of fungal infections of internal organs, such as the blood, the heart, or the brain, potent drugs such as fluconazole and itraconazole are given by mouth, or amphotericin and flucytosine are given by injection. These drugs pass into the bloodstream to fight the fungi.

HOW THEY WORK

Most antifungals alter the permeability of the fungal cell's walls. Chemicals needed for cell life leak out and the fungal cell dies.

HOW THEY AFFECT YOU

The speed with which antifungals provide benefit varies with the type of infection. Most fungal or yeast infections of the skin, mouth, and vagina improve within a week. The condition of nails affected by fungal infections improves only when new nail growth occurs, which takes months. Systemic infections of the internal organs can take weeks to cure.

CHOICE OF ANTIFUNGAL DRUG

The table below shows the range of uses for some antifungal drugs. The particular drug chosen in each case depends on the precise nature and site of the infection. The usual route of administration for each drug is also indicated.

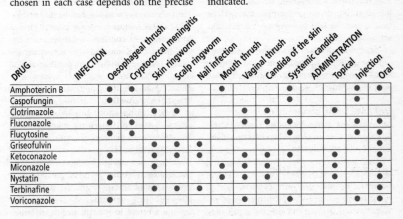

DRUG	INFECTION									ADMINISTRATION		
	Oesophageal thrush	Cryptococcal meningitis	Skin ringworm	Scalp ringworm	Nail infection	Mouth thrush	Vaginal thrush	Candida of the skin	Systemic candida	Topical	Injection	Oral
Amphotericin B	●	●				●			●		●	●
Caspofungin	●								●		●	
Clotrimazole			●	●		●	●			●		
Fluconazole	●	●				●	●		●		●	●
Flucytosine	●	●							●		●	●
Griseofulvin			●	●	●							●
Ketoconazole	●		●	●	●	●	●	●		●		●
Miconazole		●			●	●	●	●		●		●
Nystatin	●					●	●	●		●		●
Terbinafine			●	●	●							●
Voriconazole	●					●			●		●	●

Antifungal drugs applied topically rarely cause side effects, although they may irritate the skin. However, treatment by mouth or injection for systemic and nail infections may produce more serious side effects. Amphotericin, injected in cases of life-threatening systemic infections, can cause potentially dangerous effects, including kidney damage.

COMMON DRUGS

Amorolfine, Amphotericin B*, Caspofungin Clotrimazole*, Econazole, Fenticonazole, Fluconazole*, Flucytosine, Griseofulvin, Itraconazole, Ketoconazole*, Miconazole*, Nystatin*, Sulconazole, Terbinafine*, Tioconazole, Voriconazole
* See Part 2

Anthelmintic drugs

Anthelmintics are drugs that are used to eliminate the many types of worm (helminths) that can enter the body and live there as parasites, producing a general weakness in some cases and serious harm in others. The body may be host to many different worms (see Types of infestation, right). Most species spend part of their life cycle in another animal, and the infestation is often passed on to humans in food contaminated with the eggs or larvae. In some cases, such as hookworm, larvae enter the body through the skin. Larvae or adults may attach themselves to the intestinal wall and feed on the bowel contents; others feed off the intestinal blood supply, causing anaemia. Worms can also infest the bloodstream or lodge in the muscles or internal organs.

Many people have worms at some time during their life, especially during childhood; most worms can be effectively eliminated with anthelmintic drugs.

WHY THEY ARE USED

Most worms common in the United Kingdom cause only mild symptoms and usually do not pose a serious threat to general health. Anthelmintic drugs are usually necessary, however, because the body's natural defences against infection are not effective against most worm infestations. Certain types of infestation must always be treated since they can cause serious complications. In some cases, such as threadworm infestation, doctors may recommend anthelmintic treatment for the whole family to prevent reinfection. If worms have invaded tissues and formed cysts, they may have to be removed surgically. Laxatives are given with some anthelmintics to hasten expulsion of worms from the bowel. Other drugs may be prescribed to ease symptoms or to compensate for any blood loss or nutritional deficiency.

TYPES OF INFESTATION

Threadworm (*enterobiasis*) The most common worm infection in the UK, especially among young children. The worm lives in the intestine but travels to the anus at night to lay eggs, causing itching; scratching leaves eggs on the fingers, usually under the fingernails. Sucking the fingers or eating food with unwashed hands often transfers these eggs to the mouth. Keeping the nails short; good hygiene, including washing the hands after using the toilet and before each meal; and an early morning bath to remove the eggs are important in eradicating the infection.
Drugs Mebendazole, piperazine
All members of the household should be treated simultaneously.

Common roundworm (*ascariasis*) The most common worm infection worldwide. It is transmitted to humans in contaminated raw food or in soil. The worms are large, and they infect the intestine, which can be blocked by dense clusters of them.
Drugs Levamisole, mebendazole, piperazine

Tropical threadworm (*strongyloidiasis*) Occurs in the tropics and southern Europe. The larvae from contaminated soil penetrate the skin, pass into the lungs, are swallowed, and pass into the gut.
Drugs Albendazole, tiabendazole, ivermectin

Whipworm (*trichuriasis*) Mainly occurs in tropical areas of the world as a result of eating contaminated raw vegetables. The worms infest the intestines.
Drug Mebendazole

Hookworm (*uncinariasis*) Mainly found in tropical areas. The worm larvae penetrate the skin and pass via the lymphatic system and bloodstream to the lungs. They then travel up the airways, are swallowed, and attach themselves to the intestinal wall, where they feed off the intestinal blood supply.

Drug Mebendazole

Pork roundworm (*trichinosis*) Transmitted in infected undercooked pork. Initially, the worms lodge in the intestines, but larvae may invade muscle to form cysts that are often resistant to drug treatment and may require surgery.

Drugs Mebendazole, tiabendazole

Toxocariasis (*visceral larva migrans*) Usually occurs as a result of eating soil or eating with fingers contaminated with dog or cat faeces. The eggs hatch in the intestine and may travel to the lungs, liver, kidney, brain, and eyes. Treatment is not always effective.

Drugs Mebendazole, tiabendazole, diethylcarbamazine

Creeping eruption (*cutaneous larva migrans*) Mainly occurs in tropical areas and coastal areas of the southeastern US as a result of skin contact with larvae from cat and dog faeces. Infestation is usually confined to the skin.

Drugs Tiabendazole, ivermectin, albendazole

Filariasis (*including onchocerciasis and ioiasis*) Occurs in tropical areas only. It may affect the lymphatic system, blood, eyes, and skin. Infection by this group of worms is spread by the bites of insects that are carriers of worm larvae or eggs.

Drugs Diethylcarbamazine, ivermectin

Flukes Sheep liver fluke (*fascioliasis*) is indigenous to the UK. Infestation usually results from eating watercress grown in contaminated water. It mainly affects the liver and biliary tract. Other flukes only found abroad may infect the lungs, intestines, or blood.

Drug Praziquantel

Tapeworms (including beef, pork, fish, and dwarf tapeworms) Depending on the type, worms may be carried by cattle, pigs, or fish and transmitted to humans in undercooked meat. Most types affect the intestines. Larvae of the pork tapeworm may form cysts in muscle and other tissues.

Drugs Niclosamide, praziquantel

Hydatid disease (*echinococciasis*) The eggs are transmitted in dog faeces, and the larvae may form cysts over many years, commonly in the liver. Surgery is the usual treatment for cysts.

Drug Albendazole

Bilharzia (*schistosomiasis*) Occurs in polluted water in tropical areas. The larvae may be swallowed or penetrate the skin. Once inside the body, they migrate to the liver; adult worms live in the bladder.

Drug Praziquantel

HOW THEY WORK

The anthelmintic drugs act in several ways. Many of them kill or paralyse the worms, which pass out of the body in the faeces. Others, which act systemically, are used to treat infection in the tissues.

Many anthelmintics are specific for particular worms, and the doctor must identify the nature of the infection before selecting the most appropriate treatment (see Types of infestation, facing page). Most of the common intestinal infestations are easily treated, often with only one or two doses of the drug. However, tissue infections may require more prolonged treatment.

HOW THEY AFFECT YOU

Once the drug has eliminated the worms, symptoms caused by infestation rapidly disappear. Taken as a single dose or a short course, anthelmintics do not usually produce side effects. However, treatment can disturb the digestive system, causing abdominal pain, nausea, and vomiting.

COMMON DRUGS

Albendazole, Diethylcarbamazine, Ivermectin, Levamisole, Mebendazole, Niclosamide, Piperazine, Praziquantel, Tiabendazole

HORMONES AND ENDOCRINE SYSTEM

The endocrine system is a collection of glands located throughout the body that produce hormones and release them into the bloodstream. Each endocrine gland produces one or more hormones, each of which governs a particular body function, including growth and repair of tissues, sexual development and reproductive function, and the body's response to stress.

The pituitary gland produces hormones that regulate growth and sexual and reproductive development, and also stimulate other endocrine glands (see p.85).

The thyroid gland regulates metabolism. Hyperthyroidism or hypothyroidism may occur if the thyroid does not function well (see p.84).

The adrenal glands produce hormones that regulate the body's mineral and water content and reduce inflammation (see Corticosteroids, below right).

The pancreas produces insulin to regulate blood glucose levels, and glucagon, which helps the liver and muscles to store glucose (see p.82).

The kidneys produce a hormone, erythropoietin (see p.234), needed for red blood cell production. Patients with kidney failure lack this hormone and become anaemic; they may be given epoetin, a version of the hormone.

The ovaries (in women) secrete oestrogen and progesterone, responsible for female sexual and physical development (see p.88).

The testes (in men) produce testosterone, which controls the development of male sexual and physical characteristics (see p.87).

Most hormones are released continuously from birth, but the amount produced fluctuates with the body's needs. Others are produced mainly at certain times – for example, growth hormone is released mainly during childhood and adolescence. Sex hormones are produced by the testes and ovaries from puberty onwards (see p.103).

Many endocrine glands release their hormones in response to triggering hormones produced by the pituitary gland. This gland releases a variety of pituitary hormones, each of which, in turn, stimulates the appropriate endocrine gland to produce its hormone.

A "feedback" system usually regulates blood hormone levels: if the blood level rises too high, the pituitary responds by reducing the amount of stimulating hormone produced, thereby allowing the blood hormone level to return to normal.

WHAT CAN GO WRONG

Endocrine disorders, usually resulting in too much or too little of a particular hormone, have a variety of causes. Some are congenital in origin; others may be caused by autoimmune disease (including some forms of diabetes mellitus), malignant or benign tumours, injury, or certain drugs.

WHY DRUGS ARE USED

Natural hormone preparations or their synthetic versions are often prescribed to treat deficiency. Sometimes drugs are given to stimulate increased hormone production in the endocrine gland, such as oral antidiabetic drugs, which act on the insulin-producing cells of the pancreas. When too much hormone is produced, drug treatment may reduce the activity of the gland.

Hormones or related drugs are also used to treat certain other conditions. Corticosteroids related to adrenal hormones are prescribed to relieve inflammation and to suppress immune system activity (see p.99). Several types of cancer are treated with sex hormones. Female sex hormones are used as contraceptives (see p.105) and to treat menstrual disorders (see p.104).

MAJOR DRUG GROUPS
◆ Corticosteroids
◆ Drugs used in diabetes
◆ Drugs for thyroid disorders
◆ Drugs for pituitary disorders
◆ Male sex hormones
◆ Female sex hormones

Corticosteroids

Corticosteroid drugs – often simply referred to as steroids – are derived from, or are synthetic variants of, the natural corticosteroid hormones formed in the outer part (cortex) of the adrenal glands, situated on top of each kidney. Release of these hormones is governed by the pituitary gland (see p.85).

Corticosteroids may mainly have either glucocorticoid or mineralocorticoid effects. Glucocorticoid effects include the maintenance of normal levels of sugar in the blood and the promotion of recovery from injury and stress. The main mineralocorticoid effects are regulation of the balance of mineral salts and the water content of the body. When present in large amounts, corticosteroids act to reduce inflammation and suppress allergic reactions and immune system activity. They are distinct from another group of steroid hormones, the anabolic steroids (see p.88).

Although corticosteroids have broadly similar actions, they vary in their relative strength and duration of action. Their mineralocorticoid effects also vary in strength.

WHY THEY ARE USED

Corticosteroids are used primarily for their effect in controlling inflammation, whatever its cause. Topical corticosteroid preparations are often used for the treatment of many inflammatory skin disorders (see p.120). These drugs may also be injected directly into a joint or around a tendon to relieve inflammation caused by injury or disease (see p.53). However, when local administration of the drug is either not possible or not effective, corticosteroids may be given systemically, either by mouth or by intravenous injection.

Corticosteroids are commonly part of the treatment of many disorders in which inflammation is thought to be due to excessive or inappropriate activity of the immune system. These disorders include inflammatory bowel disease (p.46), rheumatoid arthritis (p.51), glomerulonephritis (a kidney disease), and some rare connective tissue disorders, such as systemic lupus erythematosus. In these conditions corticosteroids relieve symptoms and may also temporarily halt the disease.

Corticosteroids may be given regularly by mouth or inhaler to treat asthma, although they are not effective for the relief of asthma attacks in progress (see Bronchodilators, p.23 and Drugs for asthma, p.24).

An important use of oral corticosteroids is to replace the natural hormones that are deficient when adrenal gland function is reduced, as in Addison's disease. In these cases, the drugs most closely resembling the actions of the natural hormones are selected and a combination of these may be used.

Some cancers of the lymphatic system (lymphomas) and blood (leukaemias) may also respond to corticosteroid treatment. These drugs are also widely used to prevent or treat rejection of organ transplants, usually in conjunction with other drugs, such as azathioprine (see Immunosuppressants, p.99).

HOW THEY WORK

Given in high doses, corticosteroid drugs reduce inflammation by blocking the action of chemicals called prostaglandins that are responsible for triggering the inflammatory response. These drugs also temporarily depress the immune system by reducing the activity of certain types of white blood cell.

HOW THEY AFFECT YOU

Corticosteroid drugs often produce a dramatic improvement in symptoms. Given systemically, corticosteroids may also act on the brain to produce a heightened sense of wellbeing and, in some people, a sense of euphoria. Troublesome day-to-day side effects are rare. Long-term corticosteroid treatment, however, carries a number of serious risks for the patient.

RISKS AND SPECIAL PRECAUTIONS

In the treatment of Addison's disease, corticosteroids can be considered as "hormone replacement therapy", with drugs replacing the natural hormone hydrocortisone. Because replacement doses are given, the adverse effects of high-dose corticosteroids do not occur.

Drugs with strong mineralocorticoid effects, such as fludrocortisone, may cause water retention, swelling (especially of the ankles), and an increase in blood pressure. Because corticosteroids reduce the effect of insulin, they may create problems in people with diabetes and may even give rise to diabetes in susceptible people. They can also cause peptic ulcers.

Because corticosteroids suppress the immune system, they increase susceptibility to infection. They also suppress symptoms of infectious disease. People taking corticosteroids should avoid exposure to chickenpox or shingles; if they catch either disease, drugs such as aciclovir tablets may be prescribed.

With long-term use, corticosteroids may cause a variety of adverse effects, such as mood changes, acne, a moon-shaped face, increased blood pressure and fluid retention, peptic ulcers, a fat pad on the top of the back, thin skin, and easy bruising. Doctors try to avoid the long-term use of corticosteroid drugs in children because prolonged use may retard growth.

Long-term use of corticosteroids suppresses the production of the body's own corticosteroid hormones. For this reason, treatment that lasts for more than a few weeks should be withdrawn gradually to give the body time to adjust. If the drug is stopped abruptly, the lack of corticosteroid hormones may lead to sudden collapse.

People taking corticosteroids by mouth for longer than one month are advised to carry a warning card. If someone who is taking steroids long term has an accident or serious illness, his or her defences against shock may need to be quickly strengthened with extra hydrocortisone, administered intravenously.

COMMON DRUGS

Alclometastone, Beclometasone*, Betamethasone*, Budesonide*, Clobetasol*, Clobetasone, Deflazacort, Dexamethasone*, Diflucortolone, Fludrocortisone, Fludroxycortide, Flumetasone, Flunisolide, Fluocinolone, Fluocinonide, Fluocortolone, Fluticasone*, Halcinonide, Hydrocortisone*, Methylprednisolone, Mometasone*, Prednisolone*, Triamcinolone

* **See Part 2**

Drugs used in diabetes

The body obtains most of its energy from glucose, a simple form of sugar made in the intestine from the breakdown of starch and other sugars. Insulin, one of the hormones produced in the pancreas, enables body tissues to take up glucose from the blood, either to use it for energy or to store it. In diabetes mellitus (or sugar diabetes), insulin production is defective. This results in reduced uptake of glucose by the tissues and therefore the glucose level in the blood rises abnormally. A high blood glucose level is known medically as hyperglycaemia.

There are two main types of diabetes mellitus. Type 1 (insulin-dependent) diabetes usually appears in young people, with 50 per cent of cases occurring around the time of puberty. The insulin-secreting cells in the pancreas are gradually destroyed. An autoimmune condition (where the body recognizes its pancreas as "foreign" and tries to eliminate it) or a childhood viral infection is the most likely cause. Although the decline in insulin production is slow, the condition often appears suddenly, brought on by periods of stress (for example, infection or puberty) when the body's insulin requirements are high. Symptoms of Type 1 diabetes include extreme thirst, increased urination, lethargy, and weight loss. This type of diabetes is fatal if it is left untreated.

In Type 1 diabetes, insulin treatment is the only treatment option. It has to be continued for the rest of the patient's life. Several types of insulin are available, which are broadly classified by their duration of action (short-, medium-, and long-acting).

Type 2 diabetes, also known as non-insulin-dependent diabetes mellitus (NIDDM), or maturity-onset diabetes, appears at an older age (usually over 40) and tends to come on much more gradually – there may be a delay in its diagnosis for several years because of the gradual onset of symptoms. In this type of diabetes, the levels of insulin in the blood are usually high. However, the cells of the body are resistant to the effects of insulin and have a reduced glucose uptake despite the high insulin levels. This results in hyperglycaemia. Obesity is the most common cause of Type 2 diabetes.

In both types of diabetes, an alteration in diet is vital. A healthy diet consisting of a low-fat, high-fibre, low simple sugar (cakes, sweets) and high complex sugar (pasta, rice, potatoes) intake is advised. In Type 2 diabetes, a reduction in weight alone may be sufficient to lower the body's energy requirements and restore blood glucose to normal levels. If an alteration in diet fails, oral antidiabetic drugs, such as metformin, acarbose, or sulphonylureas, are prescribed. Insulin may need to be given to people with Type 2 diabetes if the above treatments fail, or in pregnancy, during severe illness, and before the patient undergoes any surgery requiring a general anaesthetic.

IMPORTANCE OF TREATING DIABETES

If diabetes is left untreated, the continuous high blood glucose levels damage various parts of the body. The major problems are caused by atherosclerosis, in which a build-up of fatty deposits in the arteries narrows them, reducing the flow of blood. This can result in heart attacks, blindness, kidney failure, reduced circulation in the legs, and even gangrene. The risk of these conditions is greatly reduced with treatment. Careful control of diabetes in young people, during puberty and afterwards, is of great importance in reducing possible long-term complications. Good diabetic control before conception reduces the chance of miscarriage or abnormalities in the baby.

HOW ANTIDIABETIC DRUGS WORK

Insulin treatment directly replaces the natural hormone that is deficient in diabetes mellitus. Human and pork insulins are the most widely available. When transferring between animal and human insulin, alteration of the dose may be required.

Insulin cannot be taken by mouth (except by inhaler, when it is delivered to the lungs) because it is broken down in the digestive tract before it reaches the bloodstream; regular injections or inhalations are necessary (see Administration of insulin, above right).

Sulphonylurea oral antidiabetics encourage the pancreas to produce insulin. They are therefore effective only when some insulin-secreting cells remain active; this is why they are ineffective in the treatment of Type 1 diabetes. Metformin alters the way in which the body metabolizes sugar. Acarbose slows digestion of starch and sugar. Both slow the increase in blood sugar that occurs after a meal. Nateglinide and repaglinide stimulate insulin release. Pioglitazone and rosiglitazone reduce the body's resistance to insulin.

ADMINISTRATION OF INSULIN

The body normally produces a background level of insulin, with additional insulin being produced as required in response to meals. The insulin delivery systems currently available cannot mimic this process precisely. In people with Type 1 diabetes, short-acting insulin is usually given before meals, and medium-acting either before the evening meal or at bedtime. Insulin pen injectors are useful for daytime administration because they are discreet and easy to carry and use. In patients with Type 2 diabetes who require insulin, a mixture of short- and medium-acting insulin may be given twice a day. Special pumps that deliver continuous subcutaneous insulin seem to have no advantage over multiple subcutaneous injections. For some adults with Type 1 or Type 2 diabetes, insulin can be taken by inhaler. Some new insulins called "insulin analogues" (such as Insulin lispro) act very rapidly and may be better at mimicking the insulin-producing behaviour of the normal pancreas.

INSULIN TREATMENT AND YOU

The insulin requirements in diabetes vary greatly between individuals and also depend on physical activity and calorie intake. Hence, insulin regimens are tailored to particular needs, and the person with diabetes is encouraged to take an active role in his or her own management.

A regular record of home blood glucose monitoring should be kept. This is the basis on which insulin doses are adjusted, preferably by the person with diabetes.

A person with diabetes should learn to recognize the warning signs of hypoglycaemia. A hypoglycaemic event may be induced by giving insulin under medical supervision. The symptoms of sweating, faintness, or palpitations are produced, but they disappear when glucose is administered. Therefore, anyone with diabetes should always carry glucose tablets or sweets with them. Recurrent "hypos" at specific times of the day or night may require a reduction of insulin dose. Rarely, undetected low glucose levels may lead to coma. The injection of glucagon (a substance that raises blood glucose) rapidly reverses this. A relative may be instructed how to perform this procedure.

Repeated injection at the same site may disturb the fat layer beneath the skin, producing either swelling or dimpling. This alters the rate of insulin absorption and can be avoided by regularly rotating injection sites. In such circumstances, insulin can be inhaled rather than injected.

Insulin requirements are increased during illness and pregnancy. During an illness, the urine should be checked for ketones, which are produced when there is insufficient insulin to permit the normal uptake of glucose by the tissues. If high ketone levels occur in the urine during an illness, urgent medical advice should be sought. The combination of high blood glucose, high urinary ketones, and vomiting is a diabetic emergency and the person should be taken to an Accident and Emergency department without delay.

Exercise increases the body's need for glucose. Therefore extra calories should be taken prior to exertion. The effects of vigorous exercise on blood glucose levels may last up to 18 hours, and the subsequent (post-exercise) doses of insulin may need to be reduced by 10–25 per cent to avoid hypoglycaemia.

It is advisable for anyone with diabetes to carry a card or bracelet detailing their condition and treatment. This may be useful in a medical emergency.

ANTIDIABETIC DRUGS AND YOU

The sulphonylureas may lower the blood glucose too much: a condition called hypoglycaemia. This can be avoided by starting treatment with low doses and ensuring a regular food intake. Rarely, these drugs cause a decrease in the blood cell count, a rash, or intestinal or liver disturbances. Interactions may occur with other drugs, so your doctor should be informed of your treatment before prescribing any medicines for you.

Unlike the sulphonylureas, metformin does not cause hypoglycaemia. Its most common side effects are nausea, weight loss, abdominal distension, and diarrhoea. It should not be used in people with liver, kidney, or heart problems. Acarbose does not cause hypoglycaemia if used on its own. The tablets must either be chewed with the first mouthful of food at meal times or swallowed whole with a little liquid immediately before food.

COMMON DRUGS

Sulphonylurea drugs Chlorpropamide, Glibenclamide*, Gliclazide*, Glimepiride, Glipizide, Gliquidone, Tolbutamide*
Other drugs Acarbose, Diazoxide, Glucagon, Insulin*, Insulin aspart*, Insulin glargine*, Insulin glulisine*, Insulin lispro*, Metformin*, Nateglinide, Pioglitazone, Repaglinide*, Rosiglitazone*
* See Part 2

Drugs for thyroid disorders

The thyroid gland produces the hormone thyroxine, which regulates the body's metabolism. Thyroxine is essential during childhood for normal physical and mental development. Calcitonin, also produced by the thyroid, regulates calcium metabolism and is used as a drug for certain bone disorders (see p.56).

HYPERTHYROIDISM

In this condition (often called thyrotoxicosis), the thyroid is overactive and produces too much thyroxine. Women are more commonly affected than men. Symptoms include anxiety, palpitations, weight loss, increased appetite, heat intolerance, diarrhoea, and menstrual disturbances. Graves' disease is the most common form of hyperthyroidism. It is an autoimmune disease in which the body produces antibodies that stimulate the thyroid to produce excess thyroxine. Patients with Graves' disease may develop abnormally protuberant eyes (exophthalmos) or a swelling involving the skin over the shins (pretibial myxoedema). Hyperthyroidism can be caused by a benign single tumour of the thyroid or a pre-existing multinodular goitre. Rarely, an overactive thyroid may follow a viral infection, a condition called thyroiditis. Inflammation of the gland leads to the release of stored thyroxine.

Goitre is a swelling of the thyroid gland. It may occur only temporarily, during puberty or pregnancy, or may be due to abnormal growth of thyroid tissue that requires surgical removal. Goitre may also, rarely, be brought about by iodine deficiency, which can be prevented or treated with iodine supplements.

MANAGEMENT OF HYPERTHYROIDISM

There are three possible treatments: anti-thyroid drugs, Radioactive iodine (radio-iodine), and surgery. The most commonly used antithyroid drug is carbimazole, which inhibits the formation of thyroid hormones and reduces their levels to normal over about 4–8 weeks. In the early stage of treatment, a beta blocker (see p.30) may be prescribed to control symptoms. This should be stopped once thyroid function returns to normal. Long-term carbimazole is usually given for 18 months to prevent relapse. A "block and replace" regimen may also be used. In this treatment, the thyroid gland is blocked by high doses of carbimazole and thyroxine is added when the level of thyroid hormone in the blood falls below normal.

Carbimazole may produce minor side effects such as nausea, vomiting, skin rashes, or headaches. Rarely, the drug may reduce the white blood cell count. Propylthiouracil may be used as an alternative antithyroid drug.

Radio-iodine is frequently chosen as a first-line therapy, especially in the elderly, and is the second choice if hyperthyroidism recurs following use of carbimazole. It acts by destroying thyroid tissue. Hypothyroidism occurs in up to 80 per cent of people within 20 years after treatment. Long-term studies show radio-iodine to be safe, but its use should be avoided during pregnancy.

Surgery is a third-line therapy. Its use may be favoured for patients with a large goitre, particularly if it causes difficulty in swallowing or breathing. Exophthalmos may require corticosteroids (see p.80) as it does not respond to other treatments.

HYPOTHYROIDISM

This is a condition resulting from too little thyroxine. Sometimes it may be caused by an autoimmune disorder, in which the body's immune system attacks the thyroid gland. Other cases may follow treatment for hyperthyroidism. In newborn babies, hypothyroidism may be the result of an inborn enzyme disorder. In the past, it also arose from a deficiency of iodine in the diet.

The symptoms of adult hypothyroidism develop slowly and include weight gain, mental slowness, dry skin, hair loss, increased sensitivity to cold, and heavy menstrual periods. In babies, low levels of thyroxine cause permanent mental and physical retardation and, for this reason, babies are tested for hypothyroidism shortly after birth.

MANAGEMENT OF HYPOTHYROIDISM

Lifelong oral treatment with the synthetic thyroid hormones levothyroxine or liothyronine is the only option. Blood tests are performed regularly to monitor treatment and permit dosage adjustments. In the elderly and people with heart disease, gradual introduction of thyroxine is used to prevent heart strain.

In severely ill patients, thyroid hormone may be given by injection. This method of administration may also be used to treat newborn infants with low levels of thyroxine.

Symptoms of thyrotoxicosis may appear if excess thyroxine replacement is given. Otherwise, no adverse events occur since treatment is adjusted to replace the natural hormone that the body should produce itself.

COMMON DRUGS

Drugs for hypothyroidism Levothyroxine (thyroxine)*, Liothyronine
Drugs for hyperthyroidism Carbimazole*, Iodine*, Nadolol, Propranolol*, Propylthiouracil*, Radioactive iodine (radio-iodine)
* See Part 2

Drugs for pituitary disorders

The pituitary gland, which lies at the base of the brain, produces a number of hormones that regulate physical growth, metabolism, sexual development, and reproductive function. Many of these hormones act indirectly by stimulating other glands, such as the thyroid, adrenal glands, ovaries, and testes, to release their own hormones.

Thyroid-stimulating hormone stimulates production and release of thyroid hormones.
Prolactin stimulates glands in the breast to produce milk in women and helps sperm production in men.
Corticotrophin (ACTH) controls production and release of adrenal corticosteroid hormones.

Gonadotrophins called follicle-stimulating hormone (FSH) and luteinizing hormone (LH) act on the sex glands to stimulate egg production and release in females and sperm production in males. They also control the output of the sex hormones oestrogen, progesterone, and testosterone.

Growth hormone promotes normal growth and development.

Melanocyte-stimulating hormone controls skin pigmentation.

Antidiuretic hormone (ADH or vasopressin) regulates the output of water in the urine.

An excess or a lack of one of the pituitary hormones may produce serious effects, the nature of which depends on the hormone involved. Abnormal levels of a particular hormone may be caused by a pituitary tumour, which may be treated with surgery, radiotherapy, or drugs. In other cases, drugs may be used to correct the hormonal imbalance.

The more common pituitary disorders that can be treated with drugs are those involving growth hormone, antidiuretic hormone, prolactin, adrenal hormones, and the gonadotrophins. The first three are discussed below. For information on the use of drugs to treat infertility arising from inadequate levels of gonadotrophins, see p.109. Lack of corticotrophin, leading to inadequate production of adrenal hormones, is usually treated with corticosteroids (see p.80).

DRUGS FOR GROWTH HORMONE DISORDERS

Growth hormone (somatotropin) is the principal hormone required for normal growth in childhood and adolescence. Lack of growth hormone impairs normal physical growth. Doctors administer hormone treatment only after tests have proven that a lack of this hormone is the cause of the disorder. If treatment is started at an early age, regular injections of somatropin, a synthetic form of natural growth hormone, administered until the end of adolescence, usually allow normal growth and development to take place.

Less often, the pituitary produces an excess of growth hormone. In children this can result in pituitary gigantism; in adults, it can produce a disorder known as acromegaly. This disorder, which is usually the result of a

pituitary tumour, is characterized by thickening of the skull, face, hands, and feet, and enlargement of some internal organs.

The pituitary tumour may either be surgically removed or destroyed by radiotherapy. In the frail or elderly, drugs such as bromocriptine and octreotide are used to reduce growth hormone levels. Octreotide is also used as an adjunctive treatment before surgery and in those with increased growth hormone levels occurring after surgery. People who have undergone surgery and/or radiotherapy may require long-term replacement with other hormones (such as sex hormones, thyroid hormone, or corticosteroids).

DRUGS FOR DIABETES INSIPIDUS

Antidiuretic hormone (also known as ADH or vasopressin) acts on the kidneys, controlling the amount of water retained in the body and returned to the blood. A lack of ADH is usually caused by damage to the pituitary; this in turn causes diabetes insipidus. In this rare condition, the kidneys cannot retain water and large quantities pass into the urine. The chief symptoms are constant thirst and the production of large volumes of urine.

Diabetes insipidus is treated with ADH or a related synthetic drug, desmopressin. These replace naturally produced ADH and may be given by mouth, injection, or as a nasal spray. Chlorpropamide may be used to treat mild cases; it works by increasing ADH release from the pituitary and by sensitizing the kidneys to the effect of ADH.

Alternatively, a thiazide diuretic (such as chlortalidone) may be prescribed for mild cases (see Diuretics, p.32). The usual effect of such drugs is to increase urine production, but in diabetes insipidus they have the opposite effect, reducing water loss from the body.

DRUGS USED TO REDUCE PROLACTIN LEVELS

Prolactin, also called lactogenic hormone, is produced in both men and women. In women, prolactin controls the secretion of breast milk following childbirth. The function of this hormone in men is not understood, although it appears to be necessary for normal sperm production.

The disorders associated with prolactin are all concerned with overproduction. High levels in women can cause galactorrhoea (lactation that is not associated with pregnancy and birth), amenorrhoea (lack of menstruation), and infertility. If excessive prolactin is produced in men, the result may be galactorrhoea, impotence, or infertility.

Some drugs, notably methyldopa, oestrogen, and the phenothiazine antipsychotics, can raise the prolactin level in the blood. More often, however, the increased prolactin results from a pituitary tumour and is usually treated with bromocriptine or cabergoline, which inhibit prolactin production.

COMMON DRUGS

Drugs for growth hormone disorders
Bromocriptine*, Lanreotide, Octreotide, Somatropin

Drugs for diabetes insipidus Carbamazepine*, Chlorpropamide, Chlortalidone, Desmopressin*, Vasopressin (ADH)

Drugs to reduce prolactin levels Bromocriptine*, Cabergoline, Quinagolide

* See Part 2

Male sex hormones

Male sex hormones, or androgens, are responsible for the development of male sexual characteristics. The principal androgen is testosterone, which in men is produced by the testes from puberty onwards. Women produce testosterone in small amounts in the adrenal glands, but its exact function in the female body is not known.

Testosterone has two major effects: an androgenic effect and an anabolic effect. Its androgenic effect is to stimulate the appearance of the secondary sexual characteristics at puberty, such as the growth of body hair, deepening of the voice, and an increase in genital size. Its anabolic effects are to increase muscle bulk and accelerate growth rate.

There are a number of synthetically produced derivatives of testosterone that produce varying degrees of the androgenic and anabolic effects mentioned above. Derivatives with a mainly anabolic effect are called anabolic steroids (see p.88).

Testosterone and its derivatives have been used under medical supervision in both men and women to treat a number of conditions.

WHY THEY ARE USED

Male sex hormones are mainly given to men to promote the development of male sexual characteristics when hormone production is deficient. This may be the result of an abnormality of the testes or of inadequate production of the pituitary hormones that stimulate the testes to release testosterone.

They are also sometimes given to adolescent boys if the onset of puberty is delayed by pituitary problems. The treatment may also help to stimulate development of secondary male sexual characteristics and to increase sex drive (libido) in adult men with inadequate testosterone levels. This has been found to reduce sperm production, however. (For information on the drug treatment of male infertility, see p.109.) An anti-androgen (a substance that inhibits the effects of androgens) may be used in the treatment of benign prostatic hyperplasia, or BPH (an enlarged prostate gland).

Androgens may also be prescribed for women to treat certain types of cancer of the breast and uterus (see Anticancer drugs, p.96). Testosterone can be given by injection, buccal tablets, capsules, patches, or surgically inserted pellets.

HOW THEY WORK

Taken in low doses as part of replacement therapy when natural production is low, male sex hormones act in the same way as the natural hormones. In adolescents suffering from delayed puberty, hormone treatment produces both androgenic and anabolic effects, initiating the development of secondary sexual characteristics over a few months; full sexual development usually takes place over three to four years. When sex hormones are given to adult men, the effects on physical appearance and libido may begin to be felt within a few weeks.

RISKS AND SPECIAL PRECAUTIONS

The main risks with these drugs occur when they are given to boys with delayed puberty and to women with breast cancer. Given to initiate the onset of puberty, they may stunt growth by prematurely sealing the growing ends of the long bones. Doctors normally try to avoid prescribing hormones in these circumstances until growth is complete. High doses given to women have various masculinizing effects, including increased facial and body hair, and a deeper voice. The drugs may also produce enlargement of the clitoris, changes in libido, and acne.

ANABOLIC STEROIDS

Anabolic steroids are synthetically produced variants that mimic the anabolic effects of the natural hormones. They increase muscle bulk and body growth.

Doctors occasionally prescribe anabolic steroids and a high-protein diet to promote recovery after serious illness or major surgery. The steroids may also help to increase the production of blood cells in some forms of anaemia and to reduce itching in chronic obstructive jaundice.

Anabolic steroids have been widely abused by athletes because these drugs speed up the recovery of muscles after a session of intense exercise. This enables the athlete to go through a more demanding daily exercise programme, which results in a significant improvement in muscle power. The use of anabolic steroids by athletes to improve their performance is condemned by doctors and athletic organizations because of the risks to health, particularly for women. The side effects range from acne and baldness to psychological changes, fluid retention, testicular atrophy and impotence (men), reduced fertility (women), hardening of the arteries, a long-term risk of liver disease, and certain forms of cancer.

COMMON DRUGS

Primarily androgenic Mesterolone, Testosterone*
Primarily anabolic Nandrolone
Anti-androgens Cyproterone, Dutasteride, Finasteride*
* See Part 2

Female sex hormones

There are two types of female sex hormones: oestrogen and progesterone. In women, these hormones are secreted by the ovaries from puberty until the menopause. Each month, the levels of oestrogen and progesterone fluctuate, producing the menstrual cycle (see p.104). During pregnancy, oestrogen and progesterone are produced by the placenta. The adrenal gland also makes small amounts of oestrogen. Production of oestrogen and progesterone is regulated by the two gonadotrophin hormones (FSH and LH) produced by the pituitary gland (see p.85).

Oestrogen is responsible for the development of female sexual characteristics, including breast development, growth of pubic hair, and widening of the pelvis. Progesterone prepares the lining of the uterus for implantation of a fertilized egg; it is also important for the maintenance of pregnancy.

Synthetic forms of these hormones, known as oestrogens and progestogens, are used medically to treat a number of conditions.

WHY THEY ARE USED

The best-known use of oestrogens and progestogens is in oral contraceptives, which are discussed on p.105. Other uses of oestrogens and progestogens include the treatment of menstrual disorders (p.104) and certain hormone-sensitive cancers (p.96). This page discusses the drug treatments that are used for natural hormone deficiency.

HORMONE DEFICIENCY

Deficiency of female sex hormones may occur as a result of deficiency of gonadotrophins caused by a pituitary disorder or by abnormal development of the ovaries (ovarian failure). This may lead to the absence of menstruation and lack of sexual development. If tests show a deficiency of gonadotrophins, preparations of these hormones may be prescribed (see p.109). These trigger the release of oestrogen and progesterone from the ovaries. If pituitary function is normal and ovarian failure is diagnosed as the cause of hormone deficiency, oestrogens and progestogens may be given as supplements. In this situation, these supplements ensure development of normal female sexual characteristics but cannot stimulate ovulation.

MENOPAUSE

A decline in the levels of oestrogen and progesterone occurs naturally following the menopause, when the menstrual cycle ceases. The sudden reduction in levels of oestrogen often causes distressing symptoms, and many doctors suggest that hormone supplements be used around the time of the menopause (see Effects of hormone replacement therapy (HRT), right). Such hormone replacement therapy may also be prescribed for those women who have undergone premature menopause as a result of surgical removal of the ovaries or radiotherapy for ovarian cancer.

HRT helps to reduce the symptoms of the menopause, including hot flushes and vaginal dryness. It is not normally recommended for long-term use or for the treatment of osteoporosis (see p.57), however, because of the increased risk of disorders such as breast cancer, stroke, and thromboembolism occurring. Oestrogen is used together with a progestogen unless the woman has had a hysterectomy, in which case oestrogen alone is used. If dryness of the vagina is a particular problem, a cream containing an oestrogen drug may be prescribed for short-term use.

HOW THEY AFFECT YOU

Hormones that are given to treat ovarian failure or delayed puberty take three to six months to produce a noticeable effect on sexual development. Taken for menopausal symptoms, they can dramatically reduce the number of hot flushes within a week.

Both oestrogens and progestogens can cause fluid retention, and oestrogens may cause nausea, vomiting, breast tenderness, headache, dizziness, and depression. Progestogens may cause "breakthrough" bleeding between menstrual periods. In the comparatively low doses used to treat these disorders, side effects are unlikely.

RISKS AND SPECIAL PRECAUTIONS

Because oestrogens increase the risk of hypertension (raised blood pressure), thrombosis (abnormal blood clotting), and breast cancer, there are risks associated with long-term HRT. Treatment is prescribed with caution for women who have heart or circulatory disorders, and in those who are overweight or who smoke. Oestrogens may also trigger the onset of diabetes mellitus or aggravate

blood glucose control in women with diabetes. Tibolone (p.406) has both oestrogenic and progestogenic properties and can be used on its own.

The use of oestrogens and progestogens as replacement therapy in ovarian failure carries few risks for young women who are otherwise healthy.

EFFECTS OF HORMONE REPLACEMENT THERAPY (HRT)

HRT is primarily used to alleviate symptoms of the menopause, such as hot flushes and vaginal dryness. It may also be used to prevent or treat osteoporosis in some women. However, the benefits of HRT must be weighed against the various increased health risks associated with its use, such as breast cancer, stroke, and thromboembolism.

Breasts There is an increased risk of breast cancer with long-term use of HRT. The increase in risk is related to the length of time for which HRT is used. If HRT is stopped, however, the risk reduces to its pre-treatment level within about five years.

Bones For women who go through premature menopause, HRT reduces the thinning of bone that occurs in osteoporosis and thus protects against fractures.

Reproductive organs Thinning of the vaginal tissues leading to painful intercourse can be prevented by HRT.

COMMON DRUGS

Oestrogens Conjugated oestrogens*, Estradiol*, Estriol, Estrone, Estropipate, Ethinylestradiol*, Tibolone*

Progestogens Desogestrel*, Dydrogesterone*, Levonorgestrel*, Medroxyprogesterone*, Norethisterone*, Norgestrel, Progesterone

Other drugs Raloxifene*

* See Part 2

NUTRITION

Food provides energy (as calories) and materials called nutrients needed for growth and renewal of tissues. Protein, carbohydrate, and fat are the three major nutrient components of food. Vitamins and minerals are found only in small amounts in food, but are very important for normal function of the body. Fibre, found only in foods from plants, is needed for the digestive system to work well.

Proteins are vital for tissue growth and repair. The moderate amounts required can be found in meat and dairy products, cereals, and pulses.

Carbohydrates are a major energy source, and are stored as fat when taken in excess. They can be found in cereals, sugar, and vegetables. Starchy foods are preferable to sugar.

Fats are a concentrated energy form needed only in small quantities. They are contained in animal products such as butter and in the oils of plants such as corn and nuts.

Vitamins and minerals are found only in small amounts in food but are very important for the normal functioning of the body.

Fibre (non-starch polysaccharides) is the indigestible part of any fruit, vegetable, or food or product derived from plants. It is needed for a healthy digestive system. Fibre contains no nutrients but adds bulk to faeces.

During digestion, large molecules of food are broken down into smaller molecules, releasing nutrients that are absorbed into the bloodstream. Carbohydrate and fat are then metabolized by body cells to produce energy. They may also be incorporated with protein into the cell structure. Each metabolic process is promoted by a specific enzyme and often requires the presence of a particular vitamin or mineral.

WHY DRUGS ARE USED

Dietary deficiency of essential nutrients can lead to illness. In poorer countries where there is a shortage of food, marasmus (resulting from lack of food energy) and kwashiorkor (from lack of protein) are common. In the developed world, however, excessive food intake leading to obesity is more common. Nutritional deficiencies in developed countries result from poor food choices and usually stem from a lack of a specific vitamin or mineral, such as in iron-deficiency anaemia.

Some nutritional deficiencies may be caused by an inability of the body to absorb nutrients from food (malabsorption) or to utilize them once they have been absorbed. Malabsorption may be caused by lack of an enzyme or an abnormality of the digestive tract. Errors of metabolism are often inborn and are not yet fully understood. They may be caused by failure of the body to produce the chemicals required to process nutrients for use.

WHY SUPPLEMENTS ARE USED

Deficiencies such as kwashiorkor or marasmus are usually treated by dietary improvement and, in some cases, food supplements rather than drugs. Vitamin and mineral deficiencies are usually treated with appropriate supplements. Malabsorption disorders may require changes in diet or long-term use of supplements. Metabolic errors are not easily treated with supplements or drugs, and a special diet may be the main treatment.

The preferred treatment of obesity is reduction of food intake, altered eating patterns, and increased exercise. When these methods are not effective, and the body mass index (BMI) is 30 or more, an anti-obesity drug may be used.

MAJOR DRUG GROUPS
◆ Vitamins
◆ Minerals

Vitamins

Vitamins are complex chemicals that are essential for a variety of body functions. With the exception of vitamin D, the body cannot manufacture these substances and therefore we need to include them in our diet. There are 13 major vitamins: A, C, D, E, K, and the B complex vitamins – thiamine (B_1), riboflavin (B_2), niacin (B_3), pantothenic acid (B_5), pyridoxine (B_6), cobalamin (B_{12}), folic acid, and biotin. Most vitamins are required in very small amounts, and each vitamin is present in one or more foods (see Main food sources of vitamins, p.92). Vitamin D is also produced in the body when the skin is exposed to sunlight. Vitamins are categorized according to whether they dissolve in fat or water.

Water-soluble vitamins Vitamin C and the B vitamins dissolve in water. Most are stored in the body for only a short period and are excreted rapidly by the kidneys if taken in higher amounts than the body needs. Vitamin B_{12} is the exception; it is stored in the liver, which may hold up to six years' supply. For these reasons, foods containing water-soluble vitamins need to be eaten daily. These vitamins are easily lost in cooking, so uncooked foods containing them should be eaten regularly. An overdose does not usually cause toxic effects, but adverse reactions to large dosages of vitamin C and pyridoxine (vitamin B_6) have been reported.

Fat-soluble vitamins Vitamins A, D, E, and K are absorbed from the intestine into the bloodstream together with fat. Deficiency of these vitamins may result from any disorder that affects fat absorption (for example, coeliac disease). These vitamins are stored in the liver and reserves of some of them may last for several years. Taking an excess of a fat-soluble vitamin for a long period may cause it to build up to a harmful level in the body. Ensuring foods rich in these vitamins are regularly included in the diet usually provides a sufficient supply without risking overdosage.

A number of vitamins (such as vitamins A, C, and E) have now been recognized as having strong antioxidant properties. Antioxidants neutralize the effect of free radicals, substances produced during the body's normal processes that may be potentially harmful if they are not neutralized.

A balanced, varied diet is likely to contain adequate amounts of all the vitamins. Inadequate intake of any vitamin over an extended period can lead to symptoms of deficiency.

A doctor may recommend vitamin supplements in various circumstances: to prevent vitamin deficiency in people considered at risk, to treat symptoms of deficiency, and in the treatment of certain medical conditions.

WHY THEY ARE USED

Preventing deficiency Most people in the UK obtain sufficient quantities of vitamins in their diet, and it is therefore not usually necessary to take additional vitamins in the form of supplements. People who are unsure if their present diet is adequate are advised to look at the table on p.92 to check that foods that are rich in vitamins are eaten regularly. Vitamin intake can often be boosted simply by increasing the quantities of fresh foods and raw fruit and vegetables in the diet. Certain groups in the population are, however, at increased risk of vitamin deficiency. These include people who have an increased need for certain vitamins that may not be met from dietary sources – in particular, women who are pregnant or breast-feeding, and infants and young children. The elderly, who may not be eating a varied diet, may also be at risk. Strict vegetarians, vegans, and others on restricted diets may not receive adequate amounts of all vitamins.

In addition, people who suffer from disorders in which absorption of nutrients from the bowel is impaired, or who need to take drugs that reduce the absorption of vitamins (for example, some types of lipid-lowering drugs), are usually given additional vitamins. In these cases, the doctor is likely to advise supplements of one or more vitamins. Although most preparations are available without prescription, it is important to seek specialist advice before starting a course of vitamin supplements to obtain a proper assessment of your individual requirements.

Vitamin supplements should not be used as a general tonic to improve wellbeing (they are not effective for this purpose) nor should they be used as a substitute for a balanced diet.

Treating deficiency It is rare for a diet to completely lack a particular vitamin. But if intake of a particular vitamin is regularly lower than requirements, over time the body's stores of vitamins may become depleted and symptoms of deficiency may appear. In Britain, vitamin deficiency disorders are most common among homeless people, alcoholics, and those on low incomes who fail to eat an adequate diet. Deficiencies of water-soluble vitamins are more likely since most are not stored in large quantities in the body.

MAIN FOOD SOURCES OF VITAMINS

The table below indicates which foods are especially good sources of particular vitamins. Ensuring that you regularly select foods from a variety of categories helps to maintain adequate intake for most people, without the need for supplements. Processed and overcooked foods are likely to contain fewer vitamins than fresh, raw, or lightly cooked foods.

Vitamins	Red meat	Poultry	Liver	Milk	Cheese	Butter/margarine	Eggs	Fish	Cereals and bread	Green vegetables	Root vegetables	Pulses/legumes	Nuts	Fruit
Biotin			●				●					●	●	
Folic acid			●				●			●				●
Niacin as nicotinic acid	●	●	●					●	●			●	●	
Pantothenic acid			●						●					
Pyridoxine	●	●	●				●	●	●					
Riboflavin			●	●	●		●		●			●	●	●
Thiamine	●		●						●			●	●	
Vitamin A			●	●	●	●	●			●	●			●
Vitamin B$_{12}$	●		●	●	●		●	●						
Vitamin C										●	●			●
Vitamin D				●		●	●	●						
Vitamin E							●	●	●	●		●	●	
Vitamin K									●	●				

Dosages of vitamins prescribed to treat vitamin deficiency are likely to be larger than those used to prevent deficiency. Medical supervision is required when correcting vitamin deficiency.

Other medical uses of vitamins Various claims have been made for the value of vitamins in the treatment of disorders other than vitamin deficiency. High doses of vitamin C have been said to be effective in preventing and treating the common cold, but such claims are not yet proved; zinc, however, may be helpful for this purpose. Vitamin and mineral supplements do not improve IQ in well-nourished children, but quite small dietary deficiencies can cause poor academic performance.

Certain vitamins have recognized medical uses apart from their nutritional role. Vitamin D has long been used to treat bone-wasting disorders (p.56). Niacin is sometimes used (in the form of nicotinic acid) as a lipid-lowering drug (p.37). Derivatives of vitamin A (retinoids) are an established part of the treatment for severe acne (p.123). Many women who suffer from premenstrual syndrome take pyridoxine (vitamin B$_6$) supplements to relieve symptoms. See also Drugs for menstrual disorders, p.104.

VITAMIN REQUIREMENTS

Normal daily vitamin requirements are usually based on the Recommended Daily Allowance (RDA). This measurement is the amount of the nutrient thought to be enough for about 97 per cent of people. Deficiency usually needs much higher doses, which should be determined by your doctor.

Biotin No RDA established; 10–200 micrograms is safe.

Folic acid (as folate) 50 micrograms (birth–1 year); 70 micrograms (1–3 years); 100 micrograms (4–6 years); 150 micrograms (7–10 years); 200 micrograms (11 years and over). For women planning pregnancy, 400 micrograms per day, before conception and during first 12 weeks of pregnancy (to prevent first occurrence of neural tube defects). To prevent recurrence of a neural tube defect, 5mg a day before conception and during first 12 weeks of pregnancy. Daily requirements increase by 60 micrograms during breast-feeding.

Niacin 3mg (birth–6 months); 4mg (7–9 months); 5mg (10–12 months); 8mg (1–3 years); 11mg (4–6 years); 12mg (7–10 years and females 11–14 years); 15mg (males 11–14 years); 18mg (males 15–18 years); 14mg (females 15–18 years); 17mg (males 19–50 years);

13mg (females 19–50 years); 16mg (males 51 years and over); 12mg (females 51 years and over); 2mg extra during breast-feeding.

Pantothenic acid No RDA established; adults require 3–7mg daily.

Pyridoxine 0.2mg (birth–6 months); 0.3mg (7–9 months); 0.4mg (10 months–1 year); 0.7mg (1–3 years); 0.9mg (4–6 years); 1mg (7–10 years and females 11–14 years); 1.2mg (males 11–14 years); 1.5mg (males 15–18 years); 1.2mg (females 15 and over); 1.4mg (males 19 and over).

Riboflavin 0.4mg (birth–1 year); 0.6mg (1–3 years); 0.8mg (4–6 years); 1mg (7–10 years); 1.2mg (males 11–14 years); 1.1mg (females 11 and over); 1.3mg (males 15 and over); extra 0.3mg in pregnancy and 0.5mg during breast-feeding.

Thiamine 0.2mg (birth–9 months); 0.3mg (10–12 months); 0.5mg (1–3 years); 0.7mg (4–10 years and females 11–14 years); 0.9mg (males 11–14 years); 1.1mg (males 15–18 years); 0.8mg (females 15 and over); 1mg (males 19–50 years); 0.9mg (males 51 and over). Extra 0.1mg in last three months of pregnancy; 0.2mg during breast-feeding.

Vitamin A 350 micrograms (up to 1 year); 400 micrograms (1–6 years); 500 micrograms (7–10 years); 600 micrograms (males 11–14 years, females 11 years and over); 700 micrograms (males 15 and over, and pregnant women); 950 micrograms (breast-feeding).

Vitamin B$_{12}$ Only minute quantities required. 0.3 micrograms (birth–6 months); 0.4 micrograms (7–12 months); 0.5 micrograms (1–3 years); 0.8 micrograms (4–6 years); 1 microgram (7–10 years); 1.2 micrograms (11–14 years); 1.5 micrograms (15 years and over); extra 0.5 micrograms during breast-feeding.

Vitamin C 25mg (birth–1 year); 30mg (1–10 years); 35mg (11–14 years); 40mg (15 years and over); extra 50mg in pregnancy; 70mg during breast-feeding.

Vitamin D 8.5 micrograms (birth–6 months); 7 micrograms (7 months–3 years); 10 micrograms (over 65 years, pregnancy, and breast-feeding). Most people outside these groups do not require supplements.

Vitamin E No UK recommendations. Requirement depends on intake of polyunsaturated fatty acid, which varies widely; 3–12mg (approx.) recommended.

Vitamin K Newborn infants may be given 1mg by single injection or they may receive the vitamin orally; 2 doses of 2mg are given in the first week and a third dose at 1 month for breast-fed babies (omitted in formula-fed babies). No RDA has been set for other groups.

RISKS AND SPECIAL PRECAUTIONS

Vitamins are essential for health, and supplements can be taken without risk by most people. It is important not to exceed the recommended dosage, particularly for fat-soluble vitamins, which may accumulate in the body. Dosage needs to be carefully calculated, taking into account the degree of deficiency, dietary intake, and duration of treatment. Overdosage has no therapeutic value and may even be harmful. Multivitamin preparations do not usually contain large amounts of each vitamin and are not likely to be harmful unless the dose is greatly exceeded. Single vitamin supplements can be harmful (excess of one vitamin may increase requirements for others) and should be used only on medical advice.

Minerals

Minerals are chemical elements (the simplest form of substance) many of which are vital in trace amounts for normal body processes. A balanced diet usually contains all the minerals needed; mineral deficiency diseases, except iron-deficiency anaemia, are uncommon.

Dietary supplements are necessary only when a doctor has diagnosed a specific deficiency, or as part of the prevention or treatment of a disorder. Doctors often prescribe minerals for people with intestinal diseases that reduce absorption of minerals from the diet. Iron supplements are often advised for pregnant or breast-feeding women, and iron-rich foods for infants over six months.

Taking mineral supplements unless under medical direction is not advisable. Exceeding the body's daily requirements is not beneficial, and large doses may be harmful.

MINERAL REQUIREMENTS

As with vitamins, normal daily mineral requirements are usually based on the Recommended Daily Allowance (RDA).

Calcium 525mg (birth–1 year); 350mg (1–3 years); 450mg (4–6 years); 550mg (7–10 years); 1,000mg (males 11–18 years); 800mg (females 11–18 years); 700mg (19 years and older); 550mg extra during breast-feeding.

Chromium Only minute quantities needed. RDA not established; about 25 micrograms is safe for adults.

Copper 0.2mg (birth–3 months); 0.3mg (4 months–1 year); 0.4mg (1–3 years); 0.6mg (4–6 years); 0.7mg (7–10 years); 0.8mg (11–14 years); 1.0mg (15–18 years); 1.2mg (19 years and over); 0.3mg extra during breast-feeding.

Fluoride No RDA established.

Iodine 50 micrograms (birth–3 months); 60 micrograms (4–12 months); 70 micrograms (1–3 years); 100 micrograms (4–6 years); 110 micrograms (7–10 years); 130 micrograms (11–14 years); 140 micrograms (15 years and over). Slightly increased requirement during breast-feeding; one vitamin tablet with calcium and iodine is recommended.

Iron 1.7mg (birth–3 months); 4.3mg (4–6 months); 7.8mg (7–12 months); 6.9mg (1–3 years); 6.1mg (4–6 years); 8.7mg (7–10 years); 11.3mg (males 11–18 years); 14.8mg (females 11–50 years); 8.7mg (males 19 and over, and females 51 and over). Requirements may be increased during pregnancy and after childbirth.

Magnesium 55mg (birth–3 months); 60mg (4–6 months); 75mg (7–9 months); 80mg (10–12 months); 85mg (1–3 years); 120mg (4–6 years); 200mg (7–10 years); 280mg (11–14 years); 300mg (males 15 and over, and females 15–18 years); 270mg (females 19 and over); 50mg extra during breast-feeding.

Potassium 0.8g (birth–3 months); 0.85g (4–6 months); 0.7g (7–12 months); 0.8g (1–3 years); 1.1g (4–6 years); 2g (7–10 years); 3.1g (11–14 years); 3.5g (15 years and over).

Selenium 10 micrograms (birth–3 months); 13 micrograms (4–6 months); 10 micrograms (7–12 months); 15 micrograms (1–3 years); 20 micrograms (4–6 years); 30 micrograms (7–10 years); 45 micrograms (11–14 years); 70 micrograms (males 15–18 years); 60 micrograms (females 15 and over); 75 micrograms (males 19 and over); 15 micrograms extra during breast-feeding.

Sodium 0.21g (birth–3 months); 0.28g (4–6 months); 0.32g (7–9 months); 0.35g (10–12 months); 0.5g (1–3 years); 0.7g (4–6 years); 1.2g (7–10 years); 1.6g (11 years and over).

Zinc 4mg (birth–6 months); 5mg (7 months–3 years); 6.5mg (4–6 years); 7mg (7–10 years); 9mg (11–14 years); 9.5mg (males 15 years and over); 7mg (females 15 years and over); 13mg extra during first 4 months of breast-feeding and 9.5mg thereafter.

MAIN FOOD SOURCES OF MINERALS

The table below indicates foods that are especially good sources of particular minerals. A balanced diet usually contains all the minerals required by the body without the need for supplements. Some, known as trace elements, are required only in minute amounts.

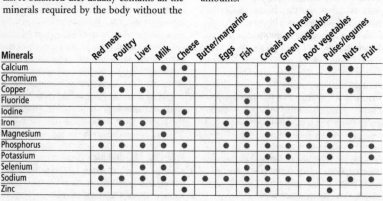

Minerals	Red meat	Poultry	Liver	Milk	Cheese	Butter/margarine	Eggs	Fish	Cereals and bread	Green vegetables	Root vegetables	Pulses/legumes	Nuts	Fruit
Calcium				●	●					●		●	●	
Chromium	●				●				●	●				
Copper	●	●	●					●	●	●		●	●	
Fluoride								●						
Iodine				●	●			●	●	●				
Iron	●	●	●				●	●	●	●				
Magnesium				●				●	●	●		●	●	
Phosphorus	●	●	●	●	●		●	●	●	●	●	●	●	●
Potassium								●	●	●	●			
Selenium	●		●					●	●					
Sodium	●	●	●	●	●	●	●	●	●	●	●	●	●	●
Zinc	●				●			●	●			●		

MALIGNANT AND IMMUNE DISEASE

New cells are continuously needed by the body to replace those that wear out and die naturally and to repair injured tissue. In normal circumstances the rate at which cells are created is carefully regulated. However, sometimes abnormal cells are formed that multiply uncontrollably. They may form lumps of abnormal tissue. These tumours are usually confined to one place and cause few problems; these are benign growths, such as warts. In other types of tumour the cells may invade or destroy the structures around the tumour, and abnormal cells may spread to other parts of the body, forming satellite or metastatic tumours. These are malignant growths, also called cancers.

Opposing the development of tumours is the body's immune system. This can recognize as foreign not only invading bacteria and viruses but also transplanted tissue and cells that have become cancerous. The immune system relies on different types of white blood cells produced in the lymph glands and the bone marrow.

TYPES OF CANCER

Uncontrolled multiplication of cells leads to the formation of tumours that may be benign or malignant. Benign tumours do not spread to other tissues; malignant (cancerous) tumours do, however.

Carcinomas affect the skin and cells in the tissue lining internal organs.
Sarcomas affect muscles, bones, and fibrous tissues and lining cells of blood vessels.
Leukaemia affects white blood cells.
Lymphomas affect the lymph glands.

WHAT CAN GO WRONG

A single cause for cancer has not been identified, and an individual's risk of developing cancer may depend both upon genetic predisposition (some families seem particularly prone to cancers of one or more types) and upon exposure to external risk factors, known as carcinogens. These include tobacco smoke, which increases the risk of lung cancer, and ultraviolet light, which makes skin cancer more likely in those who spend long periods in the sun. Long-term suppression of the immune system by disease (as in AIDS) or by drugs – for example, those given to prevent rejection of transplanted organs – also increases the risk of developing not only infections but also certain cancers. This demonstrates the importance of the immune system in removing abnormal cells with the potential to cause a tumour.

Overactivity of the immune system may also cause problems. It may respond excessively to an innocuous stimulus, as in hay fever (see Allergy, p.58), or may mount a reaction against normal tissues, leading to a variety of disorders known as autoimmune diseases. These include rheumatoid arthritis, certain inflammatory skin disorders (for example, systemic lupus erythematosus), pernicious anaemia, and some forms of hypothyroidism. Immune system activity can also be troublesome following an organ or tissue transplant, when it may lead to rejection of the foreign tissue. This shows the need for medication that can dampen the immune system and enable the body to accept the foreign tissue.

WHY DRUGS ARE USED

In cancer treatment, cytotoxic (cell-killing) drugs are used to eliminate abnormally dividing cells. These slow the growth rate of tumours and sometimes lead to their complete disappearance. Because these drugs act against all rapidly dividing cells, they also reduce the number of normal cells, including blood cells, being produced from bone marrow. This can produce serious adverse effects, such as anaemia and neutropenia in cancer patients, but it can be useful in limiting white cell activity in autoimmune disorders. Some newer anticancer drugs are more selective in the cells they target.

Other drugs that have immunosuppressant effects include corticosteroids and ciclosporin, which are used following transplant surgery. No drugs are yet available that directly stimulate the entire immune system.

However, growth factors may be used to increase the number and activity of some white blood cells, and antibody infusions may help those with deficient production or be used against specific targets in organ transplantation and cancer.

MAJOR DRUG GROUPS
◆ Anticancer drugs
◆ Immunosuppressant drugs
◆ Drugs for HIV and AIDS

Anticancer drugs

Cancer is a general term that covers a wide range of disorders, ranging from the leukaemias (blood cancers) to solid tumours of the lung, breast, and other organs. In all cancers, a group of cells escape from the normal controls on cell growth and multiplication. As a result, the malignant (cancerous) cells begin to crowd out the normal cells and a tumour develops. Cancerous cells are frequently unable to perform their usual functions, and this may lead to progressively impaired function of the organ or area concerned. Cancers may develop from cells of the blood, skin, muscle, or any other tissue.

Malignant tumours spread into nearby structures, blocking blood vessels and compressing nerves and other structures. Fragments of the tumour may become detached and carried in the bloodstream to other parts of the body, where they form secondary growths (metastases).

Many different factors, or a combination of them, can provoke cancerous changes in cells. These factors include an individual's genetic background, impairment or failure of the immune system, and exposure to cancer-causing agents (carcinogens). Known carcinogens include strong sunlight, tobacco smoke, radiation, certain chemicals, viruses, and dietary factors.

Treating cancer is a complicated process that depends on the type of cancer, its stage of development, and the patient's condition and wishes. Any of the following treatments may be used alone or in combination with the others: surgery, radiation treatment, and drug therapy.

Until recently, drug treatment of cancer relied heavily on hormonal drugs and cytotoxic agents (usually referred to as chemotherapy). Hormone treatments are suitable for only a few types of cancer and cytotoxic drugs, although valuable, can have severe side effects because of the damage that they do to normal tissues. In recent years, as understanding of cancer biology has increased, new anticancer drugs have been developed. These drugs include cytokines, such as interferon and interleukin-2, that stimulate the immune system to attack certain cancers, and monoclonal antibodies and growth-factor inhibitors that attack the cancer cells much more selectively.

WHY THEY ARE USED
Cytotoxic drugs can cure rapidly growing cancers and are the treatment of choice for leukaemias, lymphomas, and certain cancers of the testis. They are less effective against slow-growing solid tumours, such as those of the breast and bowel, but they can relieve symptoms and prolong life when given as palliative chemotherapy (treatment that relieves symptoms but does not cure the disease). Adjuvant (effect-enhancing) chemotherapy is increasingly being used after surgery, especially for breast and bowel tumours, to prevent regrowth of the cancer from cells left behind after surgery. Neoadjuvant, or primary, chemotherapy may sometimes be used before surgery to reduce the size of the tumour.

Hormone treatment is offered in cases of hormone-sensitive cancer, such as breast, uterine, and prostatic cancers, where it can be used to relieve disease symptoms or provide palliative treatment in advanced disease. Cytokines, monoclonal antibodies, and growth-factor inhibitors are used alone or alongside chemotherapy, sometimes with the aim of cure but more often to produce disease remission.

Most anticancer drug treatments, especially cytotoxic treatments, have side effects, sometimes severe, and so treatment decisions have to balance possible benefits against the risk of side effects. More aggressive treatments may be appropriate for patients who have curable cancers.

Often a combination of several drugs is used, either simultaneously or successively. Special regimes of different drugs that are used together and in succession have been devised to maximize their activity and minimize the side effects.

Certain anticancer drugs are also used for their effect in suppressing immune system activity (see p.99).

HOW THEY WORK

Anticancer drugs work in many different ways. The main groups of drugs and how they work are described in this section.

Cytotoxic drugs There are several classes of cytotoxic drugs, including the alkylating agents, antimetabolites, taxanes, and cytotoxic antibiotics. Each class has a different mechanism of action, but all act by interfering with basic processes of cell replication and division. They are particularly potent against rapidly dividing cells. These include cancer cells but also certain normal cells, especially those in the hair follicles, gut lining, and bone marrow. This explains the drugs' side effects and the need to schedule treatment carefully.

Hormone therapies Hormone treatments act by counteracting the effects of the hormone that is encouraging growth of the cancer. For example, some breast cancers are stimulated by the female sex hormone oestrogen; the action of oestrogen is opposed by the drug tamoxifen. Other cancers are damaged by very high doses of a particular sex hormone. An example is medroxyprogesterone, a progesterone that is often used to halt the spread of endometrial cancer.

Cytokines The cytokines, interferon alfa and interleukin-2, stimulate the immune system to attack certain cancers. The mechanisms responsible for this action are not entirely understood.

Monoclonal antibodies Antibodies are a fundamental building block of the immune system. They recognize and bind very specifically to "foreign" proteins on the surface of bacteria, viruses, and parasites, marking them out for destruction. Monoclonal antibodies are produced in tissue culture using cells genetically engineered to make antibodies against a particular target protein. If the target is carefully selected, the antibodies can be used to identify cancer cells for destruction by the immune system. If the target is found only on cancer cells, or on the cancer cells and the normal tissue from which it arose, the damage to healthy tissues during treatment is very limited. Once they have bound to a cell, antibodies interact with the immune system to kill cells in a variety of ways. They include attracting killer leukocytes and provoking a series of chemical reactions that dissolve the cell wall; this is called "complement fixation".

So far, three monoclonal antibodies are in routine use as cancer treatment: trastuzumab binds to a protein produced in particularly large quantities in about one-fifth of breast cancer cells; rituximab recognizes a protein found on most lymphatic cancer cells as well as some normal white blood cells; alemtuzumab recognizes and kills certain leukaemic cells in addition to some normal white blood cells. As these antibodies are so specific, they are useful only against particular cancers, in which they cause little of the toxicity of conventional chemotherapy. They do, however, often cause allergy-type reactions, especially at the beginning of treatment.

Growth-factor inhibitors It has recently been discovered that the growth of cells, including cancer cells, is controlled by a complex network of growth factors that bind very specifically to receptor sites on the cell surface. This triggers a complex series of chemical reactions that transmit the "grow" message to the nucleus, triggering cell growth and replication. In many cancers, this system is faulty and there are either too many receptors on the cell surface or other abnormalities that result in the nucleus receiving inappropriate "grow" messages. The extra or abnormal cell surface receptors can be used as targets for monoclonal antibodies (see above).

Other defects in this system are being used as the basis for other new drugs. For example, imatinib very selectively interferes with an abnormal version of an enzyme found in certain leukaemic cells. This abnormal enzyme results in the cell nucleus receiving a "grow" signal continuously, resulting in the uncontrolled growth of cancer. By stopping the enzyme working, it is possible to selectively "turn off" the growth of the abnormal cells. Imatinib is proving successful in treating certain types of leukaemia, with few serious side effects.

HOW THEY AFFECT YOU

Cytotoxic drugs are generally associated with more side effects than other anticancer drugs. At the start of treatment, adverse effects of the drugs may be more noticeable than benefits. The most common side effect is nausea and vomiting, for which an anti-emetic drug (see p.21) will usually be prescribed. Effects on the blood are also common. Many cytotoxic drugs cause hair loss because of their effect on the hair follicle cells, but the hair usually starts to grow back after chemotherapy has been completed. Individual drugs may produce other side effects.

Cytotoxic drugs are, in most cases, administered in the highest doses that can be tolerated in order to kill as many cancer cells as quickly as possible.

The unpleasant side effects of intensive chemotherapy, combined with a delay of several weeks before any beneficial effects are seen and the seriousness of the underlying disease, often lead to depression in those who are receiving anticancer drugs. Specialist counselling, support from family and friends, and, in some cases, treatment with antidepressant drugs may be helpful.

SUCCESSFUL CHEMOTHERAPY

Not all cancers respond to treatment with anticancer drugs. Some cancers can be cured by drug treatment. In other cancers, drug treatment can slow or temporarily halt the disease's progress. In certain cases, drug treatment has no beneficial effect but other treatments, such as surgery, often produce significant benefits. The main cancers that fall into each of the first two groups are described here:

Cancers that can often be cured by drugs
◆ Some cancers of the lymphatic system (including Hodgkin's disease)
◆ Acute leukaemias (forms of blood cancer)
◆ Choriocarcinoma (cancer of the placenta)
◆ Germ cell tumours (cancers affecting sperm and egg cells)

◆ Wilms' tumour (a rare form of kidney cancer that affects children)
◆ Cancer of the testis

Cancers in which drugs may produce worthwhile benefits
◆ Breast cancer
◆ Ovarian cancer
◆ Some leukaemias
◆ Multiple myeloma (a bone marrow cancer)
◆ Many types of lung cancer
◆ Head and neck cancers
◆ Cancer of the stomach
◆ Cancer of the prostate
◆ Some cancers of the lymphatic system
◆ Bladder cancer
◆ Endometrial cancer (cancer affecting the lining of the uterus)
◆ Cancer of the large intestine
◆ Cancer of the oesophagus
◆ Cancer of the pancreas
◆ Cancer of the cervix

Successful drug treatment of cancer usually requires repeated courses of anticancer drugs because the treatment needs to be halted periodically to allow the blood-producing cells in the bone marrow to recover.

RISKS AND SPECIAL PRECAUTIONS

All cytotoxic anticancer drugs interfere with the activity of noncancerous cells and, for this reason, they often produce serious adverse effects during long-term treatment. In particular, these drugs often adversely affect rapidly dividing cells such as the blood-producing cells in the bone marrow. The numbers of red and white cells and the number of platelets (particles in the blood responsible for clotting) may all be reduced. In some cases, symptoms of anaemia (weakness and fatigue) and an increased risk of abnormal or excessive bleeding may develop as a result of treatment with anticancer drugs.

Reduction in the number of white blood cells may result in an increased susceptibility to infection. A simple infection such as a sore throat may be a sign of depressed white cell production in a patient taking anticancer drugs, and it must be reported to the doctor without delay. In addition, wounds may take longer to heal, and susceptible people can develop gout as a result of increased uric acid production due to cells being broken down.

Because of these problems, anticancer chemotherapy is often given in hospital, where the adverse effects can be closely monitored. Several short courses of drug treatment are usually given, thus allowing the bone marrow time to recover in the period between courses (see Successful chemotherapy, facing page). Blood tests are performed regularly. When necessary, blood transfusions, antibiotics, or other forms of treatment are used to overcome adverse effects. When relevant, contraceptive advice is given early in treatment because most anticancer drugs can damage a developing baby. In addition to general effects, individual drugs may have adverse effects on particular organs.

By contrast, other anticancer drugs, such as hormonal drugs, antibodies, and growth-factor inhibitors are much more selective in their actions and they generally have less serious side effects.

COMMON DRUGS

Alkylating agents Chlorambucil, Cyclophosphamide*, Melphalan
Antimetabolites Azathioprine*, Capecitabine, Cytarabine, Fluorouracil, Mercaptopurine*, Methotrexate*
Cytotoxic antibiotics Doxorubicin*, Epirubicin
Hormone treatments Anastrozole*, Bicalutamide, Cyproterone acetate, Flutamide*, Goserelin*, Letrozole, Leuprorelin, Medroxyprogesterone*, Megestrol, Tamoxifen*
Cytokines Interferon alfa*, Interleukin-2
Taxanes Docetaxel, Paclitaxel
Monoclonal antibodies Alemtuzumab, Rituximab, Trastuzumab*
Growth-factor inhibitors Imatinib
Other drugs Carboplatin, Cisplatin*, Etoposide, Irinotecan
* See Part 2

Immunosuppressant drugs

The body is protected against attack from bacteria, fungi, and viruses by the specialized cells and proteins in the blood and tissues that make up the immune system. White blood cells known as lymphocytes either kill invading organisms directly or produce special proteins (called antibodies) to destroy them. These mechanisms are also responsible for eliminating abnormal or unhealthy cells that could otherwise multiply and develop into a cancer.

In certain conditions it is medically necessary to dampen the activity of the immune system. These include a number of autoimmune disorders in which the immune system attacks normal body tissue. Autoimmune disorders may affect a single organ – for example, the kidneys in Goodpasture's syndrome or the thyroid gland in Hashimoto's disease – or they may result in widespread damage, for example, in rheumatoid arthritis or systemic lupus erythematosus.

Immune system activity may also need to be reduced following an organ transplant, when the body's defences would otherwise attack and reject the transplanted tissue.

Several types of drugs are used as immunosuppressants:
Anticancer drugs (see p.96) slow the production of all cells in the bone marrow.
Corticosteroids (see p.80) reduce the activity of both B- and T-lymphocytes.
Ciclosporin (see p.182) inhibits the activity of T-lymphocytes only and not B-lymphocyte activity.

WHY THEY ARE USED

Immunosuppressant drugs are given to treat autoimmune disorders, such as rheumatoid arthritis, when symptoms are severe and other treatments have not provided adequate relief. Corticosteroids are usually prescribed initially. The pronounced anti-inflammatory effect of these drugs, as well as their immunosuppressant action, helps to promote healing of tissue damaged by abnormal immune system activity. Anticancer drugs such as methotrexate may be used in addition to corticosteroids if these do not produce sufficient improvement or if their effect wanes (see also Antirheumatic drugs, p.52).

Immunosuppressant drugs are given before and after organ and other tissue transplants. Treatment may have to be continued indefinitely to prevent rejection. Various drugs and drug combinations are used, depending on which organ is being transplanted and the underlying condition of the patient. However, ciclosporin, along with the related drug tacrolimus, is now the most widely used drug for preventing organ rejection. It is also increasingly used to treat autoimmune disorders. It is often used in combination with a corticosteroid or the more specific drug mycophenolate mofetil.

Monoclonal antibodies that attack the parts of the immune system responsible for organ rejection are also used to aid transplantation.

HOW THEY WORK
Immunosuppressant drugs reduce the effectiveness of the immune system, either by depressing the production of lymphocytes or by altering their activity.

HOW THEY AFFECT YOU
When immunosuppressants are given to treat an autoimmune disorder, they reduce the severity of symptoms and may temporarily halt the progress of the disease. However, they cannot restore major tissue damage.

Immunosuppressant drugs can produce a variety of unwanted side effects. The side effects caused by corticosteroids are described in more detail on p.80. Anticancer drugs, when prescribed as immunosuppressants, are given in low doses that produce only mild side effects. They may cause nausea and vomiting, for which an anti-emetic drug (p.21) may be prescribed. Hair loss is rare and regrowth usually occurs when the drug treatment is discontinued. Ciclosporin may cause increased growth of facial hair, swelling of the gums, and tingling in the hands.

RISKS AND SPECIAL PRECAUTIONS
All of these drugs may produce potentially serious adverse effects. By reducing the activity of the patient's immune system, immunosuppressant drugs can affect the body's ability to fight invading microorganisms, thereby increasing the risk of serious infections. Because lymphocyte activity is also important for preventing the multiplication of abnormal cells, there is an increased risk of certain types of cancer. A major drawback of anticancer drugs is that, in addition to their effect on the production of lymphocytes, they interfere with the growth and division of other blood cells in the bone marrow. Reduced production of red blood cells can cause anaemia; when the production of blood platelets is suppressed, blood clotting may be less efficient.

Although ciclosporin is more specific in its action than either corticosteroids or anticancer drugs, it can cause kidney damage and, in too high a dose, may affect the brain, causing hallucinations or fits. Ciclosporin also tends to raise blood pressure, and another drug may be required to counteract this effect (see Antihypertensive drugs, p.36).

COMMON DRUGS
Anticancer drugs Azathioprine*, Chlorambucil, Cyclophosphamide*, Methotrexate*, Mycophenolate mofetil
Corticosteroids (see p.80)
Antibodies Anti-lymphocyte globulin, Basiliximab, Daclizumab
Other drugs Ciclosporin*, Tacrolimus
* **See Part 2**

Drugs for HIV and AIDS

The disease AIDS (acquired immune deficiency syndrome) is caused by infection with the human immunodeficiency virus (HIV). This virus invades certain cells of the immune system, particularly the white blood cells called T-helper lymphocytes (or CD_4 cells), which normally activate other cells in the immune system to fight infection. HIV kills T-helper lymphocytes, so that the body cannot fight the virus or subsequent infections. Over the past few years the number of drugs available to treat HIV has increased considerably, as well as the knowledge about how best to use the drugs in combination.

WHY THEY ARE USED
Drug treatments for HIV infection can be divided into treatment of the initial infection with HIV and treatment of diseases and complications associated with AIDS.

Drugs that act directly against HIV are called antiretrovirals. The two most common groups work by interfering with enzymes vital for virus replication. The first inhibit an enzyme called the reverse transcriptase

ANTIRETROVIRAL DRUGS

Drug name	Formulation	Additional information
Abacavir, lamivudine *Kivexa*	*Kivexa* contains abacavir (600mg) and lamivudine (300mg)	Abacavir can cause a severe allergic-type reaction (see additional product information)
Abacavir, lamivudine, zidovudine (AZT) *Trizivir*	*Trizivir* contains abacavir (300mg), lamivudine (150mg), and zidovudine (300mg)	The abacavir contained in *Trizivir* can cause a severe allergic-type reaction (see additional product information)
Atazanavir *Reyataz*	Capsules (200mg, 150mg, 100mg)	
Didanosine (ddI, DDI) *Videx*	Enteric-coated capsules (400mg, 250mg, 200mg, 125mg). Tablets (25mg)	See product information
Efavirenz *Sustiva*	Capsules (200mg, 50mg). Tablets (600mg)	Efavirenz can cause a severe allergic-type rash (see additional product information)
Emtricitabine *Emtriva*	Capsules (200mg). Oral solution (10mg/ml)	
Enfuvirtide *Fuzeon*	Subcutaneous injection (90mg) powder for reconstitution	Caution in liver impairment, including hepatitis B or C
Fosamprenavir *Telzir*	Tablets (700mg). Oral suspension (50mg/ml)	
Indinavir *Crixivan*	Capsules (400mg, 100mg)	Indinavir should be taken with a low-fat meal or 1 hour before or 2 hours after any other meal
Lamivudine (3TC) *Epivir*	Tablets (300mg, 150mg). Oral solution (50mg/5ml)	Lamivudine can also be used to treat hepatitis B
Lopinavir with ritonavir *Kaletra*	Tablets (200mg lopinavir, 50mg ritonavir). Capsules (133mg, 33mg). Oral solution (400mg, 100mg/5ml).	
Nelfinavir *Viracept*	Tablet (250mg). Oral powder	Doses must be taken with a meal
Nevirapine *Viramune*	Tablets (200mg). Suspension (50mg/5ml)	Nevirapine can cause a severe allergic-type reaction (see additional product information)
Ritonavir *Norvir*	Capsules (100mg). Oral solution (400mg/5ml)	Doses should be taken with food
Saquinavir *Invirase*	Capsules (200mg). Tablets (500mg)	Doses should be taken within 2 hours of a full meal
Stavudine (d4T) *Zerit*	Capsules (40mg, 30mg, 20mg). Oral solution (1mg/ml)	
Tenofovir disoproxil *Viread*	Tablets (245mg as disoproxil fumarate = 300mg tenofovir)	Tenofovir should be taken with food
Tenofovir disoproxil, emtricitabine *Truvada*	*Truvada* contains tenofovir (245mg) and emtricitabine (200mg)	
Tipranavir *Aptivus*	Tablets (250mg)	Risk of liver toxicity
Zidovudine (AZT) *Retrovir*	Capsules (250mg, 100mg). Syrup (50mg/5ml). Injection (10mg/ml)	
Zidovudine (AZT), lamivudine	*Combivir* contains zidovudine (300mg) and lamivudine (150mg)	

enzyme. These are divided according to their chemical structure into nucleotide, nucleoside, and non-nucleoside inhibitors. The second group interfere with an enzyme called protease. Entry, or fusion, inhibitors are a new group that interfere with the entry of the virus into the cell. Further groups are being developed: integrase inhibitors to prevent the virus from injecting its genetic material into the cell nucleus; and other drugs to target the receptor sites the virus relies on for entry into the cell.

Antiretrovirals are much more effective in combination. Treatment usually starts with two nucleoside transcriptase inhibitors plus a non-nucleoside drug or protease inhibitor. If combination, or highly active antiretroviral, therapy (HAART), is started before the immune system is too damaged, it can dramatically reduce the level of HIV in the body and improve the outlook for HIV-infected people, but it is not a cure for the disease and they remain infectious.

The mainstay of drug treatment for AIDS-related diseases are antimicrobial drugs for the bacterial, viral, fungal, and protozoal infections to which people with AIDS are particularly susceptible. These drugs include the antituberculous drugs (p.67), co-trimoxazole for the treatment of pneumocystis carinii pneumonia (PCP), and ganciclovir for the treatment of CMV (cytomegalovirus) infection.

COMMON DRUGS

Nucleoside reverse transcriptase inhibitors Abacavir/lamivudine, Didanosine, Emtricitabine, Stavudine, Zidovudine (AZT)/lamivudine*
Nucleotide reverse transcriptase inhibitor Tenofovir
Non-nucleoside reverse transcriptase inhibitors Efavirenz*, Nevirapine
Protease inhibitors Atazanavir, Fosamprenavir, Indinavir, Lopinavir/ritonavir*, Nelfinavir, Saquinavir, Tipranavir
Other antiretrovirals Enfuvirtide
* See Part 2

REPRODUCTIVE & URINARY TRACTS

The reproductive systems of men and women consist of those organs that produce and release sperm (male), or store and release eggs, and then nurture a fertilized egg until it develops into a baby (female).

The urinary system filters wastes and water from the blood, producing urine, which is then expelled from the body. The reproductive and urinary systems of men are partially linked, but those of women form two physically close but functionally separate systems.

The female reproductive organs comprise the ovaries, fallopian tubes, and uterus (womb). The uterus opens via the cervix (neck of the uterus) into the vagina. The principal male reproductive organs are the two sperm-producing glands, the testes (testicles), which lie within the scrotum, and the penis. Other structures of the male reproductive tract include the prostate gland and several tubular structures – the tightly coiled epididymides, the vas deferens, the seminal vesicles and the urethra.

The urinary organs in both sexes comprise the kidneys, which filter the blood and excrete urine, the ureters down which urine passes, and the bladder, where urine is stored until it is passed out of the body through the urethra.

WHAT CAN GO WRONG

The reproductive and urinary tracts are both subject to infection. Such infections (apart from those transmitted by sexual activity) are relatively uncommon in men because the long male urethra prevents bacteria and other organisms passing easily to the bladder and upper urinary tract, and to the male sex organs. The shorter female urethra allows urinary tract infections, especially of the bladder (cystitis) and of the urethra (urethritis), to occur commonly. The female reproductive tract is also vulnerable to infection, which, in some cases, is sexually transmitted.

Reproductive function may also be disrupted by hormonal disturbances that lead to reduced fertility. Women may be troubled by symptoms arising from normal activity of the reproductive organs, including menstrual disorders as well as various problems associated with childbirth.

The most common urinary problems apart from infection are those related to bladder function. Urine may be released involuntarily (incontinence) or it may be retained in the bladder. Such disorders are usually the result of abnormal nerve signals to the bladder or sphincter muscle. The filtering action of the kidneys may be affected by alteration of the composition of the blood or the hormones that regulate urine production, or by damage (from infection or inflammation) to the filtering units themselves.

WHY DRUGS ARE USED

Antibiotic drugs (p.62) are used to eliminate infections of the urinary and reproductive tracts (including sexually transmitted infections). Certain infections of the vagina are caused by fungi or yeasts and require antifungal drugs (p.76).

Hormone drugs are used both to reduce fertility deliberately (oral contraceptives) and to increase fertility in certain conditions in which it has not been possible for a couple to conceive. Hormones may also be used to regulate menstruation when it is irregular or excessively painful or heavy. Analgesic drugs (p.9) are used to treat menstrual period pain and are also widely used for pain relief in labour. Other drugs used in labour include those that increase contraction of the muscles of the uterus and those that limit blood loss after the birth. Drugs may also be employed to halt premature labour.

Drugs that alter the transmission of nerve signals to the bladder muscles have an important role in the treatment of urinary incontinence and retention. Drugs that increase the kidneys' filtering action are commonly used to reduce blood pressure and fluid retention (see Diuretics, p.32). Other drugs may alter the composition of the urine – for example, the uricosuric drugs that are used in the treatment of gout (p.53) increase the amount of uric acid.

THE MENSTRUAL CYCLE

A monthly cycle of hormone interactions allows an egg to be released and, if it is fertilized, creates the correct environment for it to implant in the uterus. Major changes occur in the body, the most obvious of which is monthly vaginal bleeding (menstruation). The menstrual cycle usually starts between the ages of 11 and 14 years and continues until the menopause, which occurs at around the age of 50. After the menopause, child-bearing is no longer possible. The cycle is usually 28 days, but this varies from one individual to another.

Menstruation If no egg is fertilized, the endometrium is shed (days 1–5).

Fertile period Conception may take place in the two days after ovulation (days 14–16).

MAJOR DRUG GROUPS

◆ Drugs used to treat menstrual disorders
◆ Oral contraceptives
◆ Drugs for infertility
◆ Drugs used in labour
◆ Drugs used for urinary disorders

Drugs used to treat menstrual disorders

The menstrual cycle results from the actions of female sex hormones that cause ovulation (the release of an egg) and thickening of the endometrium (the lining of the uterus) each month in preparation for pregnancy. Unless the egg is fertilized, the endometrium will be shed approximately two weeks later during menstruation (see also The menstrual cycle, above).

The main problems associated with menstruation that may require medical treatment are excessive blood loss (menorrhagia), pain during menstruation (dysmenorrhoea), and the distressing physical and psychological symptoms that sometimes occur before menstruation (premenstrual syndrome).

The absence of periods (amenorrhoea) is commonly due to pregnancy in women of childbearing age or to the menopause in older women; other causes are discussed under female sex hormones (p.88).

The drugs most commonly used to treat the menstrual disorders described above include oestrogens, progestogens, danazol, and analgesics (painkillers).

WHY THEY ARE USED

Drug treatment for menstrual disorders is undertaken only when the doctor has ruled out the possibility of an underlying gynaecological disorder, such as a pelvic infection or fibroids. In some cases, especially in women over the age of 35, a D and C (dilatation and curettage) may be recommended. When no underlying reason for the problem is found, drug treatment aimed primarily at the relief of symptoms is usually prescribed.

Dysmenorrhoea Painful menstrual periods are usually treated initially with a simple analgesic (see p.9). Non-steroidal anti-inflammatory drugs (NSAIDs; see p.50), are often most effective because they counter the effects of prostaglandins, chemicals that are partly responsible for transmission of pain to the brain. Diclofenac and mefenamic acid are also used to reduce the excessive blood loss of menorrhagia (see below).

When these drugs are not sufficient to provide adequate pain relief, hormonal drug treatment may be recommended. If contraception is also required, treatment may involve an oral contraceptive pill containing both an oestrogen and a progestogen, or a progestogen alone. Non-contraceptive progestogen preparations may also be prescribed. These are usually taken for only a few days during each month.

Menorrhagia Excessive loss of blood during menstruation can sometimes be reduced by some NSAIDs. Tranexamic acid, an antifibrinolytic drug, is an effective treatment for menorrhagia. Alternatively, danazol, a drug that reduces production of the female sex hormone oestrogen, may be prescribed to reduce blood loss.

Premenstrual syndrome This is a collection of psychological and physical symptoms that affect many women to some degree in the days before menstruation. Psychological symptoms include mood changes such as increased irritability, depression, and anxiety. Principal physical symptoms are bloating, headache, and breast tenderness. Combined oral contraceptives may be prescribed and, for severe premenstrual syndrome, SSRI antidepressants (p.14) are sometimes given. Other drugs sometimes used include pyridoxine (vitamin B_6), diuretics (p.32) if bloating due to fluid retention is a problem, and bromocriptine when breast tenderness is the major symptom.

Endometriosis is a condition in which fragments of endometrial tissue (uterine lining) occur outside the uterus in the pelvic cavity. It causes severe pain during menstruation, often causes pain during intercourse, and may sometimes lead to infertility. Drugs used for this disorder are similar to those prescribed for heavy periods (menorrhagia). In this case, however, the intention is to suppress endometrial development for an extended period so that the abnormal tissue eventually withers away. Progesterone supplements that suppress endometrial thickening may be prescribed throughout the menstrual cycle. Alternatively, danazol, which suppresses endometrial development by reducing oestrogen production, may be prescribed. Any drug treatment usually needs to be continued for a minimum of six months. When drug treatment is unsuccessful, surgical removal of the abnormal tissue is usually necessary.

HOW THEY WORK

Drugs used to treat menstrual disorders act in a variety of ways. Hormonal treatments are aimed at suppressing the pattern of hormonal changes that is causing troublesome symptoms. Contraceptive preparations override the woman's normal menstrual cycle. Ovulation does not occur, and the endometrium does not thicken normally. Bleeding that occurs at the end of a cycle is less likely to be abnormally heavy, to be accompanied by severe discomfort, or to be preceded by distressing symptoms.

Non-contraceptive progestogen preparations taken in the days before menstruation do not suppress ovulation. Increased progesterone during this time reduces premenstrual symptoms and prevents excessive thickening of the endometrium.

Danazol, a potent drug, prevents the thickening of the endometrium, thereby correcting excessively heavy periods. Blood loss is reduced, and in some cases menstruation ceases altogether during treatment.

COMMON DRUGS

Oestrogens and progestogens (see p.88)
NSAID analgesics Aspirin*, Dexibuprofen, Dexketoprofen, Diclofenac*, Diflunisal, Flurbiprofen, Ibuprofen*, Indometacin, Ketoprofen*, Lumiracoxib, Mefenamic acid*, Naproxen*
Diuretics (see p.32)
Other drugs Bromocriptine*, Buserelin, Danazol*, Gestrinone, Goserelin*, Leuprorelin, Nafarelin, Pyridoxine*, Tranexamic acid, Triptorelin
* **See part 2**

Oral contraceptives

There are many different methods of ensuring that conception and pregnancy do not follow sexual intercourse, but for most women the oral contraceptive is the most effective method. It has the advantage of being convenient and unobtrusive during lovemaking. About 25 per cent of the women who seek contraceptive protection in Britain choose a form of oral contraceptive.

There are three main types of oral contraceptive: the combined pill, the progestogen-only pill (POP), and the phased pill. All three types contain a progestogen (a synthetic form of the female sex hormone, progesterone). Both the combined and phased pills also contain a natural or synthetic oestrogen.

The following list indicates the number of pregnancies occurring with each method of contraception per 100 users each year. The variation that occurs with some of these methods takes into account pregnancies that occur through incorrect use of the method.
- Combined and phased pills 2–3
- Progestogen-only pill 2.5–10
- IUD (Intrauterine device) 4–9
- Condom 3–4
- Diaphragm 10–20
- Rhythm method 25–30
- Contraceptive sponge 9–27
- Vaginal spermicide alone 2–30
- Norethisterone implant Less than 1
- No contraception 80–85
- "Morning after" pill 20–25.

WHY THEY ARE USED

The combined pill This is the most widely prescribed form of oral contraceptive and has the lowest failure rate in terms of unwanted pregnancies. It is referred to as the "pill" and is the type thought most suitable for young women who want to use a hormonal form of contraception. The combined pill is particularly suitable for those women who regularly experience exceptionally painful, heavy, or prolonged periods (see Drugs used to treat menstrual disorders, p.104).

There are many different products available containing a fixed dose of an oestrogen and a progestogen drug. They are divided generally into three groups according to their oestrogen content (see table, below). Low-dose products are chosen when possible to minimize the risk of adverse effects.

Progestogen-only pill (POP) The progestogen-only pill is often recommended for women who react adversely to the oestrogen in the combined pill or for whom the combined pill is not considered suitable because of their age or medical history (see Risks and special precautions, facing page). It is also prescribed for breast-feeding women, since it does not reduce milk production. The progestogen-only pill has a higher failure rate than the combined pill and, for maximum contraceptive effect, must be taken at precisely the same time each day. It works by changing the quality of the endometrium, making implantation of a fertilized egg less likely. However, Cerazette (a brand of the progestogen, desogestrel) also inhibits ovulation, making it more reliable than other progestogen-only pills.

Phased pills The third form of oral contraceptive is a pack of pills divided into two or three groups or phases. Each phase contains a different proportion of an oestrogen and a progestogen. The aim is to provide a hormonal balance that closely resembles the fluctuations of a normal menstrual cycle. Phased pills provide effective protection for many women who suffer side effects from other available forms of oral contraceptive.

HOW THEY WORK

In a normal menstrual cycle, the ripening and release of an egg and the preparation of the uterus for implantation of the fertilized egg are the result of a complex interplay between the natural female sex hormones, oestrogen and progesterone, and the pituitary hormones, follicle-stimulating hormone (FSH) and luteinizing hormone (LH) (see also p.88). The oestrogen and progestogens in oral contraceptives disrupt the normal menstrual cycle in such a way that conception is less likely.

HORMONE CONTENT OF COMMON ORAL CONTRACEPTIVES

The oestrogen-containing forms are classified according to their oestrogen content as follows: low: 20 micrograms; standard: 30–35 micrograms; high: 50 micrograms; phased pills: 30–40 micrograms. Morning after (levonorgestrel): 1,500 micrograms.

TYPE OF PILL (oestrogen content)	BRAND NAMES
Combined (20mcg)	Evra, Loestrin 20, Femodette, Mercilon
(30–35mcg)	Brevinor, Cilest, Femodene, Femodene ED, Loestrin 30, Marvelon, Microgynon 30, Microgynon 30 ED Minulet, Norimin, Ovranette, Ovysmen, Yasmin
(50mcg)	Norinyl-1 (as Mestranol)
Phased (30–40mcg)	BiNovum, Logynon, Logynon ED, Synphase, Triadene, Tri-Minulet, Trinordiol, TriNovum
Progestogen-only (no oestrogen)	Cerazette, Femulen, Micronor, Norgeston, Noriday
Postcoital (morning after) (no oestrogen)	Levonelle 1500, Levonelle One Step

With combined and phased pills, the increased levels of oestrogen and progesterone produce similar effects to the hormonal changes of pregnancy. The actions of the hormones inhibit the production of FSH and LH, thereby preventing the egg from ripening in the ovary and from being released.

The progestogen-only pill has a slightly different effect. It does not always prevent release of an egg; its main contraceptive action may be to thicken the mucus that lines the cervix, preventing sperm from crossing it. This effect occurs to some extent with combined and phased pills. Cerazette, additionally, inhibits ovulation.

HOW THEY AFFECT YOU

Each course of combined and phased pills lasts for 21 days, followed by a pill-free seven days, during which time menstruation occurs. Some brands contain seven additional inactive pills. With these, the new course directly follows the last so that the habit of taking the pill daily is not broken. Progestogen-only pills are taken for 28 days each month. Menstruation usually occurs during the last few days of the menstrual cycle.

Women taking oral contraceptives, especially drugs that contain oestrogen, usually find that their menstrual periods are lighter and relatively pain-free. Some women cease to menstruate altogether. This is not a cause for concern in itself, provided no pills have been missed, but it may make it difficult to determine if pregnancy has occurred. An apparently missed period probably indicates a light one, rather than pregnancy. However, if you have missed two consecutive periods and you feel that you may be pregnant, it is advisable to have a pregnancy test.

All forms of oral contraceptive may cause spotting of blood in mid-cycle ("breakthrough bleeding"), especially at first, but this can be a particular problem with the progestogen-only pill.

Oral contraceptives that contain oestrogen may produce any of a large number of mild side effects, depending on the dose. Symptoms similar to those experienced early in pregnancy may occur, particularly in the first few months of pill use: some women complain of nausea and vomiting, weight gain, depression, altered libido, increased appetite, and cramps in the legs and abdomen. The pill may also affect the circulation, producing minor headaches and dizziness. All these effects usually disappear within a few months, but if they persist it may be advisable to change to a brand containing a lower dose of oestrogen or to some other contraceptive method.

RISKS AND SPECIAL PRECAUTIONS

All oral contraceptives need to be taken regularly for maximum protection against pregnancy. Contraceptive protection can be reduced by missing a pill (see What to do if you miss a pill, p.108). It may also be reduced by vomiting or diarrhoea. If you suffer from either of these, it is advisable to act as if you had missed your last pill. Many drugs may also affect the action of oral contraceptives and it is essential to tell your doctor that you are taking oral contraceptives, before taking additional prescribed medications.

Oral contraceptives, particularly those containing an oestrogen, have been found to carry a number of risks (see Balancing the risks and benefits of oral contraceptives, p.108). One of the most serious potential adverse effects of oestrogen-containing pills is development of a thrombus (blood clot) in a vein or artery. The thrombus may travel to the lungs or cause a stroke or heart attack. The risk of thrombus formation increases with age and other factors, notably obesity, high blood pressure, and smoking. Doctors assess these risk factors for each person when prescribing oral contraceptives. A woman who is over 35 may be advised against taking a combined pill, especially if she smokes or has an underlying medical condition such as diabetes. Some studies have found that women taking a combined oral contraceptive containing either desogestrel or gestogene are at greater risk of developing a venous thromboembolism. The risk is still very small, however, and is lower than the risk of developing a venous thromboembolism during pregnancy. The combined oral contraceptive pills that contain desogestrel include Marvelon, and Mercilon; those that contain gestodene include Femodene, Femodette ED, Minulet, Triadene, and Tri-Minulet.

High blood pressure is a possible complication of oral contraceptives for some women. Measurement of blood pressure before the pill is prescribed and every six months after the woman starts taking oral contraceptives is advised for all women taking oral contraceptives.

Some very rare liver cancers have occurred in pill-users, and breast cancer may be slightly more common, but cancers of the ovaries and uterus are less common.

Although there is no evidence that oral contraceptives reduce a woman's fertility or that they damage the babies conceived after the oral contraceptives are discontinued, doctors recommend that you wait for at least one normal menstrual period before you attempt to become pregnant.

BALANCING THE RISKS AND BENEFITS OF ORAL CONTRACEPTIVES

Oral contraceptives are safe for the vast majority of young women. However, every woman who is considering oral contraception should discuss with her doctor the risks and possible adverse effects of the drugs before deciding whether or not a hormonal contraception is the most suitable method in her case. A variety of factors must be taken into account, including the woman's age, her own medical history and that of her close relatives, and factors such as whether or not she is a smoker. The importance of such factors varies depending on the type of oral contraceptive. The principal advantages and disadvantages of oestrogen-containing and progestogen-only pills are listed below.

Advantages of oestrogen-containing combined and phased pills Very reliable; convenient and unobtrusive; regularize menstruation; reduce menstrual pain and blood loss; reduce risk of benign breast disease, endometriosis, ectopic pregnancy, ovarian cysts, pelvic infection, ovarian and endometrial cancer.

Advantages of progestogen-only pill Reasonably reliable; convenient and unobtrusive; suitable for use during breast-feeding; avoids any oestrogen-related side effects and risks; allows rapid return to fertility; suitable for women in whom use of oestrogen-containing contraception is not possible.

Side effects of oestrogen-containing combined and phased pills Weight gain; depression; breast swelling; reduced sex drive; headaches; increased vaginal discharge; nausea.

Side effects of progestogen-only pill Irregular menstruation; nausea; headaches; breast discomfort; depression; changes in libido; weight changes.

Risks of oestrogen-containing combined and and pills Thrombosis/embolism; heart disease; high blood pressure; liver impairment/cancer of the liver (rare); gallstones; breast cancer (risk is low).

Risks of progestogen-only pill Ectopic pregnancy; ovarian cysts; breast cancer (risk is low).

Factors that may prohibit use of oestrogen-containing combined and phased pills Previous thrombosis*; heart disease; high levels of lipid in blood; liver disease; blood disorders; high blood pressure; unexplained vaginal bleeding; migraine; otosclerosis; presence of several risk factors (see below).

Factors that may prohibit use of progestogen-only pill Previous ectopic pregnancy; heart or circulatory disease; unexplained vaginal bleeding; history of breast cancer.

Factors that increase risks of oestrogen-containing combined and phased pills Smoking*; obesity*; increasing age; diabetes mellitus; family history of heart or circulatory disease*; current treatment with other drugs.

Factors that increase risks of progestogen-only pill As for oestrogen-containing pills, but to a lesser degree.

* Products containing desogestrel or gestodene have a higher excess risk with these factors than other progestogens.

HOW TO MINIMIZE YOUR HEALTH RISKS WHILE TAKING THE PILL

◆ Do not smoke.
◆ Maintain a healthy weight and diet.
◆ Have regular blood pressure and blood lipid checks.
◆ Have regular cervical smear tests.
◆ Remind your doctor that you are taking oral contraceptives before taking other prescription drugs.
◆ Stop taking oestrogen-containing oral contraceptives four weeks before planned major surgery (use alternative contraception).

WHAT TO DO IF YOU MISS A PILL

Contraceptive protection may be reduced if blood levels of the hormones in the body fall due to missing a pill. It is particularly important to ensure that the progestogen-only pills are taken punctually. If you miss a pill, the action you take depends on the degree of lateness and type of pill being used (see below).

Combined and phased pills If you are less than 24 hours late, take the missed pill now and the next on time. If you are over 24 hours late, the pill may not work. Take the missed pill now and the next on time. If more than one pill has been missed, just take one then the next on time (even if on the same day); take additional precautions for the next 7 days. If the 7 days extends into the pill-free (or inactive pill) period, start the next packet without a break (or without taking inactive pills).

Progestogen-only pills If you are less than 3 hours late (12 for Cerazette), take the missed pill now and the next on time. If you are over 3 hours late (12 for Cerazette), take the missed pill now and the next on time. If more than one pill has been missed, just take one then the next on time (even if on the same day). In either case, you are not protected and will need to take additional precautions for the next 2 days.

POSTCOITAL CONTRACEPTION

Pregnancy following intercourse without contraception may be avoided by taking a postcoital ("morning after") pill. The preparation used for this purpose contains a progestogen and is taken as soon as possible after intercourse as a single tablet, ideally within 12 hours but no later than 72 hours after intercourse. It postpones ovulation and acts on the lining of the uterus to prevent implantation of the egg. However, The high dose needed makes it unsuitable for regular use. This method has a higher failure rate than the usual oral contraceptives.

COMMON DRUGS

Progestogens Desogestrel*, Drospirenone, Etynodiol, Gestodene, Levonorgestrel*, Norelgestromin, Norethisterone*, Norgestimate

Oestrogens Ethinyloestradiol*, Mestranol

* **See Part 2**

Drugs for infertility

Conception and the establishment of pregnancy require a healthy reproductive system in both partners. The man must be able to produce sufficient numbers of healthy sperm; the woman must be able to produce a healthy egg that is able to pass freely down the fallopian tube to the uterus. The lining of the uterus must be in a condition that allows the implantation of the fertilized egg.

The cause of infertility may sometimes remain undiscovered, but in the majority of cases it is due to one of the following factors: intercourse taking place at the wrong time during the menstrual cycle; the man producing too few or unhealthy sperm; the woman either failing to ovulate (release an egg) or having blocked fallopian tubes, perhaps as a result of previous pelvic infection. Alternatively, production of gonadotrophin hormones – follicle-stimulating hormone (FSH) and luteinizing hormone (LH) – needed for ovulation and implantation of the egg may be affected by illness or psychological stress.

If no simple explanation can be found, the man's semen will be analysed. If these tests show that abnormally low numbers of sperm are being produced, or if a large proportion of the sperm produced are unhealthy, drug treatment may be tried.

If no abnormality of sperm production is discovered, the woman will be given a thorough medical examination. Ovulation is monitored and blood tests may be performed to assess hormone levels. If ovulation does not occur, the woman may be offered drug treatment.

WHY THEY ARE USED

In men, the evidence is poor for treating low sperm production with gonadotrophins – FSH or human chorionic gonadotrophin (HCG) – or a pituitary-stimulating drug (for example, clomifene) and corticosteroids.

In women, drugs are useful in helping to achieve pregnancy only when a hormone defect inhibiting ovulation has been diagnosed. Treatment may continue for months and does not always result in pregnancy. Women in whom the pituitary gland is producing some FSH and LH may be given courses of clomifene for several days during each month. Usually, up to three courses may be tried. An effective dose produces ovulation 5 to 10 days after the last tablet is taken.

Clomifene may thicken the cervical mucus, impeding the passage of sperm, but the advantage of achieving ovulation outweighs the risk of this side effect. If treatment with clomifene fails to produce ovulation, or if a disorder of the pituitary gland prevents the production of FSH and LH, treatment with FSH and LH together, FSH alone, or HCG may be given. In menstruating women, FSH is started within the first 7 days of the menstrual cycle.

HOW THEY WORK

Ovulation (release of an egg) and implantation are governed by hormones produced by the pituitary gland. FSH stimulates ripening of the egg follicle. LH triggers ovulation and ensures that progesterone is produced to prepare the uterus for the implantation of the egg. Drugs for female infertility boost the actions of these hormones.

Fertility drugs raise the chance of ovulation by boosting levels of LH and FSH. Clomifene stimulates the pituitary gland to increase its output of these hormones. Artificially produced FSH and HCG mimic the action of naturally produced FSH and LH respectively. Both treatments, when successful, stimulate ovulation and implantation of the fertilized egg.

HOW THEY AFFECT YOU

Clomifene may produce hot flushes, nausea, headaches, and, rarely, ovarian cysts and visual disturbance, while HCG can cause tiredness, headaches, and mood changes. FSH can cause the ovaries to enlarge, producing abdominal discomfort. These drugs increase the likelihood of multiple births, usually twins.

DRUGS FOR ERECTILE DYSFUNCTION

Erectile dysfunction (commonly known as impotence) is a common male disorder defined as inability to achieve or maintain an erection. The penis contains three cylinders of erectile tissue: the two corpora cavernosa and the corpus spongiosum. Normally, when

a man is sexually aroused, the arteries in the penis relax and widen, allowing more blood than usual to flow into the organ, filling the corpora cavernosa and corpus spongiosum. As these tissues expand and harden, the veins that carry blood out of the penis are compressed, reducing outflow and resulting in an erection. In some forms of erectile dysfunction, this does not happen. Drugs can be used to increase blood flow into the penis to produce an erection.

Sildenafil, taken by mouth, not only increases the blood flow into the penis but also prevents the muscle wall from relaxing, so the blood does not drain out of the blood vessels and the penis remains erect.

Alprostadil is a prostaglandin drug that helps men achieve an erection by widening the blood vessels, but it must be injected directly into the penis, or applied into the urethra using a special pipette.

Apomorphine works indirectly through the hypothalamus.

COMMON DRUGS

Bromocriptine*, Buserelin, Cetrorelix, Chorionic gonadotrophin (HCG), Clomifene*, Follitropin (FSH), Ganirelix, Goserelin*, Lutropin (LH), Menopausal gonadotrophins (Menotrophin), Nafarelin, Tamoxifen*
Drugs for erectile dysfunction
Alprostadil, Apomorphine, Sildenafil*, Tadalafil, Papaverine, Vardenafil
* **See part 2**

Drugs used in labour

Normal labour has three stages. In the first stage, the uterus begins to contract, initially irregularly and then gradually more regularly and powerfully, while the cervix dilates until it is fully stretched. During the second stage, powerful contractions of the uterus push the baby down the mother's birth canal and out of her body. The third stage involves the delivery of the placenta.

Drugs may be required during one or more stages of labour for any of the following reasons: to induce or augment labour; to delay premature labour (see Uterine muscle relaxants, facing page); and to relieve pain. The administration of some drugs may be viewed as part of normal obstetric care; for example, the uterine stimulants ergometrine and oxytocin may be injected routinely before the third stage of labour to prevent excessive bleeding. Other drugs are administered only when the condition of the mother or baby requires intervention. The possible adverse effects of the drug on both mother and baby are always carefully balanced against the benefits.

DRUGS TO INDUCE OR AUGMENT LABOUR

Induction of labour may be advised when a doctor considers it risky for the health of the mother or baby for the pregnancy to continue – for example, if natural labour does not occur within two weeks of the due date or when a woman has pre-eclampsia. Other common reasons for inducing labour include premature rupture of the membrane surrounding the baby (breaking of the waters), slow growth of the baby due to poor nourishment by the placenta, or death of the fetus in the uterus.

When labour needs to be induced, oxytocin may be administered intravenously. Alternatively, a prostaglandin pessary may be given to soften and dilate the cervix. If these methods are ineffective or cannot be used because of potential adverse effects (see Risks and special precautions, below), a caesarean delivery may have to be performed.

Oxytocin may also be used to strengthen the force of contractions in labour that has started spontaneously but has not continued normally.

A combination of oxytocin and another uterine stimulant, ergometrine, is given to most women as the baby is being born or immediately following birth to prevent excessive bleeding after the delivery of the placenta. This combination encourages the uterus to contract after delivery, which restricts the flow of blood.

RISKS AND SPECIAL PRECAUTIONS

When oxytocin is used to induce labour, the dosage is carefully monitored throughout to prevent the possibility of excessively violent contractions. It is administered to women who have had surgery on the uterus only with careful monitoring. The drug is not known to affect the baby adversely. Ergometrine is not given to women who have suffered from high blood pressure during the course of pregnancy.

DRUGS USED FOR PAIN RELIEF

Opioid analgesics Pethidine, morphine, or other opioids may be given once active labour has been established (see Analgesics, p.9). Possible side effects for the mother include drowsiness, nausea, and vomiting. Opioid drugs may cause breathing difficulties for the new baby, but these problems may be reversed by the antidote naloxone.

Epidural anaesthesia This provides pain relief during labour and birth by numbing the nerves leading to the uterus and pelvic area. It is often used during a planned caesarean delivery, thus enabling the mother to be fully conscious for the birth.

An epidural involves the injection of a local anaesthetic drug (see p.11) into the epidural space between the spinal cord and the vertebrae. An epidural may block the mother's urge to push during the second stage, and a forceps delivery may be necessary. Headaches may occasionally occur following epidural anaesthesia.

Oxygen and nitrous oxide These gases are combined to produce a mixture that reduces the pain caused by contractions. During the first and second stages of labour, gas is self-administered by inhalation through a mouthpiece or mask. If it is used over too long a period, it may produce nausea, confusion, and dehydration in the mother.

Local anaesthetics These drugs are injected inside the vagina or near the vaginal opening and are used to numb sensation during forceps delivery, before an episiotomy (an incision made to enlarge the vaginal opening), and when stitches are necessary. Side effects are rare.

UTERINE MUSCLE RELAXANTS

When contractions of the uterus start before the 34th week of pregnancy, doctors usually advise bed rest and may also administer a drug that relaxes the muscles of the uterus, and thus halts labour. Initially, the drug is given in hospital by injection, but it may be continued orally at home. These drugs work by stimulating the sympathetic nervous system (see Autonomic nervous system, p.8) and may cause palpitations and anxiety in the mother. They have not been shown to have adverse effects on the baby.

DRUGS USED TO TERMINATE PREGNANCY

Drugs may be used in a hospital or clinic to terminate pregnancy up to 20 weeks, or to empty the uterus after the death of the baby. Mifepristone may be given first to sensitize the tissues before a prostaglandin drug is given to dilate the cervix. Before 14 weeks, the fetus is then removed under anaesthetic. After 14 weeks, labour is induced with a prostaglandin. These methods may be supplemented by oxytocin given by intravenous drip (see Drugs to induce or augment labour, previous page).

COMMON DRUGS

Prostaglandins Carboprost, Dinoprostone, Gemeprost, Misoprostol*

Pain relief Entonox® (oxygen and nitrous oxide), Fentanyl, Morphine*, Pethidine

Antiprogestogen Mifepristone

Uterine muscle relaxants Atosiban, Ritodrine, Salbutamol*, Terbutaline*

Uterine stimulants Ergometrine, Oxytocin

Local anaesthetics Bupivacaine, Lidocaine (lignocaine)

* See Part 2

Drugs used for urinary disorders

Urine is produced by the kidneys and stored in the bladder. As the urine accumulates, the bladder walls stretch and pressure within the bladder increases. Eventually, the stretching stimulates nerve endings that produce the urge to urinate. The ring of muscle (sphincter) around the bladder neck normally keeps the bladder closed until it is consciously relaxed, allowing urine to pass via the urethra out of the body.

A number of disorders can affect the urinary tract. The most common of these disorders are infection in the bladder (cystitis) or the urethra (urethritis), and loss of reliable control over urination (urinary incontinence). A less common problem is inability to expel urine (urinary retention). Drugs used to treat these problems include antibiotics and antibacterial drugs, analgesics, drugs to increase the acidity of the urine, and drugs that act on nerve control over the muscles of the bladder and sphincter.

DRUGS FOR URINARY INFECTION

Nearly all infections of the bladder are caused by bacteria. Symptoms include a continual urge to urinate, although often nothing is passed; pain on urinating; and pain in the lower abdomen.

Many antibiotics and antibacterials are used to treat urinary tract infections. Among the most widely used, because of their effectiveness, are cephalosporins, amoxicillin, and trimethoprim (see Antibiotics, p.62, and Antibacterial drugs, p.66).

Measures are also sometimes taken to increase the acidity of the urine, thereby making it hostile to bacteria. Ascorbic acid (vitamin C) and acid fruit juices have this effect, although making the urine less acidic with potassium or sodium citrate during an attack of cystitis helps to relieve the discomfort. Symptoms are commonly relieved within a few hours of the start of treatment.

For maximum effect, all drug treatments prescribed for urinary tract infections need to be accompanied by increased fluid intake.

DRUGS FOR URINARY INCONTINENCE

Urinary incontinence can occur for a several reasons. A weak sphincter muscle allows the involuntary passage of urine when abdominal pressure is raised by coughing or physical exertion. This is known as stress incontinence and commonly affects women who have had children. Urgency – the sudden need to urinate – stems from oversensitivity of the bladder muscle; small quantities of urine in the bladder stimulate the urge to urinate frequently.

Incontinence can also occur due to loss of nerve control in neurological disorders such as multiple sclerosis. In children, the inability to control urination at night (nocturnal enuresis) is also a form of urinary incontinence.

Drug treatment is not necessary or appropriate for all forms of incontinence. In stress incontinence, exercises to strengthen the pelvic floor muscles or surgery to tighten stretched ligaments may be effective. In urgency, regular emptying of the bladder can often avoid the need for medical intervention. Incontinence caused by loss of nerve control is unlikely to be helped by drug treatment. Frequency of urination in urgency may be reduced by anticholinergic and antispasmodic drugs. These drugs reduce nerve signals from the muscles in the bladder, thereby allowing greater volumes of urine to accumulate without stimulating the urge to pass urine.

Tricyclic antidepressants, such as imipramine, have a strong anticholinergic action and have been prescribed for nocturnal enuresis in children, but many doctors believe the risk of overdosage is unacceptable. Desmopressin, a synthetic derivative of antidiuretic hormone (see p.85), is also used to treat nocturnal enuresis.

DRUGS FOR URINARY RETENTION

Urinary retention is the inability to empty the bladder. This usually results from the failure of the bladder muscle to contract sufficiently to expel the accumulated urine. Possible causes include an enlarged prostate gland or tumour, or a long-standing neurological disorder. Some drugs can also cause urinary retention.

Most cases of urinary retention need to be relieved by inserting a tube (catheter) into the urethra. Surgery may be needed to prevent a recurrence of the problem.

Drugs that relax the sphincter or stimulate bladder contraction are now rarely used in the treatment of urinary retention, but two types of drug are used in the long-term management of prostatic enlargement: finasteride and alpha blockers. Finasteride prevents production of male hormones that stimulate prostatic growth, and alpha blockers, such as prazosin, tamsulosin, and terazosin, relax prostatic and urethral smooth muscle, thereby improving urine outflow. Long-term drug treatment of urinary retention can relieve symptoms and delay the need for surgery.

COMMON DRUGS

Antibiotics and antibacterials (see pp.62–66)

Anticholinergics Flavoxate, Imipramine*, Oxybutynin*, Propantheline, Propiverine, Solifenacin, Tolterodine*, Trospium

Parasympathomimetics Bethanechol, Distigmine

Alpha blockers Alfuzosin, Doxazosin*, Indoramin, Prazosin, Tamsulosin*, Terazosin

Other drugs Desmopressin*, Dimethyl sulfoxide, Duloxetine, Finasteride*, Potassium citrate, Sodium bicarbonate/citrate, Vitamin C

* See Part 2

EYES AND EARS

The eyes and ears are the two sense organs that provide us with the most information about the world around us. The eye is the organ of vision that converts light images into nerve signals, which are transmitted to the brain for interpretation. The ear not only provides the means by which sound is detected and communicated to the brain, but it also contains the organ of balance that tells the brain about the position and movement of the body. It is divided into three parts: the outer, middle, and inner ear.

WHAT CAN GO WRONG

The most common eye and ear disorders are infection and inflammation (sometimes caused by allergy). Many parts of the eye may be affected, notably the conjunctiva (the membrane that covers the front of the eye and lines the eyelids) and the iris. The middle and outer ear are more commonly affected by infection than the inner ear.

The eye may also be damaged by glaucoma, a disorder in which pressure of fluid within the eye builds up and may eventually threaten vision. Eye problems such as retinopathy (disease of the retina) or cataracts (clouding of the lens) may occur as a result of diabetes or for other reasons, but both conditions are now treatable. Disorders for which no drug treatment is appropriate are beyond the scope of this book.

Other disorders affecting the ear include build-up of wax (cerumen) in the outer ear canal and disturbances to the balance mechanism within the ear (vertigo and Ménière's disease, see Anti-emetics, p.21).

WHY DRUGS ARE USED

Doctors usually prescribe antibiotics (see p.62) to clear ear and eye infections. These may be given by mouth or topically. Topical eye and ear preparations may contain a corticosteroid (see p.80) to reduce inflammation. When inflammation has been caused by allergy, antihistamines (see p.58) may also be taken. Decongestant drugs (see p.26) are often prescribed to help clear the eustachian tube in middle-ear infections. Various drugs are used to reduce fluid pressure in glaucoma. These include diuretics (see p.32), beta blockers (see p.30), and miotics (to narrow the pupil). In other cases, the pupil may need to be widened by mydriatic drugs. (See also Drugs affecting the pupil, p.116.)

MAJOR DRUG GROUPS
◆ Drugs for glaucoma
◆ Drugs affecting the pupil
◆ Drugs for ear disorders

Drugs for glaucoma

Glaucoma is the name given to a group of conditions in which the pressure in the eye builds up to an abnormally high level. This compresses the blood vessels that supply the nerve connecting the eye to the brain (optic nerve) and may result in irreversible nerve damage and permanent loss of vision.

In the most common type, called chronic (or open-angle) glaucoma, reduced drainage of fluid from the eye causes pressure inside the eye to build up slowly. Progressive reduction in the peripheral field of vision may take months or years to be noticed.

Acute (or closed-angle) glaucoma occurs when drainage of fluid is suddenly blocked by the iris. Fluid pressure usually builds up quite suddenly, blurring vision in the affected eye. The eye becomes red and painful, and a headache and sometimes vomiting also occur. The main attack is often preceded by milder warning attacks, such as seeing haloes around lights in the previous weeks or months. Elderly far-sighted people are particularly at risk of developing acute glaucoma. The angle may also narrow suddenly following injury or after taking certain drugs such as anticholinergic drugs. Closed-angle glaucoma may develop more slowly (chronic closed-angle glaucoma).

Drugs are used in the treatment of both types of glaucoma. These include miotics (see Drugs affecting the pupil, p.116), beta blockers (p.30), and the diuretics (p.32), carbonic anhydrase inhibitors and osmotics.

WHY THEY ARE USED

Chronic (open-angle) glaucoma In this form of glaucoma, drugs are used to reduce pressure inside the eye. These drugs will prevent further deterioration of vision, but they cannot restore damage that has already been sustained and may therefore be required lifelong. In most patients, treatment is begun with eye drops containing a beta blocker to reduce fluid production inside the eye. Miotic eye drops to constrict the pupil and improve fluid drainage may be given. The prostaglandin analogues, such as latanoprost, are also used to increase fluid outflow. If none of these drugs is effective, dipivefrine, apraclonidine, or brimonidine may be tried to reduce secretion and help outflow. Sometimes a carbonic anhydrase inhibitor such as acetazolamide or dorzolamide may be given to reduce fluid production. Laser treatment and surgery may also be used to improve fluid drainage from the eye.

Acute (closed-angle) glaucoma In acute glaucoma immediate medical treatment is required in order to prevent total loss of vision. Drugs are used initially to bring down the pressure within the eye. Laser treatment or surgery is then carried out to prevent a recurrence of the problem so that long-term drug treatment is seldom required.

Acetazolamide is often the first drug administered when the condition is diagnosed. It may be injected into a vein for rapid effect and thereafter administered by mouth. Frequent applications of eye drops containing pilocarpine or carbachol are given. An osmotic diuretic such as mannitol may be administered. This draws fluid out of all body tissues, including the eye, and reduces pressure within the eye.

HOW THEY WORK

Drugs for glaucoma act in various ways to reduce the pressure of fluid in the eye. Miotics improve drainage of fluid out of the eye. In chronic glaucoma, this is achieved by increasing the outflow of aqueous humour via the drainage channel called the trabecular meshwork. In acute glaucoma, the pupil-constricting effect of miotics pulls the iris away from the drainage channel, allowing the aqueous humour to flow out in the normal way. Prostaglandin analogues act by increasing fluid flow from the eye. Beta blockers and carbonic anhydrase inhibitors act on the fluid-producing cells inside the eye to reduce output of aqueous humour. Sympathomimetics such as brimonidine and apraclonidine are also thought to act partly in this way and partly by improving fluid drainage.

HOW THEY AFFECT YOU

Drugs for acute glaucoma relieve pain and other symptoms within a few hours of their being used. The benefits of treatment in chronic glaucoma, however, may not be immediately apparent since treatment is only able to halt a further deterioration of vision.

People receiving miotic eye drops are likely to notice darkening of vision and difficulty in seeing in the dark. Increased shortsightedness may be noticeable. Some miotics also cause irritation and redness of the eyes.

Beta blocker eye drops have few day-to-day side effects but carry risks for a few people (see below). Acetazolamide usually causes increased frequency of urination and thirst. Nausea and general malaise are also common.

RISKS AND SPECIAL PRECAUTIONS

Miotics can cause alteration in vision. Beta blockers are absorbed into the body and can affect the lungs, heart, and circulation. As a result, a cardioselective beta blocker, such as betaxolol, is prescribed with caution to people with asthma or certain circulatory disorders and, in some cases, such drugs are withheld altogether. The amount of the drug absorbed into the body can be reduced by pressing on the lacrimal (tear) duct in the corner of the eye while applying the number of eye drops prescribed by your doctor. Acetazolamide may cause troublesome adverse effects, including tingling of the hands and feet, the formation of kidney stones, and, rarely, kidney damage. People with existing kidney problems are not usually given this drug.

COMMON DRUGS

Miotics Carbachol, Pilocarpine*
Carbonic anhydrase inhibitors Acetazolamide, Brinzolamide, Dorzolamide*
Prostaglandin analogues Bimatoprost, Latanoprost*, Travoprost

Beta blockers Betaxolol, Carteolol, Levobunolol, Metipranolol, Timolol*
Sympathomimetics Apraclonidine, Brimonidine, Dipivefrine, Guanethidine
* See Part 2

Drugs affecting the pupil

The pupil of the eye is the circular opening in the centre of the iris (the coloured part of the eye) through which light enters. It continually changes in size to adjust to variations in the intensity of light; in bright light it becomes quite small (constricts), but in dim light the pupil enlarges (dilates).

Eye drops containing drugs that act on the pupil are widely used by specialists. There are two categories: mydriatics, which dilate the pupil, and miotics, which constrict it.

WHY THEY ARE USED

Mydriatics are most often used to allow the doctor to view the inside of the eye – particularly the retina, the optic nerve head, and the blood vessels that supply the retina. Many of these drugs cause a temporary paralysis of the eye's focusing mechanism, a state called cycloplegia. Cycloplegia is sometimes induced to help determine the presence of any focusing errors, especially in babies and young children. By producing cycloplegia, it is possible to determine the precise optical prescription required for a small child, especially in the case of a squint.

Dilation of the pupil is part of the treatment for uveitis, an inflammatory disease of the iris and focusing muscle. In uveitis, the inflamed iris may stick to the lens, severely damaging the eye. This complication can be prevented by early dilation of the pupil so that the iris is no longer in contact with the lens.

Constriction of the pupil with miotic drugs is often required in the treatment of glaucoma (see p.114). Miotics can also be used to restore the pupil to a normal size after dilation is induced by mydriatics.

HOW THEY WORK

The size of the pupil is controlled by two separate sets of muscles in the iris, the circular muscle and the radial muscle. The two sets of muscles are governed by separate branches of the autonomic nervous system (see p.8): the radial muscle is controlled by the sympathetic nervous system, and the circular muscle is controlled by the parasympathetic nervous system.

Individual mydriatic and miotic drugs affect different branches of the autonomic nervous system, and cause the pupil to dilate or contract, depending on the type of drug.

HOW THEY AFFECT YOU

Mydriatic drugs – especially the long-acting types – impair the ability to focus the eye(s) for several hours after use. This interferes particularly with close activities such as reading. Bright light may cause discomfort. Miotics often interfere with night vision and may cause temporary short sight.

Normally, these eye drops produce few serious adverse effects.

Sympathomimetic mydriatics may raise blood pressure and are used with caution in people with hypertension or heart disease. Miotics may irritate the eyes, but rarely cause generalized effects.

ARTIFICIAL TEAR PREPARATIONS

Tears are continually produced to keep the front of the eye covered with a thin, moist film. This is essential for clear vision and for keeping the front of the eye free from dirt and other irritants. In some conditions, known collectively as dry eye syndromes (for example, Sjögren's syndrome), inadequate tear production may make the eyes feel dry and sore. Sore eyes can also occur in disorders where the eyelids do not close properly, causing the eye to become dry.

Why they are used Since prolonged deficiency of natural tears can damage the cornea, regular application of artificial tears in the form of eye drops is recommended for all of the conditions described above. Artificial tears may also be used to provide temporary relief from any feeling of discomfort and dryness in the eye caused by irritants or exposure to wind or sun, or following the initial wearing of contact lenses.

Although artificial tears are non-irritating, they often contain a preservative (such as thiomersal or benzalkonium chloride) that may cause irritation. This risk of irritation is increased for wearers of soft contact lenses, who should ask their optician for advice before using any type of eye drops.

COMMON DRUGS
Sympathomimetic mydriatics Phenylephrine
Miotics Carbachol, Pilocarpine*
Anticholinergic mydriatics Atropine*,
Cyclopentolate, Homatropine, Tropicamide
* **See Part 2**

Drugs for ear disorders

Inflammation and infection of the outer and middle ear are the most common ear disorders treated with drugs. Drug treatment for Ménière's disease, which affects the inner ear, is described under Anti-emetics, p.21.

The type of drug treatment given for ear inflammation depends on the cause of the trouble and the site affected.

INFLAMMATION OF THE OUTER EAR
Inflammation of the external ear canal (otitis externa) can be caused by eczema or by a bacterial or fungal infection. The risk of inflammation is increased by swimming in dirty water, an accumulation of wax in the ear, or scratching or poking too frequently at the ear.

Symptoms vary, but in many cases there is itching, pain (which may be severe if there is a boil in the ear canal), tenderness, and possibly some loss of hearing. If the ear is infected there will probably be a discharge.
Drug treatment A corticosteroid (see p.80) in the form of ear drops may be used to treat inflammation of the outer ear when there is no infection. Aluminium acetate solution, as drops or applied on a piece of gauze, may also be used. Relief is usually obtained within a day or two. Prolonged use of corticosteroids is not advisable because they may reduce the ear's resistance to infection.

If there is both inflammation and infection, your doctor may prescribe ear drops containing an antibiotic (see p.62) combined with a corticosteroid to relieve the inflammation. Usually, a combination of antibiotics is prescribed to make the treatment effective

against a wide range of bacteria. Commonly used antibiotics include framycetin, neomycin, and polymyxin B. These are not used if the eardrum is perforated and are not usually applied for long periods because they can irritate the skin that lines the ear canal.

Sometimes an antibiotic given as drops is not effective, and another type of antibiotic may also have to be taken by mouth.

INFECTION OF THE MIDDLE EAR
Infection of the middle ear (otitis media) often causes severe pain and hearing loss. It is particularly common in young children in whom infecting organisms are able to spread easily into the middle ear from the nose or throat via the eustachian tube.

Viral infections of the middle ear usually cure themselves and are less serious than those caused by bacteria, which are treated with antibiotics given by mouth or injection. Bacterial infections often cause the eustachian tube to swell and become blocked. When a blockage occurs, pus builds up in the middle ear and puts pressure on the eardrum, which may perforate as a result.
Drug treatment Doctors usually prescribe a decongestant (see p.26) or antihistamine (see p.58) to reduce swelling in the eustachian tube, thus allowing the pus to drain out of the middle ear. Usually, an antibiotic is also given by mouth to clear the infection.

Although antibiotics are not effective against viral infections, it is often difficult to distinguish between a viral and a bacterial infection of the middle ear, so your doctor may prescribe an antibiotic as a precautionary measure. Paracetamol, an analgesic (see p.9), may be given to relieve pain.

COMMON DRUGS
Antibiotic and antibacterial ear drops
Chloramphenicol*, Clioquinol, Clotrimazole*,
Framycetin, Gentamicin*, Neomycin
Decongestants Ephedrine*, Oxymetazoline,
Xylometazoline
Corticosteroids Betamethasone*, Dexamethasone*,
Flumetasone, Hydrocortisone*, Prednisolone*,
Triamcinolone
Other drugs Aluminium acetate, Antihistamines (see
p.58), Choline salicylate
* **See Part 2**

SKIN

The skin waterproofs, cushions, and protects the rest of the body and is, in fact, its largest organ. It provides a barrier against innumerable infections and infestations, it helps the body to retain its vital fluids, it plays a major role in temperature control, and it houses the sensory nerves of touch.

The skin consists of two main layers: a thin, tough top layer, the epidermis, and below it a thicker layer, the dermis. The epidermis also has two layers: the skin surface, or stratum corneum (horny layer) consisting of dead cells, and below, a layer of active cells. The cells in the active layer divide and eventually die, maintaining the horny layer. Living cells produce keratin, which toughens the epidermis and is the basic substance of hair and nails. Some living cells in the epidermis produce melanin, a pigment released in increased amounts following exposure to sunlight.

The dermis contains different types of nerve ending for sensing pain, pressure, and temperature; sweat glands to cool the body; sebaceous glands to lubricate and waterproof the skin; and white blood cells that help to keep the skin clear of infection.

WHAT CAN GO WRONG

Most skin complaints are not serious but may be distressing if visible. They include infection, inflammation and irritation, infestation by skin parasites, and changes in skin structure and texture (such as psoriasis, eczema, and acne).

WHY DRUGS ARE USED

Skin problems often resolve without drug treatment. Over-the-counter preparations containing drugs are available, but their use is generally discouraged without medical supervision because they could aggravate some skin conditions if used inappropriately. Prescribed drugs, including antibiotics (see p.62) for bacterial infections, antifungals (see p.76) for fungal infections, agents for skin parasites (see p.122), and topical corticosteroids (see p.120) for inflammatory conditions, are often highly effective, however. Specialized drugs are available for conditions such as psoriasis and acne.

Many drugs are topical medications, but they must be used carefully because, like oral drugs, they can also cause adverse effects.

MAJOR DRUG GROUPS
◆ Antipruritics
◆ Topical corticosteroids
◆ Anti-infective skin preparations
◆ Drugs to treat skin parasites
◆ Drugs used to treat acne
◆ Drugs for psoriasis
◆ Treatments for eczema
◆ Drugs for dandruff
◆ Drugs for hair loss
◆ Sunscreens

Antipruritics

Itching (irritation of the skin that creates the urge to scratch), also known as pruritus, most often occurs as a result of minor physical irritation or chemical changes in the skin caused by disease, inflammation, allergy, or exposure to irritant substances. People differ in their tolerance to itching, and a person's threshold can be altered by stress and other psychological factors.

Itching is a common symptom of many skin disorders, including eczema and psoriasis and allergic conditions such as urticaria (hives). It is also sometimes caused by a localized fungal infection or parasitic infestation. Diseases such as chickenpox may also cause itching. Less commonly, itching may also occur as a symptom of diabetes mellitus, jaundice, kidney failure, or drug reactions.

In many cases, generalized itching is caused by dry skin. Itching in particular parts of the body is often caused by a specific problem. For example, itching around the anus (pruritus ani) may result from haemorrhoids or worm infestation, while genital itching in women (pruritus vulvae) may be caused by vaginal infection or, in older women, may be the result of a hormone deficiency.

Although scratching frequently provides temporary relief, it can often increase skin inflammation and make the condition worse.

Continued scratching of an area of irritated skin may occasionally lead to a vicious cycle of scratching and itching that continues long after the original cause has been removed.

Many types of medicine, including soothing topical preparations and drugs taken by mouth, relieve irritation. The main drugs in antipruritic products are local anaesthetics (see p.11), topical corticosteroids (see p.120), and antihistamines (see p.58). Simple emollient or cooling creams or ointments, which contain no active ingredients, are often recommended, especially if there is associated dry skin.

WHY THEY ARE USED

For mild itching arising from sunburn, urticaria, or insect bites, a cooling lotion such as calamine, perhaps containing menthol, phenol, or camphor, may be the most appropriate treatment. Local anaesthetic creams are sometimes helpful for small areas of irritation, such as insect bites, but are unsuitable for widespread itching. The itching caused by dry skin is often soothed by a simple emollient. Avoiding excessive bathing and using moisturizing bath oils may also help.

Severe itching in eczema or other inflammatory skin conditions may be treated with a topical corticosteroid preparation. When the irritation prevents sleep, a doctor may prescribe an antihistamine for use at night to promote sleep as well as to relieve itching (see also sleeping drugs, p.11). Antihistamines are also often included in topical preparations for the relief of skin irritation, but their effectiveness when administered in this way is doubtful. For the treatment of pruritus ani, see drugs for rectal and anal disorders (p.47). Post-menopausal pruritus vulvae may be helped by vaginal creams containing oestrogen (see female sex hormones (p.88). Itching that is caused by an underlying illness cannot be helped by skin creams and requires treatment for the principal disorder.

HOW THEY WORK

Irritation of the skin causes the release of substances such as histamine, which cause blood vessels to dilate and fluid to accumulate under the skin; this results in itching and inflammation. Antipruritic drugs act either by reducing inflammation and thus irritation, or by numbing the nerve impulses that transmit sensation to the brain.

Corticosteroids applied to the skin reduce itching caused by allergy within a few days, but the cream's soothing effect may produce an immediate improvement. The drugs pass into the underlying tissues and blood vessels and reduce the release of histamine, the chemical that causes itching and inflammation.

Antihistamines act within a few hours to reduce allergy-related skin inflammation. Applied to the skin, they pass into the underlying tissue and block the effects of histamine on the blood vessels beneath the skin. Taken by mouth, they also act on the brain to reduce the perception of irritation.

Local anaesthetics absorbed through the skin numb the transmission of signals from the nerves in the skin to the brain.

Soothing and emollient creams such as calamine lotion, applied to the skin surface, reduce inflammation and itching by cooling the skin. Emollient creams lubricate the skin surface and prevent dryness.

RISKS AND SPECIAL PRECAUTIONS

The main risk from any antipruritic, except simple emollient and soothing preparations, is skin irritation, and therefore aggravated itching, caused by prolonged or heavy use. Antihistamine and local anaesthetic creams are especially likely to cause a reaction, and must be stopped if they do so. Antihistamines taken by mouth to relieve itching are likely to cause drowsiness. The special risks of topical corticosteroids are discussed on p.120.

Because itching can be a symptom of many underlying conditions, self-treatment should be continued for no longer than a week before seeking medical advice.

COMMON DRUGS

Antihistamines (see also p.58), Alimemazine, Chlorphenamine*, Diphenhydramine, Hydroxyzine, Mepyramine

Corticosteroids (see also p.80), Hydrocortisone*

Local anaesthetics Benzocaine, Lidocaine, Tetracaine

Emollient and cooling preparations Aqueous cream, Calamine lotion, Cold cream, Emulsifying ointment

Other drugs Colestyramine*, Crotamiton, Doxepin

* See Part 2

Topical corticosteroids

Corticosteroid drugs (which are often simply referred to as steroids) are related to the hormones that are produced by the adrenal glands. For a full description of these drugs, see p.80. Topical preparations containing a corticosteroid drug are often used to treat skin conditions in which inflammation is a prominent symptom.

WHY THEY ARE USED

Corticosteroid creams and ointments are most commonly given to relieve the itching and inflammation that are associated with skin diseases such as eczema and dermatitis. These preparations may also be prescribed for the treatment of psoriasis (see p.124). Corticosteroids do not affect the underlying cause of skin irritation, and the condition is therefore likely to recur unless the substance (allergen or irritant) that has provoked the irritation is removed, or the underlying condition is treated.

A doctor might not prescribe a corticosteroid as the initial treatment, preferring instead to try a topical medicine that has fewer adverse effects (see Antipruritics, p.118).

In most cases, treatment is started with a preparation containing a low concentration of a mild corticosteroid drug. A stronger preparation may be prescribed subsequently if the first product is ineffective.

HOW THEY WORK

Irritation of the skin, caused by exposure to allergens or irritant factors, provokes white blood cells to release substances that dilate the blood vessels, making the skin hot, red, and swollen.

Applied to the skin surface, corticosteroids are absorbed into the underlying tissue. There, they inhibit the action of the substances that cause inflammation, allowing the blood vessels to return to normal and reducing the swelling.

HOW THEY AFFECT YOU

Because corticosteroids prevent the release of chemicals that trigger inflammation, conditions that are treated with these drugs improve within a few days of starting the drug. Applied topically, corticosteroids rarely cause side effects. There are, however, certain risks associated with stronger drugs used in high concentrations.

RISKS AND SPECIAL PRECAUTIONS

Prolonged use of potent corticosteroids in high concentrations usually leads to permanent skin changes – most commonly skin thinning, sometimes resulting in permanent stretch marks. Applying them sparingly and only to the affected area minimizes this risk. Fine blood vessels under the skin surface may become prominent (a condition known as telangiectasia). Because the skin on the face is especially vulnerable to such damage, only mild corticosteroids should be prescribed for use on the face. Dark-skinned people sometimes suffer a temporary reduction in pigmentation at the site of application.

When topical corticosteroids have been used for a prolonged period, abrupt discontinuation can cause rebound erythroderma (reddening of the skin). This may be avoided by gradual dosage reduction. Corticosteroids suppress the body's immune system (see p.80), thereby increasing the risk of infection. For this reason, they are never used alone to treat skin inflammation caused by bacterial or fungal infection. However, they are sometimes included in a topical preparation also containing an antibiotic or antifungal agent (see Anti-infective skin preparations, below).

COMMON DRUGS

Very potent Clobetasol*, Halcinonide
Potent Beclometasone*, Betamethasone*, Fluocinolone, Fluocinonide, Fluticasone*, Mometasone*, Triamcinolone
Moderate Alclometasone, Clobetasone, Fludroxycortide, Fluocortolone
Mild Hydrocortisone*
* See Part 2

Anti-infective skin preparations

The skin is the body's first line of defence against infection. Yet the skin can also become infected itself, especially if the outer layer (epidermis) is damaged by a burn, cut, scrape, insect bite, or an inflammatory skin condition – for example, eczema or dermatitis.

Several different types of organism may infect the skin, including bacteria, viruses, fungi, and yeasts. This section concentrates on topical drugs for bacterial skin infections and includes antiseptics, antibiotics, and other antibacterial agents. Infection by other organisms is covered elsewhere (see Antiviral drugs, p.69, Antifungal drugs, p.76, and Drugs used to treat skin parasites, p.122).

WHY THEY ARE USED

Bacterial infection of a skin wound can usually be prevented by thorough cleansing of the damaged area and the application of antiseptic creams or lotions. If infection does occur, the wound usually becomes inflamed and swollen, and pus may form. If you develop these signs, you should see your doctor. The usual treatment for a wound infection is an antibiotic taken orally, although often an antibiotic cream is also prescribed.

An antibiotic or antibacterial skin cream may also be used to prevent infection when your doctor considers this to be a particular risk (for example, in the case of severe burns).

Other skin disorders in which topical antibiotics may be prescribed include impetigo and infected eczema, bedsores, and nappy rash.

Often, a preparation containing two or more antibiotics is used to ensure that all bacteria are eradicated. The antibiotics selected for inclusion in topical preparations are usually drugs, such as aminoglycosides, that are poorly absorbed through the skin. Thus the drug remains concentrated on the surface and in the skin's upper layers where it is intended to have its effect. However, if the infection is deep under the skin, or is causing fever and malaise, antibiotics may need to be given by mouth or injection.

RISKS AND SPECIAL PRECAUTIONS

Any topical antibiotic product can irritate the skin or cause an allergic reaction. Irritation is sometimes provoked by another ingredient of the preparation rather than the active drug, such as a preservative contained in the product. An allergic reaction causing swelling and reddening of the skin is more likely to be caused by the antibiotic itself. Any adverse reaction of this kind should be reported to your doctor, who may substitute another drug, or a different preparation.

Always follow your doctor's instructions on how long the treatment with antibiotics should be continued. Stopping too soon may cause the infection to flare up again.

Never use a skin preparation that has been prescribed for someone else since it may aggravate your condition. Always throw away any unused medication.

BASES FOR SKIN PREPARATIONS

Drugs applied to the skin are usually contained in a preparation known as a base (or vehicle), such as a cream, lotion, ointment, or paste. Many bases are beneficial on their own.

Creams Cosmetically more acceptable and easier to apply, these have an emollient effect. They are usually composed of an oil-in-water emulsion and are used in the treatment of dry skin disorders, such as psoriasis and dry eczema. They may contain other ingredients, such as camphor or menthol.

Barrier preparations These may be creams or ointments. They protect the skin against water and irritating substances, and may be used for nappy rash and to protect the skin around an open sore. They may contain powders and water-repellent substances, such as silicones.

Lotions These thin, semi-liquid preparations are often used to cool and soothe inflamed skin. They are most suitable for use on large, hairy areas. Preparations called shake lotions contain fine powder that remains on the skin surface when the liquid has evaporated. They are used to encourage scabs to form.

Ointments These are usually greasy and are suitable for treating wet (weeping) eczema and very dry chronic lesions.

Pastes These are ointments containing large amounts of finely powdered solids such as starch or zinc oxide. Pastes protect the skin and absorb unwanted moisture. They are used for skin conditions that affect clearly defined areas, such as psoriasis.

Collodions These are preparations that, when applied to damaged areas of the skin such as ulcers and minor wounds, dry to form a protective film. They are sometimes used to keep a dissolved drug in contact with the skin.

COMMON DRUGS

Antibiotics Bacitracin, Colistin, Framycetin, Fusidic acid, Gramicidin, Mupirocin, Neomycin, Polymyxin B

Antiseptics and other antibacterials Cetrimide, Chlorhexidine, Hexachlorophene, Metronidazole*, Nystatin*, Oxytetracycline, Povidone iodine, Silver sulfadiazine, Triclosan

* See Part 2

Drugs to treat skin parasites

Mites and lice are the most common parasites that live on the skin. One common mite causes the skin disease scabies. The mite burrows into the skin and lays eggs, causing intense itching. Scratching the affected area results in bleeding and scab formation, as well as increasing the risk of infection.

There are three types of lice, each of which infests a different part of the human body: the head louse, the body (or clothes) louse, and the crab louse, which often infests the pubic areas but is also sometimes found on other hairy areas such as the eyebrows. All of these lice cause itching and lay eggs (nits) that look like white grains attached to hairs.

Both mites and lice are passed on by direct contact with an infected person (during sexual intercourse in the case of pubic lice) or, particularly in the case of body lice, by contact with infected bedding or clothing.

The drugs most often used to eliminate skin parasites are insecticides that kill both the adult insects and their eggs. The most effective drugs for scabies are malathion and permethrin; benzyl benzoate is occasionally used. Very severe scabies may require oral ivermectin as well. For lice infestations, carbaryl, malathion, permethrin, and phenothrin are used.

WHY THEY ARE USED

Skin parasites do not represent a serious threat to health, but their prompt eradication is needed since they can cause severe irritation and spread rapidly if left untreated. Drugs are used to eradicate them from the body, but bedding and clothing should be disinfected to avoid the possibility of reinfestation.

ELIMINATING PARASITES FROM BEDDING AND CLOTHING

Most skin parasites may also infest bedding and clothing that has been next to an infected person's skin. To avoid reinfestation following treatment of the body, any insects and eggs lodged in the bedding or clothing must also be eradicated.

Washing Because all skin parasites are killed by heat, washing any affected items of clothing and bedding in hot water and drying them in a hot tumble dryer is an effective and convenient method of dealing with the problem.

Non-washable items Items that cannot be washed should be isolated in plastic bags. The insects and their eggs cannot survive for long without their human hosts and die within days. The length of time they can survive, and therefore the period of isolation, varies depending on the type of parasite.

HOW THEY ARE USED

Lotions for the treatment of scabies are applied to the whole body (except the head and neck) after a bath or shower. Many people find these lotions messy to use, but they should not be washed off for 12 hours (malathion) or 48 hours (benzyl benzoate), otherwise they will not be effective. It is probably most convenient to apply malathion before going to bed. The lotion may then be washed off the following morning.

Two treatments one week apart are normally sufficient to remove the scabies mites. However, the itch associated with scabies may persist after the mite has been removed, so it may be necessary to use a soothing cream or medication containing an antipruritic drug (see p.118) to ease this. People who have direct skin-to-skin contact with a sufferer from scabies, such as family members and sexual partners, should also be treated with antiparasitic preparations at the same time. Head and pubic lice infestations are usually treated by applying a preparation of one of the products and washing it off with water when and as instructed by the leaflet given with the preparation. If the skin has become infected as a result of scratching, a topical antibiotic (see Anti-infective skin preparations, p.120) may also be prescribed.

RISKS AND SPECIAL PRECAUTIONS

Lotions prescribed to control parasites can cause intense irritation and stinging if they are allowed to come into contact with the eyes, mouth, or other moist membranes. Therefore, lotions and shampoos should be applied carefully, following the instructions of your doctor or the manufacturer.

Because antiparasitic drugs are topical, they do not usually have generalized effects. Nevertheless, it is important not to apply these preparations more often than directed.

COMMON DRUGS

Benzyl benzoate, Carbaryl*, Crotamiton, Dimeticone, Ivermectin, Malathion*, Permethrin*, Phenothrin
* See Part 2

Drugs used to treat acne

Acne, known medically as acne vulgaris, is a common condition caused by excess production of the skin's natural oil (sebum), leading to blockage of hair follicles. It chiefly affects adolescents but it may occur at any age, due to certain drugs, exposure to industrial chemicals, oily cosmetics, or hot, humid conditions.

Acne primarily affects the face, neck, back, and chest. The primary symptoms are blackheads, papules (inflamed spots), and pustules (raised pus-filled spots with a white centre). Mild acne may produce only blackheads and an occasional papule or pustule. Moderate cases are characterized by larger numbers of pustules and papules. In severe cases of acne, painful, inflamed cysts also develop. These can cause permanent pitting and scarring.

Medication for acne can be divided into two groups: topical preparations applied directly to the skin and systemic treatments taken by mouth.

WHY THEY ARE USED

Mild acne usually does not need medical treatment. It can be controlled by regular washing and by moderate exposure to sunlight or ultraviolet light. Over-the-counter antibacterial soaps and lotions are limited in use and may cause irritation.

When a doctor or dermatologist thinks acne is severe enough to need medical treatment, he or she usually recommends a topical preparation containing benzoyl peroxide or salicylic acid. If this does not produce an improvement, preparations containing tretinoin (a drug related to vitamin A), azelaic acid, or the antibiotics clindamycin, erythromycin, or tetracycline may be prescribed.

If acne is severe or does not respond to topical treatments, a doctor may prescribe antibiotics by mouth (usually tetracycline or minocycline). If these are unsuccessful, the more powerful vitamin A-like drug isotretinoin, taken by mouth, may be prescribed.

Oestrogen drugs may have a beneficial effect on acne. A woman with acne who also needs contraception may be given an oestrogen-containing oral contraceptive (see p.105). In severe cases, a preparation containing an oestrogen and cyproterone (a drug that opposes male sex hormones) may be prescribed.

HOW THEY WORK

Drugs used to treat acne act in different ways. Some have a keratolytic effect – that is, they loosen the dead cells on the skin surface. Others work by countering bacterial activity in the skin or reducing sebum production.

Topical preparations, such as benzoyl peroxide, salicylic acid, and tretinoin, have a keratolytic effect. Benzoyl peroxide also has an antibacterial effect. Topical or systemic tetracyclines reduce bacteria but may also have a direct anti-inflammatory effect. Isotretinoin reduces sebum production, soothes inflammation, and helps to unblock hair follicles.

HOW THEY AFFECT YOU

Keratolytic preparations often make the skin sore, especially at the start of treatment. If this persists, a change to a milder preparation may be recommended. Day-to-day side effects are rare with antibiotics. Treatment with isotretinoin often causes dry and scaly skin, particularly on the lips. The skin may become itchy and some hair loss may occur.

RISKS AND SPECIAL PRECAUTIONS

Antibiotics in skin ointments may, in rare cases, provoke an allergic reaction requiring discontinuation of treatment. The tetracyclines, some of the most commonly used antibiotics for acne, have the advantage of being effective both topically and systemically. However, they are not suitable for use by mouth in pregnancy since they can affect the bones and teeth of the developing baby.

Isotretinoin sometimes increases blood lipid levels. More seriously, it is known to damage a developing baby if taken during pregnancy. Women taking this drug must be sure to avoid conception for one month before, during, and for one month after, treatment.

COMMON DRUGS

Topical treatments Adapalene, Azelaic acid, Benzoyl peroxide*, Isotretinoin*, Nicotinamide (Niacin)*, Salicylic acid, Tretinoin

Oral and topical antibiotics Clindamycin, Doxycycline*, Erythromycin*, Minocycline*, Tetracycline*, Trimethoprim*

Other oral drugs Co-cyprindiol (women only), Isotretinoin*

* See Part 2

Drugs for psoriasis

The skin is constantly being renewed; as fast as dead cells in the outer layer (epidermis) are shed, they are replaced by cells from the base of the epidermis. Psoriasis occurs when production of new cells increases while shedding of old cells remains normal. As a result, the live skin cells accumulate and produce patches of inflamed, thickened skin covered by silvery scales. In some cases, the affected area is extensive and causes severe embarrassment and physical discomfort. Psoriasis may occasionally be accompanied by arthritis, in which the joints become swollen and painful.

The underlying cause of psoriasis is not known. The disorder usually first occurs between the ages of 10 and 30 and recurs throughout life. Outbreaks may be triggered by stress, skin damage, drugs, and physical illness. Psoriasis can also recur as a consequence of the withdrawal of corticosteroid drugs.

There is no complete cure for psoriasis. Simple measures, including careful sunbathing or using an ultraviolet lamp, may help to clear mild psoriasis. An emollient cream (see Antipruritics, p.118) often soothes the irritation. When such measures fail to provide adequate relief, additional drug therapy is needed.

WHY THEY ARE USED

Drugs are used to decrease the size of affected skin areas and to reduce scaling and inflammation. Mild and moderate psoriasis are usually treated with a topical preparation. Coal tar preparations, which are available in the form of creams, pastes, or bath additives, are often helpful. Dithranol is also widely used. Applied to the affected areas, the preparation is left for a few minutes or overnight (depending on the product), before being washed off. Both dithranol and coal tar can stain clothes and bed linen. If these agents alone do not produce adequate benefit, ultraviolet light therapy in the form of regulated exposure to natural sunlight or to ultraviolet lamps (UVB) may be advised. Salicylic acid may be applied to help remove thick scale and crusts, especially from the scalp.

Topical corticosteroids (see p.120) may be used in difficult cases that do not respond to those treatments. They are particularly useful for the skinfold areas and may be given to counter irritation caused by dithranol. If psoriasis is very severe and other treatments have failed, specialist treatment may include more powerful drugs, such as oral vitamin A derivatives (acitretin) in courses of about six months, methotrexate (p.308), an anticancer drug, vitamin D analogues such as calcipotriol (p.167), infliximab (p.268), a monoclonal antibody (see p.97), and PUVA (below).

PUVA

PUVA is the combined use of a psoralen drug (methoxsalen) and ultraviolet A light (UVA). The psoralen is applied topically or taken by mouth; then, some hours later, the skin is exposed to UVA, which enhances the effect of the drug on skin cells. The drug is activated by exposure of the skin to the ultraviolet light; it acts on the cell's genetic material (DNA) to regulate its rate of division.

This therapy is given two to three times a week and produces an improvement within about four to six weeks. Possible adverse effects include nausea, itching, and painful reddening of normal areas of skin. More seriously, there is a risk of premature skin ageing and a long-term risk of skin cancer, particularly in fair-skinned people. For these reasons, PUVA therapy is generally recommended only for severe psoriasis, when other treatments have failed.

HOW THEY WORK

Dithranol and methotrexate slow down the rapid rate of cell division that causes skin thickening. Acitretin and calcipotriol also reduce production of keratin, the hard protein that forms in the outer layer of skin. Salicylic acid and coal tar remove the layers of dead skin cells. Corticosteroids and infliximab reduce inflammation of underlying skin.

HOW THEY AFFECT YOU

Appropriate treatment of psoriasis usually improves the skin's appearance. However, since drugs cannot cure the underlying cause of the disorder, psoriasis tends to recur, even following successful treatment of a recurrence.

Individual drugs may cause side effects. Topical preparations can cause stinging and inflammation, especially if applied to normal skin. Coal tar increases the skin's sensitivity to sunlight; excessive sunbathing or overexposure to artificial ultraviolet light may damage skin and worsen the condition.

Acitretin and methotrexate can have several serious side effects, including gastrointestinal upsets, liver damage (acitretin), and bone marrow damage (methotrexate). Both are contraindicated in pregnancy; women are advised not to become pregnant for two years after completing treatment with acitretin. Topical corticosteroids may cause rebound worsening of psoriasis when stopped.

COMMON DRUGS

Acitretin, Calcipotriol*, Calcitriol, Ciclosporin*, Coal tar, Dithranol, Efalizumab, Etanercept, Hydroxycarbamide, Infliximab*, Methotrexate*, Methoxsalen, Salicylic acid, Tacalcitol, Tazarotene, Topical corticosteroids (see p.120)

* See Part 2

Treatments for eczema

Eczema is a skin condition causing a dry, itchy rash that may be inflamed and blistered. There are several types, some of which are called dermatitis. Eczema can be triggered by allergy but often occurs for no known rea-

son. In the long term, it can thicken the skin as a result of persistent scratching.

The most common type, atopic eczema, may appear in infancy, but many children grow out of it. There is often a family history of eczema, asthma, or allergic rhinitis. Atopic eczema commonly appears on the hands, due to detergents, and the feet, due to warm, moist conditions in enclosed footwear.

Contact dermatitis, another common form of eczema, is caused by chemicals, detergents, or soap. It may appear only after repeated exposure to the substance, but strong acids or alkalis can cause a reaction within minutes. It can also result from irritation of the skin by traces of detergent on clothes and bedding.

Allergic contact dermatitis can appear days or even years after initial contact has been made with triggers such as nickel, rubber, elastic, or drugs (e.g. antibiotics, antihistamines, antiseptics, or local anaesthetics). Sunlight can also trigger contact dermatitis following use of aftershave or perfume.

Nummular eczema causes circular dry, scaly, itchy, patches to develop anywhere on the body, and bacteria are often found in these areas. The cause of nummular eczema is unknown.

Seborrhoeic dermatitis mainly affects the scalp and face (see Drugs for dandruff p.126).

WHY THEY ARE USED

Emollients soften and moisten the skin. Oral antihistamines (see p.58) may be prescribed for a particularly itchy rash (topical antihistamines make the skin more sensitive and should not be used). Coal tar or ichthammol may be used for chronic atopic eczema, but topical corticosteroids (see p.120) may be needed to help control a flare up. Rarely, severe cases that are resistant to other treatments may need to be treated with the immunosuppressant drug ciclosporin (p.182). Oral corticosteroids (see p.80) may be used to treat contact dermatitis. Nummular eczema usually requires corticosteroid treatment. If it is resistant, antibiotics (see p.62) may be prescribed because infection is likely.

HOW THEY WORK

Emollients make the skin less dry and itchy. They are available as ointments, creams, lotions, soap substitutes, or bath oils. The effect is not long-lasting, so they need to be applied frequently. Emollients do not usually contain an active drug.

Antihistamines block the action of histamine (a chemical present in all cells). Histamine dilates the blood vessels in the skin, causing redness and swelling of the surrounding tissue due to fluid leaking from the circulation. Antihistamines also prevent histamine from irritating the nerve fibres, which causes itching.

Topical corticosteroids are absorbed into the tissues to relieve itching and inflammation. The least potent one that is effective is given. Hydrocortisone 1 per cent is often used in 1 to 2-week courses.

Oral or topical antibiotics destroy the bacteria sometimes present in broken, oozing, or blistered skin.

Ciclosporin blocks the action of white blood cells, which are involved in the immune response. The drug is given in short courses when the immune system responds inappropriately to an allergen.

RISKS AND SPECIAL PRECAUTIONS

All types of eczema can become infected, and antibiotics may be necessary. Herpes virus may infect atopic eczema. Therefore, direct contact with people who have a herpes infection, such as a cold sore, should be avoided. Emollients are generally well tolerated as are short-term topical mild corticosteroids. Ciclosporin may produce some adverse effects, however.

PREVENTING ECZEMA

Trigger substances can be identified using patch testing (see below) and avoided. PVC gloves should be worn to protect the hands from detergents. Cotton clothing should be worn next to the skin. Cosmetic moisturizers should be avoided because they usually contain perfumes and other sensitizers.

PATCH TESTING

Low concentrations of suspected substances are applied to the skin of the back and held in place with non-absorbent adhesive tape. This allows a number of potential allergens (substances that can cause an allergic reaction) to be tested at the same time. After 48

hours, the adhesive tape is removed and the skin inspected for any redness, swelling, or blistering, which would indicate a positive reaction. The skin is checked after a further 24 and 48 hours, in case the reaction has taken longer to develop.

COMMON DRUGS

Emollient and cooling preparations Aqueous cream, Calamine lotion, Cold cream, Emulsifying ointment
Antihistamines (see also p.58) Alimemazine, Chlorphenamine*, Clemastine, Diphenhydramine
Corticosteroids (see also p.80) Hydrocortisone*
Other drugs Azathioprine*, Ciclosporin*, Coal tar, Ichthammol, Mycophenolate mofetil, Pimecrolimus, Tacrolimus
* **See Part 2**

Drugs for dandruff

Dandruff is an irritating, but harmless, condition that involves an acceleration in the normal shedding of skin cells from the scalp. Extensive dandruff is considered to be a mild form of a type of dermatitis known as seborrhoeic dermatitis, which is caused by an overgrowth of a yeast organism that lives in the scalp. In severe cases, a rash and reddish-yellow, scaly pimples appear along the hairline and on the face.

WHY THEY ARE USED

Frequent washing with a detergent shampoo usually keeps the scalp free of dandruff, but more persistent dandruff can be treated with a shampoo containing the antifungal drug ketoconazole (p.277), medicated shampoos containing zinc pyrithione or selenium sulphide, or shampoos containing coal tar or salicylic acid. Ointments containing coal tar and salicylic acid are also available. Corticosteroid gels and lotions may be needed to treat an itchy rash, especially in cases of severe seborrhoeic dermatitis or psoriasis on the scalp (see p.124).

HOW THEY WORK

Coal tar and salicylic acid preparations reduce the overproduction of new skin cells and break down scales which are then washed off while shampooing. Antifungals (see p.76) reduce the overgrowth of yeast on the scalp by altering the permeability of the fungal cell walls. Corticosteroids (see p.80) help to relieve an itchy rash by reducing inflammation of the underlying skin.

COMMON DRUGS

Antifungals Ketoconazole*, Pyrithione zinc
Other drugs Arachis oil, Coal tar, Corticosteroids, Salicylic acid, Selenium sulphide*
* See Part 2

Drugs for hair loss

Hair loss (alopecia) is the result of greater than normal shedding of hairs, or reduced hair production. Hair loss can be caused by a skin condition such as scalp ringworm or scalp psoriasis.

Other forms of hair loss are caused by a disorder of the follicles themselves and may be a response to illness, malnutrition, or a reaction to some drugs, such as anticancer drugs or anticoagulants. The hair loss may be diffuse or in a pattern, as in male-pattern baldness, which is caused by oversensitivity to testosterone.

WHY THEY ARE USED

If the hair loss is due to a skin disorder such as scalp ringworm, an antifungal will be used to kill the fungal growth. If male-pattern baldness is a response to the male hormone, testosterone, finasteride may be used to reduce the hormone's effect. The antihypertensive drug minoxidil (p.316) can be applied to the scalp to promote hair growth.

HOW THEY WORK

Hair loss can be reversed when the underlying illness is treated or treatment is stopped. Finasteride by mouth inhibits conversion of testosterone to its more active form and reduces sensitivity to androgens. The role of minoxidil in hair growth is not fully understood, but it is thought to stimulate the hair follicles.

RISKS AND SPECIAL PRECAUTIONS

Finasteride can lead to loss of libido or erectile dysfunction. Minoxidil can be absorbed through the skin and should not be used by women of childbearing age; and anyone

with a history of heart disease or hypertension should consult their doctor before using the drug.

COMMON DRUGS

Antifungals Griseofulvin, Ketoconazole*, Terbinafine*
Other drugs Finasteride*, Minoxidil*
* See Part 2

Sunscreens

Sunscreens and sunblocks are chemicals, usually formulated as creams or oils, that protect the skin from the damaging effects of ultraviolet radiation from the sun.

People vary in their sensitivity to sunlight. Fair-skinned people generally have the least tolerance and tend to burn easily when exposed to the sun, while those with darker skin, especially brown or black skin, can withstand exposure to the sun for longer periods.

In a few cases, the skin's sensitivity to sunlight is increased by a disease such as pellagra or herpes simplex infection. Some drugs, such as thiazide diuretics, phenothiazine antipsychotics, psoralens, sulphonamide antibacterials, tetracycline antibiotics, and nalidixic acid, can also increase the skin's sensitivity.

Apart from sunburn and premature ageing of the skin, the most serious effect from sunlight is skin cancer. Reducing the skin's exposure to sunlight can help to prevent skin cancers.

HOW THEY WORK

Sunlight consists of different wavelengths of radiation. Of these, ultraviolet (UV) radiation is particularly harmful to the skin. UV radiation ages the skin and causes burning. Excessive exposure to UV radiation also increases the risk of developing skin cancer. UV radiation is mainly composed of UVA and UVB rays, both of which age the skin. In addition, UVA rays cause tanning and UVB rays cause burning. Especially vulnerable are fair-skinned people and those being treated with immunosuppressant drugs. Sunscreens absorb some of the UVB radiation, ensuring that less of it reaches the skin. Sunscreens are graded using the Sun Protection Factor (SPF) which refers to the degree of protection given by a sunscreen against sunburn. SPF is a measure of the amount of UVB radiation a sunscreen absorbs; the higher the number, the greater the protection. This number only describes the protection against UVB radiation. Some sunscreens, which contain chemicals such as zinc oxide and titanium dioxide, protect against UVA radiation as well; these are often called sunblocks. Certain preparations carry a "star" classification for the UVA protection they give; the stars do not describe an absolute measure but indicate a ratio of UVA to UVB protection. Four stars means that the product gives balanced protection against both UVA and UVB. Ratings of 1, 2, or 3 stars mean that the sunscreen has more protection against UVB than UVA. Some preparations contain chemicals such as zinc oxide and titanium dioxide, which reflect both UVB and UVA rays; these are often called sunblocks.

A sunscreen is particularly advisable for visitors to tropical, subtropical, and mountainous areas, and for those who wish to sunbathe, because sunscreens can prevent burning while allowing the skin to tan. Sunscreens must be applied before exposure to the sun. People with fair skin should use a sunscreen with a higher SPF than people with darker skin.

RISKS AND SPECIAL PRECAUTIONS

Sunscreens form only a physical barrier to the passage of UV radiation. They do not alter the skin to make it more resistant to sunlight. Sunscreen lotions must be applied frequently during exposure to the sun for protection to be maintained. People who are very fair skinned or are known to be very sensitive to sunlight should never expose their skin to direct sunlight, even if they are using a sunscreen, because not even sunscreens with high SPF values can give complete protection.

Sunscreens can irritate the skin, and some preparations may cause an allergic rash. People who are sensitive to some drugs, such as procaine and benzocaine and some hair dyes, might develop a rash after applying a sunscreen containing aminobenzoic acid or a benzophenone derivative such as oxybenzone.

COMMON DRUGS

Ingredients in sunscreens and sunblocks
Aminobenzoic acid, Benzones, Dibenzoylmethanes, Drometizole trisiloxane, Ethylhexyl methoxy-cinnamate, Methylbenzylidene camphor, Mexenone, Octocrylene, Oxybenzone, Padimate-O, Titanium dioxide, Zinc oxide

PART 2

A–Z OF DRUGS

This part of the book contains 260 generic drugs, individually profiled, and written to a standard format to help you find specific information quickly and easily; cross-references to the relevant major drug groups are provided.

Acamprosate

Brand name Campral EC
Used in the following combined preparations None

QUICK REFERENCE

Drug group Treating alcohol dependence
Overdose danger rating Low
Dependence rating Low
Prescription needed Yes
Available as generic No

GENERAL INFORMATION

Acamprosate has a chemical structure similar to some of the neurotransmitters involved in alcohol dependence. Studies show that, together with counselling, the drug reduces the desire to drink alcohol again. It does not, however, prevent symptoms of alcohol withdrawal. Treatment with acamprosate is started after withdrawal of alcohol has been achieved. The drug should be continued if the patient relapses. If regular alcohol misuse is resumed, however, the benefits of acamprosate will be lost.

Mental health problems are frequently reported in alcohol dependent patients, and psychiatric disorders (predominantly depression) that occur while a patient is taking acamprosate may be due to his or her underlying condition.

INFORMATION FOR USERS

Your drug prescription is tailored for you. Do not alter dosage without checking with your doctor.
How taken/used Tablets.
Frequency and timing of doses 3 x daily: at breakfast, midday, and at night.
Adult dosage range For bodyweight of 60kg or more: 1,998mg daily. For bodyweight of less than 60kg: 1,332mg daily.
Onset of effect Within 2 hours. Full beneficial effect is reached in about 1 week.
Duration of action 8 hours.
Diet advice None, but taking the drug with food reduces its absorption.
Storage Keep in original container at room temperature out of the reach of children.
Missed dose Take as soon as you remember. If your next dose is due within 2 hours, take a single dose now and skip the next.

Stopping the drug If you wish to stop taking the drug, you should discuss it with your doctor first.
Exceeding the dose An occasional unintentional extra dose is unlikely to cause any problems. A large overdose may cause diarrhoea. Notify your doctor.

POSSIBLE ADVERSE EFFECTS

Adverse events associated with acamprosate tend to be mild and transient in nature. These adverse events predominantly affect the skin and gastrointestinal tract. Common adverse effects include diarrhoea, nausea, vomiting, abdominal pain, and itching; if any of these becomes severe, contact your doctor. Rarer adverse effects of acamprosate treatment include a rash, loss of libido, and depression; you should seek medical advice if any of these symptoms develops. Insomnia also sometimes occurs as a side effect of acamprosate; if this becomes severe, discuss with your doctor.

INTERACTIONS

None known.

SPECIAL PRECAUTIONS

Be sure to tell your doctor if:
◆ You have kidney problems.
◆ You have severe liver impairment.
◆ You know that you are allergic to acamprosate.
◆ You are taking other medicines.
Pregnancy Safety not established. Discuss with your doctor.
Breast-feeding Safety not established. Acamprosate passes into breast milk. Discuss with your doctor.
Infants and children Not recommended.
Over 60 Not recommended.
Driving and hazardous work No special problems.
Alcohol Alcohol is not permitted while you are taking this drug.

PROLONGED USE

The recommended treatment period for acamprosate is 1 year.
Monitoring Counselling and regular monitoring for psychiatric problems such as depression are required.

Aciclovir

Brand names Boots Avert, Soothelip, Virasorb, Zovirax
Used in the following combined preparations None

QUICK REFERENCE

Drug group Antiviral drug (p.69)
Overdose danger rating Low
Dependence rating Low
Prescription needed No (cold sore cream); Yes (other preparations)
Available as generic Yes

GENERAL INFORMATION

Aciclovir is an antiviral drug used in the treatment of herpes infections, which can cause cold sores and genital herpes. It is available as tablets, a cream, eye ointment, and injection. The cream is commonly used to treat cold sores, and can speed up the healing of the lesions, provided it is started as soon as symptoms occur and before the lesions appear. The tablets and injection are used to treat severe herpes infections, shingles, chickenpox, and genital herpes. The tablets can also be used to prevent the development of herpes infection in people who have reduced immunity. Herpes infection affecting the eye can be treated with an eye ointment.

INFORMATION FOR USERS

Follow instructions on the label. Call your doctor if symptoms worsen.
How taken/used Tablets, liquid, injection, cream, eye ointment.
Frequency and timing of doses 2–5 x daily. Start as soon as possible.
Adult dosage range *Tablets, liquid* 1–4g daily (treatment); 800mg–4g daily (prevention). *Cream, eye ointment* 5 x daily.
Onset of effect Within 24 hours.
Duration of action Up to 8 hours.
Diet advice It is necessary to drink plenty of water when taking high doses by mouth or injection.
Storage Keep in original container at room temperature out of the reach of children. Protect from light.
Missed dose *Tablets/liquid* Take as soon as you remember. *Cream, eye ointment.* Do not apply the missed dose. Apply your next dose as usual.

Stopping the drug Complete the full course as directed.
Exceeding the dose An occasional unintentional extra dose is unlikely to be a cause for concern. But if you notice any unusual symptoms, or if a large overdose has been taken, notify your doctor.

POSSIBLE ADVERSE EFFECTS

Serious adverse effects are rare. The cream may cause burning, stinging, and itching at the site of application. Taken by mouth, aciclovir may occasionally cause nausea, vomiting, headache, or dizziness. Confusion or hallucinations may rarely occur with injections. If these or a rash occur, you should stop taking the drug and consult your doctor without delay.

INTERACTIONS (by mouth or injection only)

General note Any drug that affects the kidneys increases the risk of side effects with aciclovir.
Probenecid and cimetidine These drugs may increase the level of aciclovir in the blood.
Mycophenolate mofetil Aciclovir may increase blood levels of this drug and vice versa.

SPECIAL PRECAUTIONS

Be sure to consult your doctor or pharmacist before taking this drug if:
◆ You have a long-term kidney problem.
◆ You have reduced immunity.
◆ You are taking other medicines.
Pregnancy Topical preparations carry no known risk, but oral and injectable forms are not usually prescribed, as the effects on the developing baby are unknown. Discuss with your doctor.
Breast-feeding No evidence of risk with topical forms. The drug passes into the breast milk following injection or oral administration. Discuss with your doctor.
Infants and children Reduced dose necessary in young children.
Over 60 Reduced dose may be necessary.
Driving and hazardous work No known problems.
Alcohol No known problems.

PROLONGED USE

Aciclovir is usually given as single courses of treatment and is not given long term, except for people with reduced immunity.

Alendronic acid

Brand names Fosamax, Fosamax Once Weekly
Used in the following combined preparation
Fosavance

QUICK REFERENCE

Drug group Drug for bone disorders (p.56)
Overdose danger rating Medium
Dependence rating Low
Prescription needed Yes
Available as generic Yes

GENERAL INFORMATION

Alendronic acid is used to treat osteoporosis. It is also used in the treatment and prevention of corticosteroid-induced osteoporosis and to prevent postmenopausal osteoporosis in women at risk of developing the disease. A calcium supplement and vitamin D may be prescribed with the drug if dietary amounts are not adequate, but calcium should not be taken at the same time as alendronic acid because calcium is one of many substances that reduce its absorption. Combined use of alendronic acid with HRT in postmenopausal women is more effective than either treatment alone. Alendronic acid tablets should be taken on getting up in the morning, swallowed whole with a full glass of tap water (not even mineral water is acceptable because of the minerals' possible effect on absorption). After taking the tablet(s), remain upright for at least 30 minutes; do not go back to bed. This is to prevent the drug from sticking in the oesophagus, where it could cause ulcers or irritation. Breakfast may be eaten and any other medicines taken no less than 30 minutes (preferably longer) after taking alendronic acid.

INFORMATION FOR USERS

Your drug prescription is tailored for you. Do not alter dosage without checking with your doctor.
How taken/used Tablets.
Frequency and timing of doses Once daily, first thing in the morning. Once weekly, first thing in the morning (postmenopausal women). Take with water.
Adult dosage range *Treatment*: men: 10mg daily; postmenopausal women: 10mg daily or 70mg weekly. *Prevention*: 5mg (postmenopausal women). *Prevention and treatment of corticosteroid-induced osteoporosis*: 5mg; postmenopausal women not taking HRT, 10mg.
Onset of effect It may take months to notice an improvement.
Duration of action Some effects may persist for months or years.
Diet advice Do not eat for at least 30 minutes after doses.
Storage Keep in original container at room temperature out of the reach of children.
Missed dose Take the next dose at the usual time next morning.
Stopping the drug Do not stop the drug without consulting your doctor. Stopping the drug may lead to worsening of the underlying condition.
Exceeding the dose An occasional unintentional extra dose is unlikely to cause problems. Large overdoses may cause stomach problems including heartburn, irritation, and ulcers. Notify your doctor at once, and try to remain upright.

POSSIBLE ADVERSE EFFECTS

The most frequent adverse effect caused by alendronic acid is abdominal pain as a result of irritation to the oesophagus, stomach, or the small intestine. Other adverse effects include diarrhoea or constipation; muscle, bone, or joint pain; headache; and nausea or vomiting. Discuss with your doctor if any of these get severe. If the drug causes a rash, sensitivity to light, or eye inflammation, consult your doctor. You may also experience pain or difficulty in swallowing or heartburn. If these occur, stop taking the drug and consult your doctor.

INTERACTIONS

Antacids and calcium and iron salts reduce the absorption of alendronic acid.

SPECIAL PRECAUTIONS

Be sure to tell your doctor if:
◆ You have an abnormality of the oesophagus.
◆ You have stomach problems or a history of ulcers.
◆ You are unable to stand or sit upright for at least 30 minutes.
◆ You have hypocalcaemia.

◆ You have kidney impairment.
◆ You are taking other medicines.
Pregnancy Not recommended.
Breast-feeding Not recommended.
Infants and children Not recommended.
Over 60 No special problems.
Driving and hazardous work No special problems.
Alcohol May cause further stomach irritation.

PROLONGED USE
Alendronic acid is usually prescribed indefinitely for osteoporosis without causing any problems.
Monitoring Blood and urine tests may be carried out at intervals.

Alginates

Brand names Gaviscon Infant (oral); Algisite M, Algosteril, Kaltostat, Melgisorb, Seasorb, Sorbalgon, Sorbsan (dressings)
Used in the following combined preparations
Algicon, Gastrocote, Gaviscon, Peptac, Rennie Duo, Topal (oral)

QUICK REFERENCE
Drug group Antacid (p.42)
Overdose danger rating Low
Dependence rating Low
Prescription needed No
Available as generic Yes

GENERAL INFORMATION
"Alginates" is a group term that refers to a mixture of compounds extracted from brown algae (seaweeds). When the powder extract is mixed with water, alginates become a thick viscous fluid or gel depending on the chemicals used. Alginates combined with antacids form a "raft" that floats on the surface of the stomach contents, which reduces reflux and protects the lining of the oesophagus from attack by acid regurgitated from the stomach. Many of these combined preparations of alginates are used to treat mild gastro-oesophageal reflux disease. A number of indigestion remedies on sale to the public also contain alginates. The properties of alginates are also used in wound dressings where, in the form of a woven pad, they absorb fluids from the surface of the wound, keeping it moist and allowing it to heal.

INFORMATION FOR USERS
Follow instructions on the label. Call your doctor if symptoms worsen.
How taken/used Chewable tablets, liquid, powder.
Frequency and timing of doses 4 x daily after meals and at bedtime.
Adult dosage range 800–2,000mg daily.
Onset of effect 10–20 minutes.
Duration of action 3–4 hours.
Diet advice None.
Storage Keep in original container at room temperature out of the reach of children.
Missed dose Take as soon as you remember, if you need it.
Stopping the drug Alginates can be safely stopped as soon as you no longer need them.
Exceeding the dose Overdose of alginates is likely to produce abdominal distension, without other symptoms. Notify your doctor if it is severe.

POSSIBLE ADVERSE EFFECTS
The antacid salts used in combined oral preparations of alginates may cause abdominal discomfort and distension, and, rarely nausea. Discuss with your doctor if any of these symptoms are severe.

INTERACTIONS
None.

SPECIAL PRECAUTIONS
Be sure to consult your doctor or pharmacist before taking this drug if:
◆ You are on a salt-restricted diet.
◆ You are taking other medicines.
Pregnancy No evidence of risk to developing baby. Some products can be used for heartburn in pregnancy.
Breast-feeding No evidence of risk.
Infants and children Reduced dose necessary.
Over 60 No special problems.
Driving and hazardous work No known problems.
Alcohol No known problems.

PROLONGED USE
No problems expected.

Allopurinol

Brand names Caplenal, Cosuric, Rimapurinol, Xanthomax, Zyloric
Used in the following combined preparations None

QUICK REFERENCE

Drug group Drug for gout (p.53)
Overdose danger rating Medium
Dependence rating Low
Prescription needed Yes
Available as generic Yes

GENERAL INFORMATION

Allopurinol is used to prevent gout, which is caused by deposits of uric acid crystals in joints. Allopurinol blocks an enzyme known as xanthine oxidase that is involved in the formation of uric acid. Allopurinol is also used to lower high uric acid levels (hyperuricaemia) caused by other drugs, such as anticancer drugs. Allopurinol should never be started until an acute attack is over because it may cause a further episode. Treatment with the drug should be continued indefinitely to prevent further attacks.

At the start of treatment, an acute attack may occur and colchicine or an anti-inflammatory drug may also be given, until uric acid levels are reduced. If an acute attack occurs while on allopurinol, treatment should continue along with an anti-inflammatory drug.

INFORMATION FOR USERS

Your drug prescription is tailored for you. Do not alter dosage without checking with your doctor.
How taken/used Tablets.
Frequency and timing of doses 1–3 x daily after food.
Adult dosage range 100–900mg daily.
Onset of effect Within 24–48 hours. Full effect may not be felt for several weeks.
Duration of action Up to 30 hours. Some effect may last for 1–2 weeks after the drug has been stopped.
Diet advice A high fluid intake (2 litres of fluid daily) is recommended.
Storage Keep in original container at room temperature out of the reach of children.
Missed dose If your next dose is not due for another 12 hours or more, take a dose as soon as you remember and take the next one as usual. Otherwise skip the missed dose and take your next dose on schedule.
Stopping the drug Do not stop taking the drug without consulting your doctor; symptoms may recur.
Exceeding the dose An occasional unintentional extra dose is unlikely to cause problems. Large overdoses may cause nausea, vomiting, abdominal pain, diarrhoea, and dizziness. Notify your doctor.

POSSIBLE ADVERSE EFFECTS

Adverse effects of allopurinol are not very common. The most serious are an allergic rash, sore throat, fever, and chills, which should always be reported to your doctor and may require the drug to be substituted. Nausea can be avoided by taking allopurinol after food. The drug may also cause drowsiness or dizziness, headache, a metallic taste, or visual disturbances. Discuss with your doctor if these occur.

INTERACTIONS

ACE inhibitors Allopurinol may increase the risk of toxicity from these drugs.
Aspirin Large doses of aspirin may reduce the effects of allopurinol.
Anticoagulant drugs Allopurinol may increase the effects of these drugs.
Theophylline Allopurinol may increase levels of this drug.
Mercaptopurine and azathioprine Allopurinol blocks the breakdown of these drugs, requiring a reduction in their dosage.
Chlorpropamide The hypoglycaemic effects of chlorpropamide may be increased if it is taken with allopurinol.
Ciclosporin Allopurinol may increase the effects of this drug.

SPECIAL PRECAUTIONS

Be sure to tell your doctor if:
◆ You have long-term liver or kidney problems.
◆ You have had a previous sensitivity reaction to allopurinol.
◆ You have a current attack of gout.
◆ You are taking other medicines.
Pregnancy Safety in pregnancy not established. Discuss with your doctor.

Breast-feeding The drug passes into the breast milk and may affect the baby. Discuss with your doctor.

Infants and children Reduced dose necessary.

Over 60 Reduced dose may be necessary.

Driving and hazardous work Avoid such activities until you have learned how allopurinol affects you because the drug can cause drowsiness.

Alcohol Avoid. Alcohol may worsen gout.

PROLONGED USE

Apart from an increased risk of gout in the first weeks or months, no problems are expected.

Monitoring Periodic checks on levels of uric acid in the blood are usually performed, and the dose of allopurinol is adjusted if necessary.

Aluminium hydroxide

Brand name Alu-Cap

Used in the following combined preparations
Algicon, Aludrox, Asilone, Co-magaldrox, Maalox, Mucogel, Topal, and others

QUICK REFERENCE

Drug group Antacid (p.42)

Overdose danger rating Low

Dependence rating Low

Prescription needed No

Available as generic Yes

GENERAL INFORMATION

Aluminium hydroxide is a common ingredient of many over-the-counter remedies for indigestion and heartburn. Because the drug is constipating (it is sometimes used to treat diarrhoea), it is usually combined with a magnesium-containing antacid with a balancing laxative effect. The combination is sometimes referred to by the generic name of co-magaldrox.

The prolonged action of aluminium hydroxide makes it useful in preventing the pain of stomach and duodenal ulcers or heartburn. Aluminium hydroxide can also promote the healing of ulcers. The drug may be more effective as an antacid in liquid form rather than as tablets. Some antacid preparations include large amounts of sodium and these should be used with caution by those on low-sodium diets.

In the intestine, aluminium hydroxide binds with, and thereby reduces the absorption of, phosphate. This makes it helpful in treating high blood phosphate (hyperphosphataemia), which occurs in some people with impaired kidney function. However, prolonged heavy use can lead to phosphate deficiency and a consequent weakening of the bones.

INFORMATION FOR USERS

Follow instructions on the label. Call your doctor if symptoms worsen.

How taken/used Chewable tablets, capsules, liquid (suspension). The tablets should be well chewed.

Frequency and timing of doses *As antacid* 4–6 x daily as needed, or 1 hour before and after meals. *Peptic ulcer* 6–7 x daily. *Hyperphosphataemia* 3–4 x daily with meals. *Diarrhoea* 2–6 x daily.

Dosage range *Adults* Up to 70ml daily (liquid), 2–10g daily (tablets or capsules). *Children over 6 years* Reduced dose according to age and weight.

Onset of effect Within 15 minutes.

Duration of action 2–4 hours.

Diet advice For hyperphosphataemia, a low-phosphate diet may be advised in addition to aluminium hydroxide treatment.

Storage Keep in original container at room temperature out of the reach of children.

Missed dose Do not take the missed dose. Take your next dose as usual.

Stopping the drug The drug can be safely stopped as soon as you no longer need it (indigestion). When taken as ulcer treatment or for hyperphosphataemia resulting from kidney failure, do not stop without consulting your doctor.

Exceeding the dose An occasional unintentional extra dose is unlikely to be a cause for concern. But if you notice any unusual symptoms, or if a large overdose has been taken, notify your doctor.

POSSIBLE ADVERSE EFFECTS

Constipation is common with aluminium hydroxide; nausea and vomiting may occur because of the granular, powdery nature of the drug. Bone pain may occur but usually only when large doses have been taken regularly for months or years. Vomiting or severe constipation or nausea should be reported to your doctor.

INTERACTIONS

General note Aluminium hydroxide may interfere with the absorption or excretion of many drugs. Such drugs include oral anticoagulants, digoxin, many antibiotics, penicillamine, corticosteroids, antipsychotics, and phenytoin. Aluminium hydroxide should only be taken at least 2 hours before or after other drugs.

Enteric-coated tablets Aluminium hydroxide may lead to the break-up of the enteric coating of tablets (such as bisacodyl, or enteric-coated prednisolone) before they leave the stomach, leading to stomach irritation.

SPECIAL PRECAUTIONS

Be sure to consult your doctor or pharmacist before taking this drug if:
◆ You have a long-term kidney problem.
◆ You have heart problems.
◆ You have high blood pressure.
◆ You suffer from constipation.
◆ You have a bone disease.
◆ You have porphyria.
◆ You are taking other medicines.

Pregnancy Safety in pregnancy not established. Discuss with your doctor.

Breast-feeding No evidence of risk.

Infants and children Not recommended under 6 years except on the advice of a doctor.

Over 60 Increased likelihood of adverse effects. Reduced dose may therefore be necessary.

Driving and hazardous work No known problems.

Alcohol No known problems.

PROLONGED USE

Aluminium hydroxide should not be used for longer than 4 weeks without consulting your doctor. Prolonged use of high doses of aluminium hydroxide may deplete levels of phosphate and calcium in the blood, which may lead to weakening of the bones and to fractures.

Amiloride

Brand names Amilamont, Amilospare
Used in the following combined preparations Burinex A, Co-amilofruse, Co-amilozide, Moduretic, Navispare, and others

QUICK REFERENCE

Drug group Potassium-sparing diuretic (p.32)
Overdose danger rating Low
Dependence rating Low
Prescription needed Yes
Available as generic Yes

GENERAL INFORMATION

Amiloride is a diuretic that acts on the kidneys to increase the amount of urine that is passed. The drug is used in the treatment of oedema (fluid retention), which can result from heart failure or liver disease, and for hypertension (high blood pressure).

Amiloride's effect on urine flow may last for several hours. Preferably, it should be taken in the morning and no later than about 4 pm, otherwise you may need to pass urine during the night.

Amiloride causes the kidneys to conserve potassium (potassium-sparing diuretic) and should not be used when there is a high blood level of potassium. The drug is prescribed with caution in people who are taking potassium supplements or those who have kidney disease. Amiloride is usually combined with other diuretics such as furosemide (as co-amilofruse) and hydrochlorothiazide (as co-amilozide).

INFORMATION FOR USERS

Your drug prescription is tailored for you. Do not alter dosage without checking with your doctor.

How taken/used Tablets, liquid.

Frequency and timing of doses Once daily, usually in the morning.

Adult dosage range 5–10mg daily.

Onset of effect Within 2–4 hours.

Duration of action 12–24 hours.

Diet advice Avoid foods that are high in potassium – for example, dried fruit, bananas, tomatoes, and salt substitutes.

Storage Keep in original container at room temperature out of the reach of children.

Missed dose Take as soon as you remember. However, if it is late in the day, do not take the missed dose, or you may need to get up at night to pass urine. Take the next scheduled dose as usual.

Stopping the drug Do not stop the drug without consulting your doctor; symptoms may recur.

Exceeding the dose An occasional unintentional extra dose is unlikely to be a cause for concern. But if you notice any unusual symptoms, or if a large overdose has been taken, notify your doctor.

POSSIBLE ADVERSE EFFECTS

Amiloride has few adverse effects; the main problem is the possibility that potassium may be retained by the body, causing muscle weakness and numbness. Rarely, there may be digestive disturbance, confusion, muscle weakness or cramps, dry mouth and thirst, or dizziness; discuss with your doctor if any of these occur. If a rash develops, stop taking the drug and consult your doctor.

INTERACTIONS

Lithium Amiloride may increase the blood levels of lithium, leading to an increased risk of lithium toxicity.

ACE inhibitors, angiotensin II blockers, ciclosporin, drosperinone, tacrolimus, and NSAIDs These drugs may increase the risk of potassium retention if taken with amiloride.

Chlorpropamide Taken with amiloride, this drug increases the risk of low sodium levels, which may cause confusion and drowsiness.

SPECIAL PRECAUTIONS

Be sure to tell your doctor if:
◆ You have long-term liver or kidney problems.
◆ You have diabetes.
◆ You are taking other medicines.

Pregnancy Not usually prescribed. May cause a reduction in the blood supply to the developing baby. Discuss with your doctor.

Breast-feeding Not usually prescribed during breast-feeding. Discuss with your doctor.

Infants and children Not recommended.

Over 60 Increased likelihood of adverse effects. Reduced dose necessary.

Driving and hazardous work No known problems.

Alcohol No special problems.

PROLONGED USE

Monitoring Blood tests may be carried out to monitor levels of body salts.

Amiodarone

Brand name Cordarone X
Used in the following combined preparations None

QUICK REFERENCE

Drug group Anti-arrhythmic drug (p.33)
Overdose danger rating Medium
Dependence rating Low
Prescription needed Yes
Available as generic Yes (tablets)

GENERAL INFORMATION

Amiodarone is used to treat a variety of abnormal heart rhythms (arrhythmias). It works by slowing nerve impulses in the heart muscle. Amiodarone is given to prevent recurrent atrial and ventricular fibrillation and to treat ventricular and supraventricular tachycardias and Wolff-Parkinson-White Syndrome. Often the last choice when other treatments have failed, especially for long-term use, it has serious adverse effects, including liver damage, thyroid problems, and eye and lung damage. Treatment should be started only under specialist supervision or in hospital and the dosage carefully controlled in order to achieve the desired effect using the lowest possible dose.

INFORMATION FOR USERS

Your drug prescription is tailored for you. Do not alter dosage without checking with your doctor.

How taken/used Tablets, injection.

Frequency and timing of doses 3 x daily or by injection initially, then reduced to twice daily, then once daily or every other day (maintenance dose).

Adult dosage range 600mg daily, reduced to 400mg, then 100–200mg daily.

Onset of effect By mouth, some effects may occur in 72 hours; full benefits may take some weeks to show. By injection, effects may occur within 30 minutes.

Duration of action Around 1 month.

Diet advice Grapefruit juice should be avoided.

Storage Keep in original container at room temperature out of the reach of children. Protect from light.

Missed dose Take as soon as you remember. If your next dose is due within 12 hours, do not take the missed dose. Take your next scheduled dose as usual.

Stopping the drug Do not stop the drug without consulting your doctor; symptoms may recur.

Exceeding the dose An occasional unintentional extra dose is unlikely to cause problems. But if you notice any unusual symptoms or if a large overdose has been taken, notify your doctor at once.

POSSIBLE ADVERSE EFFECTS

Amiodarone has a number of unusual side effects, including a metallic taste in the mouth, a greyish skin colour, and increased sensitivity of the skin to sunlight (photosensitivity). Patients are advised to use a high factor sun block, wear a hat, and cover exposed skin. The drug can also cause nausea and vomiting, liver damage, visual disturbances, thyroid problems, heart rate disturbances, numbness and tingling in the extremities, shortness of breath, cough, headache, weakness, and fatigue. Discuss with your doctor if nausea and vomiting are severe or if any other adverse effects occur.

INTERACTIONS

General note Amiodarone can interact with many drugs. Consult your doctor or pharmacist before taking other medications.

Diuretics The loss of potassium caused by these drugs may increase the toxic effects of amiodarone.

Other anti-arrhythmic drugs Amiodarone may increase the effects of drugs such as beta blockers, digoxin, diltiazem, or verapamil.

Warfarin Amiodarone may increase the anticoagulant effect of warfarin.

SPECIAL PRECAUTIONS

Be sure to tell your doctor if:

◆ You have long-term liver or kidney problems.

◆ You have heart disease.

◆ You have eye disease.

◆ You have a lung disorder such as asthma or bronchitis.

◆ You have a thyroid disorder.

◆ You are sensitive to iodine.

◆ You are taking other medicines.

Pregnancy Not recommended. Discuss with your doctor.

Breast-feeding The drug passes into the breast milk and may affect the baby. Discuss with your doctor.

Infants and children Not recommended.

Over 60 Increased likelihood of adverse effects. Reduced dose may therefore be necessary.

Driving and hazardous work Avoid these activities until you have learned how amiodarone affects you because the drug can cause the eyes to be dazzled by bright light.

Alcohol No known problems.

PROLONGED USE

Prolonged use of this drug may cause a number of adverse effects on the eyes, heart, skin, nervous system, lungs, thyroid gland, and liver.

Monitoring A chest X-ray may be taken before treatment starts. Blood tests are done before treatment starts and then every 6 months to check thyroid and liver function. Regular eye examinations are required.

Amisulpride/sulpiride

Brand names Solian [amisulpride] Dolmatil, Sulpitil, Sulpor [sulpiride]
Used in the following combined preparations None

QUICK REFERENCE

Drug group Antipsychotic drug (p.15)
Overdose danger rating Medium
Dependence rating Low
Prescription needed Yes
Available as generic Yes

GENERAL INFORMATION

Amisulpride and sulpiride are anti psychotic drugs used to treat acute and chronic schizophrenia, in which there are "positive" symptoms such as delusions, hallucinations, and thought disorders, and/or "negative" symptoms such as emotional and social withdrawal. Patients who have mainly positive symptoms are treated with higher doses; and patients with mainly negative symptoms are treated with lower doses. Sulpiride has also been used in the treatment of Tourette's syndrome.

An advantage of amisulpride, a so-called atypical antipsychotic drug, is that it is less likely than the older antipsychotic drugs to cause parkinsonism or tardive dyskinesia (abnormal involuntary movements, mainly of the face and tongue).

INFORMATION FOR USERS

Your drug prescription is tailored for you. Do not alter dosage without checking with your doctor.

How taken/used Tablets, liquid.

Frequency and timing of doses 1–2 x daily (doses of up to 300mg of amisulpride may be 1 x daily).

Dosage range *Amisulpride* 50–300mg daily (mainly negative symptoms); 400–1,200mg daily (mainly positive symptoms).
Sulpiride 400–800mg daily (mainly negative symptoms); 400–2,400mg daily (mainly positive symptoms).

Onset of effect 1 hour.

Duration of action 12–24 hours.

Diet advice None.

Storage Keep in original container at room temperature out of the reach of children.

Missed dose Take as soon as you remember. If your next dose is due within 2 hours, take a single dose now and skip the next dose.

Stopping the drug Do not stop taking the drug without consulting your doctor; symptoms may recur.

Exceeding the dose An occasional unintentional extra dose is unlikely to cause problems. Large overdoses may cause drowsiness and low blood pressure. Notify your doctor immediately.

POSSIBLE ADVERSE EFFECTS

Most of the side effects of antipsychotic drugs like amisulpride and sulpiride are mild. Insomnia is the most common problem, although drowsiness, and anxiety or agitation are also fairly common. Consult your doctor if they get severe. More rarely, there may be weight gain, nausea or vomiting, breast swelling, movement disorders, loss of libido, or menstrual irregularities (in women); consult your doctor if you experience any of these symptoms.

INTERACTIONS

Antihypertensive drugs Amisulpride and sulpiride may reduce the blood-pressure lowering effect of certain of these drugs.

Central nervous system depressants These drugs may all increase the sedative effects of amisulpride and sulpiride.

SPECIAL PRECAUTIONS

Be sure to tell your doctor if:
◆ You have liver or kidney problems.
◆ You have heart problems or hypertension.
◆ You have epilepsy.
◆ You have Parkinson's disease.
◆ You have a pituitary tumour or breast cancer.
◆ You have had blood problems.
◆ You are taking other medicines.

Pregnancy Safety not established. Discuss with your doctor.

Breast-feeding Safety not established. Discuss with your doctor.

Infants and children Not recommended.

Over 60 Reduced dose may be necessary.

Driving and hazardous work Avoid such activities until you have learned how amisulpride and sulpiride affect you; the drugs can slow reaction times and may occasionally cause drowsiness or loss of concentration.

Alcohol Avoid. Alcohol increases the sedative effects of these drugs.

PROLONGED USE

Tardive dyskinesia may rarely occur during long-term use.

Amitriptyline

Brand names None
Used in the following combined preparations
Triptafen, Triptafen-M

QUICK REFERENCE

Drug group Tricyclic antidepressant drug (p.14)
Overdose danger rating High
Dependence rating Low
Prescription needed Yes
Available as generic Yes

GENERAL INFORMATION

Amitriptyline is a tricyclic antidepressant drug and is used mainly for long-term depression. It elevates mood, increases physical activity, improves appetite, and restores interest in everyday activities. More sedating than similar drugs, amitriptyline is useful when depression is accompanied by anxiety or insomnia. Taken at night, the drug encourages sleep and helps to eliminate the need for additional sleeping drugs. This drug is sometimes used to treat nocturnal enuresis (bedwetting) in children. It may also be used to treat nerve pain such as postherpetic neuralgia after shingles. In overdose, amitriptyline may cause coma, fits, and abnormal heart rhythms.

INFORMATION FOR USERS

Your drug prescription is tailored for you. Do not alter dosage without checking with your doctor.

How taken/used Tablets, liquid.

Frequency and timing of doses 1–3 x daily, usually as a single dose at night.

Adult dosage range 50–200mg daily.

Onset of effect Sedation can appear within hours, although full antidepressant effect may not be felt for 2–4 weeks.

Duration of action Antidepressant effect may last for 6 weeks; common adverse effects gone within 1 week.

Diet advice None.

Storage Keep in original container at room temperature out of the reach of children. Protect from light.

Missed dose Take as soon as you remember. If your next dose is due within 3 hours, take a single dose now and skip the next.

Stopping the drug An abrupt stop can cause withdrawal symptoms and recurrence of the original trouble. Consult your doctor, who may supervise a gradual reduction in dosage over at least 4 weeks.

OVERDOSE ACTION

Seek immediate medical advice in all cases. Take emergency action if palpitations are noted or consciousness is lost.

POSSIBLE ADVERSE EFFECTS

The possible adverse effects of this drug are mainly the result of its anticholinergic action and its blocking action on the transmission of signals through the heart. It may cause drowsiness, sweating, dry mouth, constipation, and blurred vision. Discuss with your doctor if these get severe or if you have difficulty in passing urine. If you have palpitations, dizziness or fainting, or confusion, you should stop taking the drug and consult your doctor immediately.

INTERACTIONS

Monoamine oxidase inhibitors (MAOIs) In the rare cases where these drugs are given with amitriptyline, there is a possibility of serious interactions.

Antiepileptics The effects of these drugs are reduced by amitriptyline as it lowers the seizure threshold.

Sedatives All drugs that have sedative effects intensify those of amitriptyline.

Anti-arrhythmic drugs There is an increased risk of abnormal heart rhythms when these drugs are taken with amitriptyline.

SPECIAL PRECAUTIONS

Be sure to tell your doctor if:
◆ You have heart problems.
◆ You have had epileptic fits.
◆ You have long-term liver or kidney problems.
◆ You have glaucoma.
◆ You have prostate trouble.
◆ You have thyroid disease.
◆ You have had mania or a psychotic illness.
◆ You are taking other medicines.

Pregnancy Avoid if possible. Discuss with your doctor.

Breast-feeding The drug passes into the breast milk, but at normal doses adverse effects are unlikely. Discuss with your doctor.

Infants and children Not recommended under 16 years for depression, or under 6 years for enuresis.

Over 60 Reduced dose may be necessary because elderly patients are more sensitive to adverse reactions.

Driving and hazardous work Avoid such activities until you have learned how amitriptyline affects you because the drug may cause blurred vision and reduced alertness.

Alcohol Avoid. Alcohol may increase the sedative effects of this drug.

Surgery and general anaesthetics Amitriptyline treatment may need to be stopped before you have a general anaesthetic. Discuss this with your doctor or dentist before any operation.

PROLONGED USE
No problems expected.

Amlodipine

Brand names Amlostin, Istin
Used in the following combined preparations
None

QUICK REFERENCE
Drug group Anti-angina drug (p.35), antihypertensive drug (p.36)
Overdose danger rating Medium
Dependence rating Low
Prescription needed Yes
Available as generic Yes

GENERAL INFORMATION
Amlodipine belongs to a group of drugs known as calcium channel blockers, which interfere with the conduction of signals in the muscles of the heart and blood vessels.

Amlodipine is used in the treatment of angina to help prevent attacks of chest pain. Unlike some other anti-angina drugs (such as beta blockers), it can be used safely by people with asthma and non-insulin-dependent diabetes.

Amlodipine is also used to reduce raised blood pressure (hypertension).

In common with other drugs of its class, amlodipine may cause blood pressure to fall too low at the start of treatment. In rare cases, angina may become worse at the start of amlodipine treatment. The drug may sometimes cause mild to moderate leg and ankle swelling.

INFORMATION FOR USERS
Your drug prescription is tailored for you. Do not alter dosage without checking with your doctor.
How taken/used Tablets.
Frequency and timing of doses Once daily.
Adult dosage range 5–10mg daily.
Onset of effect 6–12 hours.
Duration of action 24 hours.

Diet advice None.
Storage Keep in original container at room temperature out of the reach of children.
Missed dose If you miss a dose and you remember it within 12 hours, take it as soon as you remember. However, if you do not remember until later, do not take the missed dose and do not double up the next one. Instead, go back to your regular schedule.
Stopping the drug Do not stop taking the drug without consulting your doctor; stopping the drug may lead to worsening of the underlying condition.
Exceeding the dose An occasional unintentional extra dose is unlikely to cause problems. Large overdoses may cause a marked lowering of blood pressure. Notify your doctor immediately.

POSSIBLE ADVERSE EFFECTS
Amlodipine can cause a variety of minor adverse effects, including leg and ankle swelling, headache, dizziness, fatigue, and nausea. Dizziness, especially on rising, may be the result of an excessive reduction in blood pressure. The most serious effect is the rare possibility of angina becoming worse after starting amlodipine treatment. This should be reported to your doctor immediately. If effects such as leg and ankle swelling, headache, dizziness, fatigue, and flushing get serious, discuss it with your doctor. In the case of rare effects like skin rashes or breathing difficulty, stop taking the drug and consult your doctor.

INTERACTIONS
Ketoconazole, itraconazole, and ritonavir These drugs may increase blood levels and adverse effects of amlodipine.
Alpha blockers, beta blockers, ACE inhibitors, and diuretics Amlodipine may increase the effects of these drugs and vice versa.

SPECIAL PRECAUTIONS
Be sure to tell your doctor if:
◆ You have long-term liver problems.
◆ You have heart failure.
◆ You have diabetes.
◆ You are taking other medicines.
Pregnancy Safety in pregnancy not established. Discuss with your doctor.

Breast-feeding It is not known if the drug passes into the breast milk. Discuss with your doctor.

Infants and children Not recommended.

Over 60 No special problems.

Driving and hazardous work Avoid such activities until you have learned how amlodipine affects you because the drug can cause dizziness owing to lowered blood pressure.

Alcohol Avoid. Alcohol may further reduce blood pressure, causing dizziness or other symptoms.

Surgery and general anaesthetics Amlodipine may interact with some general anaesthetics, causing a fall in blood pressure. Discuss this with your doctor or dentist before any surgery.

PROLONGED USE
No problems expected.

Amoxicillin/co-amoxiclav

Brand names Almodan, Amix, Amoram, Amoxident, Amoxil, Galenamox, Rimoxallin
Used in the following combined preparations
Augmentin, Co-amoxiclav

QUICK REFERENCE
Drug group Penicillin antibiotic (p.62)
Overdose danger rating Low
Dependence rating Low
Prescription needed Yes
Available as generic Yes

GENERAL INFORMATION
Amoxicillin is a penicillin antibiotic. It is prescribed to treat a variety of infections, but is particularly useful for treating ear, nose, and throat infections, respiratory tract infections, cystitis, uncomplicated gonorrhoea, and certain skin and soft tissue infections. The drug is absorbed well by the body when taken orally.

Amoxicillin is sometimes combined with clavulanic acid (as co-amoxiclav) to prevent bacteria from breaking down amoxicillin; this makes it effective against a wider range of bacteria than amoxicillin alone. Doses of co-amoxiclav are given as two numbers (e.g. 500/125 is 500mg amoxicillin plus 125mg clavulanic acid).

Amoxicillin/co-amoxiclav can cause minor stomach upsets and intestinal disturbances and a rash. It can also provoke a severe allergic reaction with fever, swelling of the mouth and tongue, itching, and breathing difficulties. This suggests that the patient is allergic to penicillin antibiotics.

INFORMATION FOR USERS
Your drug prescription is tailored for you. Do not alter dosage without checking with your doctor.

How taken/used Tablets, capsules, liquid, powder (dissolved in water), injection.

Frequency and timing of doses Normally 3 x daily.

Dosage range *Adults* 750mg–1.5g (of amoxicillin) daily. In some cases a short course of up to 6g (of amoxicillin) daily is given. A single dose of 3g (of amoxicillin) may be given as a preventative. However, dosage range depends on preparation and condition being treated. *Children* Reduced dose according to age and weight.

Onset of effect 1–2 hours.

Duration of action Up to 8 hours.

Diet advice None.

Storage Keep in original container at room temperature out of the reach of children.

Missed dose Take as soon as you remember. Take your next dose at the scheduled time.

Stopping the drug Take the full course. Even if you feel better, the original infection may still be present and symptoms may recur if treatment is stopped too soon.

Exceeding the dose An occasional unintentional extra dose is unlikely to be a cause for concern. But if you notice any unusual symptoms, or if a large overdose has been taken, notify your doctor.

POSSIBLE ADVERSE EFFECTS
If you develop a rash, wheezing or breathing difficulty, itching, fever, swelling of the mouth or tongue, or joint swelling, this may indicate allergy to penicillin antibiotics. Stop taking the drug and call your doctor immediately. Your doctor may prescribe a different antibiotic. Diarrhoea, nausea or vomiting, dizziness, or headache may also occur as side effects. If they are severe, discuss with your doctor.

INTERACTIONS

Anticoagulant drugs Amoxicillin and co-amoxiclav may alter the anticoagulant effect of these drugs; patients may have to be monitored more closely.

Allopurinol Amoxicillin may increase the likelihood of allergic skin reactions.

Oral contraceptives Amoxicillin and co-amoxiclav may reduce the effectiveness of the pill and also increase the risk of breakthrough bleeding. Discuss with your doctor.

SPECIAL PRECAUTIONS

Be sure to tell your doctor if:
◆ You have long-term liver or kidney problems.
◆ You have an allergy (e.g. asthma, hay fever, eczema).
◆ You have had a previous allergic reaction to a penicillin or cephalosporin antibiotic.
◆ You have ulcerative colitis.
◆ You have glandular fever.
◆ You have chronic leukaemia.
◆ You are taking other medicines.

Pregnancy No evidence of risk with amoxicillin. Discuss the use of co-amoxiclav with your doctor.

Breast-feeding The drug passes into the breast milk, but at normal doses adverse effects on the baby are unlikely. Discuss with your doctor.

Infants and children Reduced dose necessary.

Over 60 No known problems.

Driving and hazardous work No known problems.

Alcohol No known problems.

PROLONGED USE

Amoxicillin and co-amoxiclav are usually given only for short courses of treatment.

Amphotericin

Brand names Abelcet, AmBisome, Amphocil, Fungilin, Fungizone
Used in the following combined preparations None

QUICK REFERENCE

Drug group Antifungal drug (p.76)
Overdose danger rating Low (oral)
Dependence rating Low
Prescription needed Yes
Available as generic No

GENERAL INFORMATION

Amphotericin is a highly effective and powerful antifungal drug. When given by injection, it is used to treat serious systemic fungal infections. It is also given by mouth to treat candida (thrush) infections of the mouth or intestines, but it is not used in vaginal candidiasis. Treatment by injection is carefully supervised, usually in hospital, because of potentially serious adverse effects. A test dose for allergy may be given before a full injection. The newer formulations of amphotericin appear to be less toxic than the original injection. Adverse reactions to the oral forms of the drug are rare.

INFORMATION FOR USERS

Your drug prescription is tailored for you. Do not alter dosage without checking with your doctor.

How taken/used Tablets, lozenges, liquid, injection.

Frequency and timing of doses Every 6 hours (by mouth); once daily (injection).

Dosage range 400–800mg daily (tablets and liquid); 40–80mg daily (lozenges); the dosage for injection is determined on an individual basis.

Onset of effect Improvement may be noticed after 2–4 days.

Duration of action 3–6 hours.

Diet advice When it is given by injection, amphotericin may reduce the levels of potassium and magnesium in the blood. To correct this, mineral supplements may be recommended.

Storage Keep in original container at room temperature out of the reach of children. Some brands of injection should be stored in the fridge.

Missed dose Take oral dose as soon as you remember. Take your next dose when scheduled.

Stopping the drug Take the full course as prescribed. Even if symptoms improve, the original infection may still be present and symptoms may recur if treatment is stopped too soon.

Exceeding the dose An occasional unintentional extra oral dose is unlikely to be a cause for concern. But if you notice unusual symptoms, notify your doctor.

POSSIBLE ADVERSE EFFECTS

Amphotericin is given by injection only under close medical supervision. Adverse effects are thus carefully monitored and promptly treated. Adverse effects from oral administration are rare.

INTERACTIONS (INJECTION ONLY)

Digitalis drugs Amphotericin may increase the toxicity of digoxin.

Diuretics Amphotericin increases the risk of low potassium levels with diuretics.

Aminoglycoside antibiotics Taken with amphotericin, these drugs increase the likelihood of kidney damage.

Corticosteroids may increase loss of potassium from the body caused by amphotericin.

Ciclosporin and tacrolimus increase the likelihood of kidney damage.

SPECIAL PRECAUTIONS

Be sure to tell your doctor if:
◆ You have a long-term liver or kidney problem.
◆ You have previously had an allergic reaction to amphotericin.
◆ You are taking other medicines.

Pregnancy There is no evidence of risk from the oral forms of the drug. Injections of amphotericin are given only when the infection is very serious.

Breast-feeding There is no evidence of risk from oral forms of the drug. It is not known whether the drug passes into the breast milk when given by injection. Discuss with your doctor.

Infants and children Reduced dose may be necessary.

Over 60 No special problems.

Driving and hazardous work No known problems.

Alcohol No known problems.

PROLONGED USE

Given by injection, the drug may cause a reduction in blood levels of potassium and magnesium. It may also damage the kidneys and cause blood disorders.

Monitoring Regular blood tests to monitor liver and kidney function, blood cell counts, and potassium and magnesium levels are advised during treatment by injection.

Anastrozole

Brand name Arimidex
Used in the following combined preparations None

QUICK REFERENCE

Drug group Anticancer drug (p.96)
Overdose danger rating Low
Dependence rating Low
Prescription needed Yes
Available as generic No

GENERAL INFORMATION

Anastrozole is a potent non-steroidal inhibitor of the enzymes that manufacture oestradiol (natural oestrogen) in the body. It can reduce production of oestradiol by more than 80 per cent. Anastrozole is used in the treatment of breast cancer in post menopausal women and is contraindicated in pregnancy and breast-feeding. Anastrozole is generally well tolerated; adverse effects are mainly gastrointestinal or gynaecological, and are generally similar to menopausal symptoms. If there is any doubt about whether the woman to be treated is postmenopausal, a biochemical test may be performed.

INFORMATION FOR USERS

Your drug prescription is tailored for you. Do not alter dosage without checking with your doctor.

How taken/used Tablets.

Frequency and timing of doses Once daily.

Adult dosage range 1mg.

Onset of effect 30 minutes.

Duration of action 24 hours.

Diet advice None.

Storage Keep in original container at room temperature out of the reach of children.

Missed dose Take as soon as you remember. If your next dose is due within 2 hours, take a single dose now and skip the next.

Stopping the drug Do not stop the drug without consulting your doctor. Stopping the drug may lead to worsening of the underlying condition.

Exceeding the dose An occasional unintentional extra dose is unlikely to be a cause for concern. But if you notice any unusual symptoms, or if a large overdose has been taken, notify your doctor.

POSSIBLE ADVERSE EFFECTS

Anastrozole is usually well tolerated, and any side effects are relatively minor. It may cause hot flushes, headache, fatigue, and dizziness. Rarely, there may be stiffness or joint pain, vaginal dryness, rashes, thinning of hair, nausea, and diarrhoea. Consult your doctor if any of the side effects become severe.

INTERACTIONS

Tamoxifen and oestrogens oppose the effects of anastrozole.

SPECIAL PRECAUTIONS

Be sure to tell your doctor if:
◆ You are premenopausal.
◆ You have kidney or liver problems.
◆ You are allergic to anastrozole.
◆ You are taking other medicines.
Pregnancy Not prescribed in pregnancy.
Breast-feeding Not prescribed when breast-feeding.
Infants and children Not recommended.
Over 60 No special problems.
Driving and hazardous work Do not drive until you know how the drug affects you. It can cause drowsiness.
Alcohol No known problems

PROLONGED USE

No known problems.
Monitoring Women with osteoporosis or at risk of osteoporosis will have their bone mineral density assessed at the start of treatment and at regular intervals.

Apomorphine

Brand name APO-go
Used in the following combined preparations None

QUICK REFERENCE

Drug group Drug for parkinsonism (p.18)
Overdose danger rating High
Dependence rating Low
Prescription needed Yes
Available as generic No

GENERAL INFORMATION

Apomorphine is a derivative of morphine, with a chemical structure similar to dopamine.

It stimulates the vomiting centre in the brain, but is used to control the "on-off" episodes of parkinsonism. A patient will be given two to three days' treatment with the anti-emetic drug domperidone before stopping his or her existing anti-parkinsonism drugs overnight to provoke an "off" period. Increasing doses of apomorphine are then given by injection to find the lowest effective dose. Then the regular drug treatment is re-started. At the first sign of an "off" period, an apomorphine injection is given into the lower abdomen or outer thigh. Dosing is adjusted according to the patient's response. Domperidone is then normally withdrawn.

INFORMATION FOR USERS

Your drug prescription is tailored for you. Do not alter dosage without checking with your doctor.
How taken/used Injection.
Frequency and timing of doses 1–10 x daily, or continuous infusion.
Adult dosage range 3–30mg daily, up to a maximum of 100mg (injection).
Onset of effect A few minutes.
Duration of action 2 hours.
Diet advice None.
Storage Keep in original container at room temperature out of the reach of children.
Missed dose Take as soon as you need to.

OVERDOSE ACTION

An unintentional extra dose may cause vomiting. If a large overdose has been taken, seek immediate medical advice. Take emergency action if breathing problems or loss of consciousness occur.

POSSIBLE ADVERSE EFFECTS

Because injections of apomorphine have a strong emetic (causing vomiting) effect, the anti-emetic drug domperidone must be taken at the same time to counteract this. Other common adverse effects of apomorphine include irritation at the injection site, drowsiness and fatigue, and taste disturbances; discuss with your doctor if these are severe. Apomorphine may also cause dizziness or confusion and visual disturbances and you should consult your doctor if you experience any of these effects.

INTERACTIONS

Nitrates When taken with apomorphine, these drugs can cause a fall in blood pressure.

Antipsychotics and methyldopa may reduce the effects of apomorphine.

Dopaminergic drugs and memantine may increase the effects of apomorphine.

SPECIAL PRECAUTIONS

Be sure to tell your doctor if:

◆ You have kidney or liver problems or lung disease.

◆ You have any psychological problems.

◆ You have recently had heart problems.

◆ You have high or low blood pressure.

◆ You are taking other medicines.

Pregnancy Safety not established. Discuss with your doctor.

Breast-feeding Safety not established. Discuss with your doctor.

Infants and children Not recommended.

Over 60 No special problems.

Driving and hazardous work Avoid such activities until you have learned how apomorphine affects you because the drug can cause dizziness, lightheadedness, drowsiness, and fainting. If you have parkinsonism, driving is not allowed.

Alcohol No special problems.

PROLONGED USE

No known problems.

Aspirin

Brand names Angettes, Aspro, Caprin, Disprin, Nu-Seals Aspirin, and others

Used in the following combined preparations Anadin, Aspav, Codis, and others

QUICK REFERENCE

Drug group Non-opioid analgesic (p.10), antiplatelet drug (p.39), and antipyretic

Overdose danger rating High

Dependence rating Low

Prescription needed No

Available as generic Yes

GENERAL INFORMATION

In use for over 80 years, aspirin relieves pain, reduces fever, and alleviates the symptoms of arthritis. In low doses, it helps to prevent blood clots, particularly in atherosclerosis or angina caused by coronary artery disease, and it reduces the risk of heart attacks and strokes.

Aspirin is present in many medicines for colds, flu, headaches, menstrual period pains, and joint or muscular aches. It may irritate the stomach and even cause stomach ulcers or bleeding. Another drawback of aspirin is that it can provoke asthma attacks.

In children, aspirin can cause Reye's syndrome, a rare but serious brain and liver disorder. For this reason, aspirin should not be given to children under the age of 16 years, except on the advice of a doctor.

INFORMATION FOR USERS

Follow instructions on the label. Call your doctor if symptoms worsen.

How taken/used Tablets, SR-capsules, suppositories.

Frequency and timing of doses *Relief of pain or fever* Every 4–6 hours, as necessary, with or after food or milk. *Prevention of blood clots* Once daily.

Adult dosage range *Relief of pain or fever* 300–900mg per dose. *Prevention of blood clots* 75–300mg daily.

Onset of effect 30–60 minutes (regular aspirin); 1½–8 hours (coated tablets or SR-capsules).

Duration of action Up to 12 hours. Effect persists for several days when used to prevent blood clotting.

Diet advice Take with or immediately after food.

Storage Keep in original container at room temperature out of the reach of children.

Missed dose Take as soon as you remember. If your next dose is due within 2 hours, take a single dose now and skip the next.

Stopping the drug If you have been prescribed aspirin by your doctor for a long-term condition, you should seek medical advice before stopping the drug. Otherwise, the drug can be safely stopped as soon as you no longer need it.

OVERDOSE ACTION

Seek immediate advice in all cases. Take emergency action if there is restlessness, stomach pain, ringing noises in the ears, blurred vision, or vomiting.

POSSIBLE ADVERSE EFFECTS

Adverse effects are more likely to occur with high doses of aspirin, but may be reduced by taking the drug with food or in buffered or enteric coated forms. If indigestion, rash, or wheezing occur, stop taking aspirin. If you vomit blood, have black bowel movements, or experience ringing noises in the ears or dizziness, stop taking the drug and contact your doctor urgently.

INTERACTIONS

Anticoagulants Aspirin may add to the anticoagulant effect of such drugs, leading to an increased risk of abnormal bleeding.

Drugs for gout Aspirin may reduce the effect of these drugs.

NSAIDs may increase the likelihood of stomach irritation with aspirin.

Methotrexate Aspirin may increase the toxicity of this drug.

Oral antidiabetic drugs Aspirin may increase the effect of these drugs.

Corticosteroids and some SSRI antidepressants These may increase the risk of stomach bleeding with aspirin.

SPECIAL PRECAUTIONS

Be sure to consult your doctor or pharmacist before taking this drug if:
◆ You have long-term liver or kidney problems.
◆ You have asthma.
◆ You are allergic to aspirin or any NSAID.
◆ You have a blood clotting disorder.
◆ You have had a stomach ulcer.
◆ You are taking other medicines.

Pregnancy Not usually recommended. An alternative may be safer. Discuss with your doctor.

Breast-feeding The drug passes into the breast milk. Discuss with your doctor.

Infants and children Do not give to children under 16 years, except on a doctor's advice.

Over 60 Adverse effects more likely.

Driving and hazardous work No special problems.

Alcohol Avoid. Alcohol increases the likelihood of stomach irritation with this drug.

Surgery and general anaesthetics Regular treatment with aspirin may need to be stopped about one week before surgery. Discuss with your doctor or dentist before any operation.

PROLONGED USE

Except for low doses to help prevent blood clotting, aspirin should not be taken for longer than 2 days except on the advice of your doctor. Prolonged use of aspirin may lead to bleeding in the stomach and to stomach ulcers.

Atenolol

Brand names Antipressan, Atenix, Tenormin
Used in the following combined preparations
Beta-Adalat, Co-tenidone, Kalten, Tenchlor, Tenif, Tenoret, Tenoretic, Totaretic

QUICK REFERENCE

Drug group Beta blocker (p.30)
Overdose danger rating Medium
Dependence rating Low
Prescription needed Yes
Available as generic Yes

GENERAL INFORMATION

Atenolol belongs to the beta blocker group of drugs. It prevents the heart from beating too quickly and is used mainly to treat irregular heart rhythms (arrhythmias), and chest pain (angina). It is also used to treat hypertension (high blood pressure) but is not usually used to initiate treatment.

Because atenolol is cardioselective, it is less likely than other, non-cardioselective beta blockers to provoke breathing difficulties, but it is not usually given to people with asthma, bronchitis, or any other form of respiratory disease. It may also be given following a heart attack to protect the heart from further damage.

Atenolol does not cure heart disease; it only controls the symptoms, so it usually has to be taken long term.

INFORMATION FOR USERS

Your drug prescription is tailored for you. Do not alter dosage without checking with your doctor.

How taken/used Tablets, liquid, injection.
Frequency and timing of doses 1–2 x daily.
Adult dosage range 25–100mg daily.
Onset of effect 2–4 hours.
Duration of action 20–30 hours.
Diet advice None.
Storage Keep in original container in a cool, dry place out of the reach of children. Protect from light.
Missed dose Take as soon as you remember. If your next dose is due within 6 hours, do not take the missed dose but take the next scheduled dose as usual.
Stopping the drug Do not stop taking the drug without consulting your doctor; sudden withdrawal may lead to dangerous worsening of the underlying condition. It should be withdrawn gradually.
Exceeding the dose An occasional unintentional extra dose is unlikely to be a cause for concern. But if you notice any unusual symptoms, or if a large overdose has been taken, notify your doctor.

POSSIBLE ADVERSE EFFECTS

Atenolol has adverse effects that are common to most beta blockers. Symptoms are usually temporary and tend to diminish with long-term use. Muscle aches, fatigue, and dry eyes are common. Other possible effects include cold hands and feet, sleep disturbances, headaches, and dizziness. If you develop a rash or breathing difficulties, stop taking the drug and contact your doctor immediately.

INTERACTIONS

Anti-arrhythmic drugs When used together with atenolol they may increase the risk of adverse effects on the heart.
Antidiabetic drugs used with atenolol may increase the risk and/or mask many symptoms of low blood glucose.
Decongestants used with atenolol may increase blood pressure and heart rate.
Calcium channel blockers Taken with atenolol, some of these drugs may further decrease blood pressure and/or heart rate. They may also reduce the force of the heart's pumping action.
Non-steroidal anti-inflammatory drugs (NSAIDs) These drugs may reduce the antihypertensive effect of atenolol.

SPECIAL PRECAUTIONS

Be sure to tell your doctor if:
◆ You have any other heart condition.
◆ You have a long-term kidney problem.
◆ You have diabetes.
◆ You have a lung disorder such as asthma or bronchitis.
◆ You are taking other medicines.
Pregnancy Safety in pregnancy not established. Discuss with your doctor.
Breast-feeding The drug passes into the breast milk. Discuss with your doctor.
Infants and children Not recommended.
Over 60 No special problems. Reduced dose may be necessary if there is impaired kidney function.
Driving and hazardous work Avoid such activities until you have learned how atenolol affects you because the drug can cause dizziness.
Alcohol No special problems with drinking small amounts.
Surgery and general anaesthetics Treatment with atenolol may need to be stopped before you have a general anaesthetic. Discuss this with your doctor or dentist before any surgery.

PROLONGED USE

No special problems expected.

Atorvastatin

Brand name Lipitor
Used in the following combined preparations None

QUICK REFERENCE

Drug group Lipid-lowering drug (p.37)
Overdose danger rating Medium
Dependence rating Low
Prescription needed Yes
Available as generic No

GENERAL INFORMATION

Atorvastatin is a member of the statin group of lipid-lowering drugs. It is used to treat hypercholesterolaemia (high levels of cholesterol in the blood) in patients who have not responded to other treatments, such as a special diet or lifestyle changes, and who have, or are at risk of developing, heart disease. Atorvastatin is also used to treat patients with diabetes who are at high risk of heart attack or stroke. It blocks the action, in the liver, of an enzyme that is needed for the manufacture of cholesterol. As a result, blood levels of cholesterol are lowered, which can help to prevent coronary heart disease. Rarely, atorvastatin can cause muscle pain, inflammation, and muscle damage.

INFORMATION FOR USERS

Your drug prescription is tailored for you. Do not alter dosage without checking with your doctor.

How taken/used Tablets.

Frequency and timing of doses Once daily.

Adult dosage range 10–80mg; up to 80mg (inherited hypercholesterolaemia).

Onset of effect Within 2 weeks. Full beneficial effects are usually seen within 4 weeks.

Duration of action 20–30 hours.

Diet advice A low-fat diet is usually recommended. Do not drink more than 2 small glasses of grapefruit juice per day.

Storage Keep in original container at room temperature out of the reach of children.

Missed dose Take as soon as you remember. If your next dose is due within 8 hours, do not take the missed dose, but take the next one on schedule.

Stopping the drug Do not stop taking the drug without consulting your doctor. Stopping the drug may lead to a recurrence of the original condition.

Exceeding the dose An occasional unintentional extra dose is unlikely to cause problems. However, large overdoses may cause liver problems. Notify your doctor.

POSSIBLE ADVERSE EFFECTS

Adverse effects of atorvastatin, which include nausea, constipation or diarrhoea, headache, dizziness, tiredness, and insomnia, are usually mild and transient. Other adverse effects include jaundice and erectile dysfunction (impotence). Muscle damage is a rare side effect of the drug, and any muscle aching or weakness should be reported to your doctor immediately. You should also notify your doctor immediately if you develop a rash.

INTERACTIONS

Warfarin Atorvastatin may reduce the anticoagulant effect of warfarin. The dose of warfarin may need to be adjusted.

Antifungal drugs Itraconazole, ketoconazole, and possibly other antifungal drugs, may increase the risk of muscle damage with atorvastatin.

Macrolide antibiotics (for example, erythromycin, clarithromycin) Taken with atorvastatin, these drugs may increase the risk of muscle damage.

Other lipid-lowering drugs Taken with atorvastatin, these drugs may increase the risk of muscle damage.

Ciclosporin and other immunosuppressant drugs Atorvastatin is not usually prescribed with these drugs because of the increased risk of muscle damage. However, if using the drugs together is unavoidable, close monitoring is advised.

SPECIAL PRECAUTIONS

Be sure to tell your doctor if:
◆ You have had liver problems.
◆ You have kidney problems.
◆ You are a heavy drinker.
◆ You have an underactive thyroid.
◆ You or a family member have a muscle disorder.
◆ You have had muscle problems or other reactions with other lipid-lowering drugs.
◆ You are taking other medicines.

Pregnancy Not usually prescribed. Safety not established. Discuss with your doctor.

Breast-feeding Safety not established. Discuss with your doctor.

Infants and children Not recommended.

Over 60 No special problems.

Driving and hazardous work No special problems.

Alcohol Avoid excessive amounts. Alcohol may increase the risk of developing liver problems with atorvastatin.

PROLONGED USE

Long-term use of atorvastatin may affect liver function.

Monitoring Regular blood tests to check liver function are needed. In addition, tests of muscle function may be carried out if any problems are suspected.

Atropine

Brand name Minims Atropine
Used in the following combined preparations
Actonorm, Co-phenotrope, Dymotil, Isopto Atropine, Lomotil

QUICK REFERENCE

Drug group Anticholinergic drug for irritable bowel syndrome (p.45) and mydriatic drug (p.116)
Overdose danger rating High
Dependence rating Low
Prescription needed Yes (most preparations)
Available as generic Yes

GENERAL INFORMATION

Atropine is an anticholinergic drug. Because of its antispasmodic action, which relaxes the muscle wall of the intestine, the drug has been used to relieve abdominal cramps in irritable bowel syndrome. Atropine may also be prescribed in combination with diphenoxylate, an antidiarrhoeal drug. However, this combination can be dangerous in overdosage, particularly in young children.

Atropine eye drops are used to enlarge the pupil during eye examinations and are part of the treatment for inflammatory eye disorders such as uveitis. Atropine may be used as part of premedication before a general anaesthetic. The drug is occasionally injected to restore normal heart beat in heart block (see p.34).

Atropine must be used with caution in children and the elderly due to their sensitivity to the drug's effects.

INFORMATION FOR USERS

Your drug prescription is tailored for you. Do not alter dosage without checking with your doctor.
How taken/used Tablets, injection, eye ointment, eye drops.
Frequency and timing of doses Once only, or up to 4 times daily according to condition (eye drops); as directed (other forms).
Adult dosage range 1–2 drops as directed (eye drops); as directed (other forms).
Onset of effect Varies according to method of administration. 30 minutes (eye drops).
Duration of action 7 days or longer (eye drops); several hours (other forms).
Diet advice None.

Storage Keep in original container at room temperature out of the reach of children. Protect from light.
Missed dose Take as soon as you remember. If your next dose is due within 2 hours, take a single dose now and skip the next.
Stopping the drug Do not stop the drug without consulting your doctor.

OVERDOSE ACTION

Seek immediate medical advice in all cases. Take emergency action if palpitations, tremor, delirium, fits, or loss of consciousness occur.

POSSIBLE ADVERSE EFFECTS

The use of this drug is limited by the frequency of anticholinergic effects. These commonly include blurred vision, dry mouth, and constipation. There may also be difficulty passing urine, nausea, vomiting, and dizziness. If palpitations or confusion occur, you should contact your doctor immediately. The eye drops may cause stinging. If the eye drops also cause pain and irritation or if a rash develops on contact, stop using them and contact your doctor without delay.

INTERACTIONS

Anticholinergic drugs Atropine increases the risk of side effects from drugs that also have anticholinergic effects.
Ketoconazole Atropine reduces the absorption of this drug from the digestive tract. Increased dose may be necessary.

SPECIAL PRECAUTIONS

Be sure to tell your doctor if:
◆ You have long-term liver or kidney problems.
◆ You have prostate problems.
◆ You have gastro-oesophageal reflux.
◆ You have glaucoma.
◆ You have urinary difficulties.
◆ You have myasthenia gravis.
◆ You have ulcerative colitis.
◆ You wear contact lenses (eye drops).
◆ You have heart problems or high blood pressure.
◆ You are taking other medicines.
Pregnancy Safety in pregnancy not established. Discuss with your doctor.

Breast-feeding The drug may pass into the breast milk and affect the baby. Discuss with your doctor.

Infants and children Combination with diphenoxylate not recommended under 4 years; reduced dose necessary in older children.

Over 60 Increased likelihood of adverse effects.

Driving and hazardous work Avoid such activities until you have learned how atropine affects you because the drug can cause blurred vision and may impair concentration.

Alcohol Avoid. Alcohol increases the likelihood of confusion and affects your concentration when taken with atropine.

PROLONGED USE

No problems expected.

Azathioprine

Brand names Immunoprin, Imuran
Used in the following combined preparations
None

QUICK REFERENCE

Drug group Disease-modifying antirheumatic drug (p.51) and immunosuppressant drug (p.99)
Overdose danger rating Medium
Dependence rating Low
Prescription needed Yes
Available as generic Yes

GENERAL INFORMATION

Azathioprine is an immunosuppressant drug used to prevent immune-system rejection of transplanted organs. It is also used to modify, halt, or slow the underlying disease process in severe rheumatoid arthritis that has failed to respond to conventional drug therapy.

Autoimmune and collagen diseases (including systemic lupus erythematosus, polymyositis, myasthenia gravis, and dermatomyositis) may be treated with azathioprine, usually when corticosteroids have not been effective.

Azathioprine is administered only under close supervision because of the risk of serious adverse effects. These include suppression of white blood cell production, which increases the risk of infection as well as the risk of excessive or prolonged bleeding.

INFORMATION FOR USERS

Your drug prescription is tailored for you. Do not alter dosage without checking with your doctor.

How taken/used Tablets, injection.

Frequency and timing of doses Usually once daily with or after food.

Dosage range Initially according to body weight and the condition being treated and then adjusted according to response.

Onset of effect 2–4 weeks. Antirheumatic effect may not be felt for 8 weeks or more.

Duration of action Immunosuppressant effects may last for several weeks after the drug is stopped.

Diet advice None.

Storage Keep in original container at room temperature out of the reach of children. Protect from light.

Missed dose Take as soon as you remember, then return to your normal schedule. If more than 2 doses are missed, consult your doctor.

Stopping the drug Do not stop the drug without consulting your doctor. If taken to prevent transplant rejection, stopping treatment could provoke the rejection of the transplant.

Exceeding the dose An occasional unintentional extra dose is unlikely to cause problems. Large overdoses may cause nausea, vomiting, abdominal pains, and diarrhoea. Notify your doctor.

POSSIBLE ADVERSE EFFECTS

The most common adverse effects of azathioprine are nausea, loss of appetite, and hair loss. The drug may also cause unusual bleeding or bruising, jaundice, rash, fever or chills, pain in the side, and difficulty urinating. If any of these symptoms develop, contact your doctor immediately.

INTERACTIONS

Allopurinol Azathioprine increases the effects and toxicity of allopurinol; dosage of azathioprine will need to be reduced.

Warfarin Azathioprine may reduce the effect of warfarin.

Co-trimoxazole and trimethoprim These drugs may increase the risk of blood problems if taken with azathioprine.

Corticosteroids may increase the risk of infections and bowel problems.

SPECIAL PRECAUTIONS

Be sure to tell your doctor if:
◆ You have long-term liver or kidney problems.
◆ You have had a previous allergic reaction to azathioprine or 6-mercaptopurine.
◆ You have recently had shingles or chickenpox.
◆ You have an infection.
◆ You have a blood disorder.
◆ You are taking other medicines.

Pregnancy Azathioprine has been taken in pregnancy without problems. Discuss with your doctor.

Breast-feeding A small amount of the drug passes into the breast milk. Discuss with your doctor.

Infants and children No special problems.

Over 60 Increased likelihood of adverse effects. Reduced dose necessary.

Driving and hazardous work Avoid such activities until you have learned how azathioprine affects you because the drug can cause dizziness.

Alcohol No known problems.

PROLONGED USE

There may be a slightly increased risk of some cancers with the long-term use of azathioprine. Blood changes may also occur. Avoiding exposure to sunlight may help to prevent adverse skin effects.

Monitoring Regular checks on blood composition are usually carried out.

Baclofen

Brand names Baclospas, Lioresal, Lyflex
Used in the following combined preparations
None

QUICK REFERENCE

Drug group Muscle-relaxant drug (p.54)
Overdose danger rating Medium
Dependence rating Low
Prescription needed Yes
Available as generic Yes

GENERAL INFORMATION

Baclofen is a muscle-relaxant drug that acts on the central nervous system, including the spinal cord. The drug relieves the spasms, cramping, and muscle rigidity (commonly known as spasticity) caused by various disorders, including multiple sclerosis, spinal cord injury, brain injury, cerebral palsy, or stroke. Although baclofen does not cure these disorders, it increases mobility, allowing other treatment, such as physiotherapy, to be carried out.

Baclofen is less likely to cause muscle weakness than similar drugs, and its side effects, such as dizziness or drowsiness, are usually temporary. Elderly people are more susceptible to side effects, especially during early stages of treatment.

INFORMATION FOR USERS

Your drug prescription is tailored for you. Do not alter dosage without checking with your doctor.

How taken/used Tablets, liquid, injection (specialist use).

Frequency and timing of doses 3 x daily with food or milk.

Adult dosage range 15mg daily (starting dose). Daily dose may be increased by 15mg every 3 days as necessary. Maximum daily dose: 100mg.

Onset of effect Some benefits may appear after 1–3 hours, but full beneficial effects may not be felt for several weeks. A dose 1 hour before a specific task will improve mobility.

Duration of action Up to 8 hours.

Diet advice None.

Storage Keep in original container at room temperature out of the reach of children. Protect liquid from light.

Missed dose Take as soon as you remember. If your next dose is due within 2 hours, take a single dose now and skip the next.

Stopping the drug Do not stop taking the drug without consulting your doctor who will supervise a gradual reduction in dosage. Abrupt cessation may cause hallucinations, confusion, anxiety, seizures, and worsening of spasticity.

Exceeding the dose An occasional unintentional extra dose is unlikely to cause problems. Large overdoses may cause weakness, vomiting, and severe drowsiness. Notify your doctor.

POSSIBLE ADVERSE EFFECTS

The common adverse effects, such as dizziness and drowsiness, are related to the sedative effects of the drug. Such effects may be minimized by starting with a low dose that is gradually increased. Nausea and muscle weakness may also occur. Rarer adverse effects include constipation or diarrhoea, headache, and difficulty in passing urine. If any of the adverse effects are severe or if blurred vision or confusion occur, you should consult your doctor.

INTERACTIONS

Antihypertensive and diuretic drugs Baclofen may increase the blood-pressure lowering effect of such drugs.

Drugs for parkinsonism Some drugs used for parkinsonism may cause confusion and hallucinations if taken with baclofen.

Sedatives All drugs with a sedative effect on the central nervous system may increase the sedative properties of baclofen.

Tricyclic antidepressants These drugs may increase the effects of baclofen, leading to muscle weakness.

SPECIAL PRECAUTIONS

Be sure to tell your doctor if:
◆ You have long-term liver or kidney problems.
◆ You have difficulty in passing urine.
◆ You have had a peptic ulcer.
◆ You have had epileptic fits.
◆ You have diabetes.
◆ You have Parkinson's disease.
◆ You suffer with breathing problems.
◆ You are taking other medicines.

Pregnancy Safety in pregnancy not established. Discuss with your doctor.

Breast-feeding The drug passes into the breast milk, but at normal doses adverse effects on a baby are unlikely. Discuss with your doctor.

Infants and children Reduced dose necessary.

Over 60 Increased likelihood of adverse effects at start of treatment. Reduced initial dose may therefore be necessary.

Driving and hazardous work Avoid such activities until you have learned how baclofen affects you because the drug can cause drowsiness, decreased alertness, and blurred vision.

Alcohol Avoid. Alcohol may increase the sedative effects of this drug.

Surgery and general anaesthetics Be sure to inform your doctor or dentist that you are taking baclofen before you have a general anaesthetic.

PROLONGED USE

No problems expected.

Beclometasone

Brand names AeroBec, Asmabec, Beclazone, Becloforte, Beconase, Becotide, Filair, Nasobec, Propaderm, Qvar, and others
Used in the following combined preparations
None

QUICK REFERENCE

Drug group Corticosteroid (p.80) and topical corticosteroid (p.120)
Overdose danger rating Low
Dependence rating Low
Prescription needed Yes (some preparations)
Available as generic Yes

GENERAL INFORMATION

Beclometasone is a corticosteroid drug prescribed to relieve the symptoms of allergic rhinitis (as a nasal spray) and to control asthma (as an inhaler). It controls nasal symptoms by reducing inflammation and mucus production in the nose. It also helps to reduce chest symptoms, such as wheezing and coughing. Asthma sufferers may take it regularly to reduce the severity and frequency of attacks. However, once an attack has started, the drug does not relieve symptoms.

Beclometasone is given primarily to people whose asthma has not responded to bronchodilators alone (see p.23). Beclometasone is also used as the main ingredient in some skin creams and ointments to treat inflammatory conditions, particularly eczema. Being potent, the drug is not usually used on the face.

There are few serious adverse effects associated with beclometasone as it is given topically by nasal spray or inhaler. Fungal infections causing irritation of the mouth and throat are a possible side effect of inhaling beclometasone. These can be avoided to some degree by rinsing the mouth and gargling with water after each inhalation.

INFORMATION FOR USERS

Your drug prescription is tailored for you. Do not alter dosage without checking with your doctor.

How taken/used Cream, ointment, inhaler, nasal spray.

Frequency and timing of doses 2–4 x daily.

Dosage range *Adults* 1–2 puffs 2–4 x daily according to preparation used (asthma); 1–2 sprays in each nostril 2–4 x daily (allergic rhinitis); as directed but usually 1–2 x daily (skin conditions). *Children* Reduced dose according to age and weight.

Onset of effect Within 1 week (asthma); 1–3 days (allergic rhinitis). Full benefit may not be felt for up to 4 weeks (all conditions).

Duration of action Several days after stopping the drug.

Diet advice None.

Storage Keep in original container at room temperature out of the reach of children. Protect from light.

Missed dose Take as soon as you remember. If your next dose is due within 2 hours, take a single dose now and skip the next.

Stopping the drug Do not stop the drug without consulting your doctor; symptoms may recur. Sometimes a gradual reduction in dosage is recommended.

Exceeding the dose An occasional unintentional extra dose is unlikely to cause problems. But if you notice any unusual symptoms, or if a large overdose has been taken, notify your doctor. Adverse effects may occur if the recommended dose is regularly exceeded over a long period.

POSSIBLE ADVERSE EFFECTS

The main side effect of the inhaler is thrush of the throat and mouth, and irritation of the nose and throat for the nasal spray. Other possible adverse effects of the inhaler or spray are cough, hoarseness, and nosebleeds. More serious side effects, such as permanent skin changes, may occur with the ointment, which should not normally be used on the face.

INTERACTIONS

None.

SPECIAL PRECAUTIONS

Be sure to tell your doctor if:

◆ You have had tuberculosis or another nasal or respiratory infection.

◆ You have a skin infection (for treatment with cream or ointment).

◆ You have varicose ulcers (for treatment with cream or ointment).

Pregnancy No evidence of risk.

Breast-feeding No evidence of risk.

Infants and children Reduced dose necessary. Avoid prolonged use of ointment in infants and children.

Over 60 No known problems.

Driving and hazardous work No known problems.

Alcohol No known problems.

PROLONGED USE

No problems expected when used for asthma or allergic rhinitis, but high doses of the nasal spray can produce systemic (whole-body) effects. Prolonged use of beclometasone cream or ointment should be avoided where possible because it can cause permanent skin changes, especially on the face, and high doses can suppress the body's own corticosteroid production.

Monitoring Periodic checks to ensure that the adrenal glands are functioning healthily may be required if large doses are being used.

Bendroflumethiazide (bendrofluazide)

Brand names Aprinox, Neo-NaClex
Used in the following combined preparations
Centyl K, Neo-NaClex-K, Prestim

QUICK REFERENCE

Drug group Thiazide diuretic (p.32)
Overdose danger rating Low
Dependence rating Low
Prescription needed Yes
Available as generic Yes

GENERAL INFORMATION

Bendroflumethiazide belongs to the thiazide diuretic group of drugs, which expel water from the body. It is useful for reducing oedema (water retention) caused by heart, kidney, or liver conditions, and for treating premenstrual oedema. The drug is frequently used as a treatment for high blood pressure (see Antihypertensive drugs, p.36).

As with all thiazides, this drug increases the loss of potassium in the urine, which can cause various symptoms (see Possible adverse effects, below), and increases the likelihood of irregular heart rhythms, particularly if taken with digoxin for heart failure. Although this effect is rare with low doses, potassium supplements may be given with bendroflumethiazide as a precautionary measure.

INFORMATION FOR USERS

Your drug prescription is tailored for you. Do not alter dosage without checking with your doctor.

How taken/used Tablets.

Frequency and timing of doses Once daily, early in the day. (Sometimes 1–3 x per week.)

Adult dosage range 2.5–10mg daily.

Onset of effect Within 2 hours.

Duration of action 6–18 hours.

Diet advice Use of bendroflumethiazide may reduce potassium in the body, so you should eat plenty of fresh fruit and vegetables. Discuss with your doctor the advisability of reducing your dietary salt intake as a further precaution for hypertension.

Storage Keep in original container at room temperature out of the reach of children.

Missed dose No cause for concern, but take as soon as you remember. However, if it is late in the day do not take the missed dose, or you may need to get up during the night to pass urine. You should take the next scheduled dose as usual.

Stopping the drug Do not stop taking the drug without consulting your doctor; symptoms may recur.

Exceeding the dose An occasional unintentional extra dose is unlikely to be a cause for concern. But if you notice any unusual symptoms, or if a large overdose has been taken, notify your doctor.

POSSIBLE ADVERSE EFFECTS

Some adverse effects, such as dizziness (which is common), nausea, fatigue, and leg cramps, are the result of excessive loss of potassium but can usually be corrected by taking a potassium supplement. Bendroflumethiazide may precipitate gout in susceptible people, and certain forms of diabetes may become more difficult to control. Blood cholesterol level may rise slightly. Rarely, erectile dysfunction (impotence) or rash may occur; if so, you should discuss with your doctor and, with a rash, stop taking the drug.

INTERACTIONS

Non-steroidal anti-inflammatory drugs (NSAIDs) may reduce diuretic and antihypertensive effect of bendroflumethiazide, and bendroflumethiazide may increase kidney toxicity of NSAIDs.

Digoxin The effects of digoxin may be increased if excessive potassium is lost from the body.

Terfenadine Low potassium levels with bendroflumethiazide increase the risk of irregular heart beat with this antihistamine.

Anti-arrhythmic drugs Low potassium levels may increase these drugs' toxicity.

Lithium Bendroflumethiazide may increase lithium levels in the blood.

Corticosteroids These drugs further increase potassium loss when they are taken with bendroflumethiazide. Potassium supplements may be necessary. Corticosteroid drugs may also reduce the diuretic effect of bendroflumethiazide.

SPECIAL PRECAUTIONS

Be sure to tell your doctor if:

◆ You have long-term liver or kidney problems.

◆ You have or have had gout.

◆ You have diabetes.

◆ You have Addison's disease.

◆ You have systemic lupus erythematosus.

◆ You are taking other medicines.

Pregnancy Not usually prescribed. Safety in pregnancy not established. May affect the baby adversely. Discuss with your doctor.

Breast-feeding The drug passes into the breast milk and may reduce your milk supply. The amount absorbed by the baby is usually too small to be harmful. Discuss with your doctor.

Infants and children Not usually prescribed. Reduced dose necessary.

Over 60 Reduced dose may be necessary.
Driving and hazardous work No special problems.
Alcohol No problems expected if consumption is kept low.

PROLONGED USE

Prolonged use of this drug can lead to excessive loss of potassium and imbalances of other salts.
Monitoring Blood tests may be performed periodically to check kidney function and levels of potassium and other salts.

Benzoyl peroxide

Brand names Acnecide, Brevoxyl, Panoxyl
Used in the following combined preparations
Benzamycin, Duac Once Daily, Quinoderm

QUICK REFERENCE

Drug group Drug for acne (p.123)
Overdose danger rating Low
Dependence rating Low
Prescription needed Yes (some preparations)
Available as generic No

GENERAL INFORMATION

Benzoyl peroxide is used in a variety of topical preparations for the treatment of acne. It is available over the counter and comes in concentrations of varying strengths for treating moderate acne.

Benzoyl peroxide works by softening and shedding the top layer of skin and unblocking the sebaceous glands. It can also reduce inflammation of blocked hair follicles by killing the bacteria that infect them.

Benzoyl peroxide may cause irritation due to its drying effect on the skin, but this generally diminishes with time. The drug should be applied to the affected areas as directed on the label. Washing the area prior to application greatly enhances the drug's beneficial effects. Side effects are less likely if treatment is started with a preparation containing a low concentration of benzoyl peroxide, and changed to a stronger preparation only if necessary. Marked dryness and peeling of the skin, which may occur, can usually be controlled by reducing the frequency of application. Care should be taken to avoid contact of the drug with the eyes, mouth, and mucous membranes. It is also advisable to avoid excessive exposure to sunlight. Preparations of benzoyl peroxide may bleach clothing.

INFORMATION FOR USERS

Your drug prescription is tailored for you. Do not alter dosage without checking with your doctor.
How taken/used Cream, bodywash, gel, lotion.
Frequency and timing of doses 1–2 x daily (after washing with soap and water).
Dosage range Apply sparingly to affected skin, as instructed on the label.
Onset of effect Reduces oiliness of skin immediately. Acne usually improves within 4–6 weeks.
Duration of action 24–48 hours.
Diet advice None.
Storage Keep in original container at room temperature out of the reach of children.
Missed dose Apply as soon as you remember.
Stopping the drug Can be safely stopped as soon as you no longer need it.
Exceeding the dose A single extra application is unlikely to cause problems. Regular overuse may result in extensive irritation, peeling, redness, and swelling of the skin.

POSSIBLE ADVERSE EFFECTS

Application of benzoyl peroxide may cause temporary burning or stinging of the skin. Redness, peeling, and swelling may result from excessive drying of the skin and usually clear up if the treatment is stopped or used less frequently. If severe burning, blistering, or crusting occur, stop using benzoyl peroxide and consult your doctor.

INTERACTIONS

Skin-drying preparations Medicated cosmetics, soaps, toiletries, and other anti-acne preparations increase the likelihood of dryness and irritation of the skin with benzoyl peroxide.

SPECIAL PRECAUTIONS

Be sure to consult your doctor if:
◆ You have eczema.
◆ You have sunburn.
◆ You have had a previous allergic reaction to benzoyl peroxide.

◆ You are taking other medicines.
Pregnancy No evidence of risk.
Breast-feeding No evidence of risk.
Infants and children Not usually recommended under 12 years except under medical supervision.
Over 60 Not usually required.
Driving and hazardous work No known problems.
Alcohol No known problems.

PROLONGED USE

Benzoyl peroxide usually takes 4–6 weeks to produce an effect. Continuation beyond this time should be on the advice of your doctor.

Betahistine

Brand name Serc
Used in the following combined preparations None

QUICK REFERENCE

Drug group Drug for Ménière's disease (p.22)
Overdose danger rating High
Dependence rating Low
Prescription needed Yes
Available as generic Yes

GENERAL INFORMATION

Betahistine, a drug that resembles the naturally occurring substance histamine in some of its effects, was introduced in the 1970s as a treatment for Ménière's disease, which is caused by the pressure of excess fluid in the inner ear. Taken regularly, betahistine reduces both the frequency and the severity of the nausea and vertigo attacks that characterize this condition. The drug may also be used to treat tinnitus (ringing in the ears) and hearing loss as a result of Ménière's disease. Betahistine is thought to work by reducing pressure in the inner ear. Drug treatment is not successful in all cases, and surgery may be needed.

INFORMATION FOR USERS

Your drug prescription is tailored for you. Do not alter dosage without checking with your doctor.
How taken/used Tablets.
Frequency and timing of doses 3 x daily with or after food.

Adult dosage range 24–48mg daily.
Onset of effect Usually within 1 hour, but full effect may not be reached for some time.
Duration of action 6–12 hours.
Diet advice None.
Storage Keep in original container at room temperature out of the reach of children.
Missed dose Take as soon as you remember. If your next dose is due within 2 hours, take a single dose now and skip the next.
Stopping the drug Do not stop taking the drug without consulting your doctor; symptoms may recur.

OVERDOSE ACTION

Seek immediate medical advice in all cases. Large overdoses may cause collapse requiring emergency action.

POSSIBLE ADVERSE EFFECTS

Adverse effects from betahistine are minor and rarely cause problems. Nausea, indigestion, headache, and itching may occur. Rarely, a rash may occur; if so, consult your doctor.

INTERACTIONS

Antihistamines Although unproven, there is a possibility that betahistine may reduce the effects of these drugs, and antihistamines may reduce the effects of betahistine.

SPECIAL PRECAUTIONS

Be sure to tell your doctor if:
◆ You have asthma.
◆ You have a peptic ulcer.
◆ You have phaeochromocytoma.
◆ You are taking other medicines.
Pregnancy Safety in pregnancy not established. Discuss with your doctor.
Breast-feeding The drug may pass into the breast milk, and effects on the baby are unknown; however, at normal doses adverse effects are unlikely. Discuss with your doctor.
Infants and children Not recommended.
Over 60 No special problems.
Driving and hazardous work No special problems.
Alcohol No special problems.

PROLONGED USE

No special problems.

Betamethasone

Brand names Betacap, Betnelan, Betnesol, Betnovate, Bettamousse, Diprosone, Vista-Methasone
Used in the following combined preparations
Betnesol-N, Betnovate-C, Betnovate-N, Diprosalic, FuciBET, Lotriderm

QUICK REFERENCE

Drug group Corticosteroid (p.80)
Overdose danger rating Low
Dependence rating Low
Prescription needed Yes
Available as generic Yes

GENERAL INFORMATION

Betamethasone is a corticosteroid drug used to treat a variety of conditions. When injected directly into the joints it relieves joint inflammation and the pain and stiffness of rheumatoid arthritis. It is also given by mouth or injection to treat certain endocrine conditions affecting the pituitary and adrenal glands, and some blood disorders. It is also used topically to treat skin complaints, such as eczema and psoriasis.

When taken for short periods, low or moderate doses of betamethasone rarely cause serious side effects. High dosages or prolonged use can lead to many symptoms (see right).

INFORMATION FOR USERS

Your drug prescription is tailored for you. Do not alter dosage without checking with your doctor.
How taken/used Tablets, injection, cream, ointment, rectal ointment, lotion, scalp solution, eye ointment, eye/ear/nose drops.
Frequency and timing of doses Usually once daily in the morning (systemic). Otherwise varies according to disorder being treated.
Dosage range Varies; follow your doctor's instructions.
Onset of effect Within 30 minutes (injection); within 48 hours (other forms).
Duration of action Up to 24 hours.
Diet advice A low-sodium and high-potassium diet may be recommended when the oral form of the drug is prescribed for extended periods. Follow the advice of your doctor.
Storage Keep in original container at room temperature out of the reach of children. Protect from light.
Missed dose Take as soon as you remember. If your next dose is due within 2 hours, take a single dose now and skip the next.
Stopping the drug Do not stop tablets without consulting your doctor, who may supervise a gradual reduction in dosage. Abrupt cessation after long-term use may cause problems with the pituitary and adrenal gland system.
Exceeding the dose An occasional unintentional extra dose is unlikely to cause problems. But if any unusual symptoms occur or if a large overdose has been taken, notify your doctor.

POSSIBLE ADVERSE EFFECTS

Topical preparations are unlikely to cause adverse effects unless overused. Possible adverse effects of oral betamethasone include indigestion, weight gain, acne, and mood changes. If any of these occur, discuss with your doctor. The drug may also cause bloody or black faeces; if so, stop taking the drug and call your doctor immediately. Serious adverse effects usually occur only when high doses are taken by mouth for long periods (see Prolonged use, right).

INTERACTIONS

Insulin, antidiabetic drugs, and oral anticoagulant drugs Betamethasone may alter insulin requirements and the effects of these drugs.
Vaccines Serious reactions can occur when certain vaccinations are given during betamethasone treatment.
Antifungal drugs (e.g. erythromycin) may increase the effects of betamethasone.
Antihypertensive drugs and drugs used in myasthenia gravis Betamethasone may reduce the effects of these drugs.
Anticonvulsants and barbiturates These drugs may reduce the effects of betamethasone.
Vaccines Betamethasone can interact with some vaccines. Discuss with your doctor before having any vaccinations.

SPECIAL PRECAUTIONS

Be sure to tell your doctor if:
◆ You suffer from a mental disorder.
◆ You have a heart condition.
◆ You have glaucoma.
◆ You have high blood pressure.

◆ You have a history of epilepsy.
◆ You have had a peptic ulcer.
◆ You have had tuberculosis.
◆ You have any infection.
◆ You have diabetes.
◆ You have liver or kidney problems.
◆ You are taking other medicines.

Pregnancy No evidence of risk with topical preparations. Taken as tablets in low doses, harm to the baby is unlikely. Discuss with your doctor.

Breast-feeding No risk with topical preparations. Normal doses of tablets are unlikely to have adverse effects on the baby. Discuss with your doctor.

Infants and children Reduced dose necessary.

Over 60 Reduced dose may be necessary.

Driving and hazardous work No known problems.

Alcohol Keep consumption low. Betamethasone tablets increase the risk of peptic ulcers.

Infection If on systemic treatment, avoid exposure to chickenpox, measles, or shingles.

PROLONGED USE

Prolonged use by mouth can lead to peptic ulcers, glaucoma, fragile bones, muscle weakness, and growth retardation in children. Prolonged use of topical treatment may also lead to skin thinning. People taking betamethasone tablets regularly should carry a "steroid treatment" card or wear a MedicAlert bracelet.

Bezafibrate

Brand names Bezalip, Bezalip-Mono, Zimbacol XL
Used in the following combined preparations
None

QUICK REFERENCE

Drug group Lipid-lowering drug (p.37)
Overdose danger rating Low
Dependence rating Low
Prescription needed Yes
Available as generic Yes

GENERAL INFORMATION

Bezafibrate belongs to a group of drugs, usually called fibrates, that lower lipid levels in the blood. Fibrates are particularly effective in decreasing levels of triglycerides in

the blood. They also reduce blood levels of cholesterol. Raised levels of lipids (fats) in the blood are associated with atherosclerosis (deposition of fat in blood vessel walls). This can lead to coronary heart disease (for example, angina and heart attacks) and cerebrovascular disease (for example, stroke). When bezafibrate is taken with a diet low in saturated fats, there is good evidence that the risk of coronary heart disease is reduced.

INFORMATION FOR USERS

Your drug prescription is tailored for you. Do not alter dosage without checking with your doctor.

How taken/used Tablets.

Frequency and timing of doses 1–3 x daily with a little liquid after a meal.

Adult dosage range 400–600mg daily.

Onset of effect A beneficial effect on blood fat levels may not be produced for some weeks, and it takes months or years for fat deposits in the arteries to be reduced. Treatment should be withdrawn if no adequate response is obtained within 3–4 months.

Duration of action About 6–24 hours. This may vary according to the individual.

Diet advice A low-fat diet will have been recommended. Follow the advice of your doctor.

Storage Keep in original container at room temperature out of the reach of children.

Missed dose Take as soon as you remember. If your next dose is due within 4 hours (and you take it once daily), take a single dose now and skip the next. If you take 2–3 times daily, take the next dose as normal.

Stopping the drug Do not stop the drug without consulting your doctor.

Exceeding the dose An occasional unintentional extra dose is unlikely to be a cause for concern. But if you notice unusual symptoms, notify your doctor.

POSSIBLE ADVERSE EFFECTS

The most common adverse effects are those on the gastrointestinal tract, such as loss of appetite and nausea. These effects normally diminish as treatment continues. More rarely, there may be a rash, headache, or muscle pain, cramp or weakness; if any of these occur, discuss with your doctor.

INTERACTIONS

Anticoagulants Bezafibrate may increase the effect of anticoagulants such as warfarin. Dosage of anticoagulant will be reduced.

Monoamine oxidase inhibitors (MAOIs) There is a risk of liver damage when bezafibrate is taken with an MAOI.

Antidiabetic drugs Bezafibrate may interact with these to lower blood glucose levels.

Pravastatin, simvastatin, and other lipid-lowering drugs whose names end in 'statin' There is an increased risk of muscle damage if bezafibrate is taken with these drugs.

SPECIAL PRECAUTIONS

Be sure to tell your doctor if:
◆ You have long-term liver or kidney problems.
◆ You have a history of gallbladder disease.
◆ You are taking other medicines.

Pregnancy Safety in pregnancy not established. Discuss with your doctor.

Breast-feeding The drug may pass into the breast milk and may affect the baby. Discuss with your doctor.

Infants and children Not usually prescribed.

Over 60 No special problems expected.

Driving and hazardous work Avoid such activities until you have learned how bezafibrate affects you; it can cause dizziness.

Alcohol No special problems.

PROLONGED USE

No problems expected, but patients with kidney disease will need special care as there is a high risk of muscle problems developing in such cases.

Monitoring Blood tests will be performed occasionally to monitor the effect of the drug on lipids in the blood.

Bisoprolol

Brand names Bipranix, Cardicor, Emcor, Monocor, Soloc, Vivacor

Used in the following combined preparations
None

QUICK REFERENCE

Drug group Beta blocker (p.30)

Overdose danger rating Medium

Dependence rating Low

Prescription needed Yes

Available as generic Yes

GENERAL INFORMATION

Bisoprolol belongs to the cardioselective group of beta blockers. It is used in the treatment of angina pectoris (pain in the chest caused by insufficient oxygen reaching the heart muscle) and heart failure (inability of the heart to cope with its workload), usually in combination with an ACE inhibitor and a diuretic. It is also used to treat hypertension (high blood pressure), but it is not usually used to initiate treatment. Because bisoprolol is cardioselective (see p.30), it is less likely than other, non-cardioselective, beta blockers to cause breathing difficulties. However, it is not usually given to people who have a history of asthma, chronic bronchitis, or other respiratory diseases.

INFORMATION FOR USERS

Your drug prescription is tailored for you. Do not alter dosage without checking with your doctor.

How taken/used Tablets.

Frequency and timing of doses Once daily.

Adult dosage range *Heart failure* 1.25mg per day (initial dose), increasing to 10mg. *Hypertension and angina* 5–20mg (5mg is adequate for many people).

Onset of effect 2 hours. Full antihypertensive effect seen after two weeks.

Duration of action 24 hours.

Diet advice None.

Storage Keep in original container in a dry cool place, out of the reach of children.

Missed dose Take as soon as you remember. If your next dose is due within 12 hours, take a single dose now. If more than 12 hours have passed, skip the missed dose and take the next dose at the scheduled time.

Stopping the drug Do not stop taking the drug without consulting your doctor; abrupt cessation may lead to worsening of the underlying condition. The drug should be withdrawn gradually.

Exceeding the dose An occasional unintentional dose is unlikely to be a cause for concern. But if you notice any unusual symptoms, or if a large overdose has been taken, notify your doctor.

POSSIBLE ADVERSE EFFECTS

Bisoprolol has adverse effects common to most beta blockers. The symptoms are usually temporary and tend to diminish with long-term use of the drug. Common adverse effects of bisoprolol include lethargy, fatigue, muscle ache, and cold hands and feet. More rarely, the drug may cause vivid dreams or nightmares, sexual dysfunction, and dizziness or fainting. If you experience dizziness or fainting, you should talk to your doctor. Occasionally, the drug may cause breathing difficulties; if so, you should stop taking it and consult your doctor immediately.

INTERACTIONS

Other antihypertensives may enhance bisoprolol's blood pressure-lowering effect and some may worsen heart failure.

Non-steroidal anti-inflammatory drugs (NSAIDs) may reduce the blood pressure-lowering effect of bisoprolol.

Insulin and oral antidiabetics Bisoprolol may increase the blood glucose-lowering effect of these drugs and may also mask symptoms of low blood glucose.

SPECIAL PRECAUTIONS

Be sure to tell your doctor if:
◆ You have, or have had, asthma.
◆ You have a slow heart rate.
◆ You have low blood pressure.
◆ You have liver or kidney problems.
◆ You have diabetes.
◆ You are taking other medicines.

Pregnancy Not normally prescribed. The drug may affect the developing baby. Discuss with your doctor.

Breast-feeding Not recommended. It is not known whether the drug passes into the breast milk. Discuss with your doctor.

Infants and children Not recommended.

Over 60 Increased risk of adverse effects.

Driving and hazardous work Avoid such activities until you have learned how bisoprolol affects you because the drug can cause fatigue and dizziness.

Alcohol Avoid excessive intake. Alcohol may increase the blood pressure-lowering effect of bisoprolol.

Surgery and general anaesthetics Bisoprolol may need to be stopped before you have a general anaesthetic. Discuss with your doctor or dentist before any surgery.

PROLONGED USE

No special problems.

Botulinum toxin

Brand names Botox, Dysport, NeuroBloc, Vistabel
Used in the following combined preparations None

QUICK REFERENCE

Drug group Muscle relaxant (p.54)
Overdose danger rating High
Dependence rating Low
Prescription needed Yes
Available as generic No

GENERAL INFORMATION

Botulinum toxin is a neurotoxin (nerve poison) that is produced naturally by the bacterium *Clostridium botulinum*. The toxin causes botulism, a rare but serious form of food poisoning.

Research has found that there are several slightly different components in the toxin. Two are used medically: botulinum A toxin and botulinum B toxin. They are used therapeutically to treat conditions in which there are painful muscle spasms: for example spastic foot deformity, blepharospasm (spasm of the eyelids, causing them almost to close), hemifacial spasm, and spasmodic torticollis (spasms of the neck muscles, causing the head to jerk). Toxin A is also used to treat very resistant and distressing cases of hyperhidrosis (excessive sweating). The effects produced by the toxins may last for 2–3 months, until new nerve endings have formed.

Botulinum toxin is used cosmetically to remove facial wrinkles by paralysing the muscles under the skin. However, it is not licensed in the UK for this use.

INFORMATION FOR USERS

This drug is given only under medical supervision and is not for self-administration.

How taken/used Injection.

Frequency and timing of doses Every 2–3 months, depending on response.

Adult dosage range Dose depends on the particular condition being treated. Individual injections may range from 1.25 units to 50 units. The number of injection sites depends on the size and number of the muscles to be paralysed. Specialist judgement is necessary.

Onset of effect Within 3 days to 2 weeks.

Duration of action 2–3 months.

Diet advice None.

Storage Not applicable as the drug is not normally kept in the home.

Missed dose Attend for treatment at the next possible time.

Stopping the drug Discuss with your doctor whether or not you should stop receiving the drug.

Exceeding the dose Overdose is unlikely since treatment is carefully monitored, and the drug is given intravenously only under close supervision.

POSSIBLE ADVERSE EFFECTS

Some of the adverse effects depend on the site of injection. Common adverse effects include reduced blinking and dry eyes, painful swallowing, and pain or weakness at the site of injection. Misplaced injections may paralyse unintended muscle groups. All paralyses are likely to be long lasting. Rarely, botulinum toxin may cause glaucoma or painful eyes, neck weakness, head tremor, or hypersensitivity reactions. Consult your doctor if any of the above adverse effects occur. Occasionally, the drug may cause difficulty swallowing (rather than just pain on swallowing); if so, call your doctor immediately.

INTERACTIONS

None.

SPECIAL PRECAUTIONS

Be sure to tell your doctor if:
◆ You have any difficulty in swallowing.
◆ You are taking an anticoagulant drug or have a bleeding disorder.
◆ You are allergic to botulinum toxin.
◆ You are taking other medicines.

Pregnancy Not prescribed.

Breast-feeding Not prescribed.

Infants and children Reduced dose necessary.

Over 60 No special problems.

Driving and hazardous work Do not drive until you know how botulinum toxin affects you; the drug may impair ability.

Alcohol No known problems.

PROLONGED USE

To maintain the desired effects, the drug may have to be administered at regular intervals.

Bromocriptine

Brand name Parlodel

Used in the following combined preparations None

QUICK REFERENCE

Drug group Drug for parkinsonism (p.18) and pituitary agent (p.85)

Overdose danger rating Low

Dependence rating Low

Prescription needed Yes

Available as generic Yes

GENERAL INFORMATION

By inhibiting secretion of the hormone prolactin from the pituitary gland, bromocriptine is used in the treatment of conditions associated with excessive prolactin production. Such conditions include some types of female infertility and occasionally male infertility. It is effective in treating some benign breast conditions and symptoms of menstrual disorders. The drug may also be used to suppress lactation in women who do not wish to breast-feed.

Bromocriptine also increases production of dopamine in the brain, thereby relieving the symptoms of parkinsonism, in which there is a lack of dopamine. It is widely used to treat people with advanced parkinsonism when other medications have failed or are unsuitable.

Bromocriptine also reduces the release of growth hormone, and is therefore used to treat acromegaly (see Drugs for growth hormone disorders, p.86).

Serious adverse effects are rare with low doses. Nausea and vomiting can be minimized by taking bromocriptine with meals. Bromocriptine may in rare cases cause ulceration of the stomach.

INFORMATION FOR USERS

Your drug prescription is tailored for you. Do not alter dosage without checking with your doctor.

How taken/used Tablets, capsules.

Frequency and timing of doses 1–4 x daily with food.

Adult dosage range The dose given depends on the condition being treated and your response. In most cases treatment starts with a daily dose of 1–1.25mg. This is gradually increased until a satisfactory response is achieved.

Onset of effect Variable depending on the condition.

Duration of action 8–12 hours.

Diet advice None.

Storage Keep in original container at room temperature out of the reach of children. Protect from light.

Missed dose Take as soon as you remember. If your next dose is due within 2 hours, take a single dose now and skip the next.

Stopping the drug Do not stop the drug without consulting your doctor; symptoms may recur.

Exceeding the dose An occasional unintentional extra dose is unlikely to be a cause for concern. If you notice any unusual symptoms, or if a large overdose has been taken, notify your doctor.

POSSIBLE ADVERSE EFFECTS

Adverse effects, such as nausea or vomiting and constipation, are usually dose-related. When used to treat parkinsonism, bromocriptine may cause abnormal movements. If the drug causes such movements or produces confusion, dizziness, or a headache, you should consult your doctor. If you experience sudden drowsiness when taking bromocriptine, you should stop taking the drug and call your doctor immediately.

INTERACTIONS

Antipsychotic drugs oppose the action of bromocriptine and increase the risk of parkinsonism.

Phenylpropanolamine, ephedrine, and pseudoephedrine These drugs are found in some over-the-counter cough and cold remedies. Use of these with bromocriptine may lead to severe adverse effects.

Erythromycin and other macrolide antibiotics These drugs may lead to increased levels of bromocriptine and the risk of adverse effects.

Domperidone and metoclopramide may reduce some of the effects of bromocriptine.

SPECIAL PRECAUTIONS

Be sure to tell your doctor if:
◆ You have poor circulation.
◆ You have, or have had, a stomach ulcer.
◆ You have a history of psychiatric disorders.
◆ You have high blood pressure.
◆ You have porphyria.
◆ You have heart disease.
◆ You have a history of lung disease.
◆ You have liver disease.
◆ You are taking other medicines.

Pregnancy Safety in pregnancy not established. Discuss with your doctor.

Breast-feeding The drug suppresses milk production, and prevents it completely if given within 12 hours of delivery. If you wish to breast-feed, consult your doctor.

Infants and children Not usually prescribed under 15 years.

Over 60 Reduced dose may be necessary.

Driving and hazardous work Avoid such activities until you have learned how bromocriptine affects you because the drug may cause dizziness and drowsiness.

Alcohol Avoid. Alcohol increases the likelihood of confusion and reduces tolerance to bromocriptine.

PROLONGED USE

No special problems.

Monitoring Periodic blood tests may be carried out to check hormone levels. Gynaecological tests may be carried out annually (or every six months in post menopausal women). Monitoring for other, rare, adverse effects (e.g. peptic ulcer in acromegaly) may also be carried out.

Budesonide

Brand names Budenofalk, Entocort, Novolizer, Pulmicort, Rhinocort Aqua
Used in the following combined preparation Symbicort

QUICK REFERENCE

Drug group Corticosteroid (p.80)
Overdose danger rating Low
Dependence rating Low
Prescription needed Yes
Available as generic Yes

GENERAL INFORMATION

Budesonide is a corticosteroid drug used as slow-release capsules to relieve the symptoms of Crohn's disease, as an enema to treat ulcerative colitis, and as an inhaler to prevent (but not stop existing) asthma attacks. Like other corticosteroids, it is used when asthma is not controlled by bronchodilators (see p.23) alone. It is also used as a nasal spray to relieve the symptoms of allergic rhinitis and for nasal polyps. It controls symptoms by reducing inflammation, whether it is in the nose, lungs, or intestine.

Side effects are fewer and less serious with budesonide when it is taken by inhaler or nasal spray because the drug is absorbed in much smaller quantities than with oral forms. However, fungal infection causing mouth and throat irritation can occur with the inhaler, but this can be minimized by thoroughly rinsing the mouth and gargling with water after each inhalation.

INFORMATION FOR USERS

Your drug prescription is tailored for you. Do not alter dosage without checking with your doctor.
How taken/used SR-capsules, enema, inhaler, powder for inhalation, nasal spray.
Frequency and timing of doses 1–3 x daily (capsules); once daily at bedtime (enema); twice daily (inhaler); once or twice daily (nasal spray).
Dosage range 3–9mg (capsules); 2mg (enema); 200–1,600mcg (inhaler), 100–200mcg (nasal spray).
Onset of effect *Asthma* Within 1 week. *Other conditions* 1–3 days.
Duration of action 12–24 hours.
Diet advice None.
Storage Keep in original container at room temperature out of the reach of children.
Missed dose Take as soon as you remember. If your next dose is due within 2 hours, take a single dose now and skip the next.

Stopping the drug Do not stop taking the drug without consulting your doctor; symptoms may recur. The SR-capsules used in Crohn's disease should be withdrawn gradually.
Exceeding the dose An occasional extra dose is unlikely to be a cause for concern. But if you notice any unusual symptoms, or if a large overdose has been taken, notify your doctor.

POSSIBLE ADVERSE EFFECTS

As with other corticosteroids, such as betamethasone, the main side effects of inhalers and nasal spray are confined to the nasal passages and mouth. They include cough, sore throat or hoarseness, nasal irritation, and, rarely, nosebleeds. Capsules and enemas can cause gastrointestinal disturbances, such as diarrhoea or constipation, and sometimes a rash, itching, or mood disorders. High doses of budesonide by any route can cause weight gain and other long-term side effects associated with corticosteroids.

Contact your doctor if a nosebleed, sore throat or hoarseness, rash, itching, mood disorders, or weight gain occur. If there is any pain in the eye, stop taking the drug and contact your doctor immediately.

INTERACTIONS

None.

SPECIAL PRECAUTIONS

Be sure to tell your doctor if:
◆ You have had tuberculosis or another respiratory infection.
◆ You are taking other medicines.
Pregnancy Discuss with your doctor, especially if used for Crohn's disease.
Breast-feeding Discuss with your doctor, especially if used for Crohn's disease.
Infants and children Reduced dose necessary.
Over 60 No special problems.
Driving and hazardous work No special problems.
Alcohol No special problems.
Infection Avoid exposure to chickenpox.

PROLONGED USE

Asthma prevention is the condition for which prolonged use may be required. High doses inhaled for a prolonged period can lead to peptic ulcers, fragile bones, glaucoma, muscle weakness, and growth retardation in children. Patients taking the drug long term are advised to carry a "steroid card" or wear a MedicAlert bracelet.

Monitoring If budesonide is being taken in large doses, periodic checks may be needed to make sure that the adrenal glands are working properly. Children using inhalers should have their height monitored regularly.

Bumetanide

Brand name Burinex
Used in the following combined preparations
Burinex A, Burinex K

QUICK REFERENCE

Drug group Loop diuretic (p.32)
Overdose danger rating Low
Dependence rating Low
Prescription needed Yes
Available as generic Yes

GENERAL INFORMATION

Bumetanide is a powerful, short-acting loop diuretic used to treat oedema (accumulation of fluid in tissue spaces) resulting from heart failure, nephrotic syndrome, and cirrhosis of the liver. Bumetanide is particularly useful in treating people with impaired kidney function who do not respond well to thiazide diuretics. Because it is fast acting, it is often injected in an emergency to relieve pulmonary oedema (fluid in the lungs).

Bumetanide increases potassium loss in the urine, which can result in a wide variety of symptoms. For this reason, potassium supplements or a potassium-sparing diuretic (see p.32) are often given with the drug.

INFORMATION FOR USERS

Your drug prescription is tailored for you. Do not alter dosage without checking with your doctor.

How taken/used Tablets, liquid, injection.
Frequency and timing of doses Usually once daily in the morning. In some cases, twice daily.
Dosage range 0.5–5mg daily. Dose may be increased if kidney function is impaired.
Onset of effect Within 30 minutes by mouth; more quickly by injection.

Duration of action 2–4 hours.
Diet advice Use of this drug may reduce potassium in the body. Eat plenty of fresh fruit and vegetables, such as bananas and tomatoes.
Storage Keep in original container at room temperature out of the reach of children. Protect from light.
Missed dose No cause for concern, but take as soon as you remember. However, if it is late in the day do not take the missed dose, or you may need to get up during the night to pass urine. Take the next scheduled dose as usual.
Stopping the drug Do not stop the drug without consulting your doctor; symptoms may recur.
Exceeding the dose An occasional unintentional extra dose is unlikely to be a cause for concern. But if you notice any unusual symptoms, or if a large overdose has been taken, notify your doctor.

POSSIBLE ADVERSE EFFECTS

Adverse effects are caused mainly by the rapid fluid loss produced by bumetanide, which can lead to dizziness and fainting. These diminish as the body adjusts to the drug. Bumetanide may precipitate gout in susceptible people and can affect the control of diabetes. The drug may also cause lethargy, fatigue, and muscle cramps, which should be notified to your doctor if they are severe. In all cases, you should contact your doctor if you experience a rash or photosensitivity, nausea, vomiting, or pain in the joints.

INTERACTIONS

Anti-arrhythmic drugs Low potassium levels may increase these drugs' toxicity.
Antibacterials Very high doses of bumetanide can increase the ear damage that is caused by some antibiotics.
Digoxin Excessive potassium loss may increase the adverse effects of digoxin.
Non-steroidal anti-inflammatory drugs (NSAIDs) These drugs may reduce the diuretic effect of bumetanide.
Lithium Bumetanide may increase the blood levels of lithium, leading to an increased risk of lithium toxicity.
Pimozide Low potassium levels increase the risk of abnormal heart rhythms with this antipsychotic drug.

SPECIAL PRECAUTIONS

Be sure to tell your doctor if:
◆ You have a long-term liver or kidney problem.
◆ You have diabetes.
◆ You have prostate trouble.
◆ You have gout.
◆ You are taking other medicines.

Pregnancy Not usually prescribed. May cause a reduction in blood supply to the developing baby. Discuss with your doctor.

Breast-feeding This drug may reduce your milk supply. Discuss with your doctor.

Infants and children Not usually prescribed. Reduced dose necessary.

Over 60 Dosage is often reduced.

Driving and hazardous work Avoid such activities until you have learned how bumetanide affects you because the drug may cause dizziness and faintness.

Alcohol Keep consumption low. The drug increases the likelihood of dehydration and hangovers after drinking alcohol.

PROLONGED USE

Serious problems are unlikely, but the levels of certain salts in the body may occasionally become abnormal during prolonged use.

Monitoring Regular blood tests may be performed to check on kidney function and levels of body salts.

Bupropion

Brand name Zyban
Used in the following combined preparations
None

QUICK REFERENCE

Drug group Nicotine withdrawal aid
Overdose danger rating High
Dependence rating Low
Prescription needed Yes
Available as generic No

GENERAL INFORMATION

Bupropion (also known as amfebutamone) is an antidepressant; chemically it is unrelated to other classes of antidepressant. It has been used to treat depression but is generally used as an aid to giving up tobacco smoking.

The person being treated must commit in advance to a date for stopping smoking. Treatment is started while the patient is still smoking, and the "target stop date" decided on within the first two weeks of treatment. Bupropion will be stopped after 7 weeks if the smoker has not given up smoking completely by then. The drug can be an effective aid, but nicotine replacement therapy (see p.327) is more popular.

Bupropion should not be prescribed for people with a history of seizures or eating disorders, or who are withdrawing from benzodiazepine or alcohol. Nor should the drug be used by people with manic depression or psychosis because there is a risk of mania developing.

INFORMATION FOR USERS

Your drug prescription is tailored for you. Do not alter dosage without checking with your doctor.

How taken/used SR-tablets.
Frequency and timing of doses 1–2 x daily. Tablets should be swallowed whole.
Adult dosage range 150–300mg.
Onset of effect Up to 4 weeks for full effect.
Duration of action 12 hours.
Diet advice None.
Storage Keep in original container at room temperature out of the reach of children.
Missed dose Take as soon as you remember. If your next dose is due within 2 hours, take a single dose now and skip the next.
Stopping the drug Do not stop the drug without consulting your doctor. He or she may want to reduce the dose gradually.

OVERDOSE ACTION

Seek immediate medical advice in all cases. Take emergency action if consciousness is lost.

POSSIBLE ADVERSE EFFECTS

Common adverse effects associated with bupropion include insomnia, poor concentration, headache, dizziness, tremor, nausea, vomiting, and constipation. Rash, fever, and depression are also common but should be discussed with your doctor in all cases. Some of these effects may be due to the withdrawal of nicotine rather than to the effects of bupropion itself. Rarely, jaundice, confusion, or anxiety may occur. If palpitations, fainting, chest pain, or seizures develop, stop taking the drug and consult your doctor at once.

INTERACTIONS

General note A wide range of drugs increases the likelihood of seizures when taken with bupropion. Check with your doctor if you are on other medications.

Ritonavir, amantadine, and levodopa increase the risk of adverse effects with bupropion.

Antiepileptics Phenytoin and carbamazepine may reduce the blood levels and effects of bupropion. Valproate may increase its blood levels and effects.

Monoamine oxidase inhibitors (MAOIs) Increase the risk of adverse effects from bupropion.

SPECIAL PRECAUTIONS

Be sure to tell your doctor if:
◆ You have had a head injury or have a history of seizures or epilepsy.
◆ You have an eating disorder.
◆ You have cancer of the nervous system.
◆ You have diabetes.
◆ You have manic depression or a psychosis.
◆ You have kidney or liver problems.
◆ You are withdrawing from alcohol or benzodiazepine dependence.
◆ You are taking other medicines.

Pregnancy Safety in pregnancy is not established. Try to give up smoking without using drugs.

Breast-feeding Safety not established. The drug passes into the breast milk and may affect the baby. Discuss with your doctor.

Infants and children Not recommended.

Over 60 Increased sensitivity to the drug's effects. Reduced dose may be necessary.

Driving and hazardous work Avoid until you have learned how bupropion affects you. The drug may cause impaired concentration and dizziness.

Alcohol Avoid. Alcohol will increase any sedative effects.

PROLONGED USE

Bupropion is used for up to 9 weeks for cessation of smoking.

Monitoring Progress will be reviewed after about 3–4 weeks, and the drug continued only if it is having some effect.

Calcipotriol

Brand name Dovonex
Used in the following combined preparation Dovobet

QUICK REFERENCE

Drug group Drug for psoriasis (p.124)
Overdose danger rating Low
Dependence rating Low
Prescription needed Yes
Available as generic No

GENERAL INFORMATION

Calcipotriol is used in the treatment of plaque psoriasis affecting up to 40 per cent of the patient's skin area, and also for psoriasis of the scalp.

Calcipotriol is similar to vitamin D. It is thought to work by reducing production of the skin cells that cause skin thickening and scaling, which are the most common symptoms of psoriasis. Because this drug is related to vitamin D, excessive use can lead to a rise in calcium levels in the body; otherwise calcipotriol is unlikely to cause any serious adverse effects.

Calcipotriol is applied to the affected areas in the form of cream, ointment, or scalp solution. It should not be used on the face, and it is important to wash the hands following application to the affected area to avoid accidental transfer of the drug to unaffected areas. Local irritation may occur during the early stages of treatment.

INFORMATION FOR USERS

Your drug prescription is tailored for you. Do not alter dosage without checking with your doctor.

How taken/used Cream, ointment, scalp solution.

Frequency and timing of doses 1–2 x daily.

Adult dosage range Maximum 100g each week (cream, ointment); maximum 60ml each week (scalp solution): less if both preparations are used together.

Onset of effect Improvement is seen within 2 weeks.

Duration of action One application lasts up to 12 hours. Beneficial effects are longer lasting.

Diet advice None.

Storage Store in original container at room temperature out of the reach of children.

Missed dose Apply the next dose at the scheduled time.

Stopping the drug Do not stop using the drug without consulting your doctor; symptoms may recur.

Exceeding the dose Excessive prolonged use may lead to an increase in blood calcium levels, which can cause nausea, constipation, thirst, abdominal pain, weakness, tiredness, and frequent urination. Notify your doctor.

POSSIBLE ADVERSE EFFECTS

Temporary local irritation and itching may occur when treatment is started. Other adverse effects, such as a rash (which may be light-sensitive), thirst, frequent urination, nausea, and constipation are usually due to heavy or prolonged use, leading to high calcium levels in the blood. If you develop abdominal pain, weakness, tiredness, or worsening of psoriasis, stop taking the drug and contact your doctor.

INTERACTIONS

None known.

SPECIAL PRECAUTIONS

Be sure to tell your doctor if:
◆ You have a metabolic disorder.
◆ You have previously had a hypersensitivity reaction to the drug.
◆ You are taking other medicines.

Pregnancy Safety in pregnancy not established. Discuss with your doctor.

Breast-feeding Not known if excreted into breast milk. Discuss with your doctor.

Infants and children Cream/ointment not recommended under 6 years. Scalp solution, only under specialist advice.

Over 60 No problems expected.

Driving and hazardous work No problems expected.

Alcohol No problems expected.

PROLONGED USE

No problems expected from use of calcipotriol in low doses. If the effects of the skin preparation decline after several weeks, they may be regained by suspending use for a few weeks and then recommencing treatment.

Monitoring Regular checks on calcium levels in the blood or urine are required during prolonged or heavy use.

Candesartan

Brand name Amias
Used in the following combined preparations
None

QUICK REFERENCE

Drug group Vasodilator (p.31) and antihypertensive drug (p.36)
Overdose danger rating Low
Dependence rating Low
Prescription needed Yes
Available as generic No

GENERAL INFORMATION

Candesartan belongs to the group of vasodilator drugs known as angiotensin II blockers and is used to treat hypertension (high blood pressure) and heart failure (inability of the heart muscle to cope with its workload). Candesartan works by blocking the action of angiotensin II (a hormone that constricts blood vessels). This relaxes the blood vessels, thereby lowering blood pressure and easing the heart's workload.

Unlike ACE inhibitors, candesartan does not cause a persistent dry cough and may be a useful alternative for people who have to discontinue treatment with an ACE inhibitor for this reason.

INFORMATION FOR USERS

Your drug prescription is tailored for you. Do not alter dosage without checking with your doctor.

How taken/used Tablets.

Frequency and timing of doses Once daily.

Adult dosage range 4mg initially, increased to maximum of 32mg.

Onset of effect 2 hours.

Duration of action 24 hours.

Diet advice None.

Storage Keep in original container at room temperature out of the reach of children.

Missed dose Take as soon as you remember. If your next dose is due within 8 hours, take a single dose now and skip the next.

Stopping the drug Do not stop taking the drug without consulting your doctor. Stopping the drug may lead to worsening of the underlying condition.

Exceeding the dose An occasional unintentional extra dose is unlikely to cause problems. Large overdoses may cause dizziness and fainting. Notify your doctor.

POSSIBLE ADVERSE EFFECTS

Adverse effects of candesartan are usually mild and transient; common effects include dizziness, headache, cold or flu-like symptoms. More rarely, there may be nausea, or muscle, joint, or back pain. If you develop jaundice or swelling of the face, lips, and tongue, stop taking the drug and consult your doctor immediately.

INTERACTIONS

ACE inhibitors (e.g. enalapril, captopril, lisinopril, or ramipril) may increase potassium levels when taken with candesartan.

Diuretics (e.g. bendroflumethiazide, furosemide, or amiloride) taken with candesartan may alter blood potassium and sodium levels.

NSAIDs (e.g. diclofenac or ibuprofen) may reduce candesartan's effectiveness.

Lithium Levels of this drug may be increased when it is combined with candesartan, leading to toxicity.

Ciclosporin may increase potassium levels when combined with candesartan.

Potassium salts may increase risk of high potassium levels with candesartan.

SPECIAL PRECAUTIONS

Be sure to tell your doctor if:
◆ You have kidney or liver disease.
◆ You have had a recent kidney transplant.
◆ You have suffered recently from excessive sweating, diarrhoea, or dehydration.
◆ You have Lapp lactase deficiency or glucose–galactose malabsorption.
◆ You are taking other medicines.

Pregnancy Not prescribed.

Breast-feeding Not recommended. It is not known whether the drug passes into the breast milk. Discuss with your doctor.

Infants and children Not prescribed.

Over 60 Increased risk of adverse effects. Reduced dose may therefore be necessary.

Driving and hazardous work Do not undertake such activities until you have learned how candesartan affects you because the drug can cause dizziness or weariness.

Alcohol Avoid. Combined with candesartan, alcohol may increase dizziness, especially at the start of treatment.

Surgery and general anaesthetics Candesartan may cause a drop in blood pressure; treatment may need to be stopped before any surgery. Discuss with your doctor or dentist.

PROLONGED USE

No special problems.

Monitoring Periodic checks on blood potassium levels and kidney function may be performed.

Captopril

Brand names Acepril, Capoten, Ecopace, Tensopril
Used in the following combined preparations
Acezide, Capozide

QUICK REFERENCE

Drug group ACE inhibitor vasodilator (p.31)
Overdose danger rating Medium
Dependence rating Low
Prescription needed Yes
Available as generic Yes

GENERAL INFORMATION

Captopril belongs to the class of drugs called ACE inhibitors, used to treat high blood pressure and heart failure. The drug works by relaxing the muscles around blood vessels, allowing them to dilate and thereby easing blood flow. Captopril lowers blood pressure rapidly but may require several weeks to achieve full effect. People with heart failure may be given captopril in addition to diuretics. It can achieve dramatic results, relaxing muscle in blood vessel walls and reducing the heart's workload.

The first dose is usually very small and taken while lying down as there is a risk of a sudden fall in blood pressure. Diuretics are often given at the same time.

A variety of minor side effects may occur. Some people experience loss of taste, while others get a persistent dry cough. A reduction in dose may help minimize these effects.

INFORMATION FOR USERS

Your drug prescription is tailored for you. Do not alter dosage without checking with your doctor.

How taken/used Tablets.

Frequency and timing of doses 2–3 x daily.

Adult dosage range 12.5–25mg daily initially, gradually increased to 50–150mg daily. Starting doses of 6.25mg may be used.

Onset of effect 30–60 minutes.

Duration of action 6–8 hours.

Diet advice None.

Storage Keep in original container at room temperature out of the reach of children.

Missed dose Take as soon as you remember. If your next dose is due within 2 hours, take a single dose now and skip the next.

Stopping the drug Do not stop the drug without consulting your doctor; stopping the drug may lead to worsening of the underlying condition.

Exceeding the dose An occasional unintentional extra dose is unlikely to cause any problems. Large overdoses may cause dizziness or fainting. Notify your doctor.

POSSIBLE ADVERSE EFFECTS

Captopril causes a variety of minor adverse effects, primarily rashes and gastrointestinal symptoms. These usually disappear soon after treatment has started. Dizziness on standing is likely after the first dose. A persistent dry cough is the most common adverse effect, and there may also be loss of taste and a rash. These effects may be minimized by reducing the dose. If dizziness, fainting, sore throat, or fever occur, consult your doctor. If you develop swelling of the mouth or lips, stop taking the drug and call your doctor immediately.

INTERACTIONS

Non-steroidal anti-inflammatory drugs (NSAIDs) may reduce the effectiveness of captopril. There is also a risk of kidney damage when they are taken with captopril.

Lithium Blood levels of lithium may be raised by captopril.

Vasodilators (e.g. nitrates) These drugs may reduce blood pressure even further.

Potassium supplements and potassium-sparing diuretics increase the risk of high potassium levels when taken with captopril.

Ciclosporin increases the risk of high blood levels of potassium when taken with captopril.

Diuretics Taking captopril with these drugs can cause a rapid fall in blood pressure.

SPECIAL PRECAUTIONS

Be sure to tell your doctor if:

◆ You have long-term kidney problems.

◆ You have coronary artery disease.

◆ You are on a low sodium diet.

◆ You are allergic to ACE inhibitors.

◆ You are taking other medicines.

Pregnancy Not usually prescribed. There is evidence of harm to the developing fetus. Discuss with your doctor.

Breast-feeding The drug passes into the breast milk, but at normal doses adverse effects on the baby are unlikely. Discuss with your doctor.

Infants and children Not usually prescribed. Reduced dose necessary.

Over 60 Reduced dose may be necessary.

Driving and hazardous work Avoid until you have learned how captopril affects you because it can cause dizziness and fainting.

Alcohol Avoid. Alcohol may increase the blood-pressure lowering and adverse effects of the drug.

Surgery and general anaesthetics Captopril may need to be stopped before you have a general anaesthetic. Discuss with your doctor or dentist before any operation.

PROLONGED USE

Rarely, prolonged use can lead to changes in the blood count or kidney function.

Monitoring Periodic checks on potassium levels, white blood cell count, kidney function, and urine are usually performed.

Carbamazepine

Brand names Carbagen SR, Epimaz, Tegretol, Tegretol Retard

Used in the following combined preparations None

QUICK REFERENCE

Drug group Anticonvulsant drug (p.16)

Overdose danger rating Medium

Dependence rating Low

Prescription needed Yes

Available as generic Yes

GENERAL INFORMATION

Carbamazepine is used to treat some forms of epilepsy as it reduces the likelihood of fits caused by abnormal nerve signals in the brain. Carbamazepine is also prescribed to relieve the intermittent severe pain caused by damage to the cranial nerves in trigeminal neuralgia. Carbamazepine is also occasionally prescribed to treat manic depression and diabetes insipidus and is used for pain relief in diabetic neuropathy.

In order to avoid side effects, carbamazepine therapy is usually commenced at a low dose and gradually increased. It is recommended that patients stick to the same brand of carbamazepine prescribed.

INFORMATION FOR USERS

Your drug prescription is tailored for you. Do not alter dosage without checking with your doctor.

How taken/used Tablets, chewable tablets, liquid, suppositories.

Frequency and timing of doses 1–2 x daily.

Adult dosage range *Epilepsy* 100–2,000mg daily (low starting dose that is slowly increased every 2 weeks). *Pain relief* 100–1,600mg daily. *Psychiatric disorders* 400–1,600mg daily.

Onset of effect Within 4 hours.

Duration of action 12–24 hours.

Diet advice None.

Storage Keep in original container at room temperature out of the reach of children.

Missed dose Take as soon as you remember. If your next dose is due within 2 hours, take a single dose now and skip the next.

Stopping the drug Do not stop the drug without consulting your doctor; symptoms may recur.

Exceeding the dose An occasional unintentional extra dose is unlikely to cause problems. Large overdoses may cause tremor, convulsions, and coma. Notify your doctor.

POSSIBLE ADVERSE EFFECTS

Most people experience very few adverse effects with this drug, but when blood levels get too high, adverse effects are common and the dose may need to be reduced. Dizziness or unsteadiness, drowsiness, nausea, and loss of appetite are common side effects. Blurred vision is also common; it should be reported to your doctor in all cases. Rarer effects include jaundice and swelling of the ankles. If you develop a sore throat, hoarseness, rash, fever, or abnormal bruising, contact your doctor immediately and stop taking the drug.

INTERACTIONS

General note Many drugs may increase or reduce the effects of carbamazepine. Discuss with your doctor or pharmacist before taking other medications.

Other antiepileptic drugs Complex and variable interactions can occur between these drugs and carbamazepine.

Contraceptive pill Carbamazepine may reduce the effectiveness of the contraceptive pill. Discuss this with your doctor.

SPECIAL PRECAUTIONS

Be sure to tell your doctor if:
◆ You have a long-term liver or kidney problem.
◆ You have heart problems.
◆ You have had blood problems with other drugs.
◆ You are taking other medicines.

Pregnancy Avoid if possible. Associated with abnormalities in the unborn baby. Folic acid supplements should be taken before and during pregnancy. Discuss with your doctor.

Breast-feeding The drug passes into the breast milk and can affect the baby. Discuss with your doctor.

Infants and children Reduced dose necessary.

Over 60 May cause confused or agitated behaviour in the elderly. Reduced dose may be necessary.

Driving and hazardous work Discuss with your doctor. Your underlying condition, as well as the possibility of reduced alertness while taking carbamazepine, may make such activities inadvisable.

Alcohol Avoid. Alcohol may increase the sedative effects of this drug.

PROLONGED USE

There is a slight risk of changes in liver function or of skin or blood abnormalities during prolonged use.

Monitoring Periodic blood tests are usually performed to monitor levels of the drug, blood cell counts, and liver and kidney function.

Carbaryl

Brand name Carylderm
Used in the following combined preparations
None

QUICK REFERENCE

Drug group Drugs to treat skin parasites (p.122)
Overdose danger rating Low
Dependence rating Low
Prescription needed Yes
Available as generic No

GENERAL INFORMATION

Carbaryl is an insecticide used in the treatment of head and crab lice. It kills the lice by interfering with the functioning of their nervous system, causing paralysis and death.

The drug is applied topically, either as a water-based liquid or an alcohol-based lotion. Lotion is considered unsuitable for small children and people with asthma, who may be affected by the alcoholic fumes. The lotion is also unsuitable for treating crab lice because it causes genital irritation. Because lice develop resistance to insecticides, carbaryl (or alternatives such as malathion) may not clear the lice. If the drug does not work for you, consult your pharmacist or doctor, who will recommend an alternative. You will need a prescription to obtain carbaryl.

INFORMATION FOR USERS

Your drug prescription is tailored for you. Do not alter dosage without checking with your doctor.
How taken/used Topical liquid, lotion.
Frequency and timing of doses Once, repeating after a week.
Adult dosage range As directed.
Onset of effect Lotion or liquid should be left on for 12 hours before being washed off.
Duration of action Until washed off.
Diet advice None.
Storage Keep in original container at room temperature out of the reach of children. Protect from light.
Missed dose If you forget the second application, use it as soon as you remember.
Stopping the drug Carbaryl should be applied as a single application or as a short course of treatment.

Exceeding the dose An occasional unintentional extra application is unlikely to be a cause for concern. Take emergency action if accidentally swallowed.

POSSIBLE ADVERSE EFFECTS

Used correctly, carbaryl preparations are unlikely to produce adverse effects, although skin irritation may occur. The alcoholic fumes given off by some lotions may cause wheezing in asthmatics.

INTERACTIONS

None.

SPECIAL PRECAUTIONS

Be sure to tell your doctor if:
◆ You have asthma.
Pregnancy No evidence of risk. It is unlikely that enough carbaryl would be absorbed to affect the developing fetus if it is applied occasionally and directions are followed.
Breast-feeding No evidence of risk. It is unlikely that enough carbaryl would be absorbed to affect the baby if it is applied occasionally and directions are followed properly, but discuss with your doctor or pharmacist before use.
Infants and children No special problems.
Over 60 No special problems.
Driving and hazardous work No special problems.
Alcohol No special problems.

PROLONGED USE

Carbaryl is intended for intermittent use only. It should not be used for prolonged periods.

Carbimazole

Brand name Neo-Mercazole
Used in the following combined preparations
None

QUICK REFERENCE

Drug group Antithyroid drug (p.84)
Overdose danger rating Medium
Dependence rating Low
Prescription needed Yes
Available as generic No

GENERAL INFORMATION

Carbimazole is an antithyroid drug that is used to suppress the formation of thyroid hormones in people who have an overactive thyroid gland (hyperthyroidism). In some people, particularly those who have Graves' disease (the most common form of hyperthyroidism), drug treatment alone may relieve the disorder.

Carbimazole is also used in more serious cases; for example, to restore the normal function of the thyroid gland before its partial removal by surgery, or to intensify the absorption of the cell-destroying drug radioactive iodine when that is used. Carbimazole also prevents the excessive, harmful release of thyroid hormone that can sometimes follow the use of radioactive iodine. Because the full benefits of this medication are not felt for several weeks, beta blockers may be given during this period to help control symptoms. Maintenance treatment may be continued for as long as 18 months unless surgery or radioactive iodine are used. Occasionally the carbimazole dose is kept high and thyroxine is also prescribed in order to prevent a goitre from developing.

INFORMATION FOR USERS

Your drug prescription is tailored for you. Do not alter dosage without checking with your doctor.

How taken/used Tablets.

Frequency and timing of doses 2–3 x daily (high doses); 1–2 x daily (low doses).

Adult dosage range 15–40mg daily (occasionally a larger dose may be needed). Once control is achieved, dosage is reduced gradually to a maintenance dose of 5–15mg for about 18 months.

Onset of effect Some improvement is usually felt within 1–3 weeks. Full beneficial effects usually take 4–8 weeks.

Duration of action 12–24 hours.

Diet advice Your doctor may advise you to avoid foods that are high in iodine, such as cod and mackerel.

Storage Keep in original container at room temperature out of the reach of children.

Missed dose Take as soon as you remember. If your next dose is due, take both of the doses together.

Stopping the drug Do not stop taking the drug without consulting your doctor; symptoms may recur.

Exceeding the dose An occasional unintentional extra dose is unlikely to cause any problems. Large overdoses may cause nausea, vomiting, and headache. Notify your doctor.

POSSIBLE ADVERSE EFFECTS

Headache, dizziness, joint pain, and nausea are common. Serious side effects are rare. If hair loss, rash, itching, or jaundice develop, consult your doctor. A sore throat, mouth ulcers, bruising, fever, or a general feeling of being unwell may be an indication of adverse effects on the blood and require prompt medical attention.

INTERACTIONS

None.

SPECIAL PRECAUTIONS

Be sure to tell your doctor if:
◆ You have a long-term liver problem.
◆ You are taking other medicines.

Pregnancy May be associated with defects in the baby. However, the risk to the baby of untreated hyperthyroidism is higher. Discuss with your doctor.

Breast-feeding The drug passes into the breast milk, but mothers may breast-feed as long as the lowest effective dose is used and the baby is carefully monitored. Discuss with your doctor.

Infants and children Reduced dose necessary.

Over 60 No special problems.

Driving and hazardous work Avoid such activities until you have learned how carbimazole affects you because the drug may cause dizziness.

Alcohol No known problems.

PROLONGED USE

Carbimazole may stop or reduce the production of blood cells by the bone marrow. For this reason, it is very important to report to your doctor immediately any symptoms, such as a sore throat, that suggest you may have an infection.

Monitoring Blood cell counts are carried out, and periodic tests of thyroid function are usually required.

Cefalexin

Brand names Ceporex, Keflex
Used in the following combined preparations
None

QUICK REFERENCE

Drug group Cephalosporin antibiotic (p.62)
Overdose danger rating Low
Dependence rating Low
Prescription needed Yes
Available as generic Yes

GENERAL INFORMATION

Cefalexin is a cephalosporin antibiotic that is prescribed for a variety of mild to moderate infections. The drug does not have such a wide range of uses as some other antibiotics, but it is helpful in treating respiratory tract infections, cystitis, ear infections and certain skin and soft tissue infections. In some cases cefalexin is prescribed as follow-up treatment for severe infections after a more powerful cephalosporin has been given by injection. Diarrhoea is the most common adverse effect, although this tends to be less severe than with other cephalosporin antibiotics. Some people may be allergic to cefalexin, especially if they are sensitive to penicillin.

INFORMATION FOR USERS

Your drug prescription is tailored for you. Do not alter dosage without checking with your doctor.
How taken/used Tablets, capsules, liquid.
Frequency and timing of doses 2–4 x daily.
Adult dosage range *Adults* 1–2g daily, up to a maximum of 6g. *Children* Reduced dose according to age and weight.
Onset of effect Within 1 hour.
Duration of action 6–12 hours.
Diet advice None.
Storage Keep tablets and capsules in original container at room temperature; refrigerate liquid, but do not freeze, and keep for no longer than 10 days. Keep all forms of the drug out of the reach of children and protect from light.
Missed dose Take as soon as you remember. If your next dose is due, take both of the doses now.

Stopping the drug Take the full course. Even if you feel better, the infection may still be present and may recur if treatment is stopped too soon.
Exceeding the dose An occasional unintentional extra dose is unlikely to be a cause for concern. But if you notice any unusual symptoms, or if a large overdose has been taken, notify your doctor.

POSSIBLE ADVERSE EFFECTS

Most people do not suffer serious adverse effects while taking cefalexin. Diarrhoea is common but tends not to be severe. Nausea and abdominal pain may occur. The rarer adverse effects, such as rash, itching, swelling, and wheezing are usually due to an allergic reaction and may necessitate stopping the drug. Consult your doctor at once if you experience any of these effects and do not take your next dose.

INTERACTIONS

Probenecid This drug increases the level of cefalexin in the blood. The dosage of cefalexin may need to be adjusted accordingly.
Oral contraceptives Cefalexin may reduce the contraceptive effect of these drugs. Discuss with your doctor.

SPECIAL PRECAUTIONS

Be sure to tell your doctor if:
◆ You have a long-term kidney problem.
◆ You have had a previous allergic reaction to a penicillin or cephalosporin antibiotic.
◆ You have a history of blood disorders.
◆ You are taking other medicines.
Pregnancy No evidence of risk to the developing baby.
Breast-feeding The drug passes into the breast milk but at normal doses adverse effects on the baby are unlikely. Discuss with your doctor.
Infants and children Reduced dose necessary.
Over 60 No special problems.
Driving and hazardous work No known problems.
Alcohol No known problems.

PROLONGED USE

Cefalexin is usually given only for short courses of treatment.

Celecoxib

Brand name Celebrex
Used in the following combined preparations
None

QUICK REFERENCE

Drug group Analgesic (p.9) and non-steroidal
anti-inflammatory drug (p.50)
Overdose danger rating Medium
Dependence rating Low
Prescription needed Yes
Available as generic No

GENERAL INFORMATION

Celecoxib is a type of non-steroidal anti-inflammatory drug (NSAID) called a cyclo-oxygenase-2 (COX-2) inhibitor; these drugs have a lower risk of causing irritation to the upper gastrointestinal tract than other NSAIDs. Celecoxib reduces pain, stiffness, and inflammation and is used to relieve the symptoms of both rheumatoid arthritis and osteoarthritis.

Elderly patients may be more sensitive to the drug's effects, and for this reason they are usually prescribed a low dose to begin with. Celecoxib is not prescribed to anyone who has had a heart attack or stroke, because it is thought to slightly increase the risk of recurrence, nor is it prescribed to people with peripheral artery disease (poor circulation). It is prescribed with caution to anyone at risk of any of these conditions.

INFORMATION FOR USERS

Your drug prescription is tailored for you. Do not alter dosage without checking with your doctor.
How taken/used Capsules.
Frequency and timing of doses 1–2 x daily.
Adult dosage range 200–400mg daily.
Onset of effect 1 hour.
Duration of action 8 hours.
Diet advice None.
Storage Keep in original container at room temperature out of the reach of children.
Missed dose Take as soon as you remember. If your next dose is due within 4 hours, take a single dose now and skip the next.
Stopping the drug If being used short term, the drug can safely be stopped as soon as you

no longer need it. If prescribed for long-term use, you should not stop taking the drug without consulting your doctor.
Exceeding the dose An occasional unintentional extra dose is unlikely to cause any problems. Large overdoses may cause stomach and intestinal pain and damage. Notify your doctor.

POSSIBLE ADVERSE EFFECTS

Gastrointestinal, nervous, and respiratory symptoms are the most likely adverse effects. If indigestion, abdominal pain, flatulence, nausea, dizziness, or insomnia are severe, consult your doctor. In all cases consult your doctor if a rash or swollen ankles develop, and call your doctor immediately if palpitations occur. If you experience wheezing or breathlessness, pain in the chest, groin, or leg, black or bloody vomit or faeces, or loss of consciousness, stop taking the drug and contact your doctor immediately.

INTERACTIONS

General note Celecoxib interacts with a wide range of drugs, including ACE inhibitors, SSRI antidepressants, antihypertensives, diuretics, and drugs that increase the risk of bleeding and/or peptic ulcers (e.g. aspirin and other NSAIDs).
Lithium Levels and effects of this drug are increased when taken with celecoxib.
Carbamazepine, fluconazole, rifampicin, and barbiturates These drugs reduce the effects of celecoxib.

SPECIAL PRECAUTIONS

Be sure to tell your doctor if:
◆ You have liver or kidney problems.
◆ You have epilepsy.
◆ You have asthma.
◆ You are allergic to aspirin or any other NSAID.
◆ You are allergic to sulphonamides.
◆ You have a peptic ulcer or gastrointestinal bleeding.
◆ You have high blood pressure.
◆ You have ankle swelling.
◆ You have angina.
◆ You have had a heart attack or stroke.
◆ You have inflammatory bowel disease.
◆ You are taking other medicines.

Pregnancy Not prescribed.

Breast-feeding Not prescribed.

Infants and children Not recommended.

Over 60 Elderly people may be more sensitive to the drug's effects. Lower doses may be necessary.

Driving and hazardous work Avoid until you know how the drug affects you. It can cause dizziness, vertigo, and sleepiness.

Alcohol Alcohol may increase drowsiness and the risk of stomach irritation.

PROLONGED USE

The lowest effective dose is given for the shortest duration.

Monitoring Periodic tests of kidney function may be performed.

Cetirizine/levocetirizine

Brand names Allertek, Benadryl, Hayfever & Allergy Relief, Hayfever Relief, Piriteze, Xyzal, Zirtek, Zirtek Allergy

Used in the following combined preparations None

QUICK REFERENCE

Drug group Antihistamine (p.58)

Overdose danger rating Medium

Dependence rating Low

Prescription needed Yes (levocetirizine) No (cetirizine)

Available as generic No (levocetirizine) Yes (cetirizine)

GENERAL INFORMATION

Cetirizine and levocetirizine are long-acting antihistamines. Their main use is in the treatment of allergic rhinitis, particularly hay fever. Both drugs are also used to treat a number of allergic skin conditions, such as urticaria (hives).

The principal difference between these medicines and traditional antihistamines such as chlorphenamine (chlorpheniramine) is that they have less sedative effect on the central nervous system and may therefore be suitable for people when they need to avoid sleepiness (for example, when driving). However, because these drugs can cause drowsiness in some people, you should learn how cetirizine and levocetirizine affect you before you undertake any activities that require concentration.

INFORMATION FOR USERS

Your drug prescription is tailored for you. Do not alter dosage without checking with your doctor.

How taken/used Tablets, liquid.

Frequency and timing of doses 1–2 x daily.

Dosage range *Cetirizine* 10mg daily (adults and children over 6 years); 5mg daily (children 2–5 years for hayfever only). *Levocetirizine* 5mg daily.

Onset of effect 1–3 hours. Some effects may not be felt for 1–2 days.

Duration of action Up to 24 hours.

Diet advice None.

Storage Keep in original container at room temperature out of the reach of children.

Missed dose No cause for concern, but take as soon as you remember. If your next dose is due within 8 hours, take a single dose now and skip the next.

Stopping the drug Can be safely stopped as soon as you no longer need it.

Exceeding the dose An occasional unintentional extra dose is unlikely to cause any problems. Large overdoses may cause nausea or drowsiness and have adverse effects on the heart. Notify your doctor.

POSSIBLE ADVERSE EFFECTS

The most common adverse effects are drowsiness, dry mouth, and fatigue. These adverse effects may be reduced if the dose of cetirizine is taken as 5mg twice a day. If the adverse effects are severe, discuss with your doctor.

INTERACTIONS

Anticholinergic drugs The anticholinergic effects of cetirizine and levocetirizine may be increased by all drugs that have anticholinergic effects, including antipsychotics, tricyclic antidepressants, and some drugs for parkinsonism.

Sedatives Cetirizine and levocetirizine may increase the sedative effects of anti-anxiety drugs, sleeping drugs, antidepressants, and antipsychotic drugs.

Allergy tests Antihistamines should be discontinued about 2 days before allergy skin testing. Discuss details in advance with your allergy clinic; timings of discontinuation vary from clinic to clinic.

SPECIAL PRECAUTIONS

Be sure to consult your doctor if:
◆ You have long-term liver or kidney problems.
◆ You have glaucoma.
◆ You are taking other medicines.
Pregnancy Safety in pregnancy not established. Discuss with your doctor.
Breast-feeding The drug passes into the breast milk. Discuss with your doctor.
Infants and children Not recommended under 2 years (cetirizine): not recommended under 6 years (levocetirizine).
Over 60 No problems expected.
Driving and hazardous work Avoid such activities until you have learned how cetirizine and levocetirizine affect you because the drug can cause drowsiness in some people.
Alcohol Keep consumption low.

PROLONGED USE

No problems expected.

Chloramphenicol

Brand names Chloromycetin, Kemicetine, Minims Chloramphenicol, Optrex Infected Eyes
Used in the following combined preparation Actinac

QUICK REFERENCE

Drug group Antibiotic (p.62)
Overdose danger rating Low
Dependence rating Low
Prescription needed Yes (except some eye drops)
Available as generic Yes

GENERAL INFORMATION

Chloramphenicol is an antibiotic used topically to treat eye and ear infections. Eye drops are available over the counter. Given by mouth or injection, the drug is used in the treatment of meningitis and brain abscesses. It is also effective in acute infections such as typhoid, pneumonia, epiglottitis, or meningitis caused by bacteria resistant to other antibiotics. Although most people experience few adverse effects, chloramphenicol occasionally causes serious or even fatal blood disorders. For this reason, chloramphenicol by mouth or injection is normally only given to treat life-threatening infections that do not respond to safer drugs.

INFORMATION FOR USERS

Your drug prescription is tailored for you. Do not alter dosage without checking with your doctor.
How taken/used Capsules, injection, lotion, eye ointment, eye and ear drops.
Frequency and timing of doses Every 6 hours (by mouth or injection); every 2–6 hours (eye preparations); 2–3 x daily (ear drops).
Adult dosage range Varies according to preparation and condition. Follow your doctor's instructions.
Onset of effect 1–3 days, depending on the condition and preparation.
Duration of action 6–8 hours.
Diet advice None.
Storage Keep in original container at room temperature out of the reach of children.
Missed dose Take as soon as you remember (capsules, liquid). If your next dose is due, double the dose to make up the missed dose. For skin, eye, and ear preparations, apply as soon as you remember.
Stopping the drug Take the full course. Even if you feel better the infection may still be present and may recur if treatment is stopped too soon.
Exceeding the dose An occasional unintentional extra dose is unlikely to be a cause for concern. But if you notice any unusual symptoms, or if a large overdose has been taken, notify your doctor.

POSSIBLE ADVERSE EFFECTS

Transient irritation may occur with eye or ear drops. If you are receiving the drug by mouth or injection, you may experience nausea, vomiting, diarrhoea, numbness or tingling in the hands or feet, or a rash; if so, notify your doctor. If you develop impaired vision or a painful mouth or tongue, stop taking the drug and consult your doctor immediately. A sore throat, fever, and unusual tiredness with any form of chloramphenicol may be signs of blood abnormalities and should be reported to your doctor without delay, even if treatment has been stopped; if these effects occur during treatment, stop taking the drug and contact your doctor.

INTERACTIONS

General note Chloramphenicol may increase the effect of certain other drugs, including phenytoin, oral anticoagulants, and oral antidiabetics; phenobarbital or rifampicin may reduce the effect of chloramphenicol.

Antidiabetic drugs Chloramphenicol may increase the effect of antidiabetic drugs.

Ciclosporin, tacrolimus, and sirolimus Chloramphenicol capsules, liquid, or injection may raise blood levels of these drugs.

SPECIAL PRECAUTIONS

Be sure to tell your doctor if:
◆ You have long-term liver or kidney problems.
◆ You have a blood disorder.
◆ You are taking other medicines.

Pregnancy No evidence of risk with eye or ear preparations. Safety in pregnancy, of other methods of administration, not established. Discuss with your doctor.

Breast-feeding No evidence of risk with eye or ear preparations. Taken by mouth, the drug passes into the breast milk and may increase the risk of blood disorders in the baby. Discuss with your doctor.

Infants and children Reduced dose necessary.

Over 60 No problems expected.

Driving and hazardous work Avoid such activities until you have learned how the drug affects you; chloramphenicol can cause transient burning when applied.

Alcohol No known problems.

PROLONGED USE

Prolonged or repeated use of this drug may increase the risk of serious blood disorders and eye damage.

Monitoring Periodic blood cell counts and eye tests may be performed. Blood levels of the drug are usually monitored in infants who are given chloramphenicol by mouth or injection.

Chloroquine

Brand names Avloclor, Malarivon, Nivaquine
Used in the following combined preparation
Paludrine/Avloclor

QUICK REFERENCE

Drug group Antimalarial (p.75) and disease-modifying antirheumatic drug (p.51)
Overdose danger rating High
Dependence rating Low
Prescription needed No (malaria prevention);
Yes (other uses)
Available as generic Yes

GENERAL INFORMATION

Chloroquine is used for the prevention and treatment of malaria. It usually clears an attack in three days. Injections may be given for a severe attack. To prevent malaria, a low dose is given once weekly, starting one week before visiting a high-risk area and continuing through 4 weeks after leaving. Chloroquine is not suitable for use in all parts of the world because resistance to the drug has developed in some areas. The other main use of chloroquine is as an antirheumatic drug in the treatment of autoimmune diseases such as rheumatoid arthritis and lupus erythematosus. It is used to modify, halt, or slow the disease process.

Common side effects include nausea, headache, diarrhoea, and abdominal cramps. Occasionally a rash develops. Chloroquine can damage the retina during prolonged treatment, causing blurred vision that may progress to blindness. Regular eye examinations are performed to detect early changes.

INFORMATION FOR USERS

Follow instructions on the label. Call your doctor if symptoms worsen.

How taken/used Tablets, liquid, injection.

Frequency and timing of doses *By mouth* 1 x weekly (prevention of malaria); 1–2 x daily (treatment of malaria); 1 x daily (arthritis); 1 x 2 daily (lupus erythematosus).

Adult dosage range *Prevention of malaria* 300mg (2 tablets) as a single dose on the same day each week. Start 1 week before entering endemic area and continue for 4 weeks after leaving. *Treatment of malaria* Initial dose 600mg (4 tablets) and following doses 300mg. *Rheumatoid arthritis* 150mg (1 tablet) per day.

Onset of effect 2–3 days. In rheumatoid arthritis, full effect may not be felt for up to 6 months.

Duration of action Up to 1 week.

Diet advice None.

Storage Keep in original container at room temperature out of the reach of children.

Missed dose Take as soon as you remember but if your next dose is due within 24 hours (1 x weekly schedule), or 6 hours (1–2 x daily schedule), take a single dose now and skip the next.

Stopping the drug Do not stop the drug without consulting your doctor.

OVERDOSE ACTION

Seek immediate medical advice in all cases. Take emergency action if breathing difficulties, fits, or loss of consciousness occur.

POSSIBLE ADVERSE EFFECTS

Common side effects, such as nausea, diarrhoea, and abdominal pain, may be avoided by taking the drug with food. More rarely, chloroquine may cause headache or dizziness, hearing problems, and mood changes; if so, you should consult your doctor. If you develop a rash or notice any changes in vision, stop taking the drug and consult your doctor promptly.

INTERACTIONS

Ciclosporin and digoxin Chloroquine increases blood levels of these drugs.

Antiepileptic drugs Chloroquine may reduce the effect of these drugs.

Amiodarone Chloroquine may increase the risk of abnormal heart rhythms if taken with this drug.

SPECIAL PRECAUTIONS

Be sure to consult your doctor or pharmacist before taking this drug if:
◆ You have liver or kidney problems.
◆ You have glucose-6-phosphate dehydrogenase (G6PD) deficiency.
◆ You have eye or vision problems.
◆ You have psoriasis.
◆ You have a history of epilepsy.
◆ You suffer from porphyria.
◆ You are taking other medicines.

Pregnancy No evidence of risk with low doses. High doses may affect the baby. Discuss the benefits versus the risks of malaria prevention with your doctor.

Breast-feeding The drug may pass into breast milk in small amounts. At normal doses, effects on the baby are unlikely. At high doses in the long term, discuss with your doctor.

Infants and children Reduced dose necessary.

Over 60 No special problems, except that it may be difficult to tell between changes in eyesight due to ageing, and those that are drug induced.

Driving and hazardous work Avoid such activities until you have learned how chloroquine affects you because the drug may cause dizziness and changes in vision.

Alcohol Keep consumption low.

PROLONGED USE

Prolonged use may cause eye damage and blood disorders.

Monitoring Periodic eye tests and blood counts must be carried out.

Chlorphenamine (chlorpeniramine)

Brand names Allergy Relief, Allerief, Calimal, Hayleve, Piriton, Pollease

Used in the following combined preparations Contac, Galpseud Plus, Haymine, Tixylix Cough and Cold

QUICK REFERENCE

Drug group Antihistamine (p.58)
Overdose danger rating Medium
Dependence rating Low
Prescription needed No (tablets, liquid); yes (injection)
Available as generic Yes

GENERAL INFORMATION

Chlorphenamine has been used for over 30 years to treat allergies such as hay fever, allergic conjunctivitis, urticaria (hives), insect bites and stings, and angioedema (allergic swellings). It is included in several over-the-counter cold remedies (see p.28). Like other antihistamines, chlorphenamine relieves allergic skin symptoms such as itching, swelling, and redness. It also reduces sneezing and the runny nose and itching eyes of hay fever. Chlorphenamine has a mild anticholinergic action, which suppresses mucus secretion.

Chlorphenamine may also be used to prevent or treat allergic reactions to blood transfusions or X-ray contrast material, and can be given with epinephrine (adrenaline) injections for acute allergic shock (anaphylaxis).

INFORMATION FOR USERS

Follow instructions on the label. Call your doctor if symptoms worsen.

How taken/used Tablets, liquid, injection.

Frequency and timing of doses 4–6 x daily (tablets, liquid); single dose as needed (injection).

Dosage range *Adults* 12–24mg daily (by mouth); up to 40mg daily (injection). *Children* Reduced dose according to age and weight.

Onset of effect Within 60 minutes (by mouth); within 20 minutes (injection).

Duration of action 4–6 hours (tablets, liquid, injection).

Diet advice None.

Storage Keep in original container at room temperature out of the reach of children.

Missed dose Take as soon as you remember. If your next dose is due within 2 hours, take a single dose now and skip the next.

Stopping the drug Can be safely stopped as soon as you no longer need it.

Exceeding the dose An occasional unintentional extra dose is unlikely to cause any problems. Large overdoses may cause drowsiness or agitation, fits, or heart problems. Notify your doctor.

POSSIBLE ADVERSE EFFECTS

Drowsiness is the most common adverse effect of chlorphenamine; other side effects are rare. Some of these, such as dryness of the mouth, blurred vision, and difficulty passing urine, are due to its anticholinergic effects. Gastrointestinal irritation may be reduced by taking the tablets or liquid with food or drink. Discuss with your doctor if these symptoms become severe. If you develop a rash, or if a child taking the drug becomes excitable, stop the drug and consult your doctor.

INTERACTIONS

Anticholinergic drugs All drugs that have an anticholinergic effect, including certain drugs used in the treatment of parkinsonism, are likely to increase the anticholinergic effect of chlorphenamine.

Phenytoin The effects of phenytoin may be enhanced by chlorphenamine.

Monoamine oxidase inhibitors (MAOIs) and tricyclic antidepressants These drugs may increase the side effects of chlorphenamine.

Sedatives All drugs with a sedative effect are likely to increase the sedative properties of chlorphenamine.

SPECIAL PRECAUTIONS

Be sure to consult your doctor or pharmacist before taking this drug if:
◆ You have a long-term liver problem.
◆ You have had epileptic fits.
◆ You have glaucoma.
◆ You have urinary difficulties.
◆ You are taking other medicines.

Pregnancy Safety in pregnancy not established. Discuss with your doctor.

Breast-feeding Chlorphenamine passes into the breast milk and may cause drowsiness and poor feeding in the baby. Discuss with your doctor.

Infants and children Reduced dose necessary.

Over 60 Reduced dose may be necessary. Increased likelihood of adverse effects.

Driving and hazardous work Avoid such activities until you have learned how the drug affects you because it can cause drowsiness, dizziness, and blurred vision.

Alcohol Avoid. Alcohol may increase the sedative effects of this drug.

PROLONGED USE

No problems expected.

Chlorpromazine

Brand names Chloractil, Largactil
Used in the following combined preparations None

QUICK REFERENCE

Drug group Phenothiazine antipsychotic (p.15) and anti-emetic drug (p.21)
Overdose danger rating Medium
Dependence rating Low
Prescription needed Yes
Available as generic Yes

GENERAL INFORMATION

Chlorpromazine was the first antipsychotic drug to be marketed and it is still used today. It has a calming and sedative effect that is useful in the short-term treatment of anxiety, agitation, and aggressive behaviour.

Chlorpromazine is prescribed for the treatment of schizophrenia, psychosis, and mania. Other uses of this drug include the treatment of nausea and vomiting, especially when caused by drug or radiation treatment; and treating severe, prolonged hiccoughs.

Chlorpromazine can produce a number of adverse effects, some of which may be serious. After continuous use of the drug over several years, eye changes and skin discoloration may occur.

INFORMATION FOR USERS

Your drug prescription is tailored for you. Do not alter dosage without checking with your doctor.

How taken/used Tablets, liquid, injection, suppositories (specialist manufacturers only).

Frequency and timing of doses 1–6 x daily.

Adult dosage range *Mental illness* 75–300mg daily; dose is started low and gradually increased. Some patients may need up to 1,000mg daily. *Nausea and vomiting* 40–150mg daily.

Onset of effect 30–60 minutes (by mouth); 15–20 minutes (injection); up to 30 minutes (suppository).

Duration of action 8–12 hours (by mouth or injection); 3–4 hours (suppository). Some effect may persist for up to 3 weeks when stopping the drug after regular use.

Diet advice None.

Storage Keep in original container at room temperature out of the reach of children. Protect from light.

Missed dose Take as soon as you remember. If your next dose is due within 2 hours, do not take the missed dose. Take your next scheduled dose as usual.

Stopping the drug Do not stop taking the drug without consulting your doctor; symptoms may recur.

Exceeding the dose An occasional unintentional extra dose is unlikely to cause any problems. Larger overdoses may cause unusual drowsiness, fainting, abnormal heart rhythms, muscle rigidity, and agitation. Notify your doctor if an overdose has been taken.

POSSIBLE ADVERSE EFFECTS

Chlorpromazine commonly causes mild drowsiness and has an anticholinergic effect, which can cause various symptoms. Side effects include weight gain, tremor or parkinsonism, blurred vision, dizziness or fainting. Women may also develop menstrual irregularities. If a light-sensitive rash or jaundice occur, you should stop taking the drug and consult your doctor.

INTERACTIONS

Drugs for parkinsonism Chlorpromazine may reduce the effect of these drugs.

Anticholinergic drugs These drugs may intensify the anticholinergic properties of chlorpromazine.

Sedatives All drugs that have a sedative effect on the central nervous system are likely to increase the sedative properties of chlorpromazine.

SPECIAL PRECAUTIONS

Be sure to tell your doctor if:
◆ You have long-term liver or kidney problems.
◆ You have had heart problems.
◆ You have had epileptic fits.
◆ You have any blood disorders.
◆ You have glaucoma.
◆ You are taking other medicines.

Pregnancy Occasionally prescribed by specialist centres. Taken near the time of delivery, it may cause drowsiness in the newborn baby. Discuss with your doctor.

Breast-feeding The drug passes into the breast milk and may affect the baby. Discuss with your doctor.

Infants and children Not recommended for infants under 1 year. Reduced dose necessary for older children.

Over 60 Initial dosage is low; it may be increased if there are no adverse reactions, such as abnormal limb movements or low blood pressure.

Driving and hazardous work Avoid such activities until you have learned how the drug affects you as it can cause drowsiness and slowed reactions.

Alcohol Avoid. Alcohol may increase the sedative effects of this drug.

Surgery and general anaesthetics Chlorpromazine treatment may need to be stopped before you have a general anaesthetic. Discuss this with your doctor or dentist before any operation.

PROLONGED USE

If used for many years, chlorpromazine may cause prolonged movement disorders. Occasionally, jaundice may occur.

Ciclosporin

Brand names Neoral, Sandimmun
Used in the following combined preparations
None

QUICK REFERENCE

Drug group Immunosuppressant drug (p.99)
Overdose danger rating Medium
Dependence rating Low
Prescription needed Yes
Available as generic No

GENERAL INFORMATION

Introduced in 1984, ciclosporin is one of the immunosuppressants, a group of drugs that suppress the body's natural defences against infection and foreign cells. This action is of particular use following organ transplants, when the recipient's immune system may reject the transplanted organ unless the immune system is controlled.

Ciclosporin is widely used after many types of transplant, such as heart, bone marrow, kidney, liver, and pancreas; its use has considerably reduced the risk of rejection. It is sometimes used to treat rheumatoid arthritis, some severe types of dermatitis, severe psoriasis, and a number of other conditions, often when other treatments have failed.

Because ciclosporin reduces the immune system's effectiveness, people being treated with it are more susceptible than usual to infections. Ciclosporin can also cause kidney damage. Different brands of ciclosporin may reach different levels in your blood. It is important to know which brand you are taking. Do not try to make dose changes

on your own. Ask your pharmacist for a patient information leaflet on the product you are taking.

INFORMATION FOR USERS

Your drug prescription is tailored for you. Do not alter dosage without checking with your doctor.

How taken/used Capsules, liquid, injection.
Frequency and timing of doses 1–2 x daily. The liquid can be mixed with water, apple juice, or orange juice just before taking. Do not mix with grapefruit juice.
Dosage range Dosage is calculated on an individual basis according to age and weight.
Onset of effect Within 12 hours.
Duration of action Up to 3 days.
Diet advice Avoid high-potassium foods, such as bananas and tomatoes, and potassium supplements. Avoid grapefruit juice.
Storage Capsules should be left in the blister pack until required. Keep in original container at room temperature out of the reach of children. Do not refrigerate.
Missed dose Take as soon as you remember. If your dose is more than 36 hours late, consult your doctor.
Stopping the drug Do not stop taking the drug without consulting your doctor; stopping the drug may lead to transplant rejection.
Exceeding the dose An occasional unintentional extra dose is unlikely to cause any problems. Large overdoses may cause vomiting and diarrhoea and may affect kidney function. Notify your doctor.

POSSIBLE ADVERSE EFFECTS

The most common adverse effects are gum swelling, excessive hair growth, nausea and vomiting, and tremor, especially at the start of treatment. Headache and muscle cramps may also occur. Less common effects are diarrhoea, facial swelling, flushing, "pins and needles" sensations, rash, and itching. Consult your doctor if any of these occur.

INTERACTIONS

General note Ciclosporin may interact with a large number of drugs. Check with your doctor or pharmacist before taking any new prescription or over-the-counter medications. Grapefruit juice can increase blood levels of ciclosporin. Avoid both grapefruit flesh and juice for 1 hour before taking ciclosporin.

SPECIAL PRECAUTIONS

Ciclosporin is prescribed only under close medical supervision, taking account of your present condition and medical history.

Pregnancy Use in pregnancy depends on the condition under treatment. Discuss with your doctor.

Breast-feeding Not recommended. The drug passes into the breast milk and safety has not been established. Discuss with your doctor.

Infants and children Used only by specialist children's doctors.

Over 60 Reduced dose may be necessary.

Driving and hazardous work No known problems.

Alcohol No known problems.

Sunlight Avoid prolonged, unprotected exposure; apply sunscreen or sunblock.

PROLONGED USE

Long-term use, especially in high doses, can affect kidney and/or liver function. It may reduce numbers of white blood cells, thus increasing susceptibility to infection.

Monitoring Regular blood tests should be carried out as well as tests for liver and kidney function. Ciclosporin blood levels should also be checked regularly.

Cimetidine

Brand names Dyspamet, Galenamet, Tagamet, Zita
Used in the following combined preparations
None

QUICK REFERENCE

Drug group Anti-ulcer drug (p.43)
Overdose danger rating Low
Dependence rating Low
Prescription needed No (some preparations)
Available as generic Yes

GENERAL INFORMATION

Introduced in the 1970s, cimetidine was the first of a new group of anti-ulcer drugs. Cimetidine reduces the secretion of gastric acid and of pepsin, an enzyme that helps in the digestion of protein. By reducing levels of acid and pepsin, it promotes ulcer healing in the stomach and duodenum. It is also used for reflux oesophagitis, in which acid stomach contents may flow up the oesophagus. Treatment is usually given in 4-8-week courses, with further short courses if symptoms recur. Cimetidine also affects the actions of certain enzymes in the liver, where many drugs are broken down. It is therefore prescribed with caution to people taking other drugs, particularly anticoagulants and anticonvulsants, whose levels need to be carefully controlled. Since cimetidine promotes healing of the stomach lining, it may mask the symptoms of stomach cancer and delay diagnosis. It is therefore prescribed with caution to patients whose symptoms change or persist, and in middle-aged and older people.

INFORMATION FOR USERS

Follow instructions on the label. Call your doctor if symptoms worsen.

How taken/used Tablets, liquid, injection.
Frequency and timing of doses 1–4 x daily (after meals and at bedtime).
Adult dosage range 800–1,600mg daily (occasionally increased to 2,400mg daily).
Onset of effect Within 90 minutes.
Duration of action 2–6 hours.
Diet advice None.
Storage Keep in original container at room temperature out of the reach of children. Protect from light.
Missed dose Do not take the missed dose. Take your next dose as usual.
Stopping the drug If prescribed by your doctor, do not stop taking the drug without consulting him or her because symptoms may recur.
Exceeding the dose An occasional unintentional extra dose is unlikely to be a cause for concern. But if you notice any unusual symptoms, or if a large overdose has been taken, notify your doctor.

POSSIBLE ADVERSE EFFECTS

Adverse effects are uncommon with cimetidine, but they include diarrhoea, dizziness, confusion, and tiredness. They are usually related to dosage level and almost always disappear when the drug is stopped. Muscle pain may occur. Men may suffer from erectile dysfunction and breast enlargement. If any of these symptoms occur, seek medical advice. If you develop a rash, stop taking the drug and consult your doctor.

INTERACTIONS

Benzodiazepines Cimetidine may increase the blood levels of some of these drugs, increasing the risk of adverse effects.

Theophylline/aminophylline Cimetidine may increase the blood levels of these drugs and their dose may need to be reduced.

Sildenafil Cimetidine may increase the blood level of this drug.

Beta blockers and anti-arrhythmic drugs Cimetidine may increase the blood levels of these drugs.

Anticonvulsant drugs Cimetidine may increase the blood levels of these drugs, and their dose may need to be reduced.

Anticoagulant drugs Cimetidine may increase the effect of anticoagulants and their dose may need to be reduced.

SPECIAL PRECAUTIONS

Be sure to consult your doctor or pharmacist before taking this drug if:
◆ You have long-term liver or kidney problems.
◆ You are taking other medicines.

Pregnancy Safety in pregnancy not established. Discuss with your doctor.

Breast-feeding The drug passes into the breast milk, but at normal doses adverse effects on the baby are unlikely. Discuss with your doctor.

Infants and children Reduced dose necessary.

Over 60 No special problems unless kidney function is reduced. The risk of stomach cancer is higher in elderly people and it must be excluded before cimetidine is prescribed.

Driving and hazardous work Avoid such activities until you have learned how cimetidine affects you because the drug may cause dizziness and confusion.

Alcohol Avoid. Alcohol may aggravate the underlying condition and counter the beneficial effects of cimetidine.

PROLONGED USE

Courses of longer than 8 weeks are not usually necessary.

Cinnarizine

Brand names Cinaziere, Stugeron
Used in the following combined preparations
None

QUICK REFERENCE

Drug group Antihistamine anti-emetic drug (p.21)
Overdose danger rating Medium
Dependence rating Low
Prescription needed No
Available as generic Yes

GENERAL INFORMATION

Introduced in the 1970s, cinnarizine is an antihistamine used mainly to control nausea and vomiting, especially motion (travel) sickness. The drug is also used to control the symptoms (nausea and vertigo) of inner ear disorders such as labyrinthitis and Ménière's disease. Taken in high doses, cinnarizine has a vasodilator effect and is used to improve circulation in Raynaud's disease and peripheral vascular disease.

Cinnarizine has adverse effects that are similar to those of most other antihistamines. Drowsiness is the most common problem, but it is usually less severe than with other antihistamines.

INFORMATION FOR USERS

Follow instructions on the label. Call your doctor if symptoms worsen.

How taken/used Tablets, capsules.

Frequency and timing of doses 2–3 x daily. For the prevention of motion sickness, the first dose should be taken 2 hours before travel.

Dosage range *Adults* 90mg daily (nausea/vomiting); 150–225mg daily (circulatory disorders); 30mg, then 15mg every 8 hours as needed (motion sickness). *Children* aged 5–12, 15mg, then 7.5mg every 8 hours as needed (motion sickness).

Onset of effect Within 2 hours. Several weeks (circulation disorders).

Duration of action Up to 8 hours.

Diet advice None.

Storage Keep in original container at room temperature out of the reach of children.

Missed dose Take as soon as you remember. If your next dose is due within 2 hours, take a single dose now and skip the next.

Stopping the drug If you are taking cinnarizine for an inner ear disorder or a circulatory condition, do not stop the drug without consulting your doctor; symptoms may recur. However, when taken for motion sickness, the drug can be safely stopped as soon as you no longer need it.

Exceeding the dose An occasional unintentional extra dose is unlikely to cause any problems. However, large overdoses may cause drowsiness or agitation. Notify your doctor.

POSSIBLE ADVERSE EFFECTS

Drowsiness is the main adverse effect of this drug. Anticholinergic effects such as blurred vision and dry mouth may also occur occasionally. Rarely, cinnarizine may cause gastrointestinal problems. If these side effects become severe, notify your doctor. If you develop a rash, stop taking the drug and consult your doctor.

INTERACTIONS

General note All drugs that have a sedative effect on the central nervous system may increase the sedative properties of cinnarizine. Such drugs include sleeping drugs, antidepressants, anti-anxiety drugs, and opioid analgesics.

SPECIAL PRECAUTIONS

Be sure to consult your doctor or pharmacist before taking this drug if:
◆ You have low blood pressure.
◆ You have Parkinson's disease.
◆ You have glaucoma.
◆ You have porphyria.
◆ You have an enlarged prostate.
◆ You are taking other medicines.

Pregnancy Safety in pregnancy not established. Discuss with your doctor.

Breast-feeding Safety not established. Discuss with your doctor.

Infants and children Reduced dose necessary.

Over 60 No special problems.

Driving and hazardous work Avoid such activities until you have learned how cinnarizine affects you because the drug can cause drowsiness.

Alcohol Avoid. Alcohol may increase the sedative effects of this drug.

PROLONGED USE

Development or aggravation of extrapyramidal symptoms (abnormal movements) may occur rarely in the elderly after prolonged use of cinnarizine, and treatment should be discontinued.

Ciprofloxacin

Brand name Ciproxin
Used in the following combined preparations
None

QUICK REFERENCE

Drug group Antibacterial (p.66)
Overdose danger rating Medium
Dependence rating Low
Prescription needed Yes
Available as generic Yes

GENERAL INFORMATION

Ciprofloxacin, a quinolone antibacterial, is used to treat several types of bacteria resistant to other commonly used antibiotics. It is especially useful for chest, intestine, and urinary tract infections. When taken by mouth, ciprofloxacin is well absorbed by the body and works quickly and effectively. In more severe systemic bacterial infections, however, it may be necessary to administer the drug by injection. Ciprofloxacin has a long duration of action and needs to be taken only once or twice daily. Its most common side effect is gastrointestinal disturbance.

INFORMATION FOR USERS

Your drug prescription is tailored for you. Do not alter dosage without checking with your doctor.

How taken/used Tablets, liquid, injection.

Frequency and timing of doses 2 x daily with plenty of fluids.

Adult dosage range 500mg–1.5g daily (tablets); 200–400mg daily (injection).

Onset of effect The drug begins to work within a few hours, although full beneficial effect may not be felt for several days.

Duration of action About 12 hours.

Diet advice Do not become dehydrated. Avoid dairy products because they may reduce the drug's absorption.

Storage Keep in original container at room temperature out of the reach of children. The injection must be protected from light.

Missed dose Take as soon as you remember, and take your next dose as usual.

Stopping the drug Take the full course. Even if you feel better the original infection may still be present, and symptoms may recur if treatment is stopped too soon.

Exceeding the dose An occasional unintentional extra dose is unlikely to cause any problems. Large overdoses may cause kidney problems, mental disturbance, and fits. Notify your doctor.

POSSIBLE ADVERSE EFFECTS

Most side effects are rare, except when very high doses are given. Nausea, vomiting, abdominal pain, diarrhoea, rash, and itching are the most common adverse effects. Others include dizziness, headache, joint pain, sleep disturbances, sensitivity to light, jaundice, and confusion. If convulsions or painful, inflamed tendons occur, you should stop taking the drug, contact your doctor immediately, and rest affected limbs.

INTERACTIONS

Oral iron preparations and antacids containing magnesium or aluminium hydroxide interfere with absorption of ciprofloxacin. Do not take antacids within 2 hours of taking ciprofloxacin tablets.

Anticoagulants and oral antidiabetics Blood levels of these drugs may be increased; their dosage may need adjusting.

Theophylline Ciprofloxacin may increase blood levels of this drug; its dose may need adjusting and its blood levels monitored.

Phenytoin Ciprofloxacin may raise or lower the blood levels of this drug.

Non-steroidal anti-inflammatory drugs These drugs increase the risk of epileptic fits.

SPECIAL PRECAUTIONS

Be sure to tell your doctor if:
◆ You have long-term liver or kidney problems.
◆ You have had epileptic fits.
◆ You have glucose-6-phosphate dehydrogenase (G6PD) deficiency.
◆ You have myasthenia gravis.
◆ You are taking other medicines.

Pregnancy Safety in pregnancy not established. Discuss with your doctor.

Breast-feeding The drug passes into the breast milk and may affect the baby adversely. Discuss with your doctor.

Infants and children Not usually recommended.

Over 60 The drug may make the elderly more susceptible to tendinitis.

Driving and hazardous work Avoid such activities until you have learned how ciprofloxacin affects you because the drug can cause dizziness and confusion.

Alcohol Avoid. Alcohol may increase the sedative effects of this drug.

Sunlight Avoid direct exposure to sunlight or sunlamps; increased risk of a photosensitivity reaction.

PROLONGED USE

No problems expected.

Monitoring Blood tests may be necessary to monitor kidney and liver function.

Cisplatin

Brand name Platinex
Used in the following combined preparations None

QUICK REFERENCE

Drug group Anticancer drug (p.96)
Overdose danger rating High
Dependence rating Low
Prescription needed Yes
Available as generic Yes

GENERAL INFORMATION

Cisplatin is one of the most effective drugs available to treat a wide variety of cancers including those of the ovaries, testes, head, neck, bladder, cervix, and lung. It is also used in treating certain children's cancers and some cancers of the blood. It is usually given along with other anticancer drugs.

The most common and serious adverse effect of cisplatin is impaired kidney function. To reduce the risk of permanent kidney damage, the drug is usually given only once every 3 weeks, allowing the kidneys time to recover between courses of treatment. Plenty of fluid must be taken to dilute the drug in the kidneys. Nausea and vomiting may occur after administration of cisplatin. These symptoms usually start within an hour and last for up to 24 hours, in some case persisting for up to a week. Because nausea and vomiting may be quite severe, anti-emetic drugs are given.

Damage to hearing is common and may be more severe in children. Use of cisplatin may also increase the risk of anaemia, blood clotting disorders, and infection during treatment.

INFORMATION FOR USERS

This drug is given only under medical supervision and is not for self-administration.
How taken/used Injection.
Frequency and timing of doses Every 3 weeks for up to 5 days; it may be given alone or in combination with other anticancer drugs.
Adult dosage range Dosage is determined individually according to body height, weight, and response.
Onset of effect Some adverse effects, such as nausea and vomiting, may appear within 1 hour of starting treatment.
Duration of action Some adverse effects may last for up to 1 week after treatment has stopped.
Diet advice Prior to treatment it is important that the body is well hydrated. Therefore, 1–2 litres of fluid are usually given by infusion over 8–12 hours.
Storage Not applicable. The drug is not normally kept in the home.
Missed dose Not applicable. The drug is given only in hospital under medical supervision.
Stopping the drug Not applicable. The drug will be stopped under medical supervision.
Exceeding the dose Overdosage is unlikely since treatment is carefully monitored, and the drug is given intravenously only under close supervision.

POSSIBLE ADVERSE EFFECTS

The most common adverse effects include loss of appetite or taste, nausea, vomiting, and ringing in the ears or hearing loss. More rarely, there may be wheezing or breathing difficulty, abnormal sensations, rash, or facial swelling. Most adverse effects appear within a few hours of injection and are carefully monitored in hospital after each dose. Some

effects wear off within 24 hours. Nausea and loss of appetite may last for up to a week.

INTERACTIONS

General note A number of drugs (for example, antibacterials such as gentamicin) increase the adverse effects of cisplatin. Because the drug is given only under close medical supervision, these interactions are carefully monitored and the dosage adjusted accordingly.

SPECIAL PRECAUTIONS

Cisplatin is prescribed only under close medical supervision, taking account of your present condition and your medical history.
Pregnancy Not usually prescribed. Cisplatin may cause birth defects or premature birth. Discuss with your doctor.
Breast-feeding Not advised. The drug passes into the breast milk and may affect the baby adversely. Discuss with your doctor.
Infants and children The risk of hearing loss is increased. Reduced dose used.
Over 60 Reduced dose may be necessary. Increased likelihood of adverse effects.
Driving and hazardous work No known problems.
Alcohol No known problems.

PROLONGED USE

Prolonged use of this drug increases the risk of damage to the kidneys, nerves, and bone marrow, and to hearing.
Monitoring Hearing tests and blood checks to monitor kidney function and bone marrow activity are carried out regularly.

Citalopram/escitalopram

Brand name Cipralex (escitalopram), Cipramil (citalopram)
Used in the following combined preparations
None

QUICK REFERENCE

Drug group Antidepressant drug (p.14)
Overdose danger rating Medium
Dependence rating Low
Prescription needed Yes
Available as generic Yes (citalopram); No (escitalopram)

GENERAL INFORMATION

Citalopram and escitalopram are selective serotonin re-uptake inhibitor (SSRI) anti-depressants used for depressive illness and panic disorder; escitalopram is also used for social and generalized anxiety disorders. The drugs gradually improve mood, increase physical activity, and restore interest in everyday pursuits.

Both drugs are generally well tolerated, and any gastrointestinal adverse effects, such as nausea, vomiting, or diarrhoea, are dose related and usually diminish with continued use of the drugs. Like other SSRIs, citalopram and escitalopram cause fewer anticholinergic side effects and are less sedating than tricyclic antidepressants. They are also less likely to be harmful in overdose, but can cause drowsiness and impair performance of tasks such as driving.

INFORMATION FOR USERS

Your drug prescription is tailored for you. Do not alter dosage without checking with your doctor.

How taken/used Tablets, oral drops.

Frequency and timing of doses Once daily in the morning or evening.

Adult dosage range *Depressive illness* 20–60mg (citalopram); 10–20mg (escitalopram). *Panic attacks* 10–60mg (citalopram); 5–20mg (escitalopram). *Social anxiety disorder* 5–20mg (escitalopram). *Generalized anxiety disorder* 10–20mg (escitalopram).

Onset of effect Some benefit may appear within 7 days, but full benefits may not be felt for 2–6 weeks (panic attacks may take longer to resolve).

Duration of action Antidepressant effect may persist for some weeks following prolonged treatment.

Diet advice None.

Storage Keep in original container at room temperature out of the reach of children.

Missed dose Take as soon as you remember. If your next dose is due within 8 hours, take a single dose now and skip the next.

Stopping the drug Do not stop taking the drug without consulting your doctor. Stopping abruptly can cause withdrawal symptoms.

Exceeding the dose An occasional unintentional extra dose is unlikely to be a cause for concern. If you notice any unusual symptoms, or if a large overdose has been taken, notify your doctor.

POSSIBLE ADVERSE EFFECTS

Common adverse effects include nausea, vomiting, indigestion, diarrhoea or constipation, sexual dysfunction, anxiety, insomnia, headache, tremor, dizziness or drowsiness, dry mouth, and sweating. Most such effects usually diminish with reduction in dosage. If convulsions or a rash occur, consult your doctor immediately. Also, if there are suicidal thoughts or attempts, stop taking the drug and seek urgent medical help.

INTERACTIONS

Sumatriptan, other 5HT$_1$ agonists, and lithium There is an increased risk of adverse effects when citalopram and escitalopram are taken with these drugs.

St. John's Wort may increase the adverse effects of citalopram and escitalopram.

Monoamine oxidase inhibitors (MAOIs) may cause a severe reaction if taken with citalopram and escitalopram; avoid if MAOIs have been taken in the last 14 days.

Anticoagulants The effect of these drugs may be increased by citalopram and escitalopram.

SPECIAL PRECAUTIONS

Be sure to tell your doctor if:
◆ You have epilepsy.
◆ You have diabetes.
◆ You have liver or kidney problems.
◆ You have had a manic-depressive illness.
◆ You have had heart problems.
◆ You have been taking monoamine oxidase inhibitors (MAOIs) or other antidepressants.
◆ You are taking other medicines.

Pregnancy Safety in pregnancy not established. Discuss with your doctor.

Breast-feeding The drug may pass into breast milk and may affect the baby. Discuss with your doctor.

Infants and children Not recommended.

Over 60 Reduced dose may be necessary.

Driving and hazardous work Such activities should be avoided until you have learned how citalopram/escitalopram affect you because they can cause drowsiness.

Alcohol No special problems.

PROLONGED USE

No problems expected. However, mild withdrawal symptoms may occur if the drug is not stopped gradually.

Monitoring Any person who experiences drowsiness, confusion, muscle cramps, or convulsions should be monitored for low sodium levels in the blood.

Clarithromycin

Brand names Clarosip, Klaricid, Klaricid XL
Used in the following combined preparation
Heliclear

QUICK REFERENCE

Drug group Antibiotic (p.62)
Overdose danger rating Low
Dependence rating Low
Prescription needed Yes
Available as generic No

GENERAL INFORMATION

Clarithromycin is a macrolide antibiotic similar to erythromycin (see p.233), from which it is derived. It has similar actions and uses to erythromycin, but is slightly more active. Clarithromycin is used for upper respiratory tract infections, such as middle ear infections, sinusitis, and pharyngitis, and lower respiratory tract infections, including whooping cough, bronchitis, and pneumonia, as well as for skin and soft tissue infections. Given with anti-ulcer drugs (see p.43) and other antibiotics, it is used to eradicate *Helicobacter pylori*, the bacterium that causes many peptic ulcers. Prolonged use of clarithromycin is not usually necessary.

INFORMATION FOR USERS

Your drug prescription is tailored for you. Do not alter dosage without checking with your doctor.

How taken/used Tablets, liquid, granules, injection.
Frequency and timing of doses 2 x daily, up to 14 days; 1 x daily (XL preparation).
Adult dosage range 500mg–1g daily.
Onset of effect 1–4 hours.
Duration of action 1–12 hours; 24 hours (XL preparation).

Diet advice None.
Storage Keep in original container at room temperature out of the reach of children. Protect from light.
Missed dose Take as soon as you remember. If your next dose is due within 2 hours, take a single dose now and skip the next.
Stopping the drug Take the full course. Even if you feel better, the infection may still be present and symptoms may recur if treatment is stopped too soon.
Exceeding the dose An occasional unintentional extra dose is unlikely to be a cause for concern. But if you notice any unusual symptoms, or if a large overdose has been taken, notify your doctor.

POSSIBLE ADVERSE EFFECTS

Clarithromycin is generally well tolerated. Gastrointestinal disturbances, such as nausea, vomiting, diarrhoea, and indigestion, are the most common problems encountered. Hearing loss is a rare possibility, but is usually reversible on stopping the drug. If an altered sense of smell or taste, anxiety, insomnia, confusion, or hallucinations occur, discuss with your doctor. If jaundice or a rash develops, stop taking the drug and consult your doctor.

INTERACTIONS

Warfarin, midazolam, disopyramide, lovastatin, rifabutin, phenytoin, ciclosporin, tacrolimus, sildenafil, and valproate Blood levels and effects of these drugs are increased by clarithromycin.
Zidovudine Blood levels of zidovudine are reduced if this drug is taken at the same time as clarithromycin.
Ergot derivatives There is an increased risk of ergot toxicity with clarithromycin.
Carbamazepine, theophylline, digoxin, and colchicine Blood levels and toxicity of these drugs are increased if clarithromycin is taken at the same time.
Pimozide, terfenadine, disopyramide, and quinidine may cause cardiac arrhythmias if taken with clarithromycin.
Lipid-lowering drugs whose names end in "statin" There is a risk of rhabdomyolysis (muscle damage) if these drugs are taken with clarithromycin.

SPECIAL PRECAUTIONS

Be sure to tell your doctor if:
◆ You have liver or kidney problems.
◆ You have had an allergic reaction to erythromycin or clarithromycin.
◆ You have a heart problem.
◆ You have porphyria.
◆ You are taking other medicines.

Pregnancy Safety has not been established. Discuss with your doctor.

Breast-feeding Clarithromycin passes into the breast milk and may affect the baby. Discuss with your doctor.

Infants and children Reduced dose necessary.

Over 60 No special problems.

Driving and hazardous work No known problems.

Alcohol No known problems.

PROLONGED USE

In courses of over 14 days, there is a risk of developing antibiotic-resistant infections.

Clobetasol

Brand names Clarelux, Dermovate
Used in the following combined preparation
Dermovate-NN

QUICK REFERENCE

Drug group Topical corticosteroid (p.120)
Overdose danger rating Low
Dependence rating Low
Prescription needed Yes
Available as generic No

GENERAL INFORMATION

Clobetasol is a potent corticosteroid drug (see p.80) used for the short-term treatment of inflammatory skin conditions that have not responded to treatment with a less potent corticosteroid. Clobetasol is used to treat conditions such as resistant eczema or psoriasis, discoid lupus erythematosus, lichen planus, and lichen simplex.

Because clobetasol is one of the strongest topical corticosteroids, it should be applied thinly and sparingly only to affected areas, and for the shortest possible duration. This is to prevent skin damage and to avoid rare systemic side effects, which can occur from the drug's absorption through the skin. Such side effects include pituitary or adrenal gland suppression and Cushing's syndrome. In addition, the drug should not be used on untreated bacterial, fungal, or viral skin infections.

Treatment of psoriasis with clobetasol must only be carried out under specialist care and supervision.

INFORMATION FOR USERS

Your drug prescription is tailored for you. Do not alter dosage without checking with your doctor.

How taken/used Cream, ointment, scalp application.

Frequency and timing of doses 1 x 2 times daily. If treating the face, use for no more than 5 days.

Dosage range No more than 50g weekly.

Onset of effect 12 hours. Full beneficial effect after 48 hours.

Duration of action Up to 24 hours.

Diet advice None.

Storage Keep in original container at room temperature out of the reach of children.

Missed dose Use as soon as you remember. If your next application is due within 8 hours, apply the usual amount now and skip the next application.

Stopping the drug Do not stop using the drug without consulting your doctor; symptoms may recur.

Exceeding the dose An occasional unintentional extra application is unlikely to cause problems. But if you notice any unusual symptoms, notify your doctor.

POSSIBLE ADVERSE EFFECTS

Most people who use clobetasol as directed do not have problems. Adverse effects mainly affect the skin; they include thinning of the skin, stretch marks, thread veins, increased size of blood capillaries in the skin, acne, dermatitis, and loss of pigmentation. Some of these effects cannot be reversed and you should talk to your doctor if any of them develop. Rarely, clobetasol may cause growth of unwanted hair.

INTERACTIONS

None.

SPECIAL PRECAUTIONS

Be sure to tell your doctor if:

◆ You have a cold sore or chickenpox.
◆ You have any other infection.
◆ You have psoriasis.
◆ You have acne or rosacea.
◆ You are taking other medicines.

Pregnancy Safety in pregnancy not established. Discuss with your doctor.

Breast-feeding The drug passes into the breast milk and may affect the baby. Discuss with your doctor.

Infants and children Not recommended for infants under 1 year. Used only with great caution for short periods in older children because overuse increases the risk of side effects.

Over 60 No special problems.

Driving and hazardous work No special problems.

Alcohol No special problems.

PROLONGED USE

Clobetasol is not normally used for more than 4 weeks. If the condition has not improved in 2 to 4 weeks, you should notify your doctor.

Clomifene

Brand name Clomid
Used in the following combined preparations
None

QUICK REFERENCE

Drug group Drug for infertility (p.109)
Overdose danger rating Low
Dependence rating Low
Prescription needed Yes
Available as generic Yes

GENERAL INFORMATION

Clomifene is used to treat female infertility. The drug stimulates ovulation by increasing the production of hormones by the pituitary gland.

Tablets are taken within about 5 days of the onset of each menstrual cycle. If clomifene does not stimulate ovulation after several months, other drugs may be prescribed. Multiple pregnancies (usually twins) occur more commonly in women

treated with clomifene than in those who have not been treated. Adverse effects of clomifene include an increased risk of ovarian cysts and ectopic pregnancy.

INFORMATION FOR USERS

Your drug prescription is tailored for you. Do not alter dosage without checking with your doctor.

How taken/used Tablets.

Frequency and timing of doses Once daily for 5 days during each menstrual cycle.

Dosage range 50mg daily initially; dose may be increased up to 100mg daily.

Onset of effect Ovulation occurs 11–12 days after the last dose in any cycle. However, ovulation may not occur for several months.

Duration of action 5 days.

Diet advice None.

Storage Keep in original container at room temperature out of the reach of children. Protect from light.

Missed dose Take as soon as you remember. If your next dose is due at this time, take the missed dose and the next scheduled dose together.

Stopping the drug Take as directed by your doctor. Stopping the drug will reduce the chances of conception.

Exceeding the dose An occasional unintentional extra dose is unlikely to be a cause for concern. But if you notice any unusual symptoms, or if a large overdose has been taken, notify your doctor.

POSSIBLE ADVERSE EFFECTS

Most side effects are related to the dose taken. These include hot flushes, nausea, vomiting, "breakthrough" bleeding, abdominal discomfort and bloating, breast tenderness, dry skin, hair loss, rash, and dizziness. Ovarian enlargement and cyst formation can occur. If this happens the problem usually resolves within a few weeks of stopping the drug. If blurred vision, convulsions, or severe pain in the chest or abdomen occur, stop taking the drug and consult your doctor.

INTERACTIONS

None.

SPECIAL PRECAUTIONS

Be sure to tell your doctor if:
◆ You have a long-term liver problem.
◆ You are taking other medicines.

Pregnancy Not prescribed. The drug is stopped as soon as pregnancy occurs.

Breast-feeding Not prescribed.

Infants and children Not prescribed.

Over 60 Not prescribed.

Driving and hazardous work Avoid such activities until you have learned how clomifene affects you because the drug can cause blurred vision.

Alcohol Keep consumption low.

PROLONGED USE

Prolonged use of clomifene may cause visual impairment. Also, no more than 6 courses of treatment are recommended since this may lead to an increased risk of ovarian cancer.

Monitoring Eye tests may be recommended if symptoms of visual impairment are noticed. Monitoring of body temperature and blood or urine hormone levels is performed to detect signs of ovulation and pregnancy.

Clomipramine

Brand names Anafranil, Anafranil SR
Used in the following combined preparations
None

QUICK REFERENCE

Drug group Tricyclic antidepressant (p.14)
Overdose danger rating High
Dependence rating Low
Prescription needed Yes
Available as generic Yes

GENERAL INFORMATION

Clomipramine belongs to the class of antidepressant drugs known as the tricyclics. It is used mainly in the long-term treatment of depression. It elevates mood, improves appetite, increases physical activity, and restores interest in everyday pursuits. Clomipramine is particularly useful in the treatment of obsessive and phobic disorders. In this case, the drug has to be taken for many months to achieve its full effect. Clomipramine has similar adverse effects to other tricyclic drugs,

such as drowsiness, dizziness, dry mouth, and constipation. In overdose, clomipramine may cause coma and dangerously abnormal heart rhythms.

INFORMATION FOR USERS

Your drug prescription is tailored for you. Do not alter dosage without checking with your doctor.

How taken/used SR-tablets, capsules.

Frequency and timing of doses 1–3 x daily.

Adult dosage range 10–250mg daily. (100mg is the usual minimum effective dose).

Onset of effect Some effects, a few days; full antidepressant effect, up to 6 weeks; phobic and obsessional disorders, full effect up to 12 weeks.

Duration of action During prolonged treatment antidepressant effect may last up to 2 weeks.

Diet advice None.

Storage Keep in original container at room temperature out of the reach of children.

Missed dose Take as soon as you remember. If your next dose is due within 3 hours, take a single dose now and skip the next.

Stopping the drug Stopping abruptly can cause withdrawal symptoms and a recurrence of the original trouble. Consult your doctor, who will supervise a gradual reduction in dosage.

OVERDOSE ACTION

Seek immediate medical advice in all cases. Take emergency action if palpitations are noted or consciousness is lost.

POSSIBLE ADVERSE EFFECTS

The possible adverse effects of clomipramine are mainly the result of its anticholinergic action; they include drowsiness and dizziness, dry mouth, sweating and flushing, blurred vision, and constipation. Weight gain may also occur. If you experience difficulty in passing urine, stop taking the drug and talk to your doctor. If you have palpitations, stop taking the drug and consult your doctor urgently.

INTERACTIONS

Sedatives All drugs that have a sedative effect may intensify those of clomipramine.

Anticonvulsant drugs Clomipramine may reduce the effects of anticonvulsant drugs and vice versa.

Monoamine oxidase inhibitors (MAOIs) A serious reaction may occur if these drugs are given with clomipramine.

Antihypertensives Clomipramine may enhance the effect of some of these drugs.

SPECIAL PRECAUTIONS

Be sure to tell your doctor if:
◆ You have heart problems.
◆ You have had epileptic fits.
◆ You have long-term liver or kidney problems.
◆ You have glaucoma.
◆ You have had prostate trouble.
◆ You have had mania or a psychotic illness.
◆ You are taking other medicines.

Pregnancy Safety in pregnancy not established. Discuss with your doctor.

Breast-feeding The drug passes into the breast milk and may affect the baby. Discuss with your doctor.

Infants and children Not recommended.

Over 60 Increased likelihood of adverse effects. Reduced dose may therefore be necessary.

Driving and hazardous work Avoid such activities until you have learned how the drug affects you because it may cause blurred vision, drowsiness, and dizziness.

Alcohol Avoid. Alcohol may increase the sedative effects of this drug.

Surgery and general anaesthetics Clomipramine treatment may need to be stopped before you have a general anaesthetic. You should discuss this with your doctor or dentist before any operation.

PROLONGED USE

No problems expected.

Monitoring Regular checks on heart and liver function are recommended.

Clonazepam

Brand name Rivotril
Used in the following combined preparations
None

QUICK REFERENCE

Drug group Benzodiazepine anticonvulsant drug (p.16)
Overdose danger rating Medium
Dependence rating Medium
Prescription needed Yes
Available as generic No

GENERAL INFORMATION

Clonazepam belongs to a group of drugs known as the benzodiazepines, which are mainly used in the treatment of anxiety (see p.13) and insomnia. However, clonazepam is usually used as an anticonvulsant to prevent and treat epileptic fits. It is particularly useful for the prevention of brief muscle spasms (myoclonus) and absence seizures (petit mal) in children but other forms of epilepsy, such as sudden flaccidity or fits induced by flashing lights, also respond to clonazepam treatment. Being a benzodiazepine, the drug also has sedative effects. Clonazepam is used either alone or together with other anticonvulsant drugs. Its anticonvulsant effect may begin to wear off after some months.

INFORMATION FOR USERS

Your drug prescription is tailored for you. Do not alter dosage without checking with your doctor.

How taken/used Tablets, injection.
Frequency and timing of doses 1–4 x daily.
Dosage range *Adults* 1mg daily at night (starting dose), increased gradually to 4–8mg daily (maintenance dose). *Children* Reduced dose according to age and weight.
Onset of effect 1–4 hours.
Duration of action Approximately 30 hours.
Diet advice None.
Storage Keep in original container at room temperature out of the reach of children.
Missed dose No cause for concern, but take as soon as you remember. Take your next dose when it is due.
Stopping the drug Do not stop taking the drug without consulting your doctor because symptoms may recur, and withdrawal symptoms may occur.
Exceeding the dose An occasional unintentional extra dose is unlikely to cause any problems. However, larger overdoses may cause excessive drowsiness and confusion. Notify your doctor.

POSSIBLE ADVERSE EFFECTS

The principal adverse effects of this drug are related to its sedative and tranquillizing properties and include daytime drowsiness, dizziness, unsteadiness, altered behaviour, forgetfulness, confusion, and muscle weakness. These effects normally diminish after the first few days of treatment and can often be reduced by medically supervised adjustment of dosage.

INTERACTIONS

Sedatives All drugs that have a sedative effect on the central nervous system are likely to increase the sedative properties of clonazepam. Such drugs include anti-anxiety and sleeping drugs, antihistamines, opioid analgesics, antidepressants, and antipsychotics.

Other anticonvulsants Clonazepam may alter the effects of other anticonvulsants you are taking, or they may alter their effect. Dosage adjustment or change of drug may be necessary.

SPECIAL PRECAUTIONS

Be sure to tell your doctor if:
◆ You have severe respiratory disease.
◆ You have long-term liver or kidney problems.
◆ You have had problems with drug or alcohol abuse.
◆ You are taking other medicines.

Pregnancy Safety in pregnancy not established. Discuss with your doctor.

Breast-feeding The drug passes into the breast milk and may affect the baby adversely. Discuss with your doctor.

Infants and children Reduced dose necessary.

Over 60 Reduced dose may be necessary.

Driving and hazardous work Your underlying condition, as well as the possibility of drowsiness while taking clonazepam, may make such activities inadvisable. Discuss with your doctor.

Alcohol Avoid. Alcohol may increase the sedative effects of this drug.

PROLONGED USE

Both beneficial and adverse effects of clonazepam may become less marked during prolonged treatment as the body adapts. Prolonged use may also result in dependence and difficulty in withdrawing.

Clopidogrel

Brand name Plavix
Used in the following combined preparations
None

QUICK REFERENCE

Drug group Antiplatelet drug (p.39)
Overdose danger rating Medium
Dependence rating Low
Prescription needed Yes
Available as generic No

GENERAL INFORMATION

Clopidogrel is an antiplatelet drug that is used to prevent blood clots from forming. It is prescribed to patients who have a tendency to form clots in the fast-flowing blood of the arteries and heart, or those who have had a stroke or a heart attack.

Clopidogrel may be suitable for people who cannot take aspirin for its antiplatelet effects. It reduces the tendency of platelets to stick together when blood flow is disrupted. However, this can lead to abnormal bleeding. You should, therefore, report any unusual bleeding to your doctor at once, and, if you require dental treatment, you should tell your dentist that you are taking clopidogrel.

Adverse effects are common with clopidogrel and are usually associated with bleeding.

INFORMATION FOR USERS

Your drug prescription is tailored for you. Do not alter dosage without checking with your doctor.

How taken/used Tablets.

Frequency and timing of doses Once daily.

Dosage range 75mg; up to 300mg as initial dose in hospital.

Onset of effect 1 hour.

Duration of action 24 hours.

Diet advice None.

Storage Keep in original container at room temperature out of the reach of children.

Missed dose Take as soon as you remember. If your next dose is due within 4 hours, take a single dose now and skip the next.

Stopping the drug Do not stop taking the drug without consulting your doctor. Stopping the drug may lead to a recurrence of the original condition.

Exceeding the dose An occasional unintentional extra dose is unlikely to be a cause for concern. But if you notice any unusual symptoms, or if a large overdose has been taken, notify your doctor.

POSSIBLE ADVERSE EFFECTS
The most frequent adverse effects of clopidogrel are bruising and bleeding, such as nosebleeds or, less commonly, gastrointesinal bleeding or blood in the urine. More rarely, there may be nausea, vomiting, headache, dizziness, constipation, rash, or itching. You should report any unusual bleeding or bruising, rash or itching to your doctor. If you develop a sore throat, you should stop taking the drug and consult your doctor urgently.

INTERACTIONS
Aspirin and other non-steroidal anti-inflammatory drugs (NSAIDs) Clopidogrel increases the effect of aspirin on platelets. The risk of gastrointestinal bleeding is increased when clopidogrel is used with these drugs.
Anticoagulant drugs (e.g. warfarin) The anticoagulant effect of these drugs is increased if they are taken with clopidogrel.

SPECIAL PRECAUTIONS
Be sure to tell your doctor if:
◆ You have liver or kidney problems.
◆ You have a condition, such as a peptic ulcer, that makes you more likely to bleed.
◆ You are taking other medicines.
Pregnancy Safety in pregnancy not established. Discuss with your doctor.
Breast-feeding The drug passes into the breast milk and may affect the baby. Discuss with your doctor.
Infants and children Not recommended.
Over 60 No special problems.
Driving and hazardous work No special problems.
Alcohol Excessive intake of alcohol may irritate the stomach and increase the risk of bleeding.
Surgery and general anaesthetics Clopidogrel may need to be stopped a week before surgery. Discuss with your doctor or dentist.

PROLONGED USE
No special problems.

Clotrimazole

Brand names Abtrim, Candiden, Canesten, Masnoderm
Used in the following combined preparations
Canesten HC, Lotriderm

QUICK REFERENCE
Drug group Antifungal drug (p.76)
Overdose danger rating Low
Dependence rating Low
Prescription needed Yes (for combined preparations)
Available as generic Yes

GENERAL INFORMATION
Clotrimazole is an antifungal drug that is commonly used to treat fungal and yeast infections. It is used for treating tinea (ringworm) infections of the skin, and candida (thrush) infections of the ear, mouth, vagina, or penis. The drug is applied in the form of a cream, spray, topical solution, or dusting powder to the affected area and inserted as pessaries or cream for vaginal conditions such as candida.

Adverse effects from clotrimazole are very rare, although some people may experience burning and irritation on the skin surface in the area where the drug has been applied.

INFORMATION FOR USERS
Your drug prescription is tailored for you. Do not alter dosage without checking with your doctor.
How taken/used Pessaries, cream, topical solution, spray, dusting powder.
Frequency and timing of doses 2–3 x daily (skin cream, spray, solution); once daily at bedtime (pessaries); once daily at bedtime (vaginal cream).
Dosage range *Vaginal infections* One applicatorful (5g) per dose (vaginal cream); 100–500mg per dose (pessaries). *Skin infections* (skin cream, spray, solution) as directed.
Onset of effect Within 2–3 days.
Duration of action Up to 12 hours.
Diet advice None.
Storage Keep in original container at room temperature out of the reach of children.
Missed dose No cause for concern, but make up the missed dose or application as soon as you remember.

Stopping the drug Apply the full course. Even if symptoms disappear, the original infection may still be present and symptoms may recur if treatment is stopped too soon.

Exceeding the dose An occasional unintentional extra dose is unlikely to cause any problems. But if you notice unusual symptoms or if a large amount of the drug has been swallowed, notify your doctor.

POSSIBLE ADVERSE EFFECTS

Clotrimazole rarely causes adverse effects. Skin preparations and vaginal applications may occasionally cause localized burning and irritation. If a rash appears, stop using the drug and discuss with your doctor.

INTERACTIONS

Latex contraceptives Damage may occur to these; additional precautions are needed during use of clotrimazole and for at least 5 days after.

SPECIAL PRECAUTIONS

Be sure to tell your doctor if:
◆ You are taking other medicines.
Pregnancy No evidence of risk to the developing baby, but use only with the advice of your doctor.
Breast-feeding No evidence of risk.
Infants and children No special problems, but use of pessaries not recommended.
Over 60 No special problems.
Driving and hazardous work No known problems.
Alcohol No known problems.

PROLONGED USE

No problems expected.

Clozapine

Brand names Clozaril, Denzapine, Zaponex
Used in the following combined preparations
None

QUICK REFERENCE

Drug group Antipsychotic drug (p.15)
Overdose danger rating Medium
Dependence rating Low
Prescription needed Yes
Available as generic No

GENERAL INFORMATION

Clozapine is an atypical antipsychotic drug for schizophrenia. It is given to patients who have not responded to other treatments or who have experienced intolerable side effects with other drugs. Clozapine helps control severe resistant schizophrenia, helping the patient to re-establish a more normal lifestyle. The improvement is gradual, and relief of severe symptoms can take several weeks to months.

All treatment is started and supervised by a consultant psychiatrist, and the patient must be registered with the appropriate drug manufacturer. The drug can cause a very serious side effect: agranulocytosis (a large decrease in white blood cells). Blood tests are performed before and during treatment; the drug is supplied only if the test results are normal.

Clozapine is less likely than other antipsychotics to cause parkinsonism.

INFORMATION FOR USERS

This drug is given only under strict medical supervision and continual monitoring.
How taken/used Tablets, liquid.
Frequency and timing of doses 1–2 x daily; a larger dose may be given at night.
Adult dosage range 25–900mg daily.
Onset of effect Gradual. Some effect may appear within 3–5 days of starting the drug, but the full beneficial effect may not be felt for some months.
Duration of action Up to 16 hours.
Diet advice None.
Storage Keep in original container at room temperature out of the reach of children.
Missed dose Take as soon as you remember. If your next dose is due within 2 hours, take a single dose now and skip the next. If you miss more than 2 days of tablets, notify your doctor because you may need to restart at a lower dose.
Stopping the drug Do not stop the drug without consulting your doctor because symptoms may recur.
Exceeding the dose An occasional unintentional extra dose is unlikely to cause problems. Large overdoses may cause unusual drowsiness, fits, and agitation. Notify your doctor.

POSSIBLE ADVERSE EFFECTS

Unlike other antipsychotics, clozapine is less likely to cause parkinsonian side effects (tremor and stiffness). The most serious side effect is agranulocytosis, and strict monitoring of the white blood cell count is necessary. Common adverse effects include drowsiness, tiredness, dry mouth or excess saliva production, weight gain, a fast heartbeat, dizziness, fainting, constipation, and blurred vision. Rarely, clozapine may cause fever, a sore throat, or fits. If any of these occur, seek urgent medical advice.

INTERACTIONS

General note A number of drugs increase the risk of adverse effects on the blood. Do not take other medication without checking with your doctor or pharmacist. Smoking lowers clozapine levels, which may reduce its effect.

Sedatives All drugs that have a sedative effect on the central nervous system are likely to increase the sedative properties of clozapine.

SPECIAL PRECAUTIONS

Be sure to tell your doctor if:
◆ You have long-term liver or kidney problems.
◆ You have a history of blood disorders.
◆ You have had epileptic fits.
◆ You have heart problems.
◆ You have colon problems or have had bowel surgery.
◆ You have diabetes.
◆ You have glaucoma.
◆ You have prostate problems.
◆ You are taking other medicines.

Pregnancy Not usually prescribed. Safety not established. Discuss with your doctor.

Breast-feeding The drug passes into the breast milk and may affect the baby adversely. Discuss with your doctor.

Infants and children Not prescribed.

Over 60 Adverse effects are more likely. Initial dose is low and is slowly increased.

Driving and hazardous work Avoid such activities until you know how clozapine affects you because the drug can cause blurred vision, drowsiness, and dizziness.

Alcohol Avoid. Alcohol may increase the sedative effects of this drug.

PROLONGED USE

Agranulocytosis may occur, and occasionally liver function may be upset. Significant weight gain may also occur.

Monitoring Blood tests are carried out weekly for 18 weeks, fortnightly until the end of the first year, and, if blood counts are stable, every 4 weeks thereafter. Liver function tests, weighing, and tests for diabetes are performed every 3–6 months.

Codeine

Used in the following combined preparations
Benylin with Codeine, Co-codamol, Codafen Continus, Codis, Cuprofen, Feminax, Migraleve, Panadol Ultra, Paracodol, Solpadeine, Solpadol, Syndol, Tylex, Veganin, and others

QUICK REFERENCE
Drug group Opioid analgesic (p.9), antidiarrhoeal drug (p.44), and cough suppressant (p.27)
Overdose danger rating High
Dependence rating Medium
Prescription needed Yes (some preparations)
Available as generic Yes

GENERAL INFORMATION

Codeine is a mild opioid analgesic that is similar to, but weaker than, morphine. It has been in common medical use since the beginning of the previous century.

Codeine is prescribed primarily to relieve mild to moderate pain, and is often combined with a non-opioid analgesic such as paracetamol. It is also an effective cough suppressant and, for this reason, is included as an ingredient in many non-prescription cough syrups and cold relief preparations.

Like the other opioid drugs, codeine is constipating, a characteristic that sometimes makes it useful in the short-term control of diarrhoea.

Although codeine is habit-forming, addiction seldom occurs if the drug is used for a limited period of time and the recommended dosage is followed.

Constipation is common with codeine. Other, rare, adverse effects include breathing difficulties, which should be reported to your doctor without delay.

INFORMATION FOR USERS

Your drug prescription is tailored for you. Do not alter dosage without checking with your doctor.

How taken/used Tablets, liquid, injection.

Frequency and timing of doses 4–6 x daily (for pain); 3–4 x daily when necessary (for cough); every 6–8 hours when necessary (for diarrhoea).

Adult dosage range 120–240mg daily (pain); 45–120mg daily (cough); 30–120mg daily (diarrhoea).

Onset of effect 30–60 minutes.

Duration of action 4–6 hours.

Diet advice None.

Storage Keep in original container at room temperature out of the reach of children. Protect from light.

Missed dose Take as soon as you remember if the drug is needed for relief of symptoms. If not needed, do not take the missed dose, and return to your normal dose schedule when necessary.

Stopping the drug Can be safely stopped as soon as you no longer need it.

OVERDOSE ACTION

Seek immediate medical advice in all cases. Take emergency action if there are symptoms such as slow or irregular breathing, severe drowsiness, or loss of consciousness.

POSSIBLE ADVERSE EFFECTS

Serious adverse effects are rare with codeine. Constipation occurs especially with prolonged use, but other side effects, such as nausea, vomiting, drowsiness, and dizziness are not usually troublesome at the recommended doses and usually disappear if the dose is reduced. If you experience agitation or restlessness, stop taking the drug. If you develop a rash, hives, wheezing, or breathlessness, stop taking the drug and seek urgent medical attention.

INTERACTIONS

Sedatives All drugs, including alcohol, that have a sedative effect on the central nervous system are likely to increase sedation with codeine. Such drugs include sleeping drugs, antidepressant drugs, antihistamines, and antipsychotics.

SPECIAL PRECAUTIONS

Be sure to tell your doctor if:
◆ You have long-term liver or kidney problems.
◆ You have a lung disorder such as asthma or bronchitis.
◆ You are taking other medicines.

Pregnancy No evidence of risk, but may adversely affect the baby's breathing if taken during labour.

Breast-feeding The drug passes into the breast milk, but at normal doses adverse effects on the baby are unlikely to occur. Discuss with your doctor.

Infants and children Reduced dose necessary.

Over 60 Reduced dose may be necessary.

Driving and hazardous work Avoid such activities until you have learned how codeine affects you because the drug may cause dizziness and drowsiness.

Alcohol Avoid. Alcohol may increase the sedative effects of this drug.

PROLONGED USE

Codeine is normally used only for short-term relief of symptoms. It can be habit-forming if taken for prolonged periods, especially if higher-than-average doses are taken.

Colchicine

Brand names None
Used in the following combined preparations None

QUICK REFERENCE

Drug group Drug for gout (p.53)
Overdose danger rating High
Dependence rating Low
Prescription needed Yes
Available as generic Yes

GENERAL INFORMATION

Colchicine, a drug originally extracted from the autumn crocus flower and later synthesized, has been used since the 18th century for gout. It has now, to an extent, been superseded by newer drugs, but is still often used to relieve joint pain and inflammation in flare-ups of gout. Colchicine is most effective when taken at the first sign of symptoms, and almost always produces an improvement. Its use is limited by the development of side effects, such as nausea, vomiting, and diarrhoea, at high doses. The drug may also be given at a lower dose during the first few months of treatment with allopurinol or probenecid (other drugs for gout), because these may at first increase the frequency of gout attacks.

Colchicine is occasionally prescribed for the relief of symptoms of familial Mediterranean fever (a rare congenital condition).

INFORMATION FOR USERS

Your drug prescription is tailored for you. Do not alter dosage without checking with your doctor.

How taken/used Tablets.

Frequency and timing of doses *Prevention of gout attacks* 2–3 x daily. *Relief of gout attacks* Every 4 hours.

Adult dosage range *Prevention of gout attacks* 1–1.5mg daily. *Relief of gout attacks* 1mg initially, followed by 0.5mg every 4 hours, until relief of pain, vomiting, or diarrhoea occurs, or until a total dose of 6mg is reached. This course must not be repeated within 3 days.

Onset of effect Relief of symptoms in an attack of gout may be felt in 6–24 hours. Full effect in gout prevention may not be felt for several days.

Duration of action Up to 2 hours. Some effect may last longer.

Diet advice Certain foods are known to make gout worse. Discuss with your doctor.

Storage Keep in original container at room temperature out of the reach of children. Protect from light.

Missed dose Take as soon as you remember. If your next dose is due within 30 minutes, take a single dose now and skip the next.

Stopping the drug When taking colchicine frequently during an acute attack of gout, stop if diarrhoea or abdominal pain develop. In other cases, do not stop without consulting your doctor.

OVERDOSE ACTION

Seek immediate medical advice in all cases; some reactions can be fatal. Take emergency action if severe nausea, vomiting, bloody diarrhoea, severe abdominal pain, or loss of consciousness occur.

POSSIBLE ADVERSE EFFECTS

The appearance of any symptom that may be an adverse effect of colchicine is a sign that you should stop the drug until you have received further medical advice. The more common adverse effects are nausea, vomiting, diarrhoea, and abdominal pain but, more rarely, colchicine may also cause numbness and tingling, unusual bleeding or bruising, and a rash.

INTERACTIONS

Ciclosporin Taking ciclosporin with colchicine may lead to adverse effects on the kidneys and muscles.

Antibiotics Erythromycin and clarithromycin may increase the adverse effects of colchicine.

SPECIAL PRECAUTIONS

Be sure to tell your doctor if:
◆ You have long-term liver or kidney problems.
◆ You have heart problems.
◆ You have a blood disorder.
◆ You have stomach ulcers.
◆ You have chronic inflammation of the bowel.
◆ You are taking other medicines.

Pregnancy Not usually prescribed. May cause defects in the unborn baby. Discuss with your doctor.

Breast-feeding The drug passes into the breast milk and may affect the baby. Discuss with your doctor.

Infants and children Not recommended.

Over 60 Increased likelihood of adverse effects.

Driving and hazardous work No special problems.

Alcohol Avoid. Alcohol may increase stomach irritation caused by colchicine.

PROLONGED USE

Prolonged use of this drug may lead to hair loss, rashes, tingling in the hands and feet, muscle pain and weakness, and blood disorders.

Monitoring Periodic checks on the blood are usually required.

Colestyramine

Brand names Questran, Questran Light
Used in the following combined preparations
None

QUICK REFERENCE

Drug group Lipid-lowering drug (p.37)
Overdose danger rating Low
Dependence rating Low
Prescription needed Yes
Available as generic Yes

GENERAL INFORMATION

Colestyramine is a resin that binds bile acids in the intestine, preventing their reabsorption. Cholesterol in the body is normally converted to bile acids. Therefore, colestyramine reduces cholesterol levels in the blood. This action on the bile acids makes bowel movements bulkier, creating an anti-diarrhoeal effect (hence its use in diarrhoea associated with, for example, Crohn's disease). Colestyramine is used to treat hyperlipidaemia (high levels of fat in the blood) in people who have not responded to dietary changes. In liver disorders such as primary biliary cirrhosis, bile salts sometimes accumulate in the bloodstream, and colestyramine may be prescribed to alleviate any accompanying itching.

Taken in large doses, colestyramine often causes bloating, mild nausea, and constipation. It may also interfere with the body's ability to absorb fat and certain fat-soluble vitamins, which may cause pale, bulky, foul-smelling faeces.

INFORMATION FOR USERS

Your drug prescription is tailored for you. Do not alter dosage without checking with your doctor.

How taken/used Powder mixed with water, juice, or soft food.
Frequency and timing of doses 1–6 x daily before meals and at bedtime.
Adult dosage range 4–36g daily.
Onset of effect May take several weeks to achieve full beneficial effects.
Duration of action 12–24 hours.
Diet advice A low-fat, low-calorie diet may be advised for patients who are overweight. Use

of this drug may deplete levels of certain vitamins. Supplements may be advised.
Storage Keep in original container at room temperature out of the reach of children.
Missed dose Take as soon as you remember.
Stopping the drug Do not stop taking the drug without consulting your doctor.
Exceeding the dose An occasional unintentional extra dose is unlikely to cause problems. But if you notice any unusual symptoms, or if a large overdose has been taken, notify your doctor.

POSSIBLE ADVERSE EFFECTS

Adverse effects are more likely if large doses are taken by people over 60. Minor side effects, such as indigestion and abdominal discomfort, are rarely a cause for concern. Nausea, vomiting, and constipation may also occur. High doses may cause diarrhoea. More serious adverse effects, such as bruising or increased bleeding, are usually the result of vitamin deficiency.

INTERACTIONS

General note Colestyramine reduces the body's ability to absorb other drugs. If you are taking other medicines, you should tell either your doctor or pharmacist so that they can discuss with you the best way to take all your drugs. To avoid any problems, take other drugs at least 1 hour before, or 4–6 hours after, colestyramine. The dosage of other drugs may need to be adjusted.

SPECIAL PRECAUTIONS

Be sure to tell your doctor if:
◆ You have jaundice.
◆ You have a peptic ulcer.
◆ You suffer from haemorrhoids.
◆ You are taking other medicines.
Pregnancy Safety in pregnancy not established. Discuss with your doctor.
Breast-feeding Safety not established. The drug binds fat-soluble vitamins long term and may cause vitamin deficiency in the baby. Discuss with your doctor.
Infants and children Not recommended for children under 6 years old. A reduced dose is necessary in older children.
Over 60 Increased likelihood of adverse effects.

Driving and hazardous work No special problems.
Alcohol Although this drug does not interact with alcohol, your underlying condition may make it inadvisable to take alcohol.

PROLONGED USE

As this drug reduces vitamin absorption, supplements of vitamins A, D, and K and folic acid may be advised.
Monitoring Periodic blood checks are usually required to monitor the level of cholesterol in the blood.

Conjugated oestrogens

Brand name Premarin
Used in the following combined preparations
Premique, Prempak-C

QUICK REFERENCE

Drug group Female sex hormone (p.88)
Overdose danger rating Low
Dependence rating Low
Prescription needed Yes
Available as generic Yes

GENERAL INFORMATION

Preparations of conjugated oestrogens consist of naturally occurring oestrogens similar to those found in the urine of pregnant mares. Taken by mouth, they are used to relieve menopausal symptoms such as hot flushes and sweating, but they are usually only advised for short-term use around the menopause and are not normally recommended for long-term use or for treatment of osteoporosis.

As replacement therapy, they are usually taken on a cyclic dosing schedule, in conjunction with a progestogen, to simulate the hormonal changes of a normal menstrual cycle. On their own, they are not recommended for women with an intact uterus. They are also available as a vaginal cream to relieve vaginal or vulval pain and dryness after the menopause.

Conjugated oestrogens do not provide contraception. Pregnancy is still possible for 2 years after a woman's last period (if she is under 50 years) or 1 year after the end of menstruation (if she is over 50).

INFORMATION FOR USERS

Your drug prescription is tailored for you. Do not alter dosage without checking with your doctor.
How taken/used Tablets, cream.
Frequency and timing of doses Once daily (tablets). Once daily (cream).
Adult dosage range *Replacement therapy* 0.625–1.25mg daily (tablets); 1–2g daily (cream).
Onset of effect 5–20 days.
Duration of action 1–2 days.
Diet advice None.
Storage Keep in original container at room temperature out of the reach of children.
Missed dose Take as soon as you remember.
Stopping the drug Do not stop the drug without consulting your doctor; symptoms may recur.
Exceeding the dose An occasional unintentional extra dose is unlikely to be a cause for concern. But if you notice any unusual symptoms, or if a large overdose has been taken, notify your doctor.

POSSIBLE ADVERSE EFFECTS

The most common adverse effects are similar to symptoms that occur in the early stages of pregnancy, such as nausea, vomiting, breast swelling or tenderness, weight changes, and abdominal bloating or pain. These generally diminish or disappear after 2–3 months of treatment. The drugs may also reduce sex drive. Women on a cyclic schedule will have a menstrual bleed towards the end of each cycle. If headache, migraine, depression, or vaginal bleeding occur, notify your doctor. Sudden, sharp pain in the chest, groin, or legs may indicate an abnormal blood clot that requires urgent medical attention.

INTERACTIONS

Tobacco smoking increases the risk of serious adverse effects on the heart and circulation with conjugated oestrogens.
Oral anticoagulant drugs Conjugated oestrogens reduce the anticoagulant effect of these drugs.

SPECIAL PRECAUTIONS

Be sure to tell your doctor if:
◆ You have heart disease or high blood pressure.

◆ You have had blood clots or a stroke.
◆ You have porphyria or diabetes.
◆ You have a history of breast disease.
◆ You have had fibroids in the uterus.
◆ You suffer from migraine or epilepsy.
◆ You have long-term liver or kidney problems.
◆ You are taking other medicines.

Pregnancy Not prescribed. May affect the baby adversely. Discuss with your doctor.

Breast-feeding Not prescribed. The drug passes into the breast milk and may inhibit its flow. Discuss with your doctor.

Infants and children Not prescribed.

Over 60 No special problems.

Driving and hazardous work No known problems.

Alcohol No known problems.

Surgery and general anaesthetics Conjugated oestrogens may need to be stopped several weeks before you have surgery. Discuss with your doctor or dentist.

PROLONGED USE

Conjugated oestrogens are normally only recommended for short-term use around the menopause (see General information, previous page).

Monitoring Regular physical examinations (e.g. mammograms) and blood pressure checks are advised.

Co-phenotrope

Brand names Dymotil, Lomotil
Used in the following combined preparations
None

QUICK REFERENCE

Drug group Opioid antidiarrhoeal drug (p.44)
Overdose danger rating Medium
Dependence rating Medium
Prescription needed Yes
Available as generic Yes

GENERAL INFORMATION

Co-phenotrope is an antidiarrhoeal drug that contains diphenoxylate and atropine. It reduces bowel contractions and, therefore, the fluidity and frequency of bowel movements. Co-phenotrope is used for the relief of sudden or recurrent bouts of diarrhoea. It may also be used to control consistency of faeces following colostomy or ileostomy.

Co-phenotrope is not suitable for treating diarrhoea caused by infections, poisons, or antibiotics as it may delay recovery by slowing expulsion of harmful substances from the bowel. The drug can cause toxic megacolon, which is a dangerous dilation of the bowel that shuts off the blood supply to the wall of the bowel and increases the risk of perforation.

At recommended doses, serious adverse effects are rare. However, if taken in excessive amounts, the atropine will cause highly unpleasant anticholinergic effects. This drug is especially dangerous for young children and should be stored out of their reach.

INFORMATION FOR USERS

Your drug prescription is tailored for you. Do not alter dosage without checking with your doctor.

How taken/used Tablets.

Frequency and timing of doses 3–4 x daily.

Dosage range *Adults* 10mg initially, followed by 5mg every 6 hours until diarrhoea is controlled. *Children* Reduced dose necessary according to age (not recommended under 4 years).

Onset of effect Within 1 hour. Control of diarrhoea may take some hours.

Duration of action 3–4 hours (single dose).

Diet advice Always drink plenty of water during an attack of diarrhoea.

Storage Keep in original container at room temperature out of the reach of children. Protect from light.

Missed dose Take as soon as you remember. If your next dose is due within 3 hours, take a single dose now and skip the next.

Stopping the drug Can be safely stopped as soon as you no longer need it.

Exceeding the dose An occasional unintentional extra dose is unlikely to cause problems. Large overdoses may cause unusual drowsiness, dryness of the mouth and skin, restlessness, and in extreme cases, loss of consciousness. Symptoms of overdose may be delayed. Notify your doctor.

POSSIBLE ADVERSE EFFECTS

Drowsiness is the most common side effect of co-phenotrope. Other adverse effects, such as restlessness, headache, rash, itching, and dizziness, are infrequent. If abdominal pain or distension, nausea, or vomiting occur, stop taking the drug and contact your doctor immediately.

INTERACTIONS

Sedatives All drugs that have a sedative effect on the central nervous system may increase co-phenotrope's sedative effect. They include anti-anxiety and sleeping drugs, antihistamines, opioid analgesics, antidepressants, and antipsychotics.

Monoamine oxidase inhibitors (MAOIs) There is a risk of a dangerous rise in blood pressure if MAOIs are taken together with co-phenotrope.

SPECIAL PRECAUTIONS

Be sure to tell your doctor if:
◆ You have a long-term liver problem.
◆ You have severe abdominal pain.
◆ You have bloodstained diarrhoea.
◆ You have recently taken antibiotics.
◆ You have ulcerative colitis.
◆ You have recently travelled abroad.
◆ You are taking other medicines.

Pregnancy Safety in pregnancy not established. Discuss with your doctor.

Breast-feeding The drug passes into the breast milk and may cause drowsiness in the baby. Discuss with your doctor.

Infants and children Not recommended under 4 years. A reduced dose is necessary for older children.

Over 60 Reduced dose may be necessary.

Driving and hazardous work Avoid such activities until you have learned how co-phenotrope affects you because the drug may cause drowsiness and dizziness.

Alcohol Avoid. Alcohol may increase the sedative effects of this drug.

PROLONGED USE

Not usually recommended.

Co-trimoxazole

Brand names Fectrim, Septrin
Used in the following combined preparations
(Co-trimoxazole is a combination of two drugs)

QUICK REFERENCE

Drug group Antibacterial drug (p.66)
Overdose danger rating Medium
Dependence rating Low
Prescription needed Yes
Available as generic Yes

GENERAL INFORMATION

Co-trimoxazole is a mixture of two anti-bacterial drugs: trimethoprim and sulfa-methoxazole. It is prescribed for serious respiratory and urinary tract infections only when they cannot be treated with other drugs. Co-trimoxazole is also used to treat pneumocystis pneumonia, toxoplasmosis, and the bacterial infection nocardiasis. The drug may also be used for otitis media in children if no safer drug is suitable. Although co-trimoxazole was widely prescribed in the past, its use has greatly declined in recent years with the introduction of new, more effective, and safer drugs.

Rare but serious adverse effects may occur with co-trimoxazole treatment. These include skin rashes, blood disorders, and liver or kidney damage.

INFORMATION FOR USERS

Your drug prescription is tailored for you. Do not alter dosage without checking with your doctor.

How taken/used Tablets, liquid, injection.

Frequency and timing of doses Normally 2 x daily, preferably with food.

Adult dosage range Usually 4 tablets daily (each standard tablet is 480mg). Higher doses may be used to treat pneumocystis pneumonia, toxoplasmosis, and nocardiasis.

Onset of effect 1–4 hours.

Duration of action 12 hours.

Diet advice Drink plenty of fluids, particularly in warm weather.

Storage Keep in original container at room temperature out of the reach of children. Protect from light.

Missed dose Take as soon as you remember. If your normal dose is 480mg, double this; if it is more than 480mg, take one dose only.

Stopping the drug Take the full course. Even if you feel better, the original infection may still be present and symptoms may recur if treatment is stopped too soon.

Exceeding the dose An occasional unintentional extra dose is unlikely to be a cause for concern. Large overdoses may cause nausea, vomiting, dizziness, and confusion. Notify your doctor.

POSSIBLE ADVERSE EFFECTS

The most common problems are nausea, diarrhoea, headache, rash, and itching. If either of the last two occur, you should stop taking the drug and consult your doctor without delay. Other, less common, adverse effects include sore tongue and jaundice. If the latter occurs, stop taking the drug and seek urgent medical advice.

INTERACTIONS

Warfarin Co-trimoxazole may increase its anticoagulant effect; the dose of warfarin may have to be reduced. Blood-clotting status may have to be checked.

Ciclosporin Taking ciclosporin together with co-trimoxazole can impair kidney function.

Phenytoin Co-trimoxazole may cause a build-up of phenytoin in the body; the dose of phenytoin may have to be reduced.

Amiodarone Co-trimoxazole may increase the risk of irregular heart beats when given with amiodarone.

SPECIAL PRECAUTIONS

Be sure to tell your doctor if:
◆ You have long-term liver or kidney problems.
◆ You have a blood disorder.
◆ You have asthma.
◆ You have glucose-6-phosphate dehydrogenase (G6PD) deficiency.
◆ You are allergic to sulphonamide drugs.
◆ You suffer from porphyria.
◆ You are taking other medicines.

Pregnancy Not usually prescribed. It may cause defects in the baby. Discuss with your doctor.

Breast-feeding The drug passes into the breast milk, but at normal levels adverse effects on the baby are unlikely. Discuss with your doctor.

Infants and children Not recommended in infants under 6 weeks old. Reduced dose necessary in older children.

Over 60 Side effects are more likely. Used only when necessary.

Driving and hazardous work No known problems.
Alcohol No known problems.

PROLONGED USE

Long-term use of this drug may lead to folic acid deficiency, which can cause anaemia. Folic acid supplements may be needed.

Monitoring Regular blood tests are recommended.

Cyclophosphamide

Brand name Endoxana
Used in the following combined preparations
None

QUICK REFERENCE

Drug group Anticancer drug (p.96)
Overdose danger rating Medium
Dependence rating Low
Prescription needed Yes
Available as generic Yes

GENERAL INFORMATION

Cyclophosphamide belongs to a group of anticancer drugs known as alkylating agents. It is used for a wide range of cancers, including lymphomas (lymph gland cancers), leukaemias, and solid tumours, particularly of the breast and lung. It is commonly given together with radiotherapy or other drugs. Cyclophosphamide has also been used for autoimmune diseases.

Cyclophosphamide causes nausea, vomiting, and hair loss, and can affect the heart, lungs, and liver. It can also cause bladder damage in susceptible people because it produces a toxic substance called acrolein. To reduce toxicity, people considered to be at risk may be given a drug called mesna before and after each dose of cyclophosphamide. Also, because the drug often reduces production of blood cells, it may lead to abnormal bleeding, increased risk of infection, and reduced fertility in men.

INFORMATION FOR USERS

Your drug prescription is tailored for you. Do not alter dosage without checking with your doctor.

How taken/used Tablets, injection.

Frequency and timing of doses Varies from once daily to every 3 weeks, depending on the condition being treated.

Dosage range Dosage is determined individually according to the nature of the condition, body weight, and response.

Onset of effect Some effects may appear within hours of starting treatment. Full beneficial effects may not be felt for many weeks.

Duration of action Several weeks.

Diet advice High fluid intake with frequent bladder emptying is recommended. This will usually prevent the drug causing bladder irritation.

Storage Keep in original container at room temperature out of the reach of children. Protect from light.

Missed dose Injections are given only in hospital. If you are taking tablets, take the missed dose as soon as you remember. If your next dose is due within 6 hours, take a single dose now and skip the next. Tell your doctor that you missed a dose.

Stopping the drug The drug will be stopped under medical supervision (injection). Do not stop taking the drug without consulting your doctor (tablets); stopping the drug may lead to worsening of the underlying condition.

Exceeding the dose An occasional unintentional extra dose is unlikely to cause problems. Large overdoses may cause nausea, vomiting, and bladder damage. Notify your doctor.

POSSIBLE ADVERSE EFFECTS

Cyclophosphamide often causes nausea and vomiting, which usually diminish as your body adjusts. Hair loss is a common indication that the drug is having an effect on growing cells. Mouth ulcers may occur, and women often experience irregular periods. Blood in the urine may be a sign of bladder damage and requires prompt medical attention. Those thought to be at risk of bladder damage may be given mesna before and after doses of cyclophosphamide.

INTERACTIONS

General note A number of drugs reduce the effects of cyclophosphamide and increase the risk of side effects. Such drugs include allopurinol, chloramphenicol, chloroquine, imipramine, and phenothiazines (e.g. chlorpromazine).

SPECIAL PRECAUTIONS

Cyclophosphamide is prescribed only under close medical supervision, taking account of your present condition and medical history.

Pregnancy Not usually prescribed. Cyclophosphamide may cause birth defects. Pregnancy should be avoided during, and for 3 months after, treatment. Discuss with your doctor.

Breast-feeding Not advised. The drug passes into the breast milk and may affect the baby adversely. Discuss with your doctor.

Infants and children Reduced dose necessary.

Over 60 No special problems.

Driving and hazardous work No known problems.

Alcohol No problems expected, but avoid excessive amounts.

PROLONGED USE

Prolonged use of this drug may reduce the production of blood cells.

Monitoring Periodic checks on blood composition and on all effects of the drug are usually required.

Desmopressin

Brand names DDAVP, Desmospray, Desmotabs, Nocutil, Octim
Used in the following combined preparations None

QUICK REFERENCE

Drug group Drug for diabetes insipidus (p.82)
Overdose danger rating Medium
Dependence rating Low
Prescription needed Yes
Available as generic Yes

GENERAL INFORMATION

Desmopressin is a synthetic form of the hormone vasopressin. Low levels of vasopressin in the body can lead to diabetes insipidus, which causes excess urine production and continual thirst.

Desmopressin can be used to correct the deficiency of vasopressin. It is also used to test for diabetes insipidus, to check kidney function, and to treat nocturnal enuresis (bedwetting) in both children and adults. When given by injection, it helps to boost clotting factors in haemophilia.

Side effects of the drug include low blood sodium and fluid retention (which sometimes requires monitoring of body weight and blood pressure to check the body's water balance).

Desmopressin should not be taken during an episode of vomiting and diarrhoea because the body's fluid balance may be upset.

INFORMATION FOR USERS

Your drug prescription is tailored for you. Do not alter dosage without checking with your doctor.

How taken/used Tablets, injection, nasal solution, nasal spray.

Frequency and timing of doses *Diabetes insipidus* 3 x daily (tablets); 1–2 x daily (nasal spray/solution). *Nocturnal enuresis* At bedtime (tablets, nasal spray/solution). Avoid fluids from 1 hour before bedtime to 8 hours afterwards.

Dosage range Diabetes insipidus: *Adults* 300–600mcg daily (tablets); 1–4 puffs (nasal spray); 10–40mcg daily (nasal solution). *Children* 300–600mcg daily (tablets); up to 2 puffs (nasal spray); 20mcg (nasal solution). Nocturnal enuresis: 200–400mcg for adults and children over 5 years only (tablets); 20–40mcg (nasal solution); 2–4 puffs (nasal spray).

Onset of effect A few minutes: full effects, a few hours (injection, nasal solution/spray); 30–90 minutes (tablets).

Duration of action Tablets 6–12 hours; injection, nasal solutions, and nasal spray 5–21 hours.

Diet advice Your doctor may advise you to avoid excessive fluid intake.

Storage Keep in original container at room temperature (tablets) or in a refrigerator, without freezing (nasal solution and nasal spray), out of the reach of children. Protect from light.

Missed dose Take as soon as you remember. If your next dose is due within 2 hours, take a single dose now and skip the next.

Stopping the drug Do not stop the drug without consulting your doctor; symptoms of diabetes insipidus may recur.

Exceeding the dose An occasional unintentional extra dose is unlikely to cause problems. Large overdoses may prevent the kidneys from eliminating fluid, with ensuing problems including convulsions. Notify your doctor immediately.

POSSIBLE ADVERSE EFFECTS

Desmopressin can cause fluid retention and low blood sodium, especially if fluid intake is too high. In serious cases, this can lead to convulsions; if so, stop taking the drug and call your doctor immediately. Headache, nausea, vomiting, nasal congestion, nosebleeds, weight gain, and stomach pain may also occur.

INTERACTIONS

Antidepressants, chlorpropamide, chlorpromazine, fludrocortisone, and carbamazepine These drugs may increase the effects of desmopressin.

Indometacin and ibuprofen These drugs may increase the body's response to desmopressin.

SPECIAL PRECAUTIONS

Be sure to tell your doctor if:
◆ You have heart problems.
◆ You have high blood pressure.
◆ You have kidney problems.
◆ You have cystic fibrosis.
◆ You have asthma or allergic rhinitis.
◆ You have epilepsy.
◆ You are taking other medicines.

Pregnancy Safety in pregnancy not established. Discuss with your doctor.

Breast-feeding The drug passes into breast milk, in small amounts, but adverse effects on the baby are unlikely.

Infants and children No special problems in children; infants may need monitoring to ensure that fluid balance is correct.

Over 60 May need monitoring to ensure that fluid balance is correct.

Driving and hazardous work No known problems.

Alcohol Your doctor may advise on fluid intake.

PROLONGED USE

Diabetes insipidus: no problems expected.

Nocturnal enuresis: the drug will be withdrawn for at least a week after 3 months for assessment of the need to continue treatment.

Desogestrel

Brand name Cerazette
Used in the following combined preparations
Marvelon, Mercilon

QUICK REFERENCE
Drug group Female sex hormone (p.88) and oral contraceptive (p.105)
Overdose danger rating Low
Dependence rating Low
Prescription needed Yes
Available as generic No

GENERAL INFORMATION
Desogestrel is a synthetic hormone that is similar to the natural female sex hormone progesterone. It is used alone as a progestogen-only pill, or POP (see p.106) and is especially helpful as contraception in women who cannot tolerate oestrogens or are breast-feeding. Desogestrel works by thickening the mucus at the neck of the cervix, making it difficult for sperm to enter. Unlike other POPs, the drug also works by preventing ovulation. In addition, it changes the quality of the endometrium (lining of the uterus), preventing implantation of a fertilized egg.

Desogestrel is also used in combination with the oestrogen ethinylestradiol as an oral contraceptive and to treat menstrual symptoms.

Desogestrel rarely causes serious side effects. When it is taken without an oestrogen, irregular vaginal bleeding may occur in the form of slight spotting, heavier bleeding, or no bleeding at all.

INFORMATION FOR USERS
Your drug prescription is tailored for you. Do not alter dosage without checking with your doctor.
How taken/used Tablets.
Frequency and timing of doses One tablet at the same time each day.
Adult dosage range 75mcg daily.
Onset of effect Within a few hours.
Duration of action 24 hours.
Diet advice None.
Storage Keep in original container at room temperature out of the reach of children. Protect from light.
Missed dose If a tablet is delayed by 12 hours or more, regard it as a missed pill. See What to do if you miss a pill (p.109).
Stopping the drug It can be safely stopped as soon as contraception is no longer required. For treatment of menstrual symptoms, consult your doctor before stopping the drug.

Exceeding the dose An occasional unintentional extra dose is unlikely to be a cause for concern. But if you notice any unusual symptoms, or if a large overdose has been taken, notify your doctor.

POSSIBLE ADVERSE EFFECTS
Irregular vaginal bleeding is the most common side effect of desogestrel taken alone. If you experience heavy or prolonged bleeding, consult your doctor. Other common side effects include nausea, vomiting, headache, breast discomfort or tenderness, weight changes, and mood changes. Discuss with your doctor if any of these becomes severe.

INTERACTIONS
General note The beneficial effects of many drugs, including oral anticoagulants, anticonvulsants, and antihypertensive and antidiabetic drugs may be affected by desogestrel. Many other drugs may reduce the contraceptive effect of desogestrel. These include anticonvulsants, antituberculous drugs, antidepressants, and the herbal remedy St John's wort.

SPECIAL PRECAUTIONS
Be sure to tell your doctor if:
◆ You have a liver problem.
◆ You have diabetes.
◆ You have jaundice.
◆ You have had an ectopic pregnancy.
◆ You have unexplained abnormal vaginal bleeding.
◆ You have had epileptic seizures.
◆ You have had blood clots or a stroke.
◆ You are taking other medicines.
Pregnancy Not prescribed. May cause defects in the developing baby. Discuss with your doctor.
Breast-feeding The drug passes into the breast milk, but at normal doses adverse effects on the baby are unlikely. Discuss with your doctor.
Infants and children Not prescribed.
Over 60 Not prescribed.
Driving and hazardous work No known problems.
Alcohol No known problems.

PROLONGED USE
Problems are rare.
Monitoring Regular blood pressure checks may be carried out.

Dexamethasone

Brand name Decadron
Used in the following combined preparations
Dexa-Rhinaspray, Maxidex, Maxitrol, Otomize,
Sofradex, Tobradex, and others

QUICK REFERENCE
Drug group Corticosteroid (p.80)
Overdose danger rating Low
Dependence rating Low
Prescription needed Yes
Available as generic Yes

GENERAL INFORMATION
Dexamethasone is a long-acting corticosteroid drug that is prescribed to suppress
inflammatory and allergic disorders, such as
rheumatoid arthritis, shock, and brain swelling (as a result of injury or tumour). It is also
used in conjunction with other drugs to alleviate the nausea and vomiting associated
with chemotherapy.

Low doses of dexamethasone taken for
short periods rarely cause serious side effects.
However, as with other corticosteroids, long-
term treatment with high doses of
dexamethasone can cause unpleasant or dangerous side effects.

INFORMATION FOR USERS
Your drug prescription is tailored for you.
Do not alter dosage without checking with
your doctor.
How taken/used Tablets, liquid, injection, eye
ointment, eye/ear drops, ear/nasal spray.
Frequency and timing of doses 1–4 x daily with
food (by mouth); 1–6 hourly (eye drops);
1–4 x daily (ear drops/spray, eye ointment);
2–6 x daily (nasal spray).
Dosage range Usually 0.5–10mg daily (by
mouth).
Onset of effect 1–4 days.
Duration of action Some effects may last for
several days.
Diet advice None.
Storage Keep in original container at room
temperature out of the reach of children.
Protect from light.
Missed dose Take as soon as you remember. If
your next dose is due within 2 hours, take a
single dose now and skip the next.

Stopping the drug Do not stop taking the drug
without consulting your doctor. It may be
necessary to withdraw the drug gradually.
Exceeding the dose An occasional unintentional extra dose is unlikely to be a cause for
concern. But if you notice any unusual symptoms, or if a large overdose has been taken,
notify your doctor.

POSSIBLE ADVERSE EFFECTS
Indigestion is the most common adverse effect of dexamethasone. More rarely, there may
also be weight gain. The more serious adverse
effects occur only with high doses taken for
long periods. These include acne and other
skin changes, fluid retention, muscle weakness, and mood changes. These are carefully
monitored during prolonged treatment.

INTERACTIONS
Antidiabetic drugs Dexamethasone reduces
the action of these drugs. Dosage may need
to be adjusted accordingly to prevent abnormally high blood glucose.
**Barbiturates, phenytoin, rifampicin, and car-
bamazepine** These drugs may reduce the
effectiveness of dexamethasone. The dosage
may need to be adjusted accordingly.
Oral anticoagulant drugs Dexamethasone may
increase the effects of these drugs.
Non-steroidal anti-inflammatory drugs These
drugs may increase the likelihood of indigestion from dexamethasone.
Antacids These drugs may reduce the effectiveness of, and should be taken at least
2 hours apart from, dexamethasone.
Vaccines Dexamethasone can interact with
some vaccines. Discuss with your doctor
before having any vaccinations.

SPECIAL PRECAUTIONS
Be sure to tell your doctor if:
◆ You have had a peptic ulcer.
◆ You have glaucoma.
◆ You have high blood pressure.
◆ You have diabetes.
◆ You have epilepsy.
◆ You have had tuberculosis.
◆ You have suffered from depression or
mental illness.
◆ You have a herpes infection.
◆ You are taking other medicines.

Pregnancy Safety in pregnancy not established. Discuss with your doctor.
Breast-feeding Safety not established. The drug passes into the breast milk. Discuss with your doctor.
Infants and children Reduced dose necessary.
Over 60 No known problems.
Driving and hazardous work No known problems.
Alcohol Avoid. Alcohol may increase the risk of indigestion and peptic ulcer with this drug.
Surgery and general anaesthetics You must tell your doctor or anaesthetist that you are taking dexamethasone; close monitoring is required during surgery.
Infection Avoid exposure to chickenpox or shingles if you are on systemic treatment.

PROLONGED USE
Prolonged use by mouth can lead to peptic ulcers, glaucoma, fragile bones, muscle weakness, and growth retardation in children. Prolonged use of topical treatment may also lead to skin thinning. People receiving long-term treatment are advised to carry a "steroid treatment" card.

Diazepam/lorazepam

Brand names [diazepam] Dialar, Diazemuls, Diazepam Rectubes, Rimapram, Stesolid, Tensium, Valclair, [lorazepam] Ativan
Used in the following combined preparations None

QUICK REFERENCE
Drug group Benzodiazepine anti-anxiety drug (p.13), muscle relaxant (p.54), and anticonvulsant (p.16)
Overdose danger rating Medium
Dependence rating High
Prescription needed Yes
Available as generic Yes

GENERAL INFORMATION
Introduced in the early 1960s, diazepam is the best known and most widely used benzodiazepine, and lorazepam is closely related to it. Benzodiazepines help to relieve tension and nervousness, relax muscles, and encourage sleep. Their actions and adverse effects are described more fully on page 13.

Diazepam and lorazepam have a wide range of uses. Besides being commonly used in the treatment of anxiety and anxiety-related insomnia, they are given in the treatment of alcohol withdrawal and for the relief of epileptic fits. Diazepam is also given as a muscle relaxant. Given intravenously, they are used to sedate people undergoing certain uncomfortable medical procedures.

Diazepam and lorazepam can be habit-forming if taken regularly over a long period. Their effects may also diminish with time. For these reasons, courses of treatment are limited to 2 weeks whenever possible.

INFORMATION FOR USERS
Your drug prescription is tailored for you. Do not alter dosage without checking with your doctor.
How taken/used Tablets, liquid, injection, suppositories, rectal solution.
Frequency and timing of doses 1–4 x daily.
Adult dosage range *Anxiety* 2–30mg daily (diazepam); 1–4mg daily (lorazepam). *Muscle spasm* 2–60mg daily (diazepam).
Onset of effect Immediate effect (injection); 30 minutes–2 hours (other methods of administration).
Duration of action Up to 24 hours; some effect for up to 4 days.
Diet advice None.
Storage Keep in the original container at room temperature; keep out of the reach of children.
Missed dose Take as soon as you remember. If your next dose is due within 2 hours, take a single dose now and skip the next.
Stopping the drug If you have been taking the drug continuously for less than 2 weeks, it can be safely stopped as soon as you no longer need it. However, if you have been taking it for longer, consult your doctor, who will supervise a gradual reduction in dosage. Stopping abruptly may lead to withdrawal symptoms, such as anxiety, restlessness, and nightmares.
Exceeding the dose An occasional unintentional extra dose is unlikely to cause problems. Larger overdoses may cause excessive drowsiness and could cause deep coma. Notify your doctor in all cases.

POSSIBLE ADVERSE EFFECTS

The principal adverse effects of this drug are related to its sedative properties. They include daytime drowsiness, dizziness, unsteadiness, headache, blurred vision, and forgetfulness or confusion. These effects normally diminish after a few days and can often be reduced by adjusting the dosage. If a rash develops, stop taking the drug and consult your doctor.

INTERACTIONS

Sedatives All drugs that have a sedative effect on the central nervous system can increase the sedative properties of diazepam and lorazepam. Such drugs include anti-anxiety drugs, sleeping drugs, antihistamines, opioid analgesics, antidepressants, and antipsychotics.

Omeprazole (diazepam), cimetidine, isoniazid, and ritonavir These drugs may inhibit the breakdown of diazepam and lorazepam, leading to increased levels in the blood and risk of adverse effects.

Rifampicin (diazepam) may reduce the effects of diazepam.

SPECIAL PRECAUTIONS

Be sure to tell your doctor if:
◆ You have severe respiratory disease.
◆ You have long-term liver or kidney problems.
◆ You have had problems with alcohol or drug abuse.
◆ You have myasthenia gravis or muscle weakness.
◆ You have a marked personality disorder.
◆ You have porphyria.
◆ You are taking other medicines.

Pregnancy Safety in pregnancy not established. Not usually recommended; may cause adverse effects to the fetus. Discuss with your doctor.

Breast-feeding The drugs pass into the breast milk and may affect the baby. Discuss with your doctor.

Infants and children Reduced dose necessary.

Over 60 Increased likelihood of adverse effects. Reduced dose may therefore be necessary.

Driving and hazardous work Avoid such activities until you have learned how diazepam and lorazepam affect you because the drugs can cause reduced alertness, slowed reactions, and increased aggression.

Alcohol Avoid. Alcohol may increase the sedative effects of these drugs.

PROLONGED USE

Regular use of these drugs over several weeks can lead to a reduction in their effect as the body adapts. They may also be habit-forming when taken for extended periods, and severe withdrawal reactions can occur.

Diclofenac

Brand names Diclomax SR, Motifene, Rhumalgan, Volraman, Voltarol, and others
Used in the following combined preparation Arthrotec

QUICK REFERENCE

Drug group Non-steroidal anti-inflammatory drug (p.50), analgesic (p.9), and drug for gout (p.53)
Overdose danger rating Medium
Dependence rating Low
Prescription needed Yes
Available as generic Yes

GENERAL INFORMATION

Taken as a single dose, diclofenac has analgesic properties similar to those of paracetamol. It is taken to relieve mild to moderate headache, menstrual pain, and pain following minor surgery. When given regularly over a long period, it has an anti-inflammatory effect and is used to relieve pain and stiffness associated with rheumatoid arthritis and advanced osteoarthritis. It may also be prescribed to treat acute gout attacks, and is given as eye drops to relieve eye inflammation.

The combined preparation, Arthrotec, contains diclofenac and misoprostol (see p.319). Misoprostol helps prevent gastroduodenal ulceration, which is sometimes caused by diclofenac, and may be particularly useful in patients at risk of developing this problem.

INFORMATION FOR USERS

Your drug prescription is tailored for you. Do not alter dosage without checking with your doctor.

How taken/used Tablets, SR-tablets, dispersible tablets, capsules, SR-capsules, injection, suppositories, gel, eye drops.

Frequency and timing of doses 1–3 x daily with food.

Adult dosage range 75–150mg daily.

Onset of effect Around 1 hour (pain relief); full anti-inflammatory effect may take 2 weeks.

Duration of action Up to 12 hours; up to 24 hours (SR-preparations).

Diet advice None.

Storage Keep in original container at room temperature out of the reach of children.

Missed dose Take as soon as you remember. If your next dose is due within 2 hours, take a single dose now and skip the next.

Stopping the drug When taken for short-term pain relief, diclofenac can be safely stopped as soon as you no longer need it. If prescribed for long-term treatment (e.g. for arthritis), speak to your doctor before stopping the drug.

Exceeding the dose An occasional unintentional extra dose is unlikely to be a cause for concern. But if you notice any unusual symptoms or if a large overdose has been taken, notify your doctor.

POSSIBLE ADVERSE EFFECTS

The most common adverse effects are gastrointestinal disturbances. More rarely, headache, dizziness, or drowsiness may occur. If you develop swelling of the feet and/or ankles, you should talk to your doctor. If you develop a rash, wheezing, breathlessness, or have black or bloodstained vomit or faeces, stop taking the drug and consult your doctor without delay.

INTERACTIONS

General note Interacts with other NSAIDs, oral anticoagulants, corticosteroids, and antidepressants to increase the risk of bleeding and/or ulcers.

Antihypertensive drugs and diuretics The beneficial effects of these drugs may be reduced with diclofenac.

Ciclosporin and tacrolimus Diclofenac may increase the risk of kidney problems.

Lithium, digoxin, and methotrexate Diclofenac may increase the blood levels of these drugs to an undesirable extent.

Indigestion remedies These should not be taken at the same time of day as enteric coated diclofenac preparations as they disrupt this coating.

SPECIAL PRECAUTIONS

Be sure to tell your doctor if:
◆ You have long-term liver or kidney problems.
◆ You have a bleeding disorder.
◆ You have had a peptic ulcer or oesophagitis.
◆ You have porphyria.
◆ You suffer from indigestion.
◆ You are allergic to aspirin or other NSAIDs.
◆ You suffer from asthma.
◆ You have heart problems or high blood pressure.
◆ You are taking other medicines.

Pregnancy Not usually prescribed in the last 3 months of pregnancy as it may increase the risk of adverse effects on the baby's heart and may prolong labour. Discuss with your doctor.

Breast-feeding Small amounts of the drug pass into breast milk, but adverse effects on the baby are unlikely. Discuss with your doctor.

Infants and children Reduced dose necessary.

Over 60 Increased risk of adverse effects. Reduced dose may therefore be necessary.

Driving and hazardous work Avoid such activities until you have learned how diclofenac affects you; the drug can cause dizziness, drowsiness, and vertigo.

Alcohol Keep consumption low. Alcohol may increase the risk of stomach irritation.

Surgery and general anaesthetics Discuss with your doctor or dentist before any surgery.

PROLONGED USE

Increased risk of bleeding from peptic ulcers and in the bowel. The lowest effective dose is given for the shortest duration.

Dicycloverine (dicyclomine)

Brand name Merbentyl
Used in the following combined preparation
Kolanticon

QUICK REFERENCE

Drug group Drug for irritable bowel syndrome (p.45)
Overdose danger rating Medium
Dependence rating Low
Prescription needed No (doses of 10mg or less)
Yes (doses of more than 10mg)
Available as generic No

GENERAL INFORMATION

Dicycloverine is a mild anticholinergic anti-spasmodic drug that relieves painful abdominal cramps occurring in the gastro-intestinal tract. It can be used to treat irritable bowel syndrome, indigestion not associated with ulcers, and colicky conditions in babies (only over 6 months).

Because the drug has anticholinergic properties, it is also included in some combined preparations used to treat flatulence, indigestion, and diarrhoea. Dicycloverine relieves symptoms but does not cure the underlying condition. Additional treatment with other drugs and self-help measures, such as dietary changes, may be recommended by your doctor.

Side effects with dicycloverine are rare, but they include headaches, constipation, urinary difficulties, and palpitations.

INFORMATION FOR USERS

Follow instructions on the label. Call your doctor if symptoms worsen.
How taken/used Tablets, liquid.
Frequency and timing of doses 3–4 x daily before or after meals.
Dosage range *Adults* 30–60mg daily. *Children* Reduced dose according to age and weight.
Onset of effect Within 1–2 hours.
Duration of action 4–6 hours.
Diet advice None.
Storage Keep in original container at room temperature out of the reach of children. Protect from light.
Missed dose Take as soon as you remember. If your next dose is due within 2 hours, take a single dose now and skip the next.
Stopping the drug The drug can be stopped without causing problems when it is no longer needed.
Exceeding the dose An occasional unintentional extra dose is unlikely to cause problems. Large overdoses may cause drow-

siness, dizziness, and difficulty in swallowing. Notify your doctor.

POSSIBLE ADVERSE EFFECTS

Most people do not notice any adverse effects when taking dicycloverine. Those that do occur are related to the anticholinergic properties of the drug and include drowsiness, dry mouth, constipation, headache, and blurred vision. Such symptoms may be overcome by adjusting the dosage, or they may disappear after a few days of usage as your body adjusts to the drug. If you experience difficulty in passing urine or palpitations, consult your doctor.

INTERACTIONS

Sedatives All drugs that have a sedative effect on the central nervous system may increase the sedative properties of dicycloverine.
Anticholinergic drugs These drugs may increase the adverse effects of dicycloverine.

SPECIAL PRECAUTIONS

Be sure to consult your doctor or pharmacist before taking this drug if:
◆ You have glaucoma.
◆ You have urinary problems.
◆ You have a hiatus hernia.
◆ You have any heart condition.
◆ You have myasthenia gravis
◆ You are taking other medicines.
Pregnancy No evidence of risk.
Breast-feeding The drug passes into the breast milk, but at normal doses adverse effects on the baby are unlikely. Discuss with your doctor.
Infants and children A reduced dose is necessary. Not recommended in infants under 6 months.
Over 60 Reduced dose may be necessary. The elderly are more susceptible to anticholinergic side effects.
Driving and hazardous work Avoid such activities until you have learned how dicycloverine affects you; the drug can cause drowsiness and blurred vision.
Alcohol Caution. Alcohol may increase the sedative effects of this drug.

PROLONGED USE

No problems expected.

Digoxin

Brand name Lanoxin
Used in the following combined preparations
None

QUICK REFERENCE

Drug group Digitalis drug (p.29)
Overdose danger rating High
Dependence rating Low
Prescription needed Yes
Available as generic Yes

GENERAL INFORMATION

Digoxin is the most widely used extract of digitalis, a compound that is obtained from the leaves of the foxglove plant. It is given in the treatment of irregular heart rhythms such as atrial fibrillation or atrial flutter; it may also sometimes be used to treat congestive heart failure.

Digoxin increases the force of the heart beat, making the heart more effective in pumping blood around the body. This in turn helps to control breathlessness, fluid retention, and tiredness.

The effective dose of digoxin can be close to the toxic dose and, therefore, treatment needs careful monitoring to prevent toxic doses from being reached. A number of adverse effects (see below) may indicate that the toxic level is close and should be reported to your doctor.

INFORMATION FOR USERS

Your drug prescription is tailored for you. Do not alter dosage without checking with your doctor.
How taken/used Tablets, liquid, injection.
Frequency and timing of doses Up to 3 x daily (starting dose); once daily, or divided to reduce nausea (maintenance dose).
Adult dosage range Usually 0.0625–0.25mg daily (by mouth), but doses of up to 0.5mg are occasionally used.
Onset of effect Within a few minutes (injection); within 1–2 hours (by mouth).
Duration of action Up to 4 days.
Diet advice Drug may be more toxic if potassium levels are low. Include potassium-rich fruit and vegetables, such as bananas and tomatoes, in your diet.

Storage Keep in original container at room temperature out of the reach of children. Protect from light.
Missed dose Take as soon as you remember. If your next dose is due within 8 hours, take a dose now and skip the next.
Stopping the drug Do not stop the drug without consulting your doctor; stopping the drug may lead to worsening of the underlying condition.

OVERDOSE ACTION

Seek immediate medical advice in all cases. Take emergency action if palpitations, severe weakness, chest pain, or loss of consciousness occur.

POSSIBLE ADVERSE EFFECTS

The possible adverse effects of digoxin are usually due to increased levels of the drug in the blood. Common effects include tiredness, nausea, and loss of appetite. More rarely, confusion, visual disturbance, and palpitations may occur. Any symptoms should be reported to your doctor without delay. If you do experience palpitations and/or visual disturbances, you should also stop taking the drug.

INTERACTIONS

General note Many drugs interact with digoxin. Do not take any medication without consulting your doctor or pharmacist.
Diuretics may increase the risk of adverse effects from digoxin if they lower potassium levels.
Calcium channel blockers may increase the blood levels of digoxin.
Antacids may reduce the effects of digoxin. The effect of digoxin may increase when antacids are stopped.
Anti-arrhythmic drugs (e.g. amiodarone and quinidine) may increase the blood levels of digoxin.
Ciclosporin may increase the blood levels of digoxin.

SPECIAL PRECAUTIONS

Be sure to tell your doctor if:
◆ You have kidney problems.
◆ You have thyroid trouble.
◆ You are taking other medicines.

Pregnancy No evidence of risk, but adjustment in dose may be necessary.

Breast-feeding The drug passes into the breast milk, but at normal doses adverse effects on the baby are unlikely. Discuss with your doctor.

Infants and children Reduced dose necessary.

Over 60 Increased likelihood of adverse effects. A reduced dose may therefore be necessary.

Driving and hazardous work Special problems are unlikely, but do not undertake these activities until you know how digoxin affects you because it can cause tiredness and visual disturbances.

Alcohol No special problems.

PROLONGED USE
No problems expected.

Monitoring Periodic checks on blood levels of digoxin and body salts may be advised.

Dihydrocodeine

Brand names DF118 Forte, DHC Continus
Used in the following combined preparations
Co-dydramol, Remedeine

QUICK REFERENCE
Drug group Opioid analgesic (p.9)
Overdose danger rating High
Dependence rating Medium
Prescription needed Yes (most preparations)
Available as generic Yes

GENERAL INFORMATION
Dihydrocodeine is an opioid analgesic that is related to codeine and of similar potency. It is used mainly for the relief of moderately severe pain but has also been used as a cough suppressant. As with codeine, side effects limit the dose that can be taken; dihydrocodeine causes constipation, nausea, and vomiting.

Dihydrocodeine is also used in combination with paracetamol; in this way, a lower dose of the opioid can be used to give pain relief with fewer side effects. A combined preparation containing dihydrocodeine and paracetamol is available under the name of co-dydramol.

INFORMATION FOR USERS
Your drug prescription is tailored for you. Do not alter dosage without checking with your doctor.

How taken/used Tablets, SR-tablets, liquid, injection.

Frequency and timing of doses 2–6 x daily.

Adult dosage range 120–240mg daily.

Onset of effect 30–60 minutes (tablets, liquid); 3–4 hours (SR-tablets).

Duration of action 4–6 hours (tablets, liquid); 12 hours (SR-tablets).

Diet advice None.

Storage Keep in original container at room temperature out of the reach of children.

Missed dose Take as soon as you remember if needed for relief of symptoms. If not needed, do not take the missed dose, and return to your normal dosage schedule when necessary.

Stopping the drug Can be safely stopped as soon as you no longer need it.

OVERDOSE ACTION
Seek immediate medical advice in all cases. Take emergency action if slow or irregular breathing, severe drowsiness, or loss of consciousness occur.

POSSIBLE ADVERSE EFFECTS
The most common adverse effects are constipation, nausea, vomiting, drowsiness or dizziness, headache, and vertigo. More rarely, abdominal pain may occur. If rash, itching, confusion, or hallucinations occur, seek medical advice. If you have breathing difficulties, stop taking the drug and consult your doctor urgently. Tolerance and dependence may develop with long-term use of the drug.

INTERACTIONS
Sedatives All drugs that have a sedative effect on the central nervous system increase dihydrocodeine's sedative properties. They include other opioid analgesics, sleeping drugs, antihistamines, antipsychotics, and antidepressants.

Monoamine oxidase inhibitors (MAOIs) may cause a dangerous rise in blood pressure. Avoid using together and for 14 days after stopping MAOI treatment.

SPECIAL PRECAUTIONS

Be sure to tell your doctor if:
◆ You have liver or kidney problems.
◆ You have a phaeochromocytoma.
◆ You have a lung disorder such as asthma or bronchitis.
◆ You have a problem with alcohol abuse.
◆ You have an enlarged prostate.
◆ You have low blood pressure.
◆ You have an underactive thyroid.
◆ You are taking other medicines.

Pregnancy Safety in pregnancy not established. The drug may affect the baby's breathing in labour.

Breast-feeding Safety not established. Discuss with your doctor.

Infants and children Not recommended for children under 4 years. In children over 4 years a reduced dose is necessary.

Over 60 Reduced dose necessary.

Driving and hazardous work Avoid such activities until you have learned how dihydrocodeine affects you because the drug may cause drowsiness, dizziness, and confusion.

Alcohol Avoid. Alcohol may increase the sedative effects of the drug.

PROLONGED USE

Dihydrocodeine is generally used only in the short term since it can be habit-forming if used long term.

Diltiazem

Brand names Adizem, Calcicard, Dilzem, Slozem, Tildiem, and others
Used in the following combined preparations None

QUICK REFERENCE

Drug group Calcium channel blocker anti-angina drug (p.35) and antihypertensive drug (p.36)
Overdose danger rating Medium
Dependence rating Low
Prescription needed Yes
Available as generic Yes

GENERAL INFORMATION

Diltiazem belongs to the group of drugs known as calcium channel blockers. These drugs interfere with the conduction of signals in the muscles of the heart and blood vessels.

Diltiazem is used in the treatment of angina, and longer-acting formulations are used to treat high blood pressure. When this drug is taken regularly, it reduces the frequency of angina attacks but does not work quickly enough to reduce the pain of an angina attack that is already in progress.

Diltiazem does not adversely affect breathing and is valuable for people who suffer from asthma, for whom other anti-angina drugs may not be suitable.

Different brands of sustained-release (SR) diltiazem may not be equivalent, so you should always take the same brand.

INFORMATION FOR USERS

Your drug prescription is tailored for you. Do not alter dosage without checking with your doctor.

How taken/used Tablets, SR-tablets, capsules, SR-capsules.

Frequency and timing of doses 3 x daily (tablets/capsules); 1–2 x daily (SR-tablets/SR-capsules).

Adult dosage range 180–480mg daily.

Onset of effect 2–3 hours.

Duration of action 6–8 hours.

Diet advice None.

Storage Keep in original container at room temperature out of the reach of children.

Missed dose Take as soon as you remember. If your next dose is due within 2 hours, take a single dose now and skip the next.

Stopping the drug Do not stop taking the drug without consulting your doctor; symptoms may recur. Stopping suddenly may worsen angina.

Exceeding the dose An occasional unintentional extra dose is unlikely to cause any problems. However, large overdoses may cause dizziness or collapse. Notify your doctor urgently.

POSSIBLE ADVERSE EFFECTS

Diltiazem can cause a variety of minor symptoms that are also common to other calcium channel blockers. These include headache, nausea, and a dry mouth. If you develop swelling of the legs or ankles, consult your doctor. The most serious effect is the possibility of a slowed heart beat, which may cause tiredness or dizziness. These effects can sometimes be controlled by an adjustment in dosage. If you develop a rash, stop taking the drug and contact your doctor urgently.

INTERACTIONS

Antihypertensive drugs Diltiazem increases the effects of these drugs, leading to a further reduction in blood pressure.

Anticonvulsant drugs Levels of these drugs may be altered by diltiazem.

Anti-arrhythmic drugs There is a risk of side effects on the heart if these are taken with diltiazem.

Digoxin Blood levels and adverse effects of this drug may be increased if it is taken with diltiazem. The dosage of digoxin may need to be reduced.

Theophylline/aminophylline Diltiazem may increase the levels of this drug.

Beta blockers These drugs increase the risk of the heart slowing.

SPECIAL PRECAUTIONS

Be sure to tell your doctor if:
◆ You have long-term liver or kidney problems.
◆ You have heart failure.
◆ You are taking other medicines.

Pregnancy Not usually prescribed. Discuss with your doctor.

Breast-feeding The drug passes into the breast milk and may affect the baby. Discuss with your doctor.

Infants and children Not recommended.

Over 60 Increased likelihood of adverse effects. A reduced dose may therefore be necessary.

Driving and hazardous work Avoid such activities until you have learned how diltiazem affects you because the drug can cause dizziness as a result of lowered blood pressure.

Alcohol Avoid excessive amounts. Alcohol may lower blood pressure, causing dizziness, when it is taken in combination with diltiazem.

PROLONGED USE

No problems expected.

Dipyridamole

Brand name Persantin
Used in the following combined preparation
Asasantin Retard

QUICK REFERENCE

Drug group Antiplatelet drug (p.39)
Overdose danger rating Medium
Dependence rating Low
Prescription needed Yes
Available as generic Yes

GENERAL INFORMATION

Dipyridamole was introduced in the late 1970s as an anti-angina drug to improve the capability of people with angina to exercise. More effective drugs are now available to help with this problem, but dipyridamole is still prescribed as an antiplatelet drug. It acts by "thinning" the blood, which reduces the likelihood of clots forming in the bloodstream. This is especially important in people who have had a stroke or transient ischaemic attacks (TIAs) or have undergone heart valve replacement surgery.

Dipyridamole is usually given together with other drugs such as warfarin or aspirin. The drug can also be given by injection during certain types of diagnostic test on the heart.

Side effects may occur, especially during the early days of treatment. If they persist, your doctor may advise a reduction in dosage.

INFORMATION FOR USERS

Your drug prescription is tailored for you. Do not alter dosage without checking with your doctor.

How taken/used Tablets, capsules, MR-capsules, liquid, injection (for diagnostic tests only).

Frequency and timing of doses 3–4 x daily, 1 hour before meals (tablets, capsules, liquid). 2 x daily with food (MR-capsules).

Adult dosage range 300–600mg daily.

Onset of effect Within 1 hour. Full therapeutic effect may not be reached for 2–3 weeks.

Duration of action Up to 8 hours. Up to 12 hours (MR-capsules).

Diet advice None.

Storage Keep in original container at room temperature out of the reach of children. Protect from light.

Missed dose Take as soon as you remember. If your next dose is due within 2 hours, take a single dose now and skip the next.

Stopping the drug Do not stop taking the drug without consulting your doctor; withdrawal of the drug could lead to abnormal clotting.

Exceeding the dose An occasional unintentional extra dose is unlikely to be a cause for concern. Large overdoses may cause dizziness or vomiting. Notify your doctor.

POSSIBLE ADVERSE EFFECTS

Adverse effects are rare. Possible symptoms include stomach upsets, nausea, diarrhoea, headache, dizziness, and fainting. If a rash, breathing difficulty, or swollen lips occur, stop taking the drug and consult your doctor. In rare cases, the drug may aggravate angina.

INTERACTIONS

Anticoagulant drugs The effect of these drugs may be increased by dipyridamole, increasing the risk of uncontrolled bleeding. The anticoagulant dosage may need to be adjusted.

Antacids may reduce the effectiveness of dipyridamole.

SPECIAL PRECAUTIONS

Be sure to tell your doctor if:
◆ You have low blood pressure.
◆ You suffer from migraine.
◆ You have angina.
◆ You have myasthenia gravis.
◆ You have had a recent heart attack.
◆ You are taking other medicines.

Pregnancy Safety in pregnancy not established. Discuss with your doctor.

Breast-feeding The drug passes into the breast milk but at normal doses adverse effects on the baby are unlikely. Discuss with your doctor.

Infants and children Reduced dose necessary.

Over 60 No special problems.

Driving and hazardous work Avoid until you have learned how the drug affects you because it may cause dizziness and faintness.

Alcohol Avoid until you have learned how dipyridamole affects you because the drug may cause dizziness and faintness when taken with alcohol.

PROLONGED USE

No known problems.

Disulfiram

Brand name Antabuse
Used in the following combined preparations
None

QUICK REFERENCE

Drug group Alcohol abuse deterrent
Overdose danger rating Medium
Dependence rating Low
Prescription needed Yes
Available as generic No

GENERAL INFORMATION

Disulfiram is used to help alcohol misusers abstain from alcohol. It does not cure alcoholism but provides a powerful deterrent to drinking. If you are taking disulfiram and drink even a small amount of alcohol, highly unpleasant reactions follow. These are due to high levels of acetaldehyde in the body because disulfiram prevents its breakdown. Flushing, throbbing headache, nausea, breathlessness, thirst, palpitations, dizziness, and fainting may be experienced. Such reactions may last from 30 minutes to several hours, leaving you feeling drowsy and fatigued. The reactions can also include unconsciousness, so it is wise to carry a card stating the person to be notified in an emergency. It is important not to drink any alcohol for at least 24 hours before starting disulfiram, and for at least a week after stopping. Foods, medicines, and even toiletries that contain alcohol should also be avoided. Disulfiram treatment is usually only started by specialist services and in conjunction with social support.

INFORMATION FOR USERS

Your drug prescription is tailored for you. Do not alter dosage without checking with your doctor.

How taken/used Tablets.

Frequency and timing of doses Once daily.

Adult dosage range 800mg initially, gradually reduced over 5 days to 100–200mg (maintenance dose).

Onset of effect Interaction with alcohol occurs within a few minutes of taking alcohol.

Duration of action Interaction with alcohol can occur for up to 6 days after the last dose of disulfiram.

Diet advice Avoid all alcoholic drinks, even in very small amounts. Food, fermented vinegar, medicines, mouthwashes, and lotions containing alcohol should also be avoided.

Storage Keep in original container at room temperature out of the reach of children. Protect from light.

Missed dose Take as soon as you remember. If your next dose is due within 2 hours, take a single dose now and skip the next.

Stopping the drug Do not stop taking the drug without consulting your doctor.

Exceeding the dose An occasional unintentional extra dose is unlikely to cause problems. Large overdoses may cause a temporary increase in adverse effects. Notify your doctor.

POSSIBLE ADVERSE EFFECTS

Adverse effects, such as drowsiness, fatigue, nausea, vomiting, bad breath, and reduced libido, may occur but usually disappear when you get used to taking the drug. If they persist or become severe, the dosage may need to be adjusted. The most potentially severe effects are due to interaction with alcohol (see General information, previous page).

INTERACTIONS

General note A number of drugs can produce an adverse reaction when taken with disulfiram. Check with your doctor or pharmacist before taking any other medication.

Phenytoin Disulfiram increases the blood levels of this drug.

Anticoagulant drugs Disulfiram increases the effect of these drugs.

Metronidazole A severe reaction can occur if this drug is taken with disulfiram.

Theophylline Disulfiram may increase the toxic effects of this drug.

Diazepam/chlordiazepoxide Disulfiram increases the effect of these drugs.

SPECIAL PRECAUTIONS

Be sure to tell your doctor if:
◆ You have long-term liver or kidney problems.
◆ You have heart problems, coronary artery disease, or high blood pressure.
◆ You have had epileptic fits.
◆ You have diabetes.
◆ You have breathing problems.
◆ You are taking other medicines.

Pregnancy Safety in pregnancy not established. Discuss with your doctor.

Breast-feeding The drug passes into the breast milk and may affect the baby adversely. Discuss with your doctor.

Infants and children Not recommended.

Over 60 Reduced dose may be necessary.

Driving and hazardous work Avoid such activities until you have learned how disulfiram affects you because the drug can cause drowsiness and dizziness.

Alcohol Never drink alcohol while under treatment with disulfiram, and avoid foods, medicines, and toiletries containing alcohol. This drug may interact dangerously with alcohol.

PROLONGED USE

Not usually prescribed for longer than 6 months without review. It is wise to carry a card indicating you are taking disulfiram with instructions as to who should be notified in an emergency.

Domperidone

Brand name Motilium
Used in the following combined preparation
Domperamol

QUICK REFERENCE

Drug group Anti-emetic drug (p.21)
Overdose danger rating Medium
Dependence rating Low
Prescription needed No
Available as generic Yes

GENERAL INFORMATION

Domperidone, an anti-emetic drug, was first introduced in the early 1980s. It is particularly effective for treating nausea and vomiting caused by gastroenteritis, chemotherapy or radiotherapy. It is not effective for motion sickness or nausea caused by inner ear disorders such as Ménière's disease.

The main advantage of domperidone over other anti-emetic drugs is that it does not usually cause drowsiness or other adverse effects such as abnormal movement. Domperidone is not suitable, however, for the long-term treatment of gastrointestinal disorders, for which an alternative drug treatment is often prescribed. Domperidone may also be used to relieve dyspepsia (indigestion and heartburn); and, in combination with paracetamol, it is sometimes used to treat acute attacks of migraine.

INFORMATION FOR USERS

Follow instructions on the label. Call your doctor if symptoms worsen.

How taken/used Tablets, liquid, suppositories.

Frequency and timing of doses *Nausea/vomiting* Every 4–8 hours as required. *Dyspepsia* 3 x daily with water before meals and at night (tablets only).

Adult dosage range *Nausea/vomiting* 10–20mg (by mouth); 30–60mg (rectally).

Onset of effect Within 1 hour. The effects of the drug may be delayed if taken after the onset of nausea.

Duration of action Approximately 6 hours.

Diet advice None.

Storage Keep in original container at room temperature out of the reach of children. Protect from light.

Missed dose Take as soon as you remember for dyspepsia. If your next dose is due within 4 hours, take a single dose now and skip the next. Then return to your normal dose schedule.

Stopping the drug Can be stopped when you no longer need it.

Exceeding the dose An occasional unintentional extra dose is unlikely to cause problems. Large overdoses may cause dizziness. Notify your doctor.

POSSIBLE ADVERSE EFFECTS

Adverse effects from this drug are rare. Occasionally it may cause breast enlargement or milk secretion, muscle spasms or tremors, reduced libido, and a rash. Consult your doctor if any of these effects occur.

INTERACTIONS

Anticholinergic drugs These may reduce the beneficial effects of domperidone.

Opioid analgesics These may reduce the beneficial effects of domperidone.

Bromocriptine and cabergoline Domperidone may reduce the effects of these drugs in some people.

SPECIAL PRECAUTIONS

Be sure to consult your doctor or pharmacist before taking this drug if:

◆ You have a long-term kidney problem.

◆ You have thyroid disease.

◆ You are taking other medicines.

Pregnancy Safety in pregnancy not established. Discuss with your doctor.

Breast-feeding The drug may pass into the breast milk, but at normal doses adverse effects on the baby are unlikely. Discuss with your doctor.

Infants and children Usually prescribed only to treat nausea and vomiting caused by anti-cancer drugs or radiation therapy. Reduced dose necessary.

Over 60 No special problems.

Driving and hazardous work No special problems.

Alcohol No special problems, but alcohol is best avoided in cases of nausea and vomiting.

PROLONGED USE

Treatment should be reviewed after four weeks and the need for continued treatment re-assessed.

Donepezil

Brand name Aricept
Used in the following combined preparations None

QUICK REFERENCE

Drug group Drug for dementia (p.19)
Overdose danger rating Medium
Dependence rating Low
Prescription needed Yes
Available as generic No

GENERAL INFORMATION

Donepezil is an inhibitor of the enzyme acetylcholinesterase. This enzyme breaks down the natural neurotransmitter acetylcholine to limit its effects. Blocking the enzyme raises levels of acetylcholine, which, in the brain, increases awareness and memory. Donepezil has been found to improve the symptoms of dementia of Alzheimer's disease and is used to diminish deterioration in that disease. It is not currently recommended for dementia due to other causes. Treatment with donepezil is initiated under specialist supervision. It is usual to assess those being treated at six-monthly intervals to decide whether the drug is helping.

Side effects may include bladder outflow obstruction and psychiatric problems, such as agitation and aggression, which might be due to the disease.

INFORMATION FOR USERS

Your drug prescription is tailored for you. Do not alter dosage without checking with your doctor.

How taken/used Tablets.
Frequency and timing of doses Once daily at bedtime.
Adult dosage range 5–10mg.
Onset of effect 1 hour. Full effects may take up to 3 months.
Duration of action Usually 1–2 days.
Diet advice None.
Storage Keep in original container at room temperature out of the reach of children.
Missed dose Take as soon as you remember. A carer should ensure that the maximum dose taken in 24 hours does not exceed 10mg.
Stopping the drug Do not stop taking the drug without consulting your doctor; symptoms may recur.
Exceeding the dose An occasional unintentional extra dose is unlikely to be a cause for concern. But if you notice any unusual symptoms, or if a large overdose has been taken, notify your doctor.

POSSIBLE ADVERSE EFFECTS

Adverse effects include such problems as accidents, which are common in people with dementia, even those not being treated. Other adverse effects include nausea, vomiting, diarrhoea, fatigue, insomnia, muscle cramps, and headache. If you experience urinary incontinence or difficulty passing urine, fainting, dizziness, or palpitations, consult your doctor. If you have convulsions, stop taking the drug and seek urgent medical help.

INTERACTIONS

Muscle relaxants used in surgery Donepezil may increase the effect of some muscle relaxants, but it may also block some others.

Fluoxetine, erythromycin, and ketoconazole can increase the levels and adverse effects of donepezil.

SPECIAL PRECAUTIONS

Be sure to tell your doctor if:
◆ You have liver or kidney problems.
◆ You have a heart problem.
◆ You have asthma or respiratory problems.
◆ You have had a gastric or duodenal ulcer.
◆ You are taking an NSAID regularly.
◆ You are taking other medicines.
Pregnancy Not recommended. Safety in pregnancy not established.
Breast-feeding Not recommended.
Infants and children Not recommended.
Over 60 No special problems.
Driving and hazardous work Your underlying condition may make such activities inadvisable. Discuss with your doctor.
Alcohol Avoid. Alcohol may reduce the effect of donepezil.
Surgery and general anaesthetics Treatment with donepezil may need to be stopped before you have a general anaesthetic. Discuss this with your doctor or dentist before any operation.

PROLONGED USE

May be continued for as long as there is benefit. Stopping the drug leads to a gradual loss of the improvements.
Monitoring Periodic checks (typically at six-monthly intervals) may be performed to test whether the drug is still providing some benefit.

Dorzolamide

Brand name Trusopt
Used in the following combined preparation Cosopt

QUICK REFERENCE

Drug group Drug for glaucoma (p.114)
Overdose danger rating Low
Dependence rating Low
Prescription needed Yes
Available as generic No

GENERAL INFORMATION

Dorzolamide is a carbonic anhydrase inhibitor (a kind of diuretic) that is used, in the form of eye drops only, to treat glaucoma. It is also used for ocular hypertension (high blood pressure inside the eye). The drug relieves the pressure by reducing production of aqueous humour, the fluid in the front chamber of the eye.

Dorzolamide may be used either alone or combined with a beta blocker by people who are resistant to the effects of beta blockers or for whom beta blockers are not suitable.

Most side effects of dorzolamide are local to the eye, but systemic effects may occur if enough of the drug is absorbed by the body.

INFORMATION FOR USERS

Your drug prescription is tailored for you. Do not alter dosage without checking with your doctor.

How taken/used Eye drops.
Frequency and timing of doses 3 x daily (on its own); 2 x daily (combined preparation).
Adult dosage range 1 drop in the affected eye(s) or as directed.
Onset of effect 15–30 minutes.
Duration of action 4–8 hours.
Diet advice None.
Storage Keep in original container at room temperature out of the reach of children. Protect from light. Discard eye drops 4 weeks after opening.
Missed dose Use as soon as you remember. If your next dose is due, skip the missed dose and then go back to your normal dosing schedule.
Stopping the drug Do not stop the drug without consulting your doctor; symptoms may recur.
Exceeding the dose An occasional unintentional extra application is unlikely to cause problems. Excessive use may provoke side effects as described below.

POSSIBLE ADVERSE EFFECTS

Local side effects of dorzolamide include conjunctivitis and keratitis (inflammation of the cornea, the transparent part of the eye), which may lead to burning, stinging, or watery eyes; inflammation or soreness of the eyes or blurred vision; or a bitter taste in the mouth. Systemic side effects such as headache, tiredness, nausea, and dizziness may also occur. If you develop a rash or breathing difficulties, you should consult your doctor urgently.

INTERACTIONS

General note Dorzolamide may interact with the following drugs, but there do not appear to be any published reports of problems. Consult your doctor.
Thiazide diuretics Excessive loss of potassium may occur when these drugs are taken with dorzolamide.
Aspirin and NSAIDs These drugs may increase the levels of dorzolamide and increase the risk of adverse effects.
Lithium Dorzolamide may reduce blood levels of lithium.

SPECIAL PRECAUTIONS

Be sure to tell your doctor if:
◆ You have liver or kidney problems.
◆ You are allergic to sulphonamide drugs.
◆ You are allergic to benzalkonium chloride.
◆ You are taking other medicines.
Pregnancy Not prescribed. Discuss with your doctor.
Breast-feeding Not recommended. Discuss with your doctor.
Infants and children Not recommended.
Over 60 No special problems.
Driving and hazardous work Avoid such activities until you have learned how dorzolamide affects you because the drug can cause dizziness and blurred vision.
Alcohol No special problems.

PROLONGED USE

No special problems.

Dosulepin (dothiepin)

Brand names Dothapax, Prepadine, Prothiaden
Used in the following combined preparations
None

QUICK REFERENCE

Drug group Tricyclic antidepressant drug (p.14)
Overdose danger rating High
Dependence rating Low
Prescription needed Yes
Available as generic Yes

GENERAL INFORMATION

Dosulepin belongs to the tricyclic class of antidepressant drugs, and is used in the long-term treatment of depression. The drug is particularly useful when the depression is accompanied by anxiety and insomnia. Dosulepin elevates mood, increases physical activity, improves appetite, and restores interest in everyday activities. Taken at night, dosulepin encourages sleep and helps eliminate the need for additional sleeping drugs.

Dosulepin takes several weeks to achieve its full antidepressant effect. It has adverse effects common to all tricyclics, including a risk of dangerous heart rhythms, fits, and coma, if taken in overdose. The drug should not be taken by anyone with a serious heart condition.

INFORMATION FOR USERS

Your drug prescription is tailored for you. Do not alter dosage without checking with your doctor.

How taken/used Tablets, capsules.

Frequency and timing of doses 2–3 x daily or once at night.

Adult dosage range 75–150mg daily (a maximum dose of up to 225mg may be given in some circumstances).

Onset of effect Full antidepressant effect may not be felt for 2–6 weeks, but adverse effects may be noticed within a day or two.

Duration of action Several days.

Diet advice None.

Storage Keep in the original container and store at room temperature out of the reach of children.

Missed dose Take as soon as you remember. If your next dose is due within 2 hours, take a single dose now and skip the next.

Stopping the drug Do not stop taking the drug without consulting your doctor, who may supervise a gradual reduction in dosage. Abrupt cessation of the drug may cause withdrawal symptoms and a recurrence of the original problem.

OVERDOSE ACTION

Seek immediate medical advice in all cases. Take emergency action if palpitations or loss of consciousness occur.

POSSIBLE ADVERSE EFFECTS

The adverse effects of dosulepin are mainly the result of its anticholinergic action. They include drowsiness, dry mouth, sweating, and blurred vision and are more common in the early days of treatment. The drug can also affect normal heart rhythm. If dizziness or fainting occur, you should consult your doctor. If you experience difficulty in passing urine or palpitations, you should stop taking the drug and consult your doctor urgently.

INTERACTIONS

Antiarrhythmic drugs Dosulepin should be avoided in patients who are taking amiodarone, sotalol, and other medications that can affect heart rhythms.

Monoamine oxidase inhibitors (MAOIs) In the rare cases where these drugs are given with dosulepin, serious interactions may occur.

Sedatives All drugs that have a sedative effect on the central nervous system increase the sedative properties of dosulepin.

Antiepileptic drugs Dosulepin may reduce the effectiveness of these drugs.

SPECIAL PRECAUTIONS

Be sure to tell your doctor if:
◆ You have heart problems.
◆ You have had epileptic fits.
◆ You have any long-term liver or kidney problems.
◆ You have glaucoma.
◆ You have had mania or a psychotic illness.
◆ You are taking other medicines.

Pregnancy Safety in pregnancy not established. Discuss with your doctor.

Breast-feeding The drug passes into the breast milk, but effects on the baby are unlikely. Discuss with your doctor.

Infants and children Not recommended.

Over 60 Greater risk of adverse effects. Reduced dose necessary.

Driving and hazardous work Avoid such activities until you have learned how dosulepin affects you because the drug can reduce alertness and may cause blurred vision, dizziness, and drowsiness.

Alcohol Avoid. Alcohol may increase the sedative effects of this drug.

Surgery and general anaesthetics Treatment with dosulepin may need to be stopped before you have a general anaesthetic. Discuss this with your doctor or dentist before any operation.

PROLONGED USE

No problems expected.

Doxazosin

Brand names Cardura, Cardura XL, Doxadura
Used in the following combined preparations None

QUICK REFERENCE

Drug group Vasodilator (p.31), antihypertensive drug (p.36), and drug for urinary disorders (p.112)
Overdose danger rating Medium
Dependence rating Low
Prescription needed Yes
Available as generic Yes

GENERAL INFORMATION

Doxazosin is an antihypertensive vasodilator drug that relieves hypertension (high blood pressure) by relaxing the muscles in the blood vessel walls, which, in turn, enables more blood to pass through. Because doxazosin is removed slowly from the body, it is usually given only once daily. It may be administered together with other antihypertensive drugs, including beta blockers, since its effects on blood pressure are increased when it is combined with most other antihypertensives. Doxazosin can also be given to patients with an enlarged prostate gland. It relaxes the muscles around the bladder exit and prostate gland allowing urine to flow out more easily.

Dizziness and fainting may occur at the onset of treatment with doxazosin, because the first dose may cause a marked fall in blood pressure. For this reason, the initial dose is usually low. It should be taken at home, preferably just before bedtime.

INFORMATION FOR USERS

Your drug prescription is tailored for you. Do not alter dosage without checking with your doctor.
How taken/used MR-tablets.
Frequency and timing of doses Once daily, at the same time each day.

Adult dosage range *Hypertension* 1mg (starting dose), increased gradually as necessary up to 16mg. *Enlarged prostate* 1mg (starting dose), increased gradually at 1–2-week intervals up to 8mg.
Onset of effect Within 2 hours.
Duration of action 24 hours.
Diet advice None.
Storage Keep in original container at room temperature out of the reach of children.
Missed dose If you forget to take a tablet, skip that dose completely but carry on as normal the following day.
Stopping the drug Do not stop taking the drug without consulting your doctor; stopping the drug may lead to a rise in blood pressure.
Exceeding the dose An occasional unintentional extra dose is unlikely to be a cause for concern. Larger overdoses may cause dizziness or fainting. Notify your doctor.

POSSIBLE ADVERSE EFFECTS

Nausea, weakness, drowsiness, and headache are common adverse effects of doxazosin. However, the main problem is that the drug may cause dizziness or fainting when you stand up. It may also cause a stuffy or runny nose and sleep disturbances. Consult your doctor if you develop a rash. If you experience chest pains or palpitations, consult your doctor urgently.

INTERACTIONS

Antihypertensive drugs Any drugs that can reduce blood pressure are likely to have an increased effect when taken with doxazosin. These include diuretics, beta blockers, ACE inhibitors, nitrates, calcium channel blockers, and some antipsychotics and antidepressants.

SPECIAL PRECAUTIONS

Be sure to tell your doctor if:
◆ You have long-term liver problems.
◆ You have had an allergic reaction to doxazosin in the past.
◆ You are due to have an operation.
◆ You are taking other medicines.
Pregnancy Safety in pregnancy not established. Discuss with your doctor.
Breast-feeding The drug passes into the breast milk. Discuss with your doctor.
Infants and children Not recommended.

Over 60 Reduced dose may be necessary. Take extra care when standing up until you have learned how the drug affects you.

Driving and hazardous work Avoid such activities until you have learned how doxazosin affects you because the drug can cause drowsiness, dizziness, and fainting.

Alcohol Avoid excessive amounts. Alcohol may increase some of the adverse effects of this drug, such as dizziness, drowsiness, and fainting.

Surgery and general anaesthetics A general anaesthetic may increase the blood-pressure-lowering effect of doxazosin.

PROLONGED USE
No known problems.

Doxorubicin

Brand names Caelyx, Myocet
Used in the following combined preparations
None

QUICK REFERENCE
Drug group Cytotoxic anticancer drug (p.96)
Overdose danger rating Medium
Dependence rating Low
Prescription needed Yes
Available as generic Yes

GENERAL INFORMATION
Doxorubicin is one of the most effective anticancer drugs. It is prescribed to treat a wide variety of cancers, usually in conjunction with other anticancer drugs. It is used in cancer of the lymph nodes (Hodgkin's disease), lung, breast, bladder, stomach, thyroid, and reproductive organs. It is also used to treat Kaposi's sarcoma in AIDS patients.

Nausea and vomiting after injection are the most common side effects of doxorubicin. Although these symptoms are unpleasant, they tend to be less severe as the body adjusts to treatment. The drug may stain the urine bright red, but this is not harmful. More seriously, because doxorubicin interferes with the production of blood cells, blood clotting disorders, anaemia, and infections may occur. Therefore, effects on the blood are carefully monitored. Hair loss is also a common side

effect. Rarely, heart rhythm disturbance and heart failure are dose-dependent side effects that may also occur.

The brand-name drugs Caelyx and Myocet are special formulations in which the doxorubicin is enclosed in fatty spheres. This makes the drug more suitable for treating certain types of cancers, for example AIDS-related Kaposi's sarcoma.

INFORMATION FOR USERS
This drug is given only under medical supervision and is not for self-administration.

How taken/used Injection, bladder instillation.
Frequency and timing of doses Every 1–3 weeks (injection); once a month (bladder instillation).
Adult dosage range Dosage is determined individually according to body height, weight, and response.
Onset of effect Some adverse effects may appear within 1 hour of starting treatment, but full beneficial effects may not be felt for up to 4 weeks.
Duration of action Adverse effects can persist for up to 2 weeks after stopping treatment.
Diet advice None.
Storage Not applicable. The drug is not normally kept in the home.
Missed dose The drug is administered in hospital under close medical supervision. If for some reason you skip your dose, contact your doctor as soon as you can.
Stopping the drug Discuss with your doctor. Stopping the drug prematurely may lead to a worsening of the underlying condition.
Exceeding the dose Overdose is unlikely as treatment is carefully monitored and supervised.

POSSIBLE ADVERSE EFFECTS
Nausea and vomiting generally occur within an hour of injection. Many people also experience hair loss and loss of appetite. Diarrhoea, mouth ulcers, and skin irritation or ulcers may also occur. Palpitations may indicate an adverse effect of the drug on the heart. Since treatment is closely supervised in hospital, all adverse effects are monitored.

INTERACTIONS
Ciclosporin Administration of ciclosporin while receiving doxorubicin can lead to adverse effects on the nervous system.

SPECIAL PRECAUTIONS

Doxorubicin is prescribed only under close medical supervision, taking account of your present condition and medical history.

Pregnancy Not usually prescribed. Doxorubicin may cause birth defects or premature birth. Discuss with your doctor.

Breast-feeding Not advised. The drug passes into the breast milk and may affect the baby adversely. Discuss with your doctor.

Infants and children Reduced dose necessary.

Over 60 Increased risk of adverse effects. Reduced dose may be necessary.

Driving and hazardous work No known problems.

Alcohol No known problems.

PROLONGED USE

Prolonged use of doxorubicin may reduce the activity of the bone marrow, leading to reduced production of all types of blood cell. The drug may also affect the heart adversely.

Monitoring Periodic checks on blood composition are usually required. Regular heart examinations are also carried out.

Doxycycline

Brand names Demix, Doxylar, Vibramycin, Vibramycin-D
Used in the following combined preparations None

QUICK REFERENCE

Drug group Tetracycline antibiotic (p.62)
Overdose danger rating Low
Dependence rating Low
Prescription needed Yes
Available as generic Yes

GENERAL INFORMATION

Doxycycline is a tetracycline antibiotic. It is used to treat infections of the urinary, respiratory, and gastrointestinal tracts. It is also prescribed for treatment of some sexually transmitted diseases, skin, eye, and prostate infections, acne, and malaria prevention (in some parts of the world, see p.75).

Doxycycline is less likely to cause diarrhoea than other tetracyclines, and its absorption is not significantly impaired by milk and food. It can therefore be taken with meals to reduce side effects such as nausea or indigestion. It is also safer than most other tetracyclines for people with impaired kidney function. Like other tetracyclines, it can stain developing teeth and may affect development of bone; it is therefore usually avoided in children under 12 years old and pregnant women.

INFORMATION FOR USERS

Your drug prescription is tailored for you. Do not alter dosage without checking with your doctor.

How taken/used Tablets, dispersible tablets, capsules.

Frequency and timing of doses 1–2 x daily with plenty of water, or with or after food, in a sitting or standing position, well before going to bed to avoid risk of throat irritation.

Dosage range 100–200mg daily.

Onset of effect 1–12 hours; several weeks (acne).

Duration of action Up to 24 hours; several weeks (acne).

Diet advice None.

Storage Keep in original container at room temperature out of the reach of children.

Missed dose Take as soon as you remember. If your next dose is due within 6 hours, take a single dose now and skip the next.

Stopping the drug Take the full course. Even if you feel better, the original infection may still be present and symptoms may recur if treatment is stopped too soon.

Exceeding the dose An occasional unintentional extra dose is unlikely to be a cause for concern. But if you notice any unusual symptoms, or if a large overdose has been taken, notify your doctor.

POSSIBLE ADVERSE EFFECTS

Adverse effects from doxycycline are rare, although nausea, vomiting, or diarrhoea may occur. Oesophageal ulcers (which may manifest as chest pain) may also occur; if so, you should consult your doctor without delay. If a rash, itching, or photosensitivity occur, you should stop taking the drug and talk to your doctor. If you experience headache or visual disturbances, you should stop taking the drug and consult your doctor urgently.

INTERACTIONS

Penicillin antibiotics Doxycycline interferes with the antibacterial action of these drugs.

Barbiturates, carbamazepine, and phenytoin All of these drugs reduce the effectiveness of doxycycline. Doxycycline dosage may need to be increased.

Oral contraceptives There is a slight risk of doxycycline reducing the effectiveness of oral contraceptives. Discuss with your doctor.

Oral anticoagulant drugs Doxycycline may increase the anticoagulant action of these drugs.

Antacids and preparations containing iron, calcium, or magnesium may impair absorption of this drug. Do not take within 2–3 hours of doxycycline.

Ciclosporin and lithium Doxycycline may increase levels of these drugs in the blood.

SPECIAL PRECAUTIONS

Be sure to tell your doctor if:
◆ You have a long-term liver problem.
◆ You have previously suffered an allergic reaction to a tetracycline antibiotic.
◆ You have porphyria.
◆ You have systemic lupus erythematosus.
◆ You have myasthenia gravis.
◆ You have a history of angioedema.
◆ You are taking other medicines.

Pregnancy Not used in pregnancy. May discolour the teeth of the developing baby.

Breast-feeding The drug passes into the breast milk and may lead to discoloration of the baby's teeth and may also have other adverse effects. Discuss with your doctor.

Infants and children Not recommended under 12 years. Reduced dose necessary for older children.

Over 60 No special problems. Dispersible tablets should be used as they are less likely to cause oesophageal irritation or ulceration.

Driving and hazardous work No known problems.

Alcohol Excessive amounts may decrease the effectiveness of doxycycline.

Surgery and general anaesthetics Before any operation notify your doctor or dentist that you are taking doxycycline.

PROLONGED USE

Not usually prescribed long term, except for acne.

Dydrogesterone

Brand names Duphaston, Duphaston HRT
Used in the following combined preparations
Femapak, Femoston

QUICK REFERENCE

Drug group Female sex hormone (p.88)
Overdose danger rating Low
Dependence rating Low
Prescription needed Yes
Available as generic No

GENERAL INFORMATION

Dydrogesterone is a progestogen, a synthetic hormone that is similar to the natural female sex hormone progesterone. The drug is widely used to treat a variety of menstrual disorders (see p.104) that are thought to result from a deficiency of progesterone. These include infertility, recurrent miscarriage, and absent, irregular, or painful periods.

Dydrogesterone is also prescribed together with an oestrogen as part of hormone replacement therapy (HRT) after the menopause. It may be prescribed for endometriosis (p.105).

Dydrogesterone is usually taken on selected days during the menstrual cycle, depending on the disorder that is being treated.

INFORMATION FOR USERS

Your drug prescription is tailored for you. Do not alter dosage without checking with your doctor.

How taken/used Tablets.

Frequency and timing of doses 1–3 x daily. In many conditions, this drug is taken at certain times in the menstrual cycle.

Adult dosage range 10–30mg daily.

Onset of effect Beneficial effects of this drug may not be felt for several months.

Duration of action 12 hours.

Diet advice None.

Storage Keep in original container at room temperature out of the reach of children. Protect from light.

Missed dose Take as soon as you remember. If your next dose is due within 2 hours, take a single dose now and skip the next.

Stopping the drug Do not stop the drug without consulting your doctor; symptoms may recur.

Exceeding the dose An occasional unintentional extra dose is unlikely to be a cause for concern. But if you notice any unusual symptoms, or if a large overdose has been taken, notify your doctor.

POSSIBLE ADVERSE EFFECTS

Irregular periods and "breakthrough" bleeding are the most common adverse effects of dydrogesterone. These symptoms may be helped by adjusting the dosage of the drug. Other common adverse effects include swollen feet or ankles, rash, and weight gain. More rarely, the drug may cause nausea, vomiting, and breast tenderness. You should talk to your doctor if any of these become severe or if the drug causes headache or dizziness.

INTERACTIONS

Anticonvulsants Some of these drugs may reduce the effect of dydrogesterone, and dydrogesterone may reduce the effect of the anticonvulsant lamotrigine.

Ciclosporin Dydrogesterone increases the effects of this drug.

SPECIAL PRECAUTIONS

Be sure to tell your doctor if:
◆ You have a long-term liver or kidney problem.
◆ You have heart or circulatory problems.
◆ You have diabetes.
◆ You have high blood pressure.
◆ You have porphyria.
◆ You or a member of your family have had breast cancer.
◆ You are taking other medicines.

Pregnancy No evidence of risk at normal dosage.

Breast-feeding The drug passes into the breast milk, but at normal doses adverse effects on the baby are unlikely. However, high doses of dydrogesterone may suppress milk production.

Infants and children Not prescribed.

Over 60 No special problems.

Driving and hazardous work Avoid such activities until you have learned how the drug affects you because dydrogesterone may rarely cause dizziness.

Alcohol No special problems.

PROLONGED USE

When used as part of HRT, dydrogesterone is usually advised only for short-term use around the menopause and is not normally recommended for long-term use or for treating osteoporosis.

Monitoring Blood-pressure checks and physical examinations, including regular mammograms, may be performed.

Efavirenz

Brand name Sustiva
Used in the following combined preparations
None

QUICK REFERENCE

Drug group Drug for HIV and immune deficiency (p.100)
Overdose danger rating Medium
Dependence rating Low
Prescription needed Yes
Available as generic No

GENERAL INFORMATION

Efavirenz is a non-nucleoside reverse transcriptase inhibitor, which is a type of antiretroviral drug that is used to treat HIV infection. It is used together with other antiretrovirals, for example two nucleoside analogues, as combination therapy to slow down the production of the virus. The aim of this treatment is to reduce the damage done to the immune system by the virus. Combination antiretroviral therapy is not a cure for HIV. If the drugs are taken regularly on a long-term basis, they can reduce the level of the virus in the body and improve the outlook for the HIV patient. However, the patient will remain infectious, and will suffer a relapse if treatment is stopped.

INFORMATION FOR USERS

Your drug prescription is tailored for you. Do not alter dosage without checking with your doctor.

How taken/used Tablets, capsules, liquid.

Frequency and timing of doses Once daily, usually at night to minimize adverse effects.

Adult dosage range 600mg, but may be reduced according to body weight.

Onset of effect 1 hour.

Duration of action 24 hours.

Diet advice None.

Storage Keep in the original container in a cool, dry place out of the reach of children.

Missed dose Take as soon as you remember. If your next dose is due within 2 hours, take a single dose now and skip the next. It is very important not to miss doses on a regular basis as this can lead to the development of drug-resistant HIV.

Stopping the drug Do not stop taking the drug without consulting your doctor. It may be necessary to withdraw all your drugs gradually, starting with efavirenz.

Exceeding the dose An occasional unintentional extra dose is unlikely to cause problems. But if you notice any unusual symptoms, or if a large overdose has been taken, notify your doctor.

POSSIBLE ADVERSE EFFECTS

Gastrointestinal upset, including nausea, vomiting and diarrhoea, and rash are the most common adverse effects. Efavirenz can cause vivid dreams and changes in sleep patterns, but these tend to wear off with time. If any of the symptoms are severe, or if mood changes occur, seek medical advice. If you develop a rash, contact your doctor without delay.

INTERACTIONS

General note A wide range of drugs may interact with efavirenz, causing either an increase in adverse effects or a reduction in the effect of the antiretroviral drugs. Check with your doctor or pharmacist before taking any new drugs, including those from the dentist and supermarket, and herbal medicines.

SPECIAL PRECAUTIONS

Be sure to tell your doctor if:
◆ You have liver or kidney problems.
◆ You have an infection such as hepatitis B or C.
◆ You are pregnant or planning pregnancy.
◆ You are taking other medicines.

Pregnancy Should not be used during pregnancy except on strict medical advice. Pregnancy should be avoided when taking efavirenz by using barrier methods of contraception in addition to other methods.

Breast-feeding Safety in breast-feeding not established. Breast-feeding is not recommended for HIV-positive mothers as the virus may be passed to the baby.

Infants and children Not prescribed to children under 3 years. Reduced dose necessary in older children.

Over 60 Reduced dose may be necessary.

Driving and hazardous work Avoid such activities until you have learned how efavirenz affects you because the drug can cause dizziness.

Alcohol No known problems, although some people may find the effects of alcohol are more pronounced while taking efavirenz.

PROLONGED USE

No known problems.

Monitoring Your doctor will take regular blood samples to check the drug's effects on the virus. Blood will also be checked for changes in lipid, cholesterol, and glucose levels.

Enalapril

Brand names Ednyt, Enacard, Innovace, Pralenal
Used in the following combined preparation Innozide

QUICK REFERENCE

Drug group ACE inhibitor vasodilator (p.31) and antihypertensive drug (p.36)
Overdose danger rating Medium
Dependence rating Low
Prescription needed Yes
Available as generic Yes

GENERAL INFORMATION

Enalapril belongs to the ACE inhibitor group of vasodilator drugs, which are used to treat hypertension (high blood pressure) and heart failure (inability of the heart to cope with its workload). It is also given to patients following a heart attack. Enalapril is often given with a diuretic to increase its effect.

The first dose of enalapril may cause a sudden drop in blood pressure. For this reason, you should be resting when you take your first dose and you should be able to lie down for 2 to 3 hours afterwards.

The more common adverse effects, such as dizziness and headache, usually diminish with long-term treatment. Rashes can also occur but usually disappear when the drug is stopped. In some cases, they clear up on their own despite continued treatment.

INFORMATION FOR USERS

Your drug prescription is tailored for you. Do not alter dosage without checking with your doctor.

How taken/used Tablets.

Frequency and timing of doses 1–2 x daily.

Adult dosage range 2.5–5mg daily (starting dose), increased to 10–40mg daily (maintenance dose).

Onset of effect Within 1 hour.

Duration of action 24 hours.

Diet advice None.

Storage Keep in original container below 25°C and out of the reach of children. Protect from light.

Missed dose Take as soon as you remember. If your next dose is due within 8 hours, take a single dose now and skip the next.

Stopping the drug Do not stop the drug without consulting your doctor; stopping the drug may lead to worsening of the underlying condition.

Exceeding the dose An occasional unintentional extra dose is unlikely to be a cause for concern. Large overdoses may cause dizziness or fainting. Notify your doctor.

POSSIBLE ADVERSE EFFECTS

Common adverse effects such as dizziness and headache usually diminish with long-term treatment. Less common problems may also diminish with time, but dose adjustment may be necessary. A rash may occur but usually disappears when the drug is stopped; consult your doctor if you develop a rash. A persistent dry cough is another common adverse effect; this can often be minimized by taking smaller, more frequent, doses, but alternative medication may be required; you should consult your doctor if you develop such a cough. Nausea, loss of appetite, and diarrhoea may sometimes occur; consult your doctor if they are severe. You should also consult your doctor if you experience fainting or muscle cramps. If you suffer from wheezing or swelling, stop taking the drug and seek urgent medical advice.

INTERACTIONS

Potassium supplements and potassium-sparing diuretics Enalapril may enhance the effect of these drugs, leading to raised levels of potassium in the blood.

Non-steroidal anti-inflammatory drugs (NSAIDs) Some of these drugs may reduce the effectiveness of enalapril. There is also risk of kidney damage when they are taken with enalapril.

Antihypertensive drugs These drugs are likely to enhance the blood pressure-lowering effect of enalapril.

Lithium Enalapril increases the levels of lithium in the blood, and serious adverse effects from lithium excess may occur.

Ciclosporin Taken with enalapril, this drug may increase blood levels of potassium.

SPECIAL PRECAUTIONS

Be sure to tell your doctor if:
◆ You have a long-term kidney problem.
◆ You have a liver problem.
◆ You have a heart problem.
◆ You have angioedema.
◆ You have had a previous allergic reaction to an ACE inhibitor drug.
◆ You are taking other medicines.

Pregnancy Not prescribed. May cause abnormalities in the fetus. Discuss with your doctor.

Breast-feeding The drug passes into the breast milk, but at normal doses adverse effects on the baby are unlikely. Discuss with your doctor.

Infants and children Not recommended.

Over 60 Reduced dose may be necessary.

Driving and hazardous work Avoid such activities until you have learned how enalapril affects you because the drug can cause dizziness and fainting.

Alcohol Avoid. When taken with enalapril, alcohol increases the likelihood of an excessive drop in blood pressure that may cause dizziness.

Surgery and general anaesthetics Discuss with your doctor or dentist before any operation.

PROLONGED USE

No problems expected.

Monitoring Periodic tests on blood and urine should be performed.

Ephedrine

Brand name Cam
Used in the following combined preparations
Do-Do Chesteze, Franol, Franol Plus, Haymine, and others

QUICK REFERENCE

Drug group Bronchodilator (p.23) and decongestant (p.26)
Overdose danger rating Medium
Dependence rating Low
Prescription needed No
Available as generic Yes

GENERAL INFORMATION

In use for more than 50 years, ephedrine promotes the release of norephedrine, a neurotransmitter. It was once widely prescribed as a bronchodilator to relax the muscles surrounding the airways, easing breathing difficulty caused by asthma, bronchitis, and emphysema. More effective drugs have largely replaced ephedrine for these uses. Its main use now is as a decongestant in nasal drops and cough preparations. Ephedrine injections may be used as a method of restoring normal blood pressure after anaesthetic procedures.

Adverse effects are unusual from nasal drops used in moderation, but taken by mouth or injection the drug may stimulate the heart and central nervous system, causing palpitations and anxiety. It is not recommended for the elderly, who are more sensitive to ephedrine's effects on the heart, and the drug may also cause urinary retention in elderly men.

INFORMATION FOR USERS

Follow instructions on the label. Call your doctor if symptoms worsen.
How taken/used Tablets, liquid, injection, nasal drops.
Frequency and timing of doses *By mouth* 3 x daily. *Nasal drops* 3–4 x daily.
Dosage range *Adults* 45–180mg daily (by mouth); 1–2 drops into each nostril per dose (drops); 3–6mg every 3–4 minutes to a maximum of 30mg (injection). *Children* Reduced dose according to age and weight.
Onset of effect Within 15–60 minutes.
Duration of action 3–6 hours.

Diet advice None.
Storage Keep in original container at room temperature out of the reach of children. Protect from light.
Missed dose Do not take the missed dose. Take your next dose as usual.
Stopping the drug Can be safely stopped as soon as you no longer need it.
Exceeding the dose An occasional unintentional extra dose is unlikely to cause problems. Large overdoses may cause shortness of breath, high fever, fits, or loss of consciousness. Notify your doctor immediately.

POSSIBLE ADVERSE EFFECTS

Adverse effects from ephedrine nasal drops are uncommon, although local irritation can occur. When taken by mouth, the drug may affect the central nervous system, causing anxiety, restlessness, and insomnia; however, taking the last dose before 4pm may help to prevent insomnia. Ephedrine may also affect the cardiovascular system, causing palpitations or chest pain; if these occur, stop taking the drug and seek urgent medical advice. Other adverse effects include cold hands and feet, a dry mouth, and tremor; consult your doctor if these are severe. You may also experience urinary difficulties; if so, discuss with your doctor.

INTERACTIONS

Monoamine oxidase inhibitors (MAOIs) Ephedrine may interact with these drugs to cause a dangerous rise in blood pressure.
Beta blockers Ephedrine may interact with these drugs to cause a dangerous rise in blood pressure.
Antihypertensive drugs Ephedrine may counteract the effects of some antihypertensive drugs.
Theophylline taken with ephedrine can lower potassium levels in children. The two drugs should not be given together.

SPECIAL PRECAUTIONS

Be sure to consult your doctor or pharmacist before taking this drug if:
◆ You have a long-term kidney problem.
◆ You have heart disease.
◆ You have high blood pressure.
◆ You have diabetes.

◆ You have an overactive thyroid gland.
◆ You have glaucoma.
◆ You have urinary difficulties.
◆ You are taking other medicines.

Pregnancy Safety in pregnancy not established. Discuss with your doctor.
Breast-feeding The drug passes into the breast milk and may affect the baby. Discuss with your doctor.
Infants and children Reduced dose necessary.
Over 60 Not usually prescribed.
Driving and hazardous work Avoid such activities until you have learned how ephedrine affects you. No special problems with nasal drops.
Alcohol No special problems.
Surgery and general anaesthetics Ephedrine may need to be stopped before you have a general anaesthetic. Discuss this with your doctor or dentist before surgery.

PROLONGED USE

Prolonged use (more than a week) is not recommended except on medical advice. When ephedrine is used as nasal drops, decongestant effects may lessen and rebound congestion may occur.

Epinephrine (adrenaline)

Brand names Ana-Guard, Ana-Kit, Anapen, EpiPen, Minijet
Used in the following combined preparations Ganda, several local anaesthetics (e.g. Xylocaine)

QUICK REFERENCE

Drug group Drug for cardiac resuscitation and anaphylaxis
Overdose danger rating High
Dependence rating Low
Prescription needed Yes
Available as generic Yes

GENERAL INFORMATION

Epinephrine is a neurotransmitter that is produced in the centre (medulla) of the adrenal glands, hence its original name, adrenaline. Synthetic epinephrine has been made since 1900. The drug is given in an emergency to stimulate heart activity and raise low blood pressure. It also narrows blood vessels in the skin and intestine.

Epinephrine is injected to counteract cardiac arrest, or to relieve severe allergic reactions (anaphylaxis) to drugs, food, or insect stings. For patients who are at risk of anaphylaxis, it is provided as a pre-filled syringe for immediate self-injection at the start of an attack.

Because it constricts blood vessels, epinephrine is used to control bleeding and to slow the dispersal, and thereby prolong the effect, of local anaesthetics.

INFORMATION FOR USERS

Your drug prescription is tailored for you and patients at risk of anaphylaxis will be instructed in advance about how to use their epinephrine. Do not alter dosage without checking with your doctor.
How taken/used Injection.
Frequency and timing of doses As directed; by itself, the drug is for use in emergencies.
Dosage range As directed.
Onset of effect Within 5 minutes.
Duration of action Up to 4 hours.
Diet advice None.
Storage Keep in original container at room temperature out of the reach of children. Protect from light.
Missed dose Not applicable. By itself, the drug is used for one-off emergencies.
Stopping the drug Not applicable. By itself, the drug is used for one-off emergencies.

OVERDOSE ACTION

Seek immediate medical advice in all cases. Take emergency action if palpitations, breathing difficulties, or loss of consciousness occur.

POSSIBLE ADVERSE EFFECTS

The principal adverse effects of this drug are related to its stimulant action on the heart and central nervous system. Dry mouth, nervousness, restlessness, nausea, vomiting, cold extremities, palpitations, headache, and blurred vision are common. As epinephrine by itself is used in emergency situations, medical help should always be sought after its use.

INTERACTIONS

General note Epinephrine may interact with various drugs, including some beta blockers, such as propranolol; monoamine oxidase inhibitors

(MAOIs); tricyclic antidepressants, such as amitriptyline; and antidiabetic drugs. However, because epinephrine is usually used only to treat life-threatening medical emergencies, possible drug interactions are usually of secondary importance.

SPECIAL PRECAUTIONS

Be sure to tell your doctor if:
◆ You have a heart problem.
◆ You have diabetes.
◆ You have an overactive thyroid gland.
◆ You have a nervous system problem.
◆ You have high blood pressure.
◆ You are taking other medicines.

Pregnancy Discuss with your doctor. Although the drug may cause defects in the fetus and prolong labour, epinephrine by itself is used only for medical emergencies and its use may be life-saving.

Breast-feeding Adverse effects on the baby are unlikely. Discuss with your doctor.

Infants and children Reduced dose necessary.

Over 60 Increased likelihood of adverse effects. Reduced dose may therefore be necessary.

Driving and hazardous work Not applicable. By itself, the drug is used for one-off medical emergencies.

Alcohol No known problems.

Surgery and general anaesthetics Epinephrine may interact with some general anaesthetics. If you have recently used or been treated with epinephrine alone or if it is a component of a combined medication, tell your doctor or dentist before surgery.

PROLONGED USE

Epinephrine is not normally used long term.

Ergotamine

Brand names None
Used in the following combined preparations
Cafergot, Migril

QUICK REFERENCE

Drug group Drug for migraine (p.20)
Overdose danger rating Medium
Dependence rating Medium
Prescription needed Yes
Available as generic Yes

GENERAL INFORMATION

Ergotamine is used to treat migraine attacks, but its use has largely been superseded by newer agents with fewer adverse effects. It may also be used in the prevention of cluster headaches. For migraine, it should be restricted to when other treatments are ineffective, and it should be taken only at the first sign of migraine (the "aura"); later use may be ineffective and cause stomach upset.

Ergotamine causes temporary narrowing of blood vessels and therefore should not be used by people with poor circulation. If taken too frequently, the drug can dangerously reduce circulation to the hands and feet; it should never be taken regularly. Frequent migraine attacks may indicate the need for a drug to prevent migraine.

INFORMATION FOR USERS

Your drug prescription is tailored for you. Do not alter dosage without checking with your doctor.

How taken/used Tablets, suppositories.

Frequency and timing of doses Once at the onset, repeated if needed after 30 minutes (tablets) up to the maximum dose (see below).

Adult dosage range Varies according to product. Generally, 1–2mg per dose. Take no more than 4mg in 24 hours or 8mg in 1 week. Treatment should not be repeated within 4 days or more than twice a month.

Onset of effect 15–30 minutes.

Duration of action Up to 24 hours.

Diet advice Changes in diet are unlikely to affect the action of ergotamine, but certain foods may provoke migraine attacks in some people.

Storage Keep in original container at room temperature out of the reach of children. Protect from light.

Missed dose Regular doses of this drug are not necessary and may be dangerous. Take only when you have symptoms of migraine.

Stopping the drug Can be safely stopped as soon as you no longer need it.

Exceeding the dose An occasional unintentional extra dose is unlikely to cause problems. Large overdoses may cause vomiting, thirst, diarrhoea, dizziness, fits, or coma. Notify your doctor immediately.

POSSIBLE ADVERSE EFFECTS

Digestive disturbances, abdominal pain, muscle cramps, and nausea (for which an anti-emetic may be given) are common with ergotamine treatment. Diarrhoea, dizziness, and muscle pain or stiffness may also occur. Cold or numb fingers and toes are rare but serious effects that may result from arterial spasm. If these symptoms occur, or if you experience chest pain, leg pain, or groin pain, stop taking the drug and seek immediate medical advice.

INTERACTIONS

Beta blockers These drugs may increase circulatory problems with ergotamine.

Sumatriptan and related drugs There is an increased risk of adverse effects on the blood circulation if ergotamine is used with these drugs.

Erythromycin and related antibiotics and antivirals taken with ergotamine increase the likelihood of adverse effects.

Oral contraceptives There is an increased risk of blood clotting in women taking these drugs with ergotamine.

SPECIAL PRECAUTIONS

Be sure to tell your doctor if:
◆ You have long-term liver or kidney problems.
◆ You have heart problems.
◆ You have poor circulation.
◆ You have high blood pressure.
◆ You have had a recent stroke.
◆ You have an overactive thyroid gland.
◆ You have anaemia.
◆ You are taking other medicines.

Pregnancy Not prescribed. Ergotamine can cause contractions of the uterus.

Breast-feeding Not recommended. The drug passes into the milk and may have adverse effects on the baby. It may also reduce your milk supply.

Infants and children Not usually prescribed.

Over 60 Not recommended. May aggravate existing heart or circulatory problems.

Driving and hazardous work Avoid such activities until you have learned how ergotamine affects you because the drug can cause vertigo.

Alcohol No special problems, but some spirits may provoke migraine in some people.

Surgery and general anaesthetics Notify your doctor if you have used ergotamine within 48 hours prior to surgery.

PROLONGED USE

Reduced circulation to the hands and feet may result if doses near to the maximum are taken for too long. The recommended dosage and length of treatment should not be exceeded. Rebound headache may occur if the drug is taken too frequently.

Erythromycin

Brand names Erymax, Erythrocin, Erythroped, Primacine, Rommix, Stiemycin, Tiloryth
Used in the following combined preparations Aknemycin Plus, Benzamycin, Isotrexin, Zineryt

QUICK REFERENCE
Drug group Antibiotic (p.62)
Overdose danger rating Low
Dependence rating Low
Prescription needed Yes
Available as generic Yes

GENERAL INFORMATION

One of the safest and most widely used antibiotics, erythromycin is effective against many different bacteria. The drug is commonly used as an alternative treatment in people who are allergic to penicillin and related antibiotics.

Erythromycin is used to treat infections of the throat, middle ear, and chest (including some rare types of pneumonia such as Legionnaires' disease). It is also used for sexually transmitted diseases such as chlamydial infections, and in some forms of gastroenteritis. Erythromycin may also be included as part of the treatment for diphtheria and is sometimes given to treat, and reduce the likelihood of infecting others with, pertussis (whooping cough).

When taken by mouth, erythromycin may sometimes cause nausea and vomiting. Other possible adverse effects of the drug include rash as well as a rare risk of liver disorders. Oral administration or topical application of erythromycin is sometimes helpful in treating acne.

INFORMATION FOR USERS

Your drug prescription is tailored for you. Do not alter dosage without consulting your doctor.

How taken/used Tablets, capsules, liquid, injection, topical solution.

Frequency and timing of doses Every 6–12 hours before or with meals.

Dosage range 1–4g daily.

Onset of effect 1–4 hours.

Duration of action 6–12 hours.

Diet advice None.

Storage Keep in original container at room temperature out of the reach of children.

Missed dose Take as soon as you remember. If your next dose is due within 2 hours, take a single dose now and skip the next.

Stopping the drug Take the full course. Even if you feel better, the original infection may still be present and symptoms may recur if treatment is stopped too soon.

Exceeding the dose An occasional unintentional extra dose is unlikely to be a cause for concern. But if you notice any unusual symptoms, or if a large overdose has been taken, notify your doctor.

POSSIBLE ADVERSE EFFECTS

Nausea and vomiting are common adverse effects of erythromycin and most likely with large doses taken by mouth. Diarrhoea is also common. Deafness is a rare adverse effect that may occur with high doses; if you develop impaired hearing, consult your doctor without delay. Symptoms such as rash, itching, skin blisters or ulcers, jaundice, and fever may also occur; if you develop any of these symptoms, stop taking the drug and consult your doctor immediately.

INTERACTIONS

General note Erythromycin interacts with a number of other drugs, particularly:

Mizolastine Erythromycin increases the risk of adverse effects on the heart with this drug.

Warfarin Erythromycin increases the risk of bleeding with warfarin.

Ergotamine Erythromycin increases the risk of side effects with this drug.

Carbamazepine, digoxin, and some immunosuppressants Erythromycin may increase blood levels of these drugs.

Theophylline/aminophylline Erythromycin increases the risk of adverse effects with these drugs.

Simvastatin and other drugs ending in "statin" Erythromycin should not be taken with simvastatin; increased risk of muscle aches and pains with other statins.

SPECIAL PRECAUTIONS

Be sure to tell your doctor if:
◆ You have a long-term liver problem.
◆ You have had a previous allergic reaction to erythromycin.
◆ You have porphyria.
◆ You are taking other medicines.

Pregnancy No evidence of risk to the developing fetus. Discuss with your doctor.

Breast-feeding The drug passes into the breast milk, but at normal doses adverse effects on the baby are unlikely. Discuss with your doctor.

Infants and children Reduced dose necessary.

Over 60 No special problems.

Driving and hazardous work No known problems.

Alcohol No known problems.

PROLONGED USE

Oral courses of longer than 14 days may increase the risk of liver damage.

Erythropoietin (epoetin, darbepoetin)

Brand names Aranesp, Eprex, NeoRecormon
Used in the following combined preparations
None

QUICK REFERENCE

Drug group Kidney hormone (p.80)
Overdose danger rating Low
Dependence rating Low
Prescription needed Yes
Available as generic No

GENERAL INFORMATION

Erythropoietin is a naturally occurring hormone produced by the kidneys; it stimulates the body to produce red blood cells. Epoetin and darbepoetin are manufactured forms of erythropoietin that are used to treat anaemia associated with chronic kidney disease.

Epoetin is available in two forms (alpha and beta) both of which may also be used to treat anaemia caused by certain cancer treatments. They are also used to boost the level of red blood cells before surgery. Patients donate blood before surgery and this is then used during or after the surgery. Epoetin may also be used as an alternative to blood transfusions in major orthopaedic (bone) surgery.

Darbepoetin is a derivative of epoetin and it has a longer duration of action. It can, therefore, be given less frequently.

Both epoetin and darbepoetin have been used by athletes to enhance their performance. However, this is not a recognized use of the drugs and they are banned by sport governing bodies.

INFORMATION FOR USERS

Your drug prescription is tailored for you. Do not alter dosage without checking with your doctor.

How taken/used Injection.

Frequency and timing of doses 1–3 x weekly, depending on the product and condition being treated.

Dosage range Dosage is calculated on an individual basis according to body weight. The dosage also varies depending on the product and condition being treated.

Onset of effect Active inside the body within 4 hours, but effects may not be noted for 2–3 months.

Duration of action Some effects may persist for several days.

Diet advice None, but if you have kidney failure, you may have to follow a special diet.

Storage Store at 2–8°C, out of the reach of children. Do not freeze or shake. Protect from light.

Missed dose Do not make up any missed doses.

Stopping the drug Discuss with your doctor.

Exceeding the dose A single excessive dose is unlikely to be a cause for concern. Too high a dose over a long period can increase the likelihood of adverse effects.

POSSIBLE ADVERSE EFFECTS

The most common adverse effects are increased blood pressure and problems at the site of the injection. More rarely, there may be flu-like symptoms, bone pain, seizures, rash, or a stabbing headache. All unusual symptoms should be discussed with your doctor immediately.

INTERACTIONS

ACE inhibitors These drugs may increase the level of potassium in the blood and epoetin may enhance the blood pressure-lowering effect of ACE inhibitors.

Iron supplements These may increase the effect of epoetin if you have a low level of iron in your blood.

SPECIAL PRECAUTIONS

Be sure to tell your doctor if:
◆ You have high blood pressure.
◆ You have a long-term liver problem.
◆ You have previously suffered allergic reactions to any drugs.
◆ You have peripheral vascular disease.
◆ You have had epileptic fits.
◆ You are taking other medicines.

Pregnancy Not usually prescribed. Safety in pregnancy not established. Discuss with your doctor.

Breast-feeding Safety not established. Discuss with your doctor.

Infants and children Reduced dose necessary.

Over 60 No known problems.

Driving and hazardous work Not applicable.

Alcohol Follow your doctor's advice regarding alcohol.

PROLONGED USE

The long-term effects of the drug are still under investigation, but problems are unlikely if treatment is carefully monitored.

Monitoring Regular blood tests to monitor blood composition and blood pressure monitoring are required.

Estradiol

Brand names Aerodiol, Climaval, Estraderm, FemSeven, Menorest, Oestrogel, Progynova, Zumenon, and others

Used in the following combined preparations
Climagest, Climesse, Estracombi, Femapak, Trisequens, and others

QUICK REFERENCE

Drug group Female sex hormone (p.88)
Overdose danger rating Low
Dependence rating Low
Prescription needed Yes
Available as generic Yes

GENERAL INFORMATION

Estradiol is a naturally occurring oestrogen (female sex hormone). It is used mainly as hormone replacement therapy (HRT) for menopausal and post-menopausal symptoms such as hot flushes, night sweats, and vaginal atrophy. Estradiol is often given with a progestogen, either as separate drugs or as a combined product. In certain cases, treatment is for a specific number of days each month; follow your doctor's instructions carefully.

Taken alone, estradiol is associated with an increased risk of cancer of the uterus. For this reason, it is usually combined with a progestogen to reduce the risk; it is usually used alone in women who have had a hysterectomy. HRT is usually only advised for short-term use around the menopause.

Estradiol is available in a variety of forms, including implants, skin gel, and patches. Skin patches of the drug may cause local rash and itching.

INFORMATION FOR USERS

Your drug prescription is tailored for you. Do not alter dosage without checking with your doctor.
How taken/used Tablets, implants, pessaries, vaginal rings, skin gel, patches, nasal spray.
Frequency and timing of doses Once daily (tablets, gel); every 1–7 days (skin patches); every 4–8 months (implants); every 1–7 days (pessaries); every 3 months (vaginal ring); 1–4 sprays daily (nasal spray).
Adult dosage range 1–2mg daily (tablets); 2–4 measures daily (skin gel); 25–100mcg daily (skin patches); 25–100mg per dose (implants); 25mcg per dose (pessaries); 7.5mcg daily (vaginal ring); 150–600mcg daily (nasal spray).
Onset of effect 10–20 days.
Duration of action Up to 24 hours; some effects may be longer lasting.
Diet advice None.

Storage Keep in original container at room temperature out of the reach of children.
Missed dose Take as soon as you remember. If your next daily treatment is due within 4 hours, take a single dose now and skip the next.
Stopping the drug Do not stop the drug without consulting your doctor; symptoms may recur.
Exceeding the dose An occasional unintentional extra dose is unlikely to be a cause for concern. But if you notice any unusual symptoms, or if a large overdose has been taken, notify your doctor.

POSSIBLE ADVERSE EFFECTS

The most common adverse effects of estradiol are similar to symptoms of early pregnancy, and generally diminish with time. They include nausea or vomiting, breast swelling or tenderness, and weight gain. Headache and depression may also occur. Sudden sharp pain in the chest, groin, or legs may indicate a blood clot; if you experience such pain, stop taking the drug and seek urgent medical help.

INTERACTIONS

Tobacco smoking This increases the risk of serious adverse effects on the heart and circulation with estradiol.
Anticonvulsants The effects of estradiol are reduced by topiramate, carbamazepine, phenytoin, and phenobarbital; estradiol reduces the effects of lamotrigine.
Anticoagulant drugs The effects of these drugs are reduced by estradiol.
St John's wort may reduce the effects of estradiol.
Rifampicin This drug may reduce the effects of estradiol.

SPECIAL PRECAUTIONS

Be sure to tell your doctor if:
◆ You have a long-term liver problem.
◆ You have heart or circulation problems.
◆ You have porphyria.
◆ You have had blood clots or a stroke.
◆ You have diabetes.
◆ You are a smoker.
◆ You suffer from migraine or epilepsy.
◆ You are taking other medicines.

Pregnancy Not prescribed.
Breast-feeding Not prescribed. The drug passes into breast milk and may inhibit its flow. Discuss with your doctor.
Infants and children Not usually prescribed.
Over 60 No special problems.
Driving and hazardous work No problems expected.
Alcohol No known problems.
Surgery and general anaesthetics You may need to stop taking estradiol several weeks before having major surgery. Discuss this with your doctor.

PROLONGED USE
When used as part of HRT, estradiol is usually advised only for short-term use around the menopause and is not normally recommended for long-term use or for treatment of osteoporosis.
Monitoring Blood pressure checks and physical examinations, including regular mammograms, may be performed.

Ethambutol

Brand names None
Used in the following combined preparations
None

QUICK REFERENCE
Drug group Antituberculous drug (p.67)
Overdose danger rating Medium
Dependence rating Low
Prescription needed Yes
Available as generic Yes

GENERAL INFORMATION
Ethambutol is an antibiotic used in the treatment of tuberculosis. It is combined with other antituberculous drugs to enhance its effect and reduce the risk of the infection becoming drug resistant. Ethambutol is not used in all cases of tuberculosis. It is more likely to be used in people with a history of tuberculosis; those with a low immune status; and in those in whom the infection may be caused by a resistant organism. Although the drug has few common adverse effects, it may occasionally cause optic neuritis, a type of eye damage leading to blurring and fading of vision. As a result, ethambutol is not usually prescribed for children under six years of age or for other patients who are unable to communicate their symptoms adequately. Before starting treatment, a full ophthalmic examination is recommended.

INFORMATION FOR USERS
Your drug prescription is tailored for you. Do not alter dosage without checking with your doctor.
How taken/used Tablets.
Frequency and timing of doses Once daily.
Adult dosage range Dosage is calculated according to body weight.
Onset of effect It may take several days for symptoms to improve.
Duration of action Up to 24 hours.
Diet advice None.
Storage Keep in original container at room temperature out of the reach of children.
Missed dose Take as soon as you remember. If your next dose is due within 6 hours, take a single dose now and skip the next.
Stopping the drug Take the full course. Even if you feel better, the original infection may still be present and may recur if treatment is stopped too soon.
Exceeding the dose An occasional unintentional extra dose is unlikely to cause problems. However, large overdoses may cause headache and abdominal pain. Notify your doctor.

POSSIBLE ADVERSE EFFECTS
Side effects are uncommon with this drug but are more likely after prolonged treatment at high doses. They include nausea, vomiting, dizziness, and numbness or tingling in the hands or feet. If a rash or itching develop, stop taking the drug and consult your doctor. If you develop blurred vision, eye pain, or loss of colour vision you should stop taking the drug and seek prompt medical attention.

INTERACTIONS
Antacids Those containing aluminium salts may decrease levels of ethambutol, and should be taken at least 2 hours before or after ethambutol.

SPECIAL PRECAUTIONS
Be sure to tell your doctor if:
◆ You have a kidney problem.
◆ You have cataracts or other eye problems.
◆ You have gout.
◆ You have had a previous allergic reaction to this drug.
◆ You are taking other medicines.
Pregnancy Safety in pregnancy not established. Discuss with your doctor.
Breast-feeding The drug passes into the breast milk, but at normal doses adverse effects on the baby are unlikely. Discuss with your doctor.
Infants and children Not generally prescribed under 6 years, and often not under 13 years.
Over 60 Increased likelihood of adverse effects. Reduced dose may therefore be necessary.
Driving and hazardous work Avoid such activities until you have learned how ethambutol affects you because the drug may cause dizziness.
Alcohol No known problems.

PROLONGED USE
Prolonged use of ethambutol may increase the risk of eye damage.
Monitoring Periodic eye tests usually needed.

Ethinylestradiol

Used in the following combined preparations
Co-cyprindiol, various combined oral contraceptives (e.g. Brevinor, Dianette, Eugynon 30, Femodene, Loestrin, Microgynon 30, Norimin, Ovranette, Ovysmen)

QUICK REFERENCE
Drug group Female sex hormone (p.88) and oral contraceptive (p.105)
Overdose danger rating Low
Dependence rating Low
Prescription needed Yes
Available as generic Yes

GENERAL INFORMATION
Ethinylestradiol is a synthetic oestrogen that is similar to estradiol, a natural female sex hormone. Ethinylestradiol is widely used in oral contraceptives, in combination with a synthetic progestogen.

Ethinylestradiol is sometimes given to control heavy bleeding from the uterus and to treat delayed female sexual development (hypogonadism). It is also sometimes used alone for the short-term treatment of menopausal symptoms and to prevent osteoporosis when other drugs cannot be used. Certain prostate cancers respond to it. With cyproterone, it is used to treat severe acne in women.

Women taking an oral contraceptive pill containing ethinylestradiol have an increased risk of thrombosis (a blood clot) developing. This risk increases in overweight women and smokers.

INFORMATION FOR USERS
Your drug prescription is tailored for you. Do not alter dosage without checking with your doctor.
How taken/used Tablets.
Frequency and timing of doses Once daily. Often at certain times of the menstrual cycle.
Adult dosage range *Menopausal symptoms* 10–20mcg daily. *Hormone deficiency* 10–50mcg daily. *Combined contraceptive pills* 20–40mcg daily, depending on preparation. *Acne* 35mcg daily. *Prostate cancer* 0.15–1.5mg daily.
Onset of effect 10–20 days. Contraceptive protection is effective after 7 days in most cases.
Duration of action 1–2 days.
Diet advice None.
Storage Keep in original container at room temperature out of the reach of children.
Missed dose Take as soon as you remember. If your next dose is due within 4 hours, take a single dose now and skip the next dose. If you are taking the drug for contraceptive purposes, see What to do if you miss a pill (p.109).
Stopping the drug Do not stop the drug without consulting your doctor. Contraceptive protection is lost unless an alternative is used.
Exceeding the dose An occasional unintentional extra dose is unlikely to be a cause for concern. But if you notice any unusual symptoms, or if a large overdose has been taken, notify your doctor.

POSSIBLE ADVERSE EFFECTS
The most common adverse effects include nausea, vomiting, breast swelling or tenderness, weight gain, and bleeding between

periods. They generally diminish with time. Headache and depression may also occur. Sudden, sharp pain in the chest, groin, or legs may indicate an abnormal blood clot. If you experience such pain or if you develop sudden breathlessness, itching, or jaundice, stop taking the drug and seek urgent medical attention.

INTERACTIONS

Tobacco smoking This increases the risk of serious adverse effects on the heart and circulation with ethinylestradiol.

Rifampicin and anticonvulsants These drugs significantly reduce the effectiveness of oral contraceptives containing ethinylestradiol.

Antihypertensive drugs and diuretics Ethinylestradiol may reduce the effectiveness of these drugs.

Antibiotics and St John's wort may reduce the effectiveness of oral contraceptives containing ethinylestradiol.

SPECIAL PRECAUTIONS

Be sure to tell your doctor if:
◆ You have heart failure or high blood pressure.
◆ You or a close relative have had blood clots or a stroke.
◆ You have a long-term liver problem.
◆ You have had breast or endometrial cancer.
◆ You have sickle cell anaemia.
◆ You have porphyria.
◆ You are a smoker.
◆ You have diabetes.
◆ You suffer from migraine or epilepsy.
◆ You are taking other medicines.

Pregnancy Not prescribed. High doses may adversely affect the baby. Discuss with your doctor.

Breast-feeding The drug passes into the breast milk; it may also inhibit milk flow. Discuss with your doctor.

Infants and children Not usually prescribed.

Over 60 No special problems.

Driving and hazardous work No known problems.

Alcohol No known problems.

Surgery and general anaesthetics Ethinylestradiol may need to be stopped several weeks before you have major surgery. Discuss this with your doctor.

PROLONGED USE

When used as part of HRT, ethinylestradiol is usually only advised for short-term use around the menopause and is not normally recommended for long-term use or for treatment of osteoporosis.

Monitoring Physical examinations and blood pressure checks may be performed.

Etidronate

Brand names Didronel, Didronel PMO
Used in the following combined preparations
None

QUICK REFERENCE

Drug group Drug for bone disorders (p.56)
Overdose danger rating Medium
Dependence rating Low
Prescription needed Yes
Available as generic No

GENERAL INFORMATION

Etidronate is given for the treatment of bone disorders such as Paget's disease. It acts only on the bones, reducing the activity of the bone cells and thereby stopping the progress of the disease. This action also stops calcium from being released from the bones into the bloodstream, so it reduces the amount of calcium in the blood. Etidronate is also used together with calcium tablets to treat osteoporosis in post-menopausal women and to prevent and treat steroid-induced osteoporosis.

Generally, the drug's side effects are mild. The most common is diarrhoea, which is more likely to occur with higher doses. If taken at high doses (20mg/kg body weight daily), the drug stops new bone from being formed properly, which can lead to thinning of the bones and fractures. For this reason, high doses must be carefully monitored and used for as short a time as possible. The effect is reversed on stopping the drug.

INFORMATION FOR USERS

Your drug prescription is tailored for you. Do not alter dosage without checking with your doctor.

How taken/used Tablets.

Frequency and timing of doses Once daily on an empty stomach, 2 hours before or after food (absorption of the drug is reduced by food).

Dosage range *Paget's disease* 5–20mg/kg body weight daily for a maximum of 3–6 months. Courses may be repeated after a break of at least 3 months. *Osteoporosis* 400mg daily for 2 weeks, repeated every 3 months.

Onset of effect *Paget's disease/osteoporosis* Beneficial effects of the drug may not be felt for several months.

Duration of action Some effects may persist for several weeks or months.

Diet advice Absorption of etidronate is reduced by foods, especially those containing calcium (e.g. dairy products), so the drug should be taken on an empty stomach. The diet must contain adequate calcium and vitamin D; supplements may be given.

Storage Keep in original container below 30°C out of the reach of children. Protect from light.

Missed dose Take as soon as you remember. If your next dose of the drug is due within 6 hours, take a single dose now and skip the next one.

Stopping the drug Do not stop the drug without consulting your doctor. Stopping the drug may lead to worsening of the underlying condition.

Exceeding the dose An occasional unintentional extra dose is unlikely to cause any problems. However, large overdoses may cause numbness and muscle spasm. Notify your doctor.

POSSIBLE ADVERSE EFFECTS

The most common side effect, diarrhoea, is more likely to occur if the dose of etidronate is increased above 5mg/kg daily. Other common side effects include nausea, constipation, and abdominal pain. More rarely, etidronate may cause headache, rash or itching, bone pain, bruising, fever, and sore throat. In some patients with Paget's disease, bone pain may be increased initially, but this symptom usually disappears with further treatment. However, if you experience bone pain, bruising, fever, or a sore throat, you should notify your doctor without delay.

INTERACTIONS

Antacids and products containing calcium, magnesium, or iron These products should be given at least 2 hours before or after etidronate to minimize the risk of reduced absorption of etidronate.

SPECIAL PRECAUTIONS

Be sure to tell your doctor if:
◆ You have a long-term kidney problem.
◆ You have osteomalacia.
◆ You have had a previous allergic reaction to etidronate or to other bisphosphonate drugs.
◆ You have an overactive parathyroid gland.
◆ You have a high concentration of calcium in your blood or urine.
◆ You have colitis.
◆ You are taking other medicines.

Pregnancy Safety in pregnancy not established. Discuss with your doctor.

Breast-feeding Safety in breast-feeding not established. Discuss with your doctor.

Infants and children Not recommended.

Over 60 No special problems.

Driving and hazardous work No special problems.

Alcohol No special problems.

PROLONGED USE

In patients with Paget's disease, courses of treatment longer than 3 to 6 months are not usually prescribed, but repeat courses may be required. When used to treat or prevent osteoporosis, however, etidronate may be taken long term, in cycles.

Monitoring Blood and urine tests may be carried out.

Ezetimibe

Brand name Ezetrol
Used in the following combined preparation
Inegy

QUICK REFERENCE

Drug group Lipid-lowering drug (p.37)
Overdose danger rating Low
Dependence rating Low
Prescription needed Yes
Available as generic No

GENERAL INFORMATION

Ezetimibe is a lipid-lowering drug that is used to treat hypercholesterolaemia (high levels of cholesterol in the blood) in people at risk of developing heart disease. It works in the small intestine to reduce the absorption of cholesterol.

Ezetimibe is prescribed in conjunction with a low-fat diet and usually in combination with a "statin" (a drug that blocks the action in the liver of an enzyme needed for the manufacture of cholesterol). Ezetimibe is also prescribed alone to people for whom a statin is considered inappropriate or who cannot tolerate statins.

Common side effects of ezetimibe include headache, abdominal pain, and diarrhoea. It is important to notify your doctor if you are taking over-the-counter statins. When ezetimibe is combined with statins, it can, rarely, cause marked muscle pain, weakness, or tenderness, which should be reported to your doctor immediately. These effects are less likely to occur when ezetimibe is used alone.

INFORMATION FOR USERS

Your drug prescription is tailored for you. Do not alter dosage without checking with your doctor.

How taken/used Tablets.

Frequency and timing of doses Once daily.

Adult dosage range 10mg daily.

Onset of effect Two weeks.

Duration of action 24 hours.

Diet advice A low-fat diet is usually recommended.

Storage Keep in original container at room temperature out of the reach of children.

Missed dose Take as soon as you remember. If your next dose is due within 12 hours, do not take the missed dose, but take the next one on schedule.

Stopping the drug Do not stop taking the drug without consulting your doctor. Stopping the drug may lead to a recurrence of the original condition.

Exceeding the dose An occasional unintentional extra dose is unlikely to cause problems. But if you notice any unusual symptoms or if a large overdose has been taken, notify your doctor.

POSSIBLE ADVERSE EFFECTS

The most common adverse effects of ezetimibe include headache, abdominal pain, and diarrhoea. More rarely, the drug may cause nausea, joint pain, bleeding, or bruising. If you develop a rash, swelling of the face or tongue, muscle pain, or muscle weakness, you should stop taking the drug and contact your doctor without delay.

INTERACTIONS

Fibrates (e.g. gemfibrozil, bezafibrate) These drugs, which also reduce cholesterol, may raise levels of ezetimibe.

Colestyramine This drug may reduce the effects of ezetimibe. Ezetimibe should be taken either 2 hours before or 4 hours after colestyramine.

Ciclosporin The levels of both ciclosporin and ezetimibe may be increased when they are taken together.

Warfarin If ezetimibe is added to warfarin the INR (International Normalized Ratio, a standardized measure of blood clotting) should be closely monitored.

SPECIAL PRECAUTIONS

Be sure to tell your doctor if:
◆ You have liver problems.
◆ You are taking a statin.
◆ You have Lapp lactase deficiency or glucose-galactose malabsorption.
◆ You are allergic to ezetimibe.
◆ You are taking other medicines.

Pregnancy Not usually prescribed. Safety not established. Discuss with your doctor.

Breast-feeding Not usually prescribed. It is not known whether the drug passes into the breast milk. Discuss with your doctor.

Infants and children Not recommended under 10 years.

Over 60 Increased likelihood of adverse effects.

Driving and hazardous work No special problems.

Alcohol No special problems.

PROLONGED USE

No known problems.

Monitoring Regular blood tests to check the drug's effectiveness in reducing cholesterol levels may be performed. Blood tests of liver and muscle function may also be carried out.

Felodipine

Brand names Cardioplen, Felotens, Keloc, Neloc, Plendil, Vascalpha
Used in the following combined preparation Triapin

QUICK REFERENCE

Drug group Anti-angina drug (p.35) and antihypertensive drug (p.36)
Overdose danger rating Medium
Dependence rating Low
Prescription needed Yes
Available as generic Yes

GENERAL INFORMATION

Felodipine belongs to a group of drugs known as calcium channel blockers. It is used either alone, or with another antihypertensive, such as a beta blocker, ACE inhibitor, or a diuretic, in the treatment of hypertension (high blood pressure) and angina (obstruction of blood flow to the heart muscle).

The drug works by relaxing the lining of the muscles in small blood vessels, dilating them. This enables blood to be pumped more easily throughout the body, thereby lowering blood pressure and reducing the strain on the heart.

Felodipine is not prescribed to people with unstable angina or uncontrolled heart failure. It is prescribed with caution to people whose liver function is impaired.

As with other drugs of its class, felodipine may cause the blood pressure to fall too low at the start of treatment.

INFORMATION FOR USERS

Your drug prescription is tailored for you. Do not alter dosage without checking with your doctor.
How taken/used Tablets, MR-tablets.
Frequency and timing of doses Once daily, in the morning, swallowed whole with at least half a glass of water; do not chew or crush.
Adult dosage range *Hypertension* 5mg (2.5mg for elderly people) daily (initial dose), increased to 10mg daily (maintenance dose). *Angina* 5mg daily, increased to 10mg if needed.
Onset of effect 1–2 hours.
Duration of action 24 hours.

Diet advice A low-fat diet is recommended. Avoid grapefruit juice.
Storage Keep in original container at room temperature out of the reach of children.
Missed dose Take as soon as you remember. Take the next dose as scheduled. Do not take an extra dose to make up.
Stopping the drug Do not stop taking the drug without consulting your doctor. Stopping abruptly may worsen the underlying condition.
Exceeding the dose An occasional unintentional extra dose is unlikely to cause problems. Large overdoses may cause dizziness or collapse. Notify your doctor urgently.

POSSIBLE ADVERSE EFFECTS

Flushing, headache, palpitations, and fatigue are common. They are usually transient and are most likely to occur at the start of treatment or after an increase in dosage. Other common side effects include dizziness (which may be due to excessively lowered blood pressure), ankle swelling, and tinnitus. More rarely, there may be gingivitis or worsening of angina. If you experience swelling of the face, tongue, or lips, you should consult your doctor urgently and stop taking the drug.

INTERACTIONS

Other antihypertensives may increase felodipine's blood pressure-lowering effects.
Erythromycin, itraconazole, ketoconazole, atazanavir, and ritonavir may increase the effects of felodipine.
Antiepileptics may reduce the effectiveness of felodipine.
Ciclosporin and theophylline Toxicity of these drugs may be increased with felodipine.

SPECIAL PRECAUTIONS

Be sure to tell your doctor if:
◆ You have liver problems.
◆ You are allergic to felodipine or any other calcium channel blocker.
◆ You have experienced failure of the circulation.
◆ You have angina.
◆ You have had a recent heart attack.
◆ You have heart problems.
◆ You have kidney problems.
◆ You are taking other medicines.

Pregnancy Not prescribed. May cause defects in the unborn baby.

Breast-feeding Not recommended. The drug passes into the breast milk and may affect the baby adversely.

Infants and children Not recommended. Safety not established.

Over 60 Increased likelihood of adverse effects. Reduced dose may therefore be necessary.

Driving and hazardous work Do not undertake such activities until you have learned how felodipine affects you because the drug can cause dizziness.

Alcohol Avoid. Alcohol may increase dizziness and the blood pressure-lowering effect of felodipine, especially at the start of treatment.

PROLONGED USE

No problems expected.

Filgrastim

Brand name Neupogen
Used in the following combined preparations
None

QUICK REFERENCE

Drug group Blood stimulant
Overdose danger rating Medium
Dependence rating Low
Prescription needed Yes
Available as generic No

GENERAL INFORMATION

Filgrastim is a synthetic form of G-CSF (granulocyte-colony stimulating factor), a naturally occurring protein responsible for the manufacture of white blood cells, which fight infection. Deficiency of G-CSF therefore increases the risk of infection. The drug works by stimulating bone marrow to produce white blood cells. It also causes bone marrow cells to move into the bloodstream, where they can be collected for use in the treatment of bone marrow disease, or to replace bone marrow lost during intensive cancer treatment.

Filgrastim is used to treat patients with congenital neutropenia (deficiency of G-CSF from birth), some AIDS patients, and those who have recently received high doses of chemotherapy or radiotherapy during bone-marrow transplantation or cancer treatment. Such patients are prone to frequent and severe infections.

Bone pain is a common adverse effect but it can be controlled with painkillers. There is an increased risk of leukaemia (cancer of white blood cells) if filgrastim is given to patients with certain rare blood disorders.

INFORMATION FOR USERS

Your drug prescription is tailored for you. Do not alter dosage without checking with your doctor.

How taken/used Injection.

Frequency and timing of doses Once daily.

Adult dosage range 0.5–1.2 million units/kg body weight, depending upon condition being treated and response to treatment.

Onset of effect 24 hours (increase in numbers of white blood cells); several weeks (recovery of normal numbers of white blood cells).

Duration of action Approximately 2 days.

Diet advice None.

Storage Store in a refrigerator out of the reach of children.

Missed dose Take as soon as you remember. If your next dose is due within 6 hours, do not take the missed dose. Take the next scheduled dose as usual.

Stopping the drug Do not stop taking the drug without consulting your doctor; stopping the drug may lead to worsening of the underlying condition.

Exceeding the dose An occasional unintentional extra dose is unlikely to cause problems. But if you notice any unusual symptoms or if a large overdose has been taken, notify your doctor.

POSSIBLE ADVERSE EFFECTS

Adverse effects resulting from short courses of filgrastim are unusual. The most common adverse effect is bone pain, which is probably linked to the stimulant effect of the drug on bone marrow. Muscle pain is another common side effect. More rarely, there may be difficulty in, or pain on, passing urine or a skin rash. If you experience any of these symptoms, you should consult your doctor.

INTERACTIONS

Cytotoxic chemotherapy or radiotherapy should not be administered within 24 hours of taking filgrastim because of the risk of increasing the damage these treatments inflict on the bone marrow.

SPECIAL PRECAUTIONS

Be sure to tell your doctor if:
◆ You suffer from any blood disorders.
◆ You have sickle-cell disease.
◆ You are taking other medicines.

Pregnancy Safety in pregnancy not established. Discuss with your doctor.

Breast-feeding Safety in breast-feeding not established. Discuss with your doctor.

Infants and children No special problems.

Over 60 No special problems.

Driving and hazardous work No known problems.

Alcohol No known problems.

PROLONGED USE

Prolonged use may lead to a slightly increased risk of certain leukaemias. Cutaneous vasculitis (inflammation of blood vessels of the skin), osteoporosis (weakening of the bones), hair thinning, enlargement of the spleen and liver, and bleeding due to reduction in platelet numbers may also occur.

Monitoring Blood checks and regular physical examinations are performed, as well as X-rays or bone scans to check for bone thinning.

Finasteride

Brand names Propecia, Proscar
Used in the following combined preparations
None

QUICK REFERENCE

Drug group Drug used for urinary disorders (p.112)
Overdose danger rating Low
Dependence rating Low
Prescription needed Yes
Available as generic Yes

GENERAL INFORMATION

Finasteride is an anti-androgen drug (see Male sex hormones, p.87) used to treat benign prostatic hyperplasia (BPH), in which the prostate gland, which surrounds the urethra, enlarges, making urination difficult. The drug works by gradually shrinking the prostate gland, which improves urine flow and other obstructive symptoms such as difficulty in starting urination. The symptoms of BPH are similar to those of prostate cancer and so finasteride is used only when the possibility of cancer has been ruled out.

Finasteride is also used, at a lower dose, to reverse male-pattern baldness by preventing the hair follicles from becoming inactive. Noticeable improvements may take about three months but will disappear within a year of treatment being stopped.

Because finasteride is excreted in semen and can feminize a male fetus, you should use a condom if your sexual partner may be, or is likely to become, pregnant. Also, women of childbearing age should not handle broken or crushed tablets because small quantities of the drug are absorbed through the skin.

INFORMATION FOR USERS

Your drug prescription is tailored for you. Do not alter dosage without checking with your doctor.

How taken/used Tablets.

Frequency and timing of doses Once daily.

Adult dosage range *Prostate disease* 5mg. *Male-pattern baldness* 1mg.

Onset of effect Within 1 hour, but beneficial effects may take several months.

Duration of action 24 hours.

Diet advice None.

Storage Keep in original container at room temperature out of the reach of children. Protect from light.

Missed dose Do not take the missed dose, but take your next scheduled dose as usual.

Stopping the drug Do not stop the drug without consulting your doctor; stopping may lead to worsening of the underlying condition.

Exceeding the dose An occasional unintentional extra dose is unlikely to cause problems. But if you notice any unusual symptoms or have taken a large overdose, notify your doctor.

POSSIBLE ADVERSE EFFECTS

Most people experience very few adverse effects when taking finasteride; erectile dysfunction, decreased libido, and reduced ejaculate volume are the most common. Breast swelling or tenderness and testicular pain occur more rarely. If a rash, swelling of the lips, or wheezing develop, seek urgent medical attention and stop taking the drug.

INTERACTIONS
None.

SPECIAL PRECAUTIONS
Be sure to tell your doctor if:
◆ You have liver problems.
◆ You are taking other medicines.
Pregnancy Not prescribed.
Breast-feeding Not applicable.
Infants and children Not prescribed.
Over 60 No special problems.
Driving and hazardous work No special problems.
Alcohol No special problems.

PROLONGED USE
Treatment with finasteride for benign prostatic hyperplasia and male-pattern baldness is reviewed after about 6 months to see if it has been effective.

Flucloxacillin

Brand names Floxapen, Fluclomix, Galfloxin, Ladropen
Used in the following combined preparations
Co-Fluampicil, Flu-Amp, Magnapen

QUICK REFERENCE
Drug group Penicillin antibiotic (p.62)
Overdose danger rating Low
Dependence rating Low
Prescription needed Yes
Available as generic Yes

GENERAL INFORMATION
Flucloxacillin is a penicillin antibiotic. It was developed to deal with staphylococci bacteria that are resistant to other antibiotics. Such bacteria make enzymes (penicillinases) that neutralize the antibiotics but flucloxacillin is not inactivated by penicillinases and is therefore effective for treating penicillin-resistant staphylococcal infections. The drug is used to treat ear infections, pneumonia, impetigo, cellulitis, osteomyelitis, and endocarditis.

Flucloxacillin is also available combined in equal parts with ampicillin, a preparation known as co-fluampicil. This is used for treating mixed infections of penicillinase-producing organisms.

Staphylococci have evolved so that some strains are now resistant to flucloxacillin as well. These are the so-called methicillin-resistant *Staphylococcus aureus* infections (MRSA). Only a few antibiotics held in reserve can deal with them.

INFORMATION FOR USERS
Your drug prescription is tailored for you. Do not alter dosage without checking with your doctor.
How taken/used Capsules, liquid, injection.
Frequency and timing of doses 4 x daily at least 30 minutes before food.
Adult dosage range 1–2g daily (oral); 1–8g daily (injection); 8–12g daily (endocarditis).
Onset of effect 30 minutes.
Duration of action 4–6 hours.
Diet advice None.
Storage Keep in the original container at room temperature. Keep out of the reach of children.
Missed dose Take as soon as you remember. Take your next dose of the drug at the scheduled time.
Stopping the drug Take the full course. Even if you feel better, the original infection may still be present and symptoms may recur if treatment is stopped too soon.
Exceeding the dose An occasional unintentional extra dose is unlikely to be a cause for concern. But if you notice any unusual symptoms, or if a large overdose has been taken, notify your doctor.

POSSIBLE ADVERSE EFFECTS
The most common adverse effects of flucloxacillin are gastrointestinal: diarrhoea and nausea. More rarely, the drug may cause abdominal pain, bruising, a sore throat, and fever. If you develop a rash, itching, wheezing, or swollen joints (signs of an allergic reaction), or if jaundice occurs weeks or even months after finishing treatment, consult your doctor urgently. If breathing difficulties occur, call your doctor immediately and stop taking the drug.

INTERACTIONS

Probenecid This drug reduces the excretion of flucloxacillin, thereby prolonging its effects.

SPECIAL PRECAUTIONS

Be sure to tell your doctor if:
◆ You are allergic to penicillin antibiotics.
◆ You have a history of allergy.
◆ You have liver or kidney problems.
◆ You are taking other medicines.
Pregnancy No evidence of risk.
Breast-feeding No evidence of risk.
Infants and children Reduced dose necessary.
Over 60 No known problems.
Driving and hazardous work No known problems.
Alcohol No known problems.

PROLONGED USE

Although the drug is not normally necessary for long-term use, osteomyelitis and endocarditis may require longer than usual courses of treatment.

Monitoring Regular tests of liver and kidney function will be performed if a longer course of treatment is prescribed.

Fluconazole

Brand names Canestan Oral, Diflucan
Used in the following combined preparations
None

QUICK REFERENCE

Drug group Antifungal drug (p.76)
Overdose danger rating Medium
Dependence rating Low
Prescription needed Yes (except for vaginal infection preparations)
Available as generic Yes

GENERAL INFORMATION

Fluconazole is an antifungal drug used to treat local candida infections ("thrush") affecting the vagina, mouth, and skin as well as systemic or more widespread candida infections. The drug is also used to treat some more unusual fungal infections, including cryptococcal meningitis. It may also be used to prevent fungal infections in patients with defective immunity. The dosage and length of course will depend on the condition treated.

The drug is generally well tolerated, although side effects such as nausea and vomiting, diarrhoea, and abdominal discomfort are common.

INFORMATION FOR USERS

Your drug prescription is tailored for you. Do not alter dosage without checking with your doctor.
How taken/used Capsules, liquid, injection.
Frequency and timing of doses Once daily.
Adult dosage range 50–400mg daily.
Onset of effect Within a few hours, but full beneficial effects may take several days.
Duration of action Up to 24 hours.
Diet advice None.
Storage Keep in original container at room temperature out of the reach of children. Store liquid in a refrigerator (do not freeze) for no longer than 14 days.
Missed dose Take as soon as you remember. If your next dose is due within 6 hours, take a single dose now and skip the next.
Stopping the drug Take the full course. Even if you feel better, the original infection may still be present and may recur if treatment is stopped too soon.
Exceeding the dose An occasional unintentional extra dose is unlikely to be a cause for concern. But if you notice any unusual symptoms, or if a large overdose has been taken, notify your doctor.

POSSIBLE ADVERSE EFFECTS

Fluconazole is generally well tolerated. Most side effects affect the gastrointestinal tract, and include nausea, vomiting, abdominal discomfort, diarrhoea, and flatulence. If, rarely, a rash occurs, stop taking the drug and notify your doctor without delay.

INTERACTIONS

General note Most interactions with other drugs relate to multiple doses of fluconazole. The relevance of a single dose of fluconazole is not established, but is likely to be small.
Rifampicin The effect of fluconazole may be reduced by rifampicin.
Oral antidiabetic drugs Fluconazole may increase the risk of hypoglycaemia with oral sulphonylureas, such as gliclazide, glibenclamide, chlorpropamide, and tolbutamide.

Phenytoin, bosentan, theophylline/aminophylline, ciclosporin, tacrolimus, and zidovudine Fluconazole may increase the blood levels of these drugs.

Anticoagulant drugs Fluconazole may increase the effect of oral anticoagulants such as warfarin.

Oestrogens Contraceptive failure has occasionally been reported during treatment with fluconazole.

SPECIAL PRECAUTIONS

Be sure to tell your doctor if:
◆ You have long-term liver or kidney problems.
◆ You have previously had an allergic reaction to antifungal drugs.
◆ You have diabetes.
◆ You are taking other medicines.
Pregnancy Safety in pregnancy not established. Discuss with your doctor.
Breast-feeding Not recommended. The drug passes into the breast milk. Discuss with your doctor.
Infants and children Reduced dose necessary.
Over 60 Normal dose used as long as kidney function is not impaired.
Driving and hazardous work No known problems.
Alcohol No known problems.

PROLONGED USE

Fluconazole is usually given for short courses of treatment. However, for prevention of relapse of cryptococcal meningitis in patients with defective immunity, it may be administered indefinitely.

Fluoxetine

Brand names Oxactin, Prozac
Used in the following combined preparations
None

QUICK REFERENCE

Drug group Antidepressant (p.14)
Overdose danger rating Low
Dependence rating Low
Prescription needed Yes
Available as generic Yes

GENERAL INFORMATION

Fluoxetine belongs to the group of antidepressants called selective serotonin re-uptake inhibitors (SSRIs). These drugs tend to cause less sedation and have different side effects to older antidepressants. Fluoxetine elevates mood, increases physical activity, and restores interest in everyday pursuits. Fluoxetine is broken down slowly and remains in the body for several weeks after treatment is stopped. The drug is used to treat depression, to reduce binge eating and purging activity (bulimia nervosa), and to treat obsessive-compulsive disorder.

INFORMATION FOR USERS

Your drug prescription is tailored for you. Do not alter dosage without checking with your doctor.
How taken/used Capsules, liquid.
Frequency and timing of doses Once daily in the morning.
Adult dosage range 20–60mg daily.
Onset of effect Some benefits may appear in 14 days, but full benefits may not be felt for 6 weeks or more. Obsessive-compulsive disorder and bulimia may take longer to respond.
Duration of action Beneficial effects may last for up to 6 weeks following prolonged treatment. Adverse effects may wear off within 1–2 weeks.
Diet advice None.
Storage Keep in original container at room temperature out of the reach of children.
Missed dose Take as soon as you remember. If your next dose is due within 8 hours, take a single dose now and skip the next.
Stopping the drug Do not stop the drug without consulting your doctor, who may supervise a gradual reduction in dosage.
Exceeding the dose An occasional unintentional extra dose is unlikely to cause problems. Large overdoses may cause adverse effects. Notify your doctor.

POSSIBLE ADVERSE EFFECTS

Headache, restlessness, insomnia, anxiety, and nausea and/ or diarrhoea are common. There are fewer anticholinergic (see Autonomic nervous system, p.8) side effects than with tricyclics. Rarely, sexual dysfunction may occur. If you develop a rash, of if there are suicidal thoughts or attempts, stop taking the drug and consult your doctor at once.

INTERACTIONS

Sedatives All drugs having a sedative effect may increase the sedative effects of fluoxetine.

Monoamine oxidase inhibitors (MAOIs) Fluoxetine should not be started less than 14 days after stopping an MAOI (except moclobemide) as serious adverse effects can occur. An MAOI should not be started less than 5 weeks after stopping fluoxetine.

Tricyclic antidepressants Fluoxetine reduces the breakdown of tricyclics and may increase the toxicity of these drugs.

Antipsychotics The levels and effects of some of these drugs can be increased by fluoxetine.

SPECIAL PRECAUTIONS

Be sure to tell your doctor if:
◆ You have long-term liver or kidney problems.
◆ You have a history of mania.
◆ You have diabetes.
◆ You have had epileptic fits.
◆ You have previously had an allergic reaction to fluoxetine or other SSRIs.
◆ You are taking other medicines.

Pregnancy Avoid if possible. Discuss with your doctor.

Breast-feeding The drug passes into the breast milk. Discuss with your doctor.

Infants and children Not generally recommended under 18 years, but occasionally given under specialist supervision.

Over 60 No special problems.

Driving and hazardous work Avoid such activities until you have learned how fluoxetine affects you because the drug can cause drowsiness and can affect your judgment and coordination.

Alcohol No special problems.

PROLONGED USE

No problems expected. Side effects tend to decrease with time.

Monitoring Any person experiencing drowsiness, confusion, muscle cramps, or convulsions should be monitored for low sodium levels in the blood.

Flupentixol

Brand names Depixol, Fluanxol
Used in the following combined preparations None

QUICK REFERENCE

Drug group Antipsychotic drug (p.15)
Overdose danger rating Medium
Dependence rating Low
Prescription needed Yes
Available as generic No

GENERAL INFORMATION

Flupentixol is an antipsychotic drug used to treat schizophrenia and similar illnesses. It is also occasionally used as an antidepressant for mild to moderate depression. Side effects are similar to those of the phenothiazines, but flupentixol is less sedating. It has fewer anticholinergic effects (see Autonomic nervous system, p.8) than phenothiazines but can cause side effects such as parkinsonism. It is not suitable for patients with mania because it may worsen the symptoms.

INFORMATION FOR USERS

Your drug prescription is tailored for you. Do not alter dosage without checking with your doctor.

How taken/used Tablets, injection.

Frequency and timing of doses 1–2 x daily no later than 4 pm (tablets); every 2–4 weeks (injection).

Adult dosage range *Schizophrenia and other psychoses* 6–18mg daily (tablets); from 20mg every 4 weeks: maximum of 400mg weekly (injection). *Depression* 1–3mg daily (tablets).

Onset of effect 10 days (side effects may appear much sooner).

Duration of action Up to 12 hours (by mouth); 1–2 months (by depot injection).

Diet advice None.

Storage Store at room temperature out of the reach of children. Protect injections from light.

Missed dose Take as soon as you remember. If your next dose is due within 2 hours, do not take the missed dose, but take your next scheduled dose as usual.

Stopping the drug Do not stop the drug without consulting your doctor, who will supervise gradual dosage reduction. Abrupt cessation may cause withdrawal symptoms and a recurrence of the original problem.

Exceeding the dose An occasional unintentional extra dose is unlikely to cause problems. Larger overdoses may cause severe drowsiness, fits, low blood pressure, or shock. Notify your doctor.

POSSIBLE ADVERSE EFFECTS

Flupentixol's possible adverse effects are mainly due to its anticholinergic action and blocking action on transmission of signals through the heart. Weight gain, nausea, drowsiness, sexual dysfunction, breast growth, absent periods, blurred vision, and tremors are common; report dizziness, fainting, or confusion to your doctor. If, rarely, persistent infection, sore throat, or jaundice occur, stop taking the drug and call your doctor at once.

INTERACTIONS

Antiarrhythmic drugs Flupentixol may increase the risk of arrhythmias with these drugs.

Anticholinergic drugs Flupentixol may increase the effects of these drugs.

Anticonvulsant drugs Flupentixol may reduce the effects of these drugs.

Sedatives Flupentixol enhances the effect of all sedative drugs.

SPECIAL PRECAUTIONS

Be sure to tell your doctor if:
◆ You have long-term liver or kidney problems.
◆ You have heart problems.
◆ You have had epileptic fits.
◆ You have Parkinson's disease.
◆ You have glaucoma.
◆ You are taking other medicines.

Pregnancy Not usually prescribed. May cause lethargy in the baby during labour. Discuss with your doctor.

Breast-feeding The drug passes into the breast milk and may affect the baby. Discuss with your doctor.

Infants and children Not recommended.

Over 60 Reduced dose necessary. Increased risk of late-appearing movement disorders or confusion.

Driving and hazardous work Avoid such activities until you have learned how the drug affects you; it can cause drowsiness and slowed reactions.

Alcohol Avoid. Flupentixol enhances the sedative effect of alcohol.

Surgery and general anaesthetics Treatment may need to be stopped before you have any surgery. Discuss with your doctor or dentist.

PROLONGED USE

The risk of late-appearing movement disorders increases as treatment continues. Blood disorders, as well as jaundice and other liver disorders, are occasionally seen.

Flutamide

Brand names Chimax, Drogenil
Used in the following combined preparations None

QUICK REFERENCE

Drug group Anticancer drug (p.96)
Overdose danger rating Medium
Dependence rating Low
Prescription needed Yes
Available as generic Yes

GENERAL INFORMATION

Flutamide is an anti-androgen used in the treatment of advanced prostate cancer, often in combination with drugs such as goserelin (see p.258) that control production of the male sex hormones (androgens). The drugs are effective because the cancer is dependent on androgens for its continued development. Treatment with goserelin-type drugs causes an initial increase in release of the hormone testosterone, leading to a growth spurt of the cancer ("tumour flare"), which flutamide is prescribed to stop. In the UK, flutamide treatment is begun 3 days before the goserelin-type drug. Flutamide is also used to treat prostate cancer when goserelin-type drugs are not prescribed.

Flutamide may discolour the urine amber or yellow-green, which is harmless. However, you should notify your doctor straight away if your urine becomes dark coloured, because this may be an indication of liver damage.

INFORMATION FOR USERS

Your drug prescription is tailored for you. Do not alter dosage without checking with your doctor.

How taken/used Tablets.
Frequency and timing of doses 3 x daily, starting 3 days before the goserelin-type drug and continuing for 3 weeks.
Adult dosage range 250mg.
Onset of effect 1 hour.
Duration of action 8 hours.
Diet advice None.
Storage Keep in original container at room temperature out of the reach of children.
Missed dose Take as soon as you remember. If your next dose is due within 2 hours, take a single dose now and skip the next.
Stopping the drug Do not stop taking the drug without consulting your doctor because the condition may worsen rapidly.
Exceeding the dose An occasional unintentional extra dose is unlikely to be a cause for concern. But if you notice any unusual symptoms, or if a large overdose has been taken, notify your doctor.

POSSIBLE ADVERSE EFFECTS

Breast swelling, nausea, vomiting, diarrhoea, insomnia, headache, decreased libido, and thirst are common. Rarely, dizziness, blurred vision, and stomach or chest pain occur. If a rash, dark urine, or jaundice occur, stop taking the drug and consult your doctor urgently.

INTERACTIONS

Warfarin Flutamide increases the effect of this drug.

SPECIAL PRECAUTIONS

Be sure to tell your doctor if:
◆ You have heart problems.
◆ You have liver problems.
◆ You are taking other medicines.
Pregnancy Not prescribed.
Breast-feeding Not prescribed.
Infants and children Not prescribed.
Over 60 No special problems.
Driving and hazardous work Do not undertake such activities until you have learned how flutamide affects you because the drug can cause blurred vision and dizziness.
Alcohol Avoid excessive consumption.

PROLONGED USE

Prolonged use of flutamide may cause liver damage. The drug also reduces sperm count.

Monitoring Periodic liver-function tests are usually performed.

Fluticasone

Brand names Cutivate, Flixonase, Flixotide, Nasofan
Used in the following combined preparation Seretide

QUICK REFERENCE

Drug group Corticosteroid (p.80)
Overdose danger rating Low
Dependence rating Low
Prescription needed Yes (except for nasal spray)
Available as generic No

GENERAL INFORMATION

Fluticasone is a corticosteroid used to control inflammation in asthma and allergic rhinitis. It does not produce relief immediately, so it is important to take it regularly. For allergic rhinitis, treatment with nasal spray needs to begin 2 to 3 weeks before the hay fever season starts. Fluticasone should be taken regularly by inhaler to prevent asthma attacks; proper instruction is essential to ensure correct use. An ointment or cream is also prescribed to treat dermatitis and eczema (see Topical corticosteroids, p.120).

Fluticasone has few serious adverse effects because it is administered directly into the lungs (by inhaler) or nasal mucosa (by nasal spray). Fungal infection causing irritation of the mouth and throat is a possible side effect of the inhaled form but can be minimized by thoroughly rinsing the mouth and gargling with water after each inhalation.

INFORMATION FOR USERS

Follow instructions on the label. Call your doctor if symptoms worsen.
How taken/used Ointment, cream, inhaler, nasal spray.
Frequency and timing of doses *Allergic rhinitis* 1–2 x daily; *asthma* 2 x daily.
Adult dosage range *Allergic rhinitis* 1–2 sprays into each nostril per dose; *asthma* 100–1,000mcg per dose.
Onset of effect 4–7 days (asthma); 3–4 days (allergic rhinitis).
Duration of action The effects can last for several days after stopping the drug.

Diet advice None.

Storage Keep in original container at room temperature out of the reach of children.

Missed dose Take as soon as you remember.

Stopping the drug Do not stop the drug without consulting your doctor; symptoms may recur.

Exceeding the dose An occasional unintentional extra dose is unlikely to be a cause for concern. Adverse effects may occur if the recommended dose is regularly exceeded over a prolonged period.

POSSIBLE ADVERSE EFFECTS

The main side effects are irritation of the nasal passages or, rarely, nosebleeds (spray) and sore throat or mouth or hoarseness, usually due to fungal infection of the throat and mouth (inhaler). Discuss any skin changes (ointment/cream) and disturbances in taste or smell with your doctor. If a rash or facial swelling, breathing difficulty, or wheezing develop, seek immediate medical attention.

INTERACTIONS

None.

SPECIAL PRECAUTIONS

Be sure to consult your doctor or pharmacist before taking this drug if:

◆ You have chronic sinusitis.

◆ You have had nasal ulcers or surgery.

◆ You have had tuberculosis or another respiratory infection.

◆ You have a history of angioedema.

◆ You have glaucoma.

◆ You are taking other medicines.

Pregnancy Safety in pregnancy not established. Discuss with your doctor.

Breast-feeding Safety in breast-feeding not established. Drug unlikely to pass into breast milk; discuss with your doctor.

Infants and children Not recommended under 4 years. Reduced dose necessary in older children; avoid prolonged use of ointment.

Over 60 No known problems.

Driving and hazardous work No known problems.

Alcohol No known problems.

PROLONGED USE

Long-term use can lead to peptic ulcers, glaucoma, muscle weakness, fragile bones, growth retardation in children, and, rarely, adrenal-gland suppression. Prolonged use of topical treatment may also lead to skin thinning. Long-term patients should carry a "steroid card" or wear a MedicAlert bracelet.

Monitoring Periodic checks on adrenal gland function may be required if large doses are being taken.

Furosemide (frusemide)

Brand names Froop, Frusol, Lasix, and others
Used in the following combined preparations
Co-Amilofruse, Fru-Co, Frumil, Lasikal, Lasilactone, and others

QUICK REFERENCE

Drug group Loop diuretic (p.32) and antihypertensive drug (p.36)
Overdose danger rating Low
Dependence rating Low
Prescription needed Yes
Available as generic Yes

GENERAL INFORMATION

In use for over 20 years, furosemide is a powerful, short-acting loop diuretic. Like other diuretics, it is used to treat oedema (fluid accumulation) due to heart failure, and certain lung, liver, and kidney disorders. It is fast acting and is often used in emergencies to relieve pulmonary oedema (fluid in the lungs).

Furosemide is particularly useful for people with impaired kidney function because they do not respond well to thiazides (see p.33).

Because furosemide increases potassium loss, which can produce a wide variety of symptoms, potassium supplements or a potassium-sparing diuretic are often also given.

INFORMATION FOR USERS

Your drug prescription is tailored for you. Do not alter dosage without checking with your doctor.

How taken/used Tablets, liquid, injection.

Frequency and timing of doses Once daily, usually in the morning; 4–6 x hourly (high dose therapy).

Adult dosage range 20–80mg daily. Dose may be increased to a maximum of 2g daily if kidney function is impaired.

Onset of effect Within 1 hour (by mouth); within 5 minutes (by injection).

Duration of action Up to 6 hours.

Diet advice Use of this drug may reduce potassium in the body. Eat plenty of potassium-rich fresh fruits and vegetables, such as bananas and tomatoes.

Storage Keep in original container at room temperature out of the reach of children. Protect from light.

Missed dose No cause for concern, but take as soon as you remember. However, if it is late in the day do not take the missed dose, or you may need to get up during the night to pass urine. Take the next scheduled dose as usual.

Stopping the drug Do not stop the drug without consulting your doctor; symptoms may recur.

Exceeding the dose An occasional unintentional extra dose is unlikely to be a cause for concern. But if you notice any unusual symptoms, or if a large overdose has been taken, notify your doctor.

POSSIBLE ADVERSE EFFECTS

Adverse effects of furosemide, which include nausea and lethargy, are caused mainly by the rapid fluid loss that is produced by furosemide. These effects tend to diminish as the body adjusts to the drug. The disturbance in body salts and water balance can also cause muscle cramps, headache, and dizziness. If a rash, photosensitivity, or palpitations occur, stop taking the drug and consult your doctor urgently. Ringing in the ears may occur with high doses given by injection.

INTERACTIONS

Non-steroidal anti-inflammatory drugs (NSAIDs) Some of these drugs may reduce the diuretic effect of furosemide.

Lithium Furosemide may increase blood levels of lithium, leading to an increased risk of lithium poisoning.

Digoxin Loss of potassium may lead to digoxin toxicity with furosemide.

Aminoglycoside antibiotics The risk of hearing and kidney problems may be increased when these drugs are taken with furosemide.

Angiotensin-converting enzyme inhibitors and angiotensin II blockers There is a risk of low blood pressure when these drugs are taken with furosemide.

SPECIAL PRECAUTIONS

Be sure to tell your doctor if:
◆ You have long-term liver problems.
◆ You have gout.
◆ You have diabetes.
◆ You have previously had an allergic reaction to furosemide or sulphonamides.
◆ You have prostate trouble.
◆ You are taking laxatives.
◆ You are taking other medicines.

Pregnancy Safety in pregnancy not established. Discuss with your doctor.

Breast-feeding The drug may reduce milk supply, but the amount in the milk is unlikely to affect the baby. Discuss with your doctor.

Infants and children Reduced dose necessary.

Over 60 Reduced dose may be necessary.

Driving and hazardous work Avoid such activities until you have learned how furosemide affects you because the drug may reduce mental alertness and cause dizziness.

Alcohol Keep consumption low. Furosemide increases the likelihood of dehydration and hangovers after the consumption of alcohol.

PROLONGED USE

Serious problems are unlikely, but levels of salts, such as potassium, sodium, and calcium, may become depleted. Low blood pressure, palpitations, headaches, problems passing urine, or muscle cramps may develop, particularly in the elderly.

Monitoring Periodic tests may be performed to check kidney function and levels of body salts.

Gabapentin

Brand name Neurontin
Used in the following combined preparations None

QUICK REFERENCE

Drug group Anticonvulsant drug (p.16)
Overdose danger rating Medium
Dependence rating Low
Prescription needed Yes
Available as generic Yes

GENERAL INFORMATION

Gabapentin is an anticonvulsant drug introduced in 1993 to treat epilepsy. It is used to treat partial seizures, and is often prescribed in combination with other drugs when a patient's epilepsy is not being satisfactorily controlled with the other drugs alone. Unlike some other anticonvulsants, gabapentin does not need blood level monitoring and has no interactions with other anticonvulsants.

Gabapentin is also used to relieve neuropathic pain, such as that following shingles.

Patients with impaired kidney function should be given smaller doses, and diabetic patients taking gabapentin may notice fluctuations in their blood glucose levels.

INFORMATION FOR USERS

Your drug prescription is tailored for you. Do not alter dosage without checking with your doctor.

How taken/used Tablets, capsules.
Frequency and timing of doses Dose gradually built up to 3 x daily (maintenance). No more than 12 hours should elapse between doses.
Adult dosage range *Epilepsy* 900–2,400mg daily; maintenance dose reached gradually over a few days. *Neuropathic pain* Maximum 1,800mg daily, reached gradually over a few days.
Onset of effect The full antiepileptic effect may not be seen for 48 hours.
Duration of action 6–8 hours.
Diet advice None.
Storage Keep in original container at room temperature out of the reach of children.
Missed dose Take as soon as you remember. If your next dose is due within 4 hours, take a dose now and skip the next.
Stopping the drug Gabapentin should not be stopped abruptly. Gradual withdrawal over at least 7 days is advised to reduce the risk of seizures in those being treated for epilepsy.
Exceeding the dose An occasional unintentional extra dose is unlikely to be a cause for concern. Large overdoses may lead to dizziness, double vision, and slurred speech. Notify your doctor.

POSSIBLE ADVERSE EFFECTS

Drowsiness, dizziness, and fatigue are common; discuss any muscle tremor with your doctor. Vision disturbances, indigestion, or weight gain are less common; seek medical advice. Mood changes, hallucinations, and a rash require urgent medical attention.

INTERACTIONS

Antacids containing aluminium or magnesium These may reduce the effect of gabapentin. The drug should not be taken within 2 hours of antacid preparations.
Urinary protein tests for diabetics False-positive readings have been recorded with some tests. Special procedures are required for diabetics taking gabapentin.

SPECIAL PRECAUTIONS

Be sure to tell your doctor if:
◆ You have a kidney problem.
◆ You have diabetes.
◆ You have a history of psychiatric illness.
◆ You are taking other medicines.

Pregnancy The drug is likely to reach the fetus and its effects are unknown. Discuss with your doctor.
Breast-feeding The drug passes into the breast milk, and the effects on the baby are unknown. Discuss with your doctor.
Infants and children Rarely used in children under 6 years. Reduced doses based on body weight are required in children under 12 years.
Over 60 Doses may have to be adjusted to allow for decreased kidney function.
Driving and hazardous work Avoid such activities until you have learned how the drug affects you. Gabapentin may produce drowsiness or dizziness.
Alcohol Alcohol may increase the sedative effects of gabapentin.

PROLONGED USE

No problems expected.

Gentamicin

Brand names Cidomycin, Genticin, Minims gentamicin
Used in the following combined preparation Gentisone HC

QUICK REFERENCE

Drug group Aminoglycoside antibiotic (p.62)
Overdose danger rating Low
Dependence rating Low
Prescription needed Yes
Available as generic Yes

GENERAL INFORMATION

Gentamicin is one of the aminoglycoside antibiotics. The injectable form is usually reserved for hospital treatment of serious infections. These include lung, urinary tract, bone, joint, and wound infections, as well as peritonitis, septicaemia, and meningitis. This form is also used together with a penicillin for prevention and treatment of heart valve infections (endocarditis).

In the form of drops, gentamicin is used to treat eye and ear infections. Gentamicin given by injection can have serious adverse effects on the ears and the kidneys. Damage to the ears may lead to deafness and problems with the balance mechanism in the inner ear (vertigo). Courses of treatment are, therefore, limited to 7 days when this is possible. Treatment is monitored with particular care when high doses are needed or kidney function is poor.

INFORMATION FOR USERS

Your drug prescription is tailored for you. Do not alter dosage without checking with your doctor.

How taken/used Injection, eye/ear drops.
Frequency and timing of doses 1–3 x daily (injection); 3–4 x daily or as directed (ear drops); every 2 hours or as directed (eye drops).
Adult dosage range According to condition and response (injection); according to your doctor's instructions (eye and ear drops).
Onset of effect Within 1–2 hours.
Duration of action 8–12 hours.
Diet advice None.
Storage Keep in original container at room temperature out of the reach of children.
Missed dose Apply eye/ear preparations as soon as you remember.
Stopping the drug Complete the course. Even if you feel better, the original infection may still be present and may recur if treatment is stopped too soon.
Exceeding the dose Although overdose by injection is dangerous, it is unlikely because treatment is carefully monitored. For other preparations of the drug, an occasional unintentional extra dose is unlikely to cause concern. But if you notice any unusual symptoms, notify your doctor.

POSSIBLE ADVERSE EFFECTS

Adverse effects are rare, but those that occur with the injectable form may be serious. Dizziness, vertigo, ringing in the ears (tinnitus), impaired hearing, and changes in the urine should be reported promptly. Nausea or vomiting may also occur. If the ointment or cream is applied to large areas the drug may be absorbed and could cause hearing loss. Allergic reactions, including rash and itching, may occur with all preparations that contain gentamicin. Blurred vision or eye irritation may occur with the eye preparations and should be reported to your doctor.

INTERACTIONS

General note A wide range of drugs, including furosemide, vancomycin, and cephalosporins, increase the risk of hearing loss and/or kidney failure with gentamicin injections.

SPECIAL PRECAUTIONS

Be sure to tell your doctor if:
◆ You have a long-term kidney problem.
◆ You have a hearing disorder.
◆ You have myasthenia gravis.
◆ You have Parkinson's disease.
◆ You have previously had an allergic reaction to aminoglycosides.
◆ You are taking other medicines.
Pregnancy No evidence of risk with eye or ear drops. Injections are not prescribed, as they may cause hearing defects in the baby. Discuss with your doctor.
Breast-feeding No evidence of risk (eye or ear preparations). The drug may pass into breast milk (injection). Discuss with your doctor.
Infants and children Reduced dose necessary for injections.
Over 60 Increased likelihood of adverse effects. Reduced dose may therefore be necessary.
Driving and hazardous work No known problems from preparations for the eye or ear.
Alcohol No known problems.

PROLONGED USE

Not usually given for longer than seven days. When given by injection, there is a risk of adverse effects on hearing and balance.
Monitoring Blood levels of the drug are usually checked if it is given by injection. Tests on kidney function are also usually carried out.

Glibenclamide

Brand names Daonil, Euglucon, Semi-Daonil
Used in the following combined preparations None

QUICK REFERENCE

Drug group Oral antidiabetic drug (p.82)
Overdose danger rating High
Dependence rating Low
Prescription needed Yes
Available as generic Yes

GENERAL INFORMATION

Glibenclamide is a sulphonylurea oral antidiabetic drug. Like other drugs of this type, it stimulates the production and secretion of insulin from the islet cells in the pancreas, promoting the uptake of glucose into body cells, thereby lowering blood glucose levels.

This drug is used in the treatment of Type 2 diabetes mellitus, in conjunction with exercise and a diet low in carbohydrates and fats.

In conditions of severe illness, injury, or stress, glibenclamide may lose its effectiveness, making it necessary to take insulin. Adverse effects are generally mild. Symptoms of poor diabetic control will occur if the dosage of glibenclamide is not appropriate.

INFORMATION FOR USERS

Your drug prescription is tailored for you. Do not alter dosage without checking with your doctor.
How taken/used Tablets.
Frequency and timing of doses Once daily in the morning with breakfast.
Adult dosage range 5–15mg daily.
Onset of effect Within 3 hours.
Duration of action 10–15 hours.
Diet advice A low-carbohydrate, low-fat diet must be maintained in order for the drug to be fully effective. Follow the advice of your doctor.
Storage Keep in original container at room temperature out of the reach of children. Protect from light.
Missed dose Take with next meal; do not double the dose to account for missed dose.
Stopping the drug Do not stop the drug without consulting your doctor; stopping the drug may lead to worsening of your diabetes.

OVERDOSE ACTION

Seek immediate medical advice in all cases. If any early warning symptoms of excessively low blood glucose (such as fainting, sweating, trembling, confusion, or headache) occur, eat or drink something sugary. Take emergency action if fits or loss of consciousness occur.

POSSIBLE ADVERSE EFFECTS

Serious adverse effects are rare. Symptoms such as fainting or confusion, weakness or tremor, sweating, and constipation and diarrhoea may be signs of low blood glucose due to lack of food or too high a dose of the drug. If any of these symptoms occur, eat or drink something sugary immediately and seek medical assistance. Other adverse effects include nausea or vomiting, rash and itching, and weight changes. If jaundice occurs, consult your doctor without delay.

INTERACTIONS

General note A variety of drugs, including corticosteroids, diuretics, and rifampicin, may reduce the effect of glibenclamide and raise blood glucose levels. Others, including warfarin, aspirin, sulphonamides and other antibacterials, antifungals, beta blockers, NSAIDs, and ACE inhibitors, increase the risk of low blood glucose.

SPECIAL PRECAUTIONS

Be sure to tell your doctor if:
◆ You have long-term liver or kidney problems.
◆ You are allergic to sulphonylurea drugs.
◆ You have thyroid problems.
◆ You have porphyria.
◆ You have ever had adrenal gland problems.
◆ You are taking other medicines.
Pregnancy Not usually prescribed. Insulin is generally substituted in pregnancy because it gives better diabetic control.
Breast-feeding The drug passes into the breast milk and may lower the baby's blood glucose.
Infants and children Not prescribed.
Over 60 Reduced dose may be necessary. Greater likelihood of low blood glucose exists when glibenclamide is used.
Driving and hazardous work Usually no problems. Avoid these activities if you have warning signs of low blood glucose.

Alcohol Avoid. Alcohol may upset diabetic control increasing the risk of hypoglycaemia.
Surgery and general anaesthetics Notify your doctor or dentist that you have diabetes before undergoing any surgery.
Sunlight Avoid exposure to this and tanning beds. The drug may make skin more sensitive.

PROLONGED USE

No problems expected.

Monitoring Regular monitoring of levels of glucose in the urine or blood is required. Periodic assessment of the eyes, heart, and kidneys may also be advised.

Gliclazide

Brand names DIAGLYK, Diamicron, Diamicron MR
Used in the following combined preparations None

QUICK REFERENCE

Drug group Oral antidiabetic drug (p.82)
Overdose danger rating High
Dependence rating Low
Prescription needed Yes
Available as generic Yes

GENERAL INFORMATION

Gliclazide is a sulphonylurea oral antidiabetic drug. It stimulates production and secretion of insulin from the islet cells in the pancreas, promoting uptake of glucose into body cells thereby lowering blood glucose levels.

The drug is used to treat Type 2 diabetes mellitus, in conjunction with exercise and a diet low in carbohydrates and fats.

In conditions of severe illness, injury, stress, or surgery, the drug may lose its effectiveness, necessitating the use of insulin injections. Adverse effects are generally mild. However, symptoms of poor diabetic control will occur if the dosage is not appropriate.

INFORMATION FOR USERS

Your drug prescription is tailored for you. Do not alter dosage without checking with your doctor.
How taken/used Tablets, MR-tablets.
Frequency and timing of doses 1–2 x daily (in the morning and evening with a meal).

Dosage range 40–320mg daily (doses above 160mg are divided into two doses).
Onset of effect Within 1 hour.
Duration of action 12–24 hours.
Diet advice An individual low-fat, low-carbohydrate diet must be maintained for the drug to be fully effective. Follow the advice of your doctor.
Storage Keep in original container at room temperature out of the reach of children.
Missed dose Take with next meal; do not double the dose to account for missed dose.
Stopping the drug Do not stop the drug without consulting your doctor; stopping may lead to worsening of the underlying condition.

OVERDOSE ACTION

Seek immediate medical advice in all cases. If early warning symptoms of excessively low blood glucose such as fainting, sweating, trembling, confusion, or headache occur, eat or drink something sugary at once. Take emergency action if fits or loss of consciousness occur.

POSSIBLE ADVERSE EFFECTS

Serious adverse effects are rare. Symptoms such as fainting, confusion, tremors, sweating, and weakness may be signs of low blood glucose due to lack of food or too high a dose of the drug; eat or drink something sugary immediately and seek medical advice. Constipation or diarrhoea may also occur. Rarely, nausea or vomiting, rash, itching, or weight changes may occur. If jaundice occurs, consult your doctor without delay.

INTERACTIONS

General note A variety of drugs may reduce the effect of gliclazide and may therefore raise blood glucose levels. These include corticosteroids, oestrogens, NSAIDs, diuretics, and rifampicin. Other drugs increase the risk of low blood glucose. These include warfarin, sulphonamides and other antibacterial drugs, aspirin, beta blockers, ACE inhibitors, and antifungal drugs.

SPECIAL PRECAUTIONS

Be sure to tell your doctor if:
◆ You have long-term liver or kidney problems.
◆ You are allergic to sulphonylurea drugs.

◆ You have thyroid problems.

◆ You have porphyria.

◆ You have ever had problems with your adrenal glands.

◆ You are taking other medicines.

Pregnancy Not recommended. May cause abnormally low blood glucose in the newborn baby. Insulin is generally substituted in pregnancy because it gives better diabetic control.

Breast-feeding The drug passes into the breast milk and may cause low blood glucose in the baby. Discuss with your doctor.

Infants and children Not prescribed.

Over 60 Signs of low blood glucose may be more difficult to recognize. Reduced dose may be necessary.

Driving and hazardous work Avoid such activities until you have learned how gliclazide affects you because it can cause dizziness, drowsiness, and confusion.

Alcohol Avoid. Alcoholic drinks may upset diabetic control increasing the risk of hypoglycaemia.

Surgery and general anaesthetics Notify your doctor or dentist that you have diabetes before undergoing any surgery.

Sunlight Avoid exposure to the sun and do not use a sunlamp or sunbed.

PROLONGED USE

No problems expected.

Monitoring Regular testing of glucose levels in the blood and/or urine is required. Periodic assessment of the eyes, heart, and kidneys may also be advised.

Glyceryl trinitrate

Brand names Coro-Nitro, Deponit, Minitran, Nitro-Dur, Nitrolingual, Percutol, Rectogesic, Sustac, Transiderm-Nitro, and others
Used in the following combined preparations None

QUICK REFERENCE

Drug group Anti-angina drug (p.35)
Overdose danger rating Medium
Dependence rating Low
Prescription needed No (most preparations); yes (injection)
Available as generic Yes

GENERAL INFORMATION

Introduced in the late 1800s, glyceryl trinitrate is one of the oldest drugs in continual use. It is a type of vasodilator known as a nitrate and is used to relieve the pain of angina attacks. It is available in short-acting forms (sublingual or buccal tablets, ointment, and spray) and long-acting forms (slow-release tablets and patches). The short-acting forms act very quickly to relieve angina. The drug is also given by injection in hospital for severe angina and to control blood pressure.

Glyceryl trinitrate may cause a variety of minor symptoms, such as flushing and headache; most can be controlled by adjusting the dosage. The drug is best taken for the first time while sitting, as fainting may follow the drop in blood pressure caused by the drug.

Glyceryl trinitrate may also be used for the treatment of anal fissures.

INFORMATION FOR USERS

Follow instructions on the label. Call your doctor if symptoms worsen.

How taken/used SR-tablets, buccal tablets, sublingual tablets, injection, ointment, gel, skin patches, spray.

Frequency and timing of doses *Angina prevention* 3 x daily (buccal/SR-tablets); every 3–4 hours (ointment); once daily (patches). *Angina relief* Use buccal or sublingual tablets, ointment, or spray at the onset of an attack or immediately prior to exercise. Dose may be repeated within 5 minutes if further relief required.

Adult dosage range *Angina prevention* 2.6–38.4mg daily (SR-tablets); 2–15mg daily (buccal tablets); 5–15mg daily (patches); as directed (ointment). *Angina relief* 0.3–1mg per dose (sublingual tablets); 1–3mg per dose (buccal tablets); 1–2 sprays per dose (spray).

Onset of effect Angina 1–3 minutes (buccal and sublingual tablets and spray); 30–60 minutes (SR-tablets, patches, and ointment). Anal fissure 12 hours.

Duration of action 20–30 minutes (sublingual tablets and spray); 3–5 hours (buccal tablets and ointment); 8–12 hours (SR-tablets); up to 24 hours (patches).

Diet advice None.

Storage Keep sublingual tablets in an airtight glass container fitted with a foil-lined, screw-on cap in a cool, dry place out of the reach of children. Protect from light. Do not expose to heat. Discard tablets within 8 weeks of opening. Check label of other preparations for storage conditions.

Missed dose If your next dose is due within 6 hours, skip the missed dose and take your next scheduled dose as usual (buccal and SR-tablets); take as soon as you remember, or when needed. If your next dose is due within 2 hours, take a single dose now and skip the next (other preparations).

Stopping the drug Do not stop taking the drug without consulting your doctor.

Exceeding the dose An occasional unintentional extra dose is unlikely to cause problems. Large overdoses may cause dizziness, vomiting, severe headache, sweating, fits, or loss of consciousness. Notify your doctor.

POSSIBLE ADVERSE EFFECTS

The most serious effect is lowered blood pressure, which may cause dizziness, and should be reported to your doctor. Other effects, such as headache and flushing, usually diminish after regular use but can also be controlled by dosage adjustment.

INTERACTIONS

Antihypertensive drugs and other anti-angina drugs These drugs increase the possibility of lowered blood pressure or fainting when taken with glyceryl trinitrate.

Sildenafil, tadalafil, and vardenafil The hypotensive effect of glyceryl trinitrate is increased significantly by sildenafil. The two drugs should not be used together.

SPECIAL PRECAUTIONS

Be sure to consult your doctor or pharmacist before taking this drug if:
◆ You have any other heart condition.
◆ You have a lung condition.
◆ You have long-term liver or kidney problems.
◆ You have any blood disorders.
◆ You have glaucoma.
◆ You have thyroid disease.
◆ You have low blood pressure.
◆ You have anaemia.
◆ You have had a recent head injury or stroke.
◆ You are taking other medicines.

Pregnancy Safety in pregnancy not established. Discuss with your doctor.

Breast-feeding It is not known whether the drug passes into the breast milk. Discuss with your doctor.

Infants and children Not usually prescribed.

Over 60 No special problems.

Driving and hazardous work Avoid such activities until you have learned how glyceryl trinitrate affects you because the drug can cause dizziness.

Alcohol Avoid excessive intake. Alcohol may increase the risk of lowered blood pressure, causing dizziness and fainting.

PROLONGED USE

The drug's effects usually weaken slightly as the body adapts. Timing of the doses may be changed to prevent this effect.

Monitoring Periodic checks on blood pressure are usually required.

Goserelin

Brand names Zoladex, Zoladex LA
Used in the following combined preparations None

QUICK REFERENCE

Drug group Anticancer drug (p.96)
Overdose danger rating Low
Dependence rating Low
Prescription needed Yes
Available as generic No

GENERAL INFORMATION

Goserelin is a synthetic drug chemically related to the hormone gonadorelin. Like gonadorelin, it stimulates the release of other hormones from the pituitary gland, which in turn control production of the sex hormones.

Goserelin is used to suppress production of sex hormones in breast and prostate cancer. At the start of treatment for prostate cancer, it is often given with an anti-androgen drug (see p.87) to control an initial growth spurt of the tumour ("tumour flare".)

The drug is also used in the management of fibroids, endometriosis, and assisted reproduction. The first dose is normally given during menstruation to avoid the possibility that the patient may be pregnant. Women of childbearing age are advised to use barrier methods of contraception during treatment.

Loss of bone density is an important side effect in women. Therefore, repeat courses of the drug are given only for cancerous conditions.

INFORMATION FOR USERS

Your drug prescription is tailored for you. Do not alter dosage without checking with your doctor.

How taken/used Implant injection, long-acting implant injection.

Frequency and timing of doses *Endometriosis* Every 28 days, maximum of a single 6-month treatment course only (implant). *Fibroids* Every 28 days, maximum 3 months' treatment (implant). *Breast and prostate cancer* Every 28 days. *Prostate cancer* Every 12 weeks (LA implant).

Adult dosage range 3.6mg (implant) every 28 days (endometriosis/fibroids/breast and prostate cancer); 10.8mg (LA implant) every 3 months.

Onset of effect Within 24 hours (endometriosis/fibroids/breast cancer); 1–2 weeks after tumour flare (prostate).

Duration of action 28 days (implant); 12 weeks (long-acting implant).

Diet advice None.

Storage Not applicable. The drug is not kept at home.

Missed dose No cause for concern. Treatment can be resumed when possible.

Stopping the drug Do not stop treatment without consulting your doctor.

Exceeding the dose Overdosage is unlikely since treatment is not self-administered.

POSSIBLE ADVERSE EFFECTS

Symptoms similar to those of the menopause, such as hot flushes and changes in breast size, headache, and bleeding on stopping goserelin are common. Some women have vaginal bleeding in the early stages of treatment. Rarely, dizziness, fainting, wheezing, rash, and reaction at the injection site occur and should be reported to your doctor straight away. Ovarian cysts may, rarely, also develop.

INTERACTIONS

None.

SPECIAL PRECAUTIONS

Be sure to tell your doctor if:
◆ You have osteoporosis.
◆ You have previously been treated with goserelin (or another gonadorelin analogue) for endometriosis or fibroids.
◆ You have polycystic ovarian disease.
◆ You are allergic to gonadorelin analogues.
◆ You are taking other medicines.

Pregnancy Not prescribed. Risk of harm to the fetus.

Breast-feeding Not recommended. Discuss with your doctor.

Infants and children Not recommended.

Over 60 No special problems.

Driving and hazardous work No special problems.

Alcohol No special problems.

PROLONGED USE

Only used long term for prostate or breast cancer. Bone density is lost over time in women but may be partly recoverable after treatment.

Monitoring Women are usually monitored for changes in bone density.

Haloperidol

Brand names Dozic, Haldol, Serenace
Used in the following combined preparations None

QUICK REFERENCE

Drug group Butyrophenone antipsychotic drug (p.15)
Overdose danger rating Medium
Dependence rating Low
Prescription needed Yes
Available as generic Yes

GENERAL INFORMATION

Haloperidol is an antipsychotic used to treat schizophrenia and other psychoses, mania, and to reduce agitation and violent behaviour. It is also used short term to treat severe anxiety. It does not cure the underlying disorder but relieves the distressing symptoms. The drug is also used in the control of Tourette's syndrome and to treat intractable hiccups.

The main drawback of the drug is that it can produce abnormal, involuntary movements and stiffness of the face and limbs.

INFORMATION FOR USERS

Your drug prescription is tailored for you. Do not alter dosage without checking with your doctor.

How taken/used Tablets, capsules, liquid, injection, depot injection.

Frequency and timing of doses 2–4 x daily.

Adult dosage range *Mental illness* 3–10mg daily initially, up to a maximum of 30mg daily. *Severe anxiety* 1mg daily.

Onset of effect 2–3 hours (by mouth); 20–30 minutes (by injection).

Duration of action 6–24 hours (by mouth); 2–4 hours (injection); up to 4 weeks (depot).

Diet advice None.

Storage Keep in original container at room temperature out of the reach of children.

Missed dose Take as soon as you remember. If your next dose is due within 3 hours, take a single dose now and skip the next.

Stopping the drug Do not stop the drug without consulting your doctor; symptoms may recur.

Exceeding the dose An occasional unintentional extra dose is unlikely to cause problems. Larger overdoses may cause unusual drowsiness, muscle weakness or rigidity, and/or faintness. Notify your doctor.

POSSIBLE ADVERSE EFFECTS

Various minor anticholinergic symptoms, such as dry mouth and blurred vision, can occur but often diminish with time. Drowsiness, lethargy, and sexual dysfunction can also occur. Abnormal movements of the face and limbs (parkinsonism) may be controlled by dosage adjustment. If, rarely, a high fever or confusion occur, stop taking the drug and seek immediate medical attention.

INTERACTIONS

Sedatives These are likely to increase the sedative properties of haloperidol.

Rifampicin and anticonvulsants These drugs may reduce the effects of haloperidol.

Lithium This drug may increase the risk of parkinsonism and effects on the nerves.

Methyldopa This drug may increase the risk of parkinsonism and low blood pressure.

Terfenadine This drug may have adverse effects on the heart if taken with haloperidol.

Anticholinergic drugs Haloperidol may increase the side effects of these drugs.

SPECIAL PRECAUTIONS

Be sure to tell your doctor if:

◆ You have long-term liver or kidney problems.

◆ You have heart or circulation problems.

◆ You have had epileptic fits.

◆ You have Parkinson's disease or other movement disorders.

◆ You are taking other medicines.

Pregnancy Safety in pregnancy not established. Drug is occasionally used by specialist services. Discuss with your doctor.

Breast-feeding The drug passes into the breast milk and may affect the baby. Discuss with your doctor.

Infants and children Rarely required. Reduced dose necessary.

Over 60 Reduced dose may be necessary.

Driving and hazardous work Avoid such activities until you have learned how the drug affects you; it can cause drowsiness and slowed reactions.

Alcohol Avoid. Alcohol may increase the sedative effect of this drug.

PROLONGED USE

Use of this drug for more than a few months may lead to tardive dyskinesia (abnormal, involuntary movements of the eyes, face, and tongue). Occasionally, jaundice may occur.

Heparin/Low molecular weight heparins

Brand names Calciparine, Monoparin, Multiparin; [LMWH] Alphaparin, Clexane, Clivarine, Fragmin, Innohep, Zibor
Used in the following combined preparations None

QUICK REFERENCE

Drug group Anticoagulant (p.38)
Overdose danger rating High
Dependence rating Low
Prescription needed Yes
Available as generic Yes (heparin); No (LMWH)

GENERAL INFORMATION

Heparin is an anticoagulant used to prevent formation of, and aid in dispersion of, blood clots. It acts quickly, and is particularly useful in emergencies to prevent further clotting when a clot has reached the lungs or brain, for instance. It is also used to prevent clotting in open heart surgery or kidney dialysis. A low dose is sometimes given after surgery to prevent deep vein thrombosis (clots in leg veins). Heparin is often given in conjunction with other slower-acting anticoagulants, such as warfarin. It is also used to treat unstable angina.

Several types of heparin (low molecular weight heparins, or LMWH), do not have to be administered in hospital.

INFORMATION FOR USERS

This drug is given only under medical supervision and is not for self-administration.
How taken/used Injection.
Frequency and timing of doses Every 8–12 hours or continuous intravenous infusion; once daily (LMWH).
Dosage range Dosage is determined by nature of condition being treated or prevented.
Onset of effect Within 15 minutes.
Duration of action 4–12 hours after treatment; 24 hours after treatment (LMWH).
Diet advice None.
Storage Keep in original container at room temperature out of the reach of children.
Missed dose Notify your doctor.
Stopping the drug Do not stop taking the drug without consulting your doctor. Stopping the drug may lead to clotting of blood.

OVERDOSE ACTION

Seek immediate medical advice in all cases. Take emergency action if bleeding, severe headache, or loss of consciousness occur. Overdose can be reversed under medical supervision by a drug called protamine.

POSSIBLE ADVERSE EFFECTS

Bleeding is a common adverse effect, and bruising may also occur. Call your doctor if breathing difficulties, jaundice, or vomiting of blood occur. If a rash occurs, stop taking the drug and consult your doctor urgently.

INTERACTIONS

Aspirin and other NSAIDs may increase anticoagulant effect of heparin and risk of bleeding.
ACE inhibitors and potassium supplements may increase the risk of high blood potassium.

Clopidogrel, ticlopidine, and dipyridamole Anticoagulant effect of heparin may be increased. Dosage of heparin may need to be adjusted.

SPECIAL PRECAUTIONS

Be sure to tell your doctor if:
◆ You have long-term liver or kidney problems.
◆ You have high blood pressure.
◆ You bleed easily or are currently bleeding.
◆ You have any allergies.
◆ You have stomach ulcers.
◆ You have diabetes.
◆ You have had a previous reaction to heparin.
◆ You have had a recent stroke, injury, or surgery.
◆ You are taking other medicines.
Pregnancy Careful monitoring is necessary as it may cause the mother to bleed excessively if taken near delivery. Discuss with your doctor.
Breast-feeding No evidence of risk.
Infants and children Reduced dose necessary according to age and weight.
Over 60 No special problems, but the elderly may be more prone to bleeding.
Driving and hazardous work Avoid risk of injury; excessive bruising and bleeding may occur.
Alcohol No special problems.
Surgery and general anaesthetics Heparin may need to be stopped. Discuss this with your doctor or dentist before having any surgery.

PROLONGED USE

Osteoporosis and hair loss may occur very rarely; tolerance to heparin may develop.
Monitoring Periodic blood and liver function tests will be required.

Hydrochlorothiazide

Brand names None
Used in the following combined preparations Acezide, Capozide, Cozaar Comp, Dyazide, Moducren, Moduretic, and others

QUICK REFERENCE

Drug group Thiazide diuretic (p.32)
Overdose danger rating Low
Dependence rating Low
Prescription needed Yes
Available as generic No

GENERAL INFORMATION

Hydrochlorothiazide is a thiazide diuretic that removes excess water from the body and reduces oedema (fluid retention) in people with congestive heart failure, kidney disorders, liver cirrhosis, and premenstrual syndrome. It is also used, in combination with other antihypertensives (see p.36), to treat high blood pressure. The drug increases potassium loss in the urine and increases the likelihood of irregular heart rhythms, particularly in patients taking drugs such as digoxin. For this reason, potassium supplements are often also given.

INFORMATION FOR USERS

Your drug prescription is tailored for you. Do not alter dosage without checking with your doctor.

How taken/used Tablets.

Frequency and timing of doses Once daily, or every 2 days, early in the day.

Adult dosage range *Hypertension* 25–50mg daily. *Oedema* 25–100mg daily.

Onset of effect Within 2 hours.

Duration of action 6–12 hours.

Diet advice Use of this drug may reduce potassium in the body. Eat plenty of fresh fruit and vegetables. Discuss with your doctor the advisability of reducing your salt intake.

Storage Keep in original container at room temperature out of the reach of children. Protect from light.

Missed dose No cause for concern, but take as soon as you remember. However, if it is late in the day do not take the missed dose, or you may have to get up during the night to pass urine. Take the next scheduled dose as usual.

Stopping the drug Do not stop the drug without consulting your doctor; symptoms may recur.

Exceeding the dose An occasional unintentional extra dose is unlikely to be a cause for concern. But if you notice any unusual symptoms, or if a large overdose has been taken, notify your doctor.

POSSIBLE ADVERSE EFFECTS

Muscle cramps are common. Most effects are rare and are due to excessive potassium loss, which can usually be put right by potassium supplements. They include lethargy, dizziness, headache, digestive disturbance, and temporary erectile dysfunction. Rarely, gout may occur in susceptible people, and certain forms of diabetes may become more difficult to control. Report nausea, vomiting, constipation, or diarrhoea to your doctor. If a rash occurs, stop taking the drug and consult your doctor promptly.

INTERACTIONS

Non-steroidal anti-inflammatories (NSAIDs) Some NSAIDs may reduce the diuretic effect of the drug, whose dosage may need to be adjusted.

Anti-arrhythmic and digitalis drugs increase the risk of toxicity from low blood potassium with hydrochlorothiazide.

Corticosteroids These drugs further increase loss of potassium from the body when taken with hydrochlorothiazide, and may reduce its diuretic effect.

Lithium Hydrochlorothiazide may increase lithium levels in the blood, leading to a risk of serious adverse effects.

SPECIAL PRECAUTIONS

Be sure to tell your doctor if:

◆ You have long-term liver or kidney problems.

◆ You have had gout.

◆ You have diabetes.

◆ You have porphyria.

◆ You have Addison's disease or systemic lupus erythematosus.

◆ You are taking other medicines.

Pregnancy Not usually prescribed. May cause jaundice in the newborn baby. Discuss with your doctor.

Breast-feeding The drug passes into the breast milk, but at normal doses adverse effects on the baby are unlikely. Discuss with your doctor.

Infants and children Not usually prescribed. Reduced dose necessary.

Over 60 Increased likelihood of adverse effects.

Driving and hazardous work Avoid such activities until you have learned how the drug affects you; it may reduce mental alertness and cause dizziness.

Alcohol Keep consumption low. The drug increases the likelihood of dehydration and hangovers with alcohol.

PROLONGED USE

Excessive loss of potassium and imbalances of other salts may result.

Monitoring Blood tests may be performed periodically to check kidney function and levels of potassium and other salts.

Hydrocortisone

Brand names Colifoam, Corlan, Dioderm, Efcortelan, Efcortesol, Hydrocortistab, Hydrocortone, Mildison, Solu-Cortef
Used in the following combined preparations
Alphaderm, Xyloproct, and many others

QUICK REFERENCE

Drug group Corticosteroid (p.80), and topical corticosteroid (p.120)
Overdose danger rating Low
Dependence rating Low
Prescription needed Yes (except for some topical preparations)
Available as generic Yes

GENERAL INFORMATION

Hydrocortisone is chemically identical to the hormone cortisol, produced by the adrenal glands, and is prescribed to replace natural hormones in adrenal insufficiency (Addison's disease). Its main use is in the treatment of various allergic and inflammatory conditions. Used topically, it gives prompt relief from inflammation of the skin, eye, and outer ear. It is also used orally to relieve asthma, inflammatory bowel disease, and many rheumatic and allergic disorders. Injected into the joints, it relieves pain and stiffness (see Corticosteroids for rheumatic disorders, p.53). Injections may also be given for severe asthma attacks.

Overuse of skin preparations can lead to permanent skin thinning. Long-term high-dose oral treatment may cause serious side effects.

INFORMATION FOR USERS

Your drug prescription is tailored for you. Do not alter dosage without checking with your doctor.
How taken/used Tablets, lozenges, injection, rectal foam, cream, ointment, eye/ear ointment/drops.
Frequency and timing of doses Varies according to condition and preparation.
Dosage range Varies according to condition and preparation.

Onset of effect Within 1–4 days.
Duration of action Up to 12 hours.
Diet advice Salt intake may need to be restricted when drug is taken by mouth. Potassium supplements may also be necessary.
Storage Keep in original container at room temperature out of the reach of children.
Missed dose Take as soon as you remember. If your next dose is due within 2 hours, take a single dose now and skip the next.
Stopping the drug Do not stop the drug without consulting your doctor. Gradual dosage reduction is required following prolonged treatment with oral hydrocortisone.
Exceeding the dose An occasional unintentional extra dose is unlikely to cause problems. If you notice any unusual symptoms or a large overdose has been taken, notify your doctor.

POSSIBLE ADVERSE EFFECTS

Taken by mouth, the drug may cause indigestion, weight gain, acne, and fluid retention. High doses may cause muscle weakness, mood changes, and menstrual irregularities; consult your doctor. The most serious effects occur only with high oral doses taken long term. These are carefully monitored.

INTERACTIONS (BY MOUTH ONLY)

Barbiturates, anticonvulsants, and rifampicin reduce the effectiveness of hydrocortisone.
Antidiabetic drugs Hydrocortisone reduces the action of these drugs.
Antihypertensive drugs Hydrocortisone reduces the effects of these drugs.
Vaccines Severe reactions can occur if certain vaccines are given during treatment.
Aspirin and other NSAIDs Increased risk of peptic ulcer and bleeding from the stomach.

SPECIAL PRECAUTIONS

Be sure to tell your doctor if:
◆ You have liver or kidney problems.
◆ You have had a peptic ulcer.
◆ You have had a mental illness or epilepsy.
◆ You have glaucoma.
◆ You have had tuberculosis.
◆ You have diabetes or heart problems.
◆ You are taking other medicines.
Pregnancy No evidence of risk with topical preparations. Oral doses may adversely affect the developing baby. Discuss with your doctor.

Breast-feeding The drug passes into the breast milk and may affect the baby. Discuss with your doctor.

Infants and children Reduced dose necessary.

Over 60 Reduced dose may be necessary.

Driving and hazardous work No special problems.

Alcohol Avoid. Alcohol may increase the risk of peptic ulcer when drug is taken by mouth.

Surgery and general anaesthetics Notify your doctor; you may need to have hydrocortisone by injection in hospital.

Infection If on systemic treatment, avoid exposure to chickenpox, shingles, or measles.

PROLONGED USE

Prolonged high dosage can lead to peptic ulcers, glaucoma, muscle weakness, fragile bones, and growth retardation in children. People on long-term treatment are advised to carry a "steroid treatment" card.

Monitoring Periodic checks on blood pressure are usually required (oral forms).

Hyoscine

Brand names Buscopan, Joy-Rides, Kwells, Scopoderm TTS

Used in the following combined preparations Feminax, Papaveretum and Hyoscine Injection

QUICK REFERENCE

Drug group Drug for irritable bowel syndrome (p.45), drug affecting the pupil (p.116), and anti-emetic (p.21)

Overdose danger rating Medium

Dependence rating Low

Prescription needed No (most preparations)

Available as generic Yes

GENERAL INFORMATION

Hyoscine is an anticholinergic with both an antispasmodic effect on the intestine and a calming action on the nerve pathways that control nausea and vomiting. By its anticholinergic action, it also dilates the pupil.

There are two forms: hyoscine butylbromide, to reduce spasm of the gastrointestinal tract in irritable bowel syndrome and to treat dysmenorrhoea (painful menstruation), sometimes with other drugs; and hyoscine hydrobromide, to control motion sickness and giddiness and nausea due to inner-ear disturbances such as vertigo and Ménière's disease (see p.22), which is available as skin patches or tablets. This form is also used as premedication to dry secretions before operations. Eye drops containing hyoscine hydrobromide are used to dilate the pupil during eye examinations and eye surgery.

INFORMATION FOR USERS

Follow instructions on the label. Call your doctor if symptoms worsen.

How taken/used Tablets, injection, patches.

Frequency and timing of doses *Irritable bowel syndrome* Up to 4 x daily, as required (tablets). *Motion sickness* Up to 3 x daily (tablets); every 3 days as required (patches).

Adult dosage range *Irritable bowel syndrome* 30–80mg daily (butylbromide). *Motion sickness* 0.3mg per dose (tablets); 1mg over 72 hours (hydrobromide patches).

Onset of effect Within 1 hour.

Duration of action Up to 6 hours (by mouth); up to 72 hours (patches).

Diet advice None.

Storage Keep in original container at room temperature out of the reach of children. Protect from light.

Missed dose Take when you remember. Adjust the timing of your next dose accordingly.

Stopping the drug Can be safely stopped as soon as you no longer need it.

Exceeding the dose An occasional unintentional extra dose is unlikely to cause problems. Large overdoses may cause drowsiness or agitation. Notify your doctor.

POSSIBLE ADVERSE EFFECTS

Taken by mouth or injection, hyoscine has a strong anticholinergic effect, causing various minor symptoms, such as dry mouth and drowsiness. These can sometimes be minimized by dosage reduction. If you experience blurred vision, difficulty in passing urine, or a fast heart rate, consult your doctor.

INTERACTIONS

Anticholinergic drugs Many drugs have anticholinergic effects. The risk of such side effects is increased with hyoscine.

Sedatives All drugs that have a sedative effect on the central nervous system are likely to increase the sedative properties of hyoscine. Such drugs include anti-anxiety and sleeping drugs, antidepressants, opioid analgesics, and antipsychotics.

Sublingual tablets Hyoscine can cause a dry mouth and may reduce the effectiveness of sublingual tablets.

SPECIAL PRECAUTIONS

Be sure to consult your doctor or pharmacist before taking this drug if:
◆ You have long-term liver or kidney problems.
◆ You have heart problems.
◆ You have myasthenia gravis.
◆ You have epilepsy.
◆ You have megacolon or intestinal obstruction problems.
◆ You have glaucoma.
◆ You have prostate trouble or urinary retention.
◆ You have porphyria.
◆ You are taking other medicines.

Pregnancy Safety in pregnancy not established. Discuss with your doctor.

Breast-feeding No evidence of risk. Discuss with your doctor.

Infants and children Not recommended under 4 years for motion sickness. Patches not recommended under 10 years. Other uses not recommended under 6 years. Reduced dose necessary in older children.

Over 60 Reduced dose may be necessary.

Driving and hazardous work Avoid such activities until you have learned how hyoscine affects you because the drug can cause drowsiness and blurred vision.

Alcohol Avoid. Alcohol may increase the sedative effect of this drug.

PROLONGED USE

Use of this drug for longer than a few days is unlikely to be necessary.

Ibuprofen

Brand names Arthrofen, Brufen, Calprofen, Ebufac, Fenbid, Ibugel, Ibuleve, Ibumousse, Nurofen, and many others
Used in the following combined preparations Codafen, Cuprofen Plus, Nurofen Plus, Solpaflex

QUICK REFERENCE

Drug group Analgesic (p.9) and non-steroidal anti-inflammatory drug (p.50)
Overdose danger rating Low
Dependence rating Low
Prescription needed No (some preparations)
Available as generic Yes

GENERAL INFORMATION

Ibuprofen is a non-steroidal anti-inflammatory (NSAID) that reduces pain, stiffness, and inflammation. It is used to treat the symptoms of osteoarthritis, rheumatoid arthritis, and gout. In rheumatoid arthritis, it may be prescribed with slower-acting drugs. Ibuprofen is also used for mild to moderate headache (including migraine), juvenile arthritis, menstrual and dental pain, ankylosing spondylitis, the pain of soft tissue injuries, or that which may follow surgery.

Ibuprofen has fewer side effects than many of the other NSAIDs. Unlike aspirin, it rarely causes bleeding in the stomach.

Ibuprofen is also available as a cream or gel for muscular aches and sprains.

INFORMATION FOR USERS

Follow instructions on the label. Call your doctor if symptoms worsen.

How taken/used Tablets, SR-tablets, capsules, SR-capsules, liquid, granules, cream, mousse, gel.

Frequency and timing of doses 1–2 x daily (SR-preparations); 3–4 x daily (topical preparations and other oral preparations). Take all oral preparations with or after food.

Dosage range *Adults* 600mg–2.4g daily. *Children* Varies according to age/weight.

Onset of effect Pain relief begins in 15 minutes–2 hours. Full anti-inflammatory effect in arthritic conditions may take up to 2 weeks.

Duration of action 5–10 hours.

Diet advice None.

Storage Keep in original container at room temperature out of the reach of children.

Missed dose Take as soon as you remember. If your next dose is due within 2 hours, take a single dose now and skip the next.

Stopping the drug Taken short term, the drug can be safely stopped as soon as you no longer need it. For long-term treatment of arthritis, seek medical advice before stopping.

Exceeding the dose An occasional unintentional extra dose is unlikely to be a cause for concern. But if you notice any unusual symptoms, or if a large overdose has been taken, notify your doctor.

POSSIBLE ADVERSE EFFECTS

Gastrointestinal disturbances, such as heartburn and indigestion are common. Rarely, nausea and vomiting occur. Swollen feet and ankles and ringing in the ears also occur rarely and are normally associated with too high a dose. If a rash, wheezing, breathlessness, black or bloodstained faeces, or abdominal pain occur, stop taking the drug and seek immediate medical attention.

INTERACTIONS

General note Ibuprofen interacts with many drugs, including other NSAIDs, aspirin, oral anticoagulants, and corticosteroids, to increase the risk of bleeding and/or peptic ulcers.

Ciprofloxacin Ibuprofen increases risk of seizures with this and related antibiotics.

Antihypertensive drugs and diuretics The beneficial effects of these drugs may be reduced by ibuprofen; rarely, diuretics can also increase the risk of adverse effects on the kidneys.

Ciclosporin and tacrolimus increase the risk of adverse effects on the kidneys.

SPECIAL PRECAUTIONS

Be sure to consult your doctor or pharmacist before taking this drug if:
◆ You have a long-term kidney problem.
◆ You have a long-term liver problem.
◆ You have high blood pressure.
◆ You have had a peptic ulcer, oesophagitis, or acid indigestion.
◆ You are allergic to aspirin/other NSAIDs.
◆ You have asthma.
◆ You are taking other medicines.

Pregnancy Not usually recommended. May affect the unborn baby and may prolong labour. Discuss with your doctor.

Breast-feeding The drug passes into the breast milk; at normal doses adverse effects on the baby are unlikely. Discuss with your doctor.

Infants and children Reduced dose necessary.

Over 60 Reduced dose may be necessary.

Driving and hazardous work No problems expected.

Alcohol Avoid. Alcohol may increase the risk of stomach disorders with ibuprofen.

Surgery and general anaesthetics Ibuprofen may prolong bleeding. Discuss stopping treatment temporarily with your doctor or dentist.

PROLONGED USE

Increased risk of bleeding from peptic ulcers and in the bowel. The lowest effective dose is given for the shortest duration.

Imipramine

Brand names None
Used in the following combined preparations
None

QUICK REFERENCE

Drug group Antidepressant (p.14) and drug for urinary disorders (p.112)
Overdose danger rating High
Dependence rating Low
Prescription needed Yes
Available as generic Yes

GENERAL INFORMATION

Imipramine is a tricyclic antidepressant used mainly in the long-term treatment of depression to elevate mood, improve appetite, increase physical activity, and restore interest in everyday life. Because it is less sedating than some other tricyclics, the drug is particularly useful when a depressed person has become withdrawn or apathetic. Imipramine is also prescribed to treat night-time enuresis (bedwetting) in children.

The most common adverse effects of the drug are the result of its anticholinergic action. In overdose, imipramine may cause coma and abnormal heart rhythms.

INFORMATION FOR USERS

Your drug prescription is tailored for you. Do not alter dosage without checking with your doctor.

How taken/used Tablets, liquid.

Frequency and timing of doses 1–3 x daily.

Dosage range *Adults* Usually 75–200mg daily (up to a maximum of 300mg in hospital patients). *Children* Reduced dose according to age and weight.

Onset of effect Some benefits and effects may appear within hours, but full antidepressant effect may not be felt for 2–6 weeks.

Duration of action Following prolonged treatment, antidepressant effect may persist for up to 6 weeks, common adverse effects for 1–2 weeks.

Diet advice None.

Storage Keep in original container at room temperature out of the reach of children.

Missed dose Take as soon as you remember. If your next dose is due within 3 hours, take a single dose now and skip the next.

Stopping the drug Do not stop the drug without consulting your doctor, who will supervise a gradual reduction in dosage. Stopping abruptly may cause withdrawal symptoms.

OVERDOSE ACTION

Seek immediate medical advice in all cases. Take emergency action if palpitations are noted or consciousness is lost.

POSSIBLE ADVERSE EFFECTS

Adverse effects are mainly due to the drug's anticholinergic (see Autonomic nervous system, p.8) action and its effect on heart rhythm. Sweating, flushing, dry mouth, constipation, weight gain, and blurred vision are common. Dizziness or drowsiness may also occur. If you experience confusion, stop taking the drug. If palpitations occur, stop taking the drug and seek urgent medical advice.

INTERACTIONS

Anti-arrhythmic drugs increase the risk of abnormal heart rhythms.

Sedatives Increased effect with imipramine.

Antihypertensives and anticonvulsants The effects of these are reduced by imipramine.

Monoamine oxidase inhibitors (MAOIs) are prescribed with imipramine only under strict supervision due to the possibility of a serious interaction.

Some selective serotonin reuptake inhibitors (SSRIs) can increase levels of imipramine.

SPECIAL PRECAUTIONS

Be sure to tell your doctor if:
◆ You have heart problems.
◆ You have long-term liver or kidney problems.

◆ You have had epileptic fits.
◆ You have porphyria.
◆ You have glaucoma.
◆ You have prostate trouble.
◆ You have had mania or a psychotic illness.
◆ You are taking other medicines.

Pregnancy Avoid if possible. Discuss with your doctor.

Breast-feeding The drug passes into the breast milk; at normal doses adverse effects on the baby are unlikely. Discuss with your doctor.

Infants and children Not recommended under 7 years. Reduced dose necessary in older children.

Over 60 Increased likelihood of adverse effects. Reduced dose may therefore be necessary.

Driving and hazardous work Avoid such activities until you have learned how imipramine affects you because the drug can cause reduced alertness and blurred vision.

Alcohol Avoid. Alcohol may increase the sedative effect of imipramine.

Surgery and general anaesthetics Imipramine treatment may need to be stopped before you have a general anaesthetic. Discuss this with your doctor or dentist before any operation.

PROLONGED USE

No problems expected. Not usually given for bedwetting for longer than 3 months.

Indapamide

Brand names Natrilix SR, Nindaxa
Used in the following combined preparation
Coversyl Plus

QUICK REFERENCE

Drug group Diuretic (p.32)
Overdose danger rating Low
Dependence rating Low
Prescription needed Yes
Available as generic Yes

GENERAL INFORMATION

Indapamide is related in its effects and uses to thiazide diuretics (see p.33) but is used to treat hypertension (high blood pressure). It prevents the hormone norepinephrine (noradrenaline) from constricting blood vessels, allowing them to dilate. Indapamide is sometimes combined with other antihypertensive drugs but not with other diuretics.

Indapamide's diuretic effects are slight at low doses, but susceptible people need to have blood levels of potassium and uric acid monitored. These include the elderly, those taking digitalis drugs, or those with gout or hyperaldosteronism (overproduction of the hormone aldosterone). Unlike thiazides, indapamide does not affect control of diabetes.

INFORMATION FOR USERS

Your drug prescription is tailored for you. Do not alter dosage without checking with your doctor.

How taken/used Tablets, SR-tablets.

Frequency and timing of doses Once daily in the morning.

Adult dosage range 1.5–2.5mg.

Onset of effect 1–2 hours, but the full effect may take several months.

Duration of action 12–24 hours.

Diet advice None.

Storage Keep in original container at room temperature out of the reach of children.

Missed dose Take as soon as you remember. If your next dose is due within 4 hours, take a single dose now and skip the next.

Stopping the drug Do not stop taking the drug without consulting your doctor; high blood pressure may return.

Exceeding the dose An occasional unintentional extra dose is unlikely to cause problems. If you notice unusual symptoms, or if a large overdose has been taken, notify your doctor.

POSSIBLE ADVERSE EFFECTS

Headaches, fatigue, and muscle cramps are common. Diarrhoea, constipation, nausea, and dyspepsia are less common. If you experience palpitations, dizziness, fainting, a rash on light-exposed skin, jaundice, sore throat, tingling or "pins and needles", or erectile dysfunction, seek medical advice.

INTERACTIONS

Diuretics taken with indapamide increase the risk of imbalance of salts in the blood.

Anti-arrhythmic and digitalis drugs Potassium loss with indapamide may lead to toxicity.

Lithium Blood levels of lithium are increased when it is taken with indapamide.

Mexiletine Potassium loss with indapamide use may reduce the effect of mexiletine.

SPECIAL PRECAUTIONS

Be sure to tell your doctor if:
◆ You have had a stroke.
◆ You have liver or kidney problems.
◆ You have gout.
◆ You have hyperaldosteronism or hyperparathyroidism.
◆ You are allergic to sulphonamide drugs.
◆ You are taking other medicines.

Pregnancy Safety not established. Discuss with your doctor.

Breast-feeding Safety not established. Discuss with your doctor.

Infants and children Not prescribed.

Over 60 No special problems.

Driving and hazardous work No special problems.

Alcohol No special problems.

PROLONGED USE

Long-term use of indapamide may lead to potassium loss in the elderly.

Monitoring Blood potassium and uric acid levels may be checked periodically.

Infliximab

Brand name Remicade
Used in the following combined preparations
None

QUICK REFERENCE

Drug group Drug for inflammatory bowel disease (p.46) and disease-modifying antirheumatic drug (p.51)
Overdose danger rating Low
Dependence rating Low
Prescription needed Yes
Available as generic No

GENERAL INFORMATION

Infliximab is a monoclonal antibody (see p.97) that can change the working of the body's own defence (immune) system and cut down inflammation. One of its actions is to combine with a body protein known as "tumour necrosis factor alpha" (TNF), which is overactive in many diseases, including psoriasis, rheumatoid arthritis, Crohn's disease, and ulcerative colitis, making them more severe. Given by intravenous infusion, generally into the arm, it reduces the level of TNF activity, helping to improve the conditions.

Infections, most often those of the upper respiratory and urinary tracts, are common.

INFORMATION FOR USERS

The drug is given only under medical supervision and is not for self-administration.
How taken/used Intravenous infusion.
Frequency and timing of doses Every 6–8 weeks. Infusion time is generally over a 2-hour period.
Adult dosage range Dosing is based on body weight; 3mg/kg to 5mg/kg per dose.
Onset of effect 1 hour.
Duration of action 2–8 weeks.
Diet advice None.
Storage Not applicable. The drug is not normally kept in the home.
Missed dose As infliximab is dosed every 6–8 weeks, it is important to adhere to the dosing schedule arranged by your doctor. Missed doses should be rectified as soon as possible.
Stopping the drug No adverse effects are reported when infliximab is stopped abruptly.
Exceeding the dose This is unlikely since doses are organized by healthcare professionals. Tell your doctor, nurse, or pharmacist immediately if you feel that you have received a higher dose.

POSSIBLE ADVERSE EFFECTS

Infusion reactions may occur during treatment, or within 1–2 hours, particularly with the first or second treatment. Delayed reactions, including muscle and joint pain, fever, and rash may occur 3–12 days after infusion. Nausea, vomiting, diarrhoea, headache, back pain, and infusion reactions are common. Susceptibility to infection occurs rarely. Discuss this and infusion reactions with your doctor. If you have a swollen tongue, are wheezing, or have a rash, stop taking the drug and seek immediate medical attention.

INTERACTIONS

Anakinra should not be combined with infliximab due to an increased risk of reactions.
Live vaccines Infliximab may affect the efficacy of these.

SPECIAL PRECAUTIONS

Infliximab is prescribed only under close medical supervision. However, be sure to tell your doctor if:
◆ You have active tuberculosis.
◆ You have any current, or signs of, infection (e.g. fever, malaise, wounds, dental problems).
◆ You are having surgery or dental treatment.
◆ You have liver or kidney problems.
◆ You have a central nervous system disorder such as multiple sclerosis.
◆ You have recently received, or are scheduled to receive, a vaccine.
◆ You have had heart failure.
◆ You are taking other medicines.
Pregnancy Not recommended.
Breast-feeding Not recommended during treatment or for 6 months after last dose.
Infants and children Not recommended.
Over 60 Not recommended.
Driving and hazardous work Do not undertake such activities until you have learned how infliximab affects you because the drug can cause fatigue and dizziness.
Alcohol No special problems.

PROLONGED USE

Serious problems are unlikely.
Monitoring Periodic blood and liver-function tests may be carried out. Body temperature, heart rate, and blood pressure may be monitored during the first infusion.

Insulin

Brand names Apidra, Exubera, Humalog, Human Actrapid, Human Insulatard, Human Mixtard, Human Velosulin, Humulin, Hypurin, Insuman, Lantus, NovoRapid, Pork Insulatard, Pork Mixtard, Pork Velosulin, and others

QUICK REFERENCE

Drug group Drug for diabetes (p.82)
Overdose danger rating High
Dependence rating Low
Prescription needed Yes
Available as generic No

GENERAL INFORMATION

Insulin is a hormone manufactured by the pancreas and vital to the body's ability to use glucose. It is given by injection (or, in certain cases, inhaler) to supplement or replace natural insulin in the treatment of diabetes mellitus. It is the only effective treatment in juvenile (Type 1) diabetes and may also be used in adult (Type 2) diabetes. Insulin should be used with a carefully controlled diet. Illness, vomiting, or alterations in diet or in exercise levels may require dosage adjustment. Insulin is available in a range of short-, medium-, or long-acting preparations. Combinations of types are often given. People receiving insulin should carry a warning card or tag.

INFORMATION FOR USERS

Your drug prescription is tailored for you. Do not alter dosage without checking with your doctor.

How taken/used Injection, infusion pump, pen injection, inhaler.

Frequency and timing of doses 1–4 x daily usually 15–30 minutes before meals (short-acting); some forms given directly before or after eating. Exact timing of injections and longer-acting preparations will be tailored to individual needs; follow instructions given.

Dosage range Exact timing of doses is tailored to individual needs. Follow manufacturer's instructions.

Onset of effect 15–60 minutes (short-acting); within 2 hours (medium-acting); 2–3 hours (long-acting).

Duration of action 2–8 hours (short-acting); 18–26 hours (medium-acting); 28–36 hours (long-acting); 6 hours (inhaler).

Diet advice A low-carbohydrate diet is necessary. Follow your doctor's advice.

Storage Refrigerate, but once opened may be stored at room temperature for 1 month. Do not freeze. Follow instructions on container.

Missed dose Discuss with your doctor. Appropriate action depends on dose and type of insulin.

Stopping the drug Do not stop taking the drug without consulting your doctor; confusion and coma may occur.

OVERDOSE ACTION

Seek immediate medical advice. You may notice symptoms of low blood glucose, such as faintness, hunger, sweating, and trembling.

Eat or drink something sugary. Take emergency action if fits or loss of consciousness occur.

POSSIBLE ADVERSE EFFECTS

Symptoms such as dizziness, sweating, weakness, and confusion indicate low blood glucose. Irritation at the injection site is common. Eyesight problems or dimpling at the injection site are rare; discuss with your doctor. If a rash, swelling, and shortness of breath occur, seek urgent medical attention.

INTERACTIONS

General note 1 Many drugs, including some antibiotics, monoamine oxidase inhibitors (MAOIs), and oral antidiabetic drugs, increase the risk of low blood glucose.

Corticosteroids and diuretics may oppose the effect of insulin.

General note 2 Check with your doctor or pharmacist before taking any medicines; some contain sugar and may upset control of diabetes.

Beta blockers may affect insulin needs and mask signs of low blood glucose.

SPECIAL PRECAUTIONS

Be sure to tell your doctor if:
◆ You have had a previous allergic reaction to insulin.
◆ You are taking other medicines, or your other drug treatment is changed.

Pregnancy No evidence of risk to the developing baby from insulin, but poor control of diabetes increases the risk of birth defects. Careful monitoring is required because insulin requirements may change.

Breast-feeding No evidence of risk. Adjustment in dose may be necessary while breast-feeding.

Infants and children Reduced dose necessary.

Over 60 No special problems.

Driving and hazardous work Usually no problem, but strenuous exercise alters insulin and glucose requirements. Avoid such activities if you have warning signs of low blood glucose.

Alcohol Avoid. Alcohol upsets diabetic control.

Surgery and general anaesthetics Insulin requirements may increase during surgery, and blood glucose levels will need to be monitored during and after an operation. Notify your doctor or dentist that you are diabetic before any surgery.

PROLONGED USE
No problems expected.
Monitoring Regular monitoring of glucose levels in the urine and/or blood is required.

Interferon

Brand names Avonex, Betaferon, Immukin, IntronA, Pegasys, PegIntron, Rebif, Roferon-A, Viraferon, ViraferonPeg
Used in the following combined preparations
None

QUICK REFERENCE
Drug group Antiviral drug (p.69) and anticancer drug (p.96)
Overdose danger rating Medium
Dependence rating Low
Prescription needed Yes
Available as generic No

GENERAL INFORMATION
Interferons are a group of substances normally produced in human and animal cells that have been infected with viruses or stimulated by other substances. They are thought to promote resistance to several types of viral infection. Three main types of interferon (alpha, beta, and gamma) are used to treat a range of diseases. Interferon alpha is used for leukaemias, other cancers, and chronic hepatitis B and C. Interferon beta reduces the frequency and severity of relapses in multiple sclerosis. Interferon gamma is given in conjunction with antibiotics for patients with chronic granulomatous disease.

Interferons can cause severe adverse effects (see below).

INFORMATION FOR USERS
This drug is given only under medical supervision and is not for self-administration.
How taken/used Injection.
Frequency and timing of doses Once daily 3 times a week, depending on product and condition being treated.
Adult dosage range Depends on product and condition being treated. Dosage may sometimes be calculated from body surface area.
Onset of effect Active in the body within 1 hour, but effects may not be noted for 1–2 months.

Duration of action Immediate effects last for about 12 hours.
Diet advice None.
Storage Store in a refrigerator at 2–8°C (36–46°F). Do not let it freeze, and protect from light. Keep out of the reach of children.
Missed dose Not applicable. This drug is usually given only in hospital under close medical supervision.
Stopping the drug Discuss with your doctor.
Exceeding the dose Overdosage is unlikely since treatment is carefully monitored.

POSSIBLE ADVERSE EFFECTS
Headache, lethargy, depression, dizziness, drowsiness, digestive disturbance, chills, fever, muscle-ache, poor appetite, and weight loss are common. Hair loss and vision problems are rare. Notify your doctor of all unusual symptoms without delay; some may be dose-related, requiring dosage reduction.

INTERACTIONS
General note A number of drugs increase the risk of adverse effects on the blood, heart, or nervous system. This is taken into account when prescribing an interferon with other drugs.
Vaccines Interferon may reduce the effectiveness of vaccines.
Theophylline/aminophylline The effects of this drug may be increased by interferon.
Sedatives All drugs that have a sedative effect on the central nervous system are likely to increase the sedative properties of interferon. Such drugs include opioid analgesics, anti-anxiety and sleeping drugs, antihistamines, antidepressants, and antipsychotics.

SPECIAL PRECAUTIONS
Interferon is prescribed only under close medical supervision, taking account of your present condition and medical history. However, be sure to tell your doctor if:
◆ You have long-term liver or kidney problems.
◆ You have heart disease.
◆ You have had epileptic fits.
◆ You have had any previous drug allergies.
◆ You have diabetes.
◆ You have asthma, eczema, or psoriasis.
◆ You suffer from depression.
◆ You are taking other medicines.

Pregnancy Not usually prescribed. Safety in pregnancy not established. Discuss with your doctor.

Breast-feeding It is not known whether the drug passes into the breast milk. Discuss with your doctor.

Infants and children Not usually used.

Over 60 Increased likelihood of adverse effects. Reduced dose may be necessary.

Driving and hazardous work Not applicable.

Alcohol Avoid. Alcohol may increase the sedative effects of this drug.

PROLONGED USE

Increased risk of liver damage. Blood cell production in the bone marrow may be reduced. Repeated large doses are associated with lethargy, fatigue, collapse, and coma.

Monitoring Frequent blood tests are required to monitor blood composition and liver function.

Ipratropium bromide

Brand names Atrovent, Respontin, Rinatec
Used in the following combined preparations
Combibent, Duovent, Ipramol

QUICK REFERENCE

Drug group Bronchodilator (p.23)
Overdose danger rating Low
Dependence rating Low
Prescription needed Yes
Available as generic Yes

GENERAL INFORMATION

Ipratropium bromide is a bronchodilator with an anticholinergic (see Autonomic nervous system, p.8) action that relaxes the muscles surrounding the bronchioles (airways in the lung). It is used primarily in the maintenance treatment of reversible airway disorders, particularly chronic bronchitis, and is given only by inhaler or via a nebulizer.

Although its effect lasts longer, ipratropium bromide has a slower onset of action than the sympathomimetic bronchodilators (see p.24). For this reason, it is not as effective in treating acute attacks of wheezing, or in emergency treatment of asthma, and it is usually used together with the faster-acting drugs. Ipratropium bromide is also pre-scribed as a nasal spray for the treatment of a continually runny nose due to allergy.

Unlike with other anticholinergics, side effects are rare. The drug is unlikely to affect the heart, eyes, bowel, or bladder. Eye problems may occur if the drug comes into contact with the eyes during use with the inhaler or nebulizer. Correct use of inhalers or nebulizers is important, especially if you have glaucoma.

INFORMATION FOR USERS

Your drug prescription is tailored for you. Do not alter dosage without checking with your doctor.

How taken/used Inhaler, liquid for nebulizer, nasal spray.

Frequency and timing of doses 3–4 x daily (inhaler); 2 sprays into each nostril 2–3 x daily (nasal spray).

Adult dosage range 80–320mcg daily (inhaler); 400–2,000mcg daily (nebulizer); 1–2 puffs to the affected nostril 2–3 x daily (nasal spray).

Onset of effect 3–30 minutes.

Duration of action Up to 8 hours.

Diet advice None.

Storage Keep in original container at room temperature out of the reach of children. Do not puncture or burn containers.

Missed dose Take as soon as you remember. If your next dose is due within 2 hours, take a single dose now and skip the next.

Stopping the drug Do not stop taking the drug without consulting your doctor; symptoms may recur.

Exceeding the dose An occasional unintentional extra dose is unlikely to be a cause for concern. But if you notice any unusual symptoms, or if a large overdose has been taken, notify your doctor.

POSSIBLE ADVERSE EFFECTS

Side effects are rare; the most common are dry mouth or throat, nausea, and headache. Constipation, difficulty in passing urine, and a cough are rare. Discuss a fast heart rate or palpitations with your doctor. If a rash or facial swelling occur, stop taking the drug and consult your doctor promptly.

INTERACTIONS

None.

SPECIAL PRECAUTIONS

Be sure to tell your doctor if:
◆ You have glaucoma.
◆ You have prostate problems.
◆ You have difficulty in passing urine.
◆ You have cystic fibrosis.
◆ You are taking other medicines.

Pregnancy No evidence of risk, but discuss with your doctor before using in the first 3 months of pregnancy.

Breast-feeding No evidence of risk, but discuss with your doctor.

Infants and children Reduced dose necessary.

Over 60 No special problems.

Driving and hazardous work No special problems.

Alcohol No known problems.

PROLONGED USE

No special problems.

Irbesartan

Brand name Aprovel
Used in the following combined preparation
CoAprovel

QUICK REFERENCE

Drug group Vasodilator (p.31) and antihypertensive drug (p.36)
Overdose danger rating Medium
Dependence rating Low
Prescription needed Yes
Available as generic No

GENERAL INFORMATION

Irbesartan is an angiotensin-II blocker vasodilator (see p.32) used to treat hypertension. The drug is also used to protect the kidneys in people with Type 2 diabetes who have hypertension and impaired kidney function.

Unlike ACE inhibitors, irbesartan does not cause a persistent dry cough. Along with other angiotensin-II blockers, it is being evaluated for the treatment of some of the other conditions, such as heart failure, for which ACE inhibitors are used. Irbesartan is also available in combination with a diuretic.

Irbesartan is prescribed with caution to people with renal artery stenosis (narrowing of the arteries to the kidneys) because the initial dose causes a sudden drop in blood pressure. It is important to notify your doctor if you know that you have this condition.

INFORMATION FOR USERS

Your drug prescription is tailored for you. Do not alter dosage without checking with your doctor.

How taken/used Tablets.

Frequency and timing of doses Once daily.

Adult dosage range 150mg (maintenance dose), increased to 300mg if needed; 75mg may be used in people over 75 years and those on haemodialysis.

Onset of effect Within 1 hour. Blood pressure lowered within 1–2 weeks; maximum beneficial effect 4–6 weeks from start of treatment.

Duration of action 24 hours.

Diet advice None.

Storage Keep in original container at room temperature out of the reach of children.

Missed dose Take as soon as you remember. If your next dose is due within 8 hours, take a single dose now and skip the next.

Stopping the drug Do not stop the drug without consulting your doctor. Stopping the drug may lead to worsening of the high blood pressure.

Exceeding the dose An occasional unintentional extra dose is unlikely to be a cause for concern. Large overdoses may cause dizziness, fainting, and a faint pulse or slow heart rate. Notify your doctor.

POSSIBLE ADVERSE EFFECTS

Adverse effects are usually mild. Dizziness, fatigue, and flushing are common, as are nausea and vomiting, which should be discussed with your doctor. Headaches are rare. If you experience a fast heart rate or develop a rash, consult your doctor.

INTERACTIONS

Diuretics There is a risk of a sudden fall in blood pressure if these drugs are being taken when irbesartan treatment is started.

Potassium supplements, potassium-sparing diuretics, and ciclosporin used with irbesartan may raise levels of potassium in the blood.

Antihypertensives increase irbesartan's effects.

Lithium Irbesartan increases the blood levels and toxicity of lithium.

NSAIDs Some may reduce the blood-pressure lowering effects of irbesartan, and there is a risk that they may worsen kidney function.

SPECIAL PRECAUTIONS

Be sure to tell your doctor if:
◆ You have kidney problems or renal artery stenosis.
◆ You have heart problems.
◆ You have congestive heart failure.
◆ You have primary aldosteronism.
◆ You have glucose or galactose malabsorption or galactose intolerance.
◆ You have Lapp lactase deficiency.
◆ You are taking other medicines.

Pregnancy Not prescribed. If you become pregnant during treatment, consult your doctor without delay.

Breast-feeding Safety not established. Discuss with your doctor.

Infants and children Not prescribed.

Over 60 Reduced dose may be necessary in people over 75 years.

Driving and hazardous work Avoid such activities until you have learned how irbesartan affects you because the drug can cause dizziness and fatigue.

Alcohol Avoid. Regular intake of alcohol may raise the blood pressure and reduce the effectiveness of irbesartan. Alcohol may also increase the likelihood of an excessive fall in blood pressure.

PROLONGED USE

No special problems.

Monitoring Periodic checks on blood potassium levels and kidney function may be performed.

Isoniazid

Brand names None
Used in the following combined preparations
Rifater, Rifinah, Rimactazid

QUICK REFERENCE

Drug group Antituberculous drug (p.67)
Overdose danger rating High
Dependence rating Low
Prescription needed Yes
Available as generic Yes

GENERAL INFORMATION

In use for over 30 years, isoniazid (also known as INAH and INH) remains an effective drug for tuberculosis. It is given alone to prevent tuberculosis and in combination with other drugs for its treatment. Treatment usually lasts 6 months, but courses of 9 months or a year may sometimes be prescribed.

One of isoniazid's side effects is increased loss of pyridoxine (vitamin B_6) from the body. This is more likely with high doses, and is rare in children but common among people with poor nutrition. Since pyridoxine deficiency can lead to irreversible nerve damage, supplements are usually given.

INFORMATION FOR USERS

Your drug prescription is tailored for you. Do not alter dosage without checking with your doctor.

How taken/used Tablets, liquid, injection.

Frequency and timing of doses Normally once daily.

Dosage range *Adults* 300mg daily. *Children* According to age and weight.

Onset of effect Over 2–3 days.

Duration of action Up to 24 hours.

Diet advice Take 30 minutes before food because food decreases absorption of isoniazid.

Storage Keep in original container at room temperature out of the reach of children. Protect from light.

Missed dose Take as soon as you remember. If your next dose is scheduled within 8 hours, take a single dose now and skip the next.

Stopping the drug Take the full course. Even if you feel better the infection may still be present and may recur if treatment is stopped too soon.

OVERDOSE ACTION

Seek immediate medical advice in all cases. Take emergency action if breathing difficulties, fits, or loss of consciousness occur.

POSSIBLE ADVERSE EFFECTS

Serious problems are uncommon, but all adverse effects should receive prompt medical attention due to the possibility of nerve or liver damage. Adverse effects include nausea, vomiting, fatigue, malaise, weakness, numbness, tingling, mood changes, and a rash. If blurred vision, jaundice, twitching, or muscle weakness occur, stop taking the drug and consult your doctor without delay.

INTERACTIONS

Alcohol and rifampicin Large quantities of alcohol may reduce the effectiveness of isoniazid. If the two are taken together, the likelihood of liver damage is increased; if, in addition, rifampicin is being taken, the risk of liver damage is increased further.

Theophylline Isoniazid may increase levels and effects of theophylline.

Antiepileptics The effects of these drugs may be increased with isoniazid.

Antacids These drugs may reduce the absorption of isoniazid.

Ketoconazole Isoniazid reduces the blood concentration of ketoconazole.

SPECIAL PRECAUTIONS

Be sure to tell your doctor if:
◆ You have long-term liver or kidney problems.
◆ You have had liver damage following isoniazid treatment in the past.
◆ You have problems with drug or alcohol abuse.
◆ You have diabetes.
◆ You have porphyria.
◆ You have HIV infection.
◆ You have had epileptic fits.
◆ You are taking other medicines.

Pregnancy Not known to be harmful to the fetus, but discuss with your doctor.

Breast-feeding The drug passes into the breast milk and may affect the baby. The infant should be monitored for signs of toxic effects. Discuss with your doctor.

Infants and children Reduced dose necessary.

Over 60 Increased likelihood of adverse effects.

Driving and hazardous work No special problems.

Alcohol Avoid excessive amounts.

PROLONGED USE

Pyridoxine (vitamin B_6) deficiency may occur with prolonged use and lead to nerve damage. Supplements are usually prescribed. There is also a risk of serious liver damage.

Monitoring Periodic blood tests are usually performed to monitor liver function.

Isosorbide dinitrate/ mononitrate

Brand names [Dinitrate] Angitak, Cedocard, Isoket, and others; [Mononitrate] Chemydur, Elantan, Imdur, Isib, Ismo, Isodur, Isotard, Modisal, Monomil XL, and others

Used in the following combined preparations None

QUICK REFERENCE

Drug group Nitrate vasodilator (p.31) and anti-angina drug (p.35)

Overdose danger rating Medium

Dependence rating Low

Prescription needed No (some preparations); yes (other preparations and injection)

Available as generic No

GENERAL INFORMATION

Similar to glyceryl trinitrate, isosorbide dinitrate and mononitrate are vasodilators usually used to treat patients with angina. They are also used in some cases of heart failure.

Unlike glyceryl trinitrate, both of these drugs are stable and can be stored for long periods without losing their effectiveness.

Headache, flushing, and dizziness are common at the start of treatment; initially, small doses can help to minimize these. The drugs' effectiveness may be reduced after a few months; dosage change may be used to allow low drug levels for some hours in the day.

INFORMATION FOR USERS

Follow instructions on the label. Call your doctor if symptoms worsen.

How taken/used *Dinitrate* Tablets, SR-tablets, injection, spray. *Mononitrate* Tablets, SR-tablets, SR-capsules.

Frequency and timing of doses *Relief of angina attacks* As required (spray). *Heart failure/prevention of angina* 2–4 x daily; 1–2 x daily (SR-tablets, capsules).

Adult dosage range *Prevention of angina* 30–120mg daily (divided doses). *Treatment of angina* 1–3 doses under the tongue (spray). *Heart failure* 40–240mg daily (divided doses).

Onset of effect 2–3 minutes (spray); 20–30 minutes (SR-tablets, capsules).

Duration of action 4–6 hours (dinitrate tablets); 8–10 hours (mononitrate tablets); up to 17 hours (SR-tablets); up to 10 hours (SR-capsules); 1–2 hours (spray).

Diet advice None.

Storage Keep in original container at room temperature out of the reach of children. Protect from light.

Missed dose Take as soon as you remember. If your next dose is due within 2 hours, take a single dose now and skip the next.

Stopping the drug Do not stop the drug without consulting your doctor. Doing so may lead to worsening of the underlying condition.

Exceeding the dose An occasional unintentional extra dose is unlikely to cause problems. Large doses may cause dizziness, headache, or shortness of breath. Notify your doctor.

POSSIBLE ADVERSE EFFECTS

Flushing and headache are common. The most serious problem is excessively lowered blood pressure, which may produce dizziness, fainting, or weakness. These, and fast or slow heart rate, should be discussed with your doctor. Other effects of both forms usually improve with regular use; dosage adjustment may help.

INTERACTIONS

Sildenafil, tadalafil, and vardenafil significantly enhance the blood-pressure lowering effect of nitrates; they should not be used together.

Antihypertensives taken with nitrates cause further lowering of blood pressure.

SPECIAL PRECAUTIONS

Be sure to consult your doctor or pharmacist before taking this drug if:
◆ You have long-term liver or kidney problems.
◆ You have any blood disorders or anaemia.
◆ You have glaucoma.
◆ You have low blood pressure.
◆ You have ever had a heart attack.
◆ You have an underactive thyroid.
◆ You have G6PD deficiency.
◆ You have had a recent head injury.
◆ You are taking other medicines.

Pregnancy Safety in pregnancy not established. Discuss with your doctor.

Breast-feeding Safety not established. Discuss with your doctor.

Infants and children Not usually prescribed.

Over 60 No special problems.

Driving and hazardous work Avoid such activities until you have learned how the drugs affect you because they can cause dizziness.

Alcohol Avoid. Alcohol may further lower blood pressure, depressing the heart and causing dizziness and fainting.

PROLONGED USE

The initial adverse effects may disappear with prolonged use. The effects of the drug become weaker as the body adapts. This may be overcome by a change in the dose to allow a period of low drug level during each day.

Isotretinoin

Brand names Isotrex Gel, Roaccutane
Used in the following combined preparation Isotrexin

QUICK REFERENCE

Drug group Drug for acne (p.123)
Overdose danger rating Medium
Dependence rating Low
Prescription needed Yes
Available as generic Yes

GENERAL INFORMATION

Chemically related to vitamin A, isotretinoin is prescribed for the treatment of severe acne that has failed to respond to other treatments.

The drug reduces production of the skin's natural oils (sebum) and the horny protein (keratin) in the outer layers of skin, making it useful in conditions such as ichthyosis where abnormally thickened skin causes scaling.

A single 16-week course of treatment often clears the acne. The skin may be very dry, flaky, and itchy at first, but usually improves with time. Serious adverse effects include liver damage and bowel inflammation.

INFORMATION FOR USERS

Your drug prescription is tailored for you. Do not alter dosage without checking with your doctor.

How taken/used Capsules, gel.

Frequency and timing of doses 1–2 x daily (take capsules with food or milk).

Adult dosage range Dosage is determined individually.

Onset of effect 2–4 weeks (capsules); 6–8 weeks (gel). Acne may worsen initially in some people but usually improves in 7–10 days.

Duration of action Effects persist for several weeks after the drug is stopped.

Diet advice None.

Storage Keep in original container at room temperature out of the reach of children. Protect from light.

Missed dose Take as soon as you remember. If your next dose is due within 4 hours, take a single dose now and skip the next.

Stopping the drug Can be safely stopped as soon as you no longer need it.

Exceeding the dose An occasional unintentional extra dose is unlikely to cause problems. Large overdoses may cause headaches, vomiting, dizziness, abdominal pain, flushing, and incoordination. Notify your doctor.

POSSIBLE ADVERSE EFFECTS

The most serious effects occur with the capsules. Dry nose, mouth, and eyes, inflamed lips, nosebleeds, and flaking skin often occur. Mood changes, skin pigment changes, muscle or joint pains, and temporary hair loss or increase may also occur. If headache, nausea, vomiting, blood in the faeces, visual impairment, or a rash or bruising occur, consult your doctor promptly. If abdominal pain or diarrhoea occur, stop taking the drug and consult your doctor immediately.

INTERACTIONS

Tetracycline antibiotics increase the risk of high pressure in the skull, leading to headaches, nausea, and vomiting.

Skin-drying preparations Medicated cosmetics, soaps, and toiletries, and anti-acne or abrasive skin preparations increase the likelihood of dry, irritated skin with isotretinoin.

Vitamin A supplements increase the risk of adverse effects from isotretinoin.

Progestogen-only contraceptives work poorly during isotretinoin treatment. Alternative contraception should be used 1 month before, during, and 1 month after, treatment.

SPECIAL PRECAUTIONS

Do not donate blood during, or for at least a month after, taking oral isotretinoin. Be sure to tell your doctor if:

◆ You have long-term liver or kidney problems.

◆ You suffer from arthritis or gout.

◆ You have diabetes.

◆ You have a history of depression.

◆ You have fructose intolerance.

◆ You have high blood fat levels.

◆ You wear contact lenses.

◆ You are taking other medicines.

Pregnancy Must not be prescribed. The drug is known to cause abnormalities in the developing baby. Effective contraception must be used during treatment and for at least a month before and after.

Breast-feeding The drug is likely to pass into the breast milk and may affect the baby. Discuss with your doctor.

Infants and children Not prescribed.

Over 60 Not usually prescribed.

Driving and hazardous work Avoid such activities until you have learned how the drug affects you because it can cause vision problems in dim light or darkness.

Alcohol Avoid heavy consumption.

Sunlight Avoid exposure: use a sunscreen or sunblock; do not use a sunlamp or sunbed.

PROLONGED USE

Treatment rarely exceeds 16 weeks. Prolonged use may raise blood fat levels, and increase the risk of heart and blood vessel disease. Bone changes may occur.

Monitoring Liver function tests and checks on blood fat levels are performed.

Ketoconazole

Brand names Daktarin Gold, Nizoral
Used in the following combined preparations None

QUICK REFERENCE

Drug group Antifungal drug (p.76)
Overdose danger rating Medium
Dependence rating Low
Prescription needed Yes (except for some shampoos)
Available as generic No

GENERAL INFORMATION

Ketoconazole is prescribed for severe, internal systemic fungal infections. It is also given to treat serious infections of the skin and mucous membranes caused by the *Candida* yeast. People with rare fungal diseases (for example, paracoccidioidomycosis, histoplasmosis, and coccidioidomycosis) may also be given this antifungal drug.

Ketoconazole is also available as cream to treat fungal skin infections, and shampoo for the treatment of scalp infections and seborrhoeic dermatitis.

The most common side effect of oral ketoconazole is nausea, which can reduced by taking the drug at bedtime or with meals. Ketoconazole may also cause liver damage.

INFORMATION FOR USERS

Your drug prescription is tailored for you. Do not alter dosage without checking with your doctor.

How taken/used Tablets, liquid, cream, shampoo.

Frequency and timing of doses Once daily with food (by mouth); 1–2 x daily (cream); 1–2 times weekly (shampoo used for seborrhoeic dermatitis).

Dosage range *Adults* 200–400mg daily (by mouth). *Children* Reduced dose according to age and weight.

Onset of effect Within a few hours; full beneficial effect may take several days (or weeks in severe infections).

Duration of action Up to 24 hours.

Diet advice None.

Storage Keep in original container at room temperature out of the reach of children.

Missed dose (oral) Take as soon as you remember. If your next dose is due within 6 hours, take a single dose now and skip the next.

Stopping the drug Take the full course. Even if you feel better, the infection may still be present; symptoms may recur if treatment is stopped too soon.

Exceeding the dose An occasional unintentional extra dose is unlikely to be a cause for concern. Large overdoses may cause gastric problems. Notify your doctor.

POSSIBLE ADVERSE EFFECTS

Nausea and vomiting are common; abdominal pain and headache may also occur. If itching or a rash occur, or (in men) you develop painful breasts, stop taking the drug

and consult your doctor. Liver damage is rare, but serious, and causes jaundice (yellowing of the skin and whites of the eyes) that may necessitate stopping the drug.

INTERACTIONS (ADMINISTRATION BY MOUTH ONLY)

General note Ketoconazole interacts with a wide range of drugs to increase their effects (including side effects). Such drugs include warfarin, ciclosporin, domperidone, tacrolimus, some calcium channel blockers, and corticosteroids.

Eletriptan Use of this drug with ketoconazole is not recommended.

Antiviral drugs Dosage adjustment of these drugs may be necessary with ketoconazole.

Antimalarials Artemether with lumefantrine should be avoided with ketoconazole.

Antacids, cimetidine, and ranitidine taken within 2 hours before or after ketoconazole may reduce its effectiveness.

Rifampicin, rifabutin, carbamazepine, isoniazid, and phenytoin may reduce the effect of ketoconazole.

Simvastatin and possibly other "statins" taken with ketoconazole increase the risk of muscle damage.

Pimozide, sertindole, mizolastine, quinidine taken with ketoconazole increase the risk of adverse effects on the heart.

SPECIAL PRECAUTIONS

Be sure to tell your doctor if:
◆ You have liver or kidney problems.
◆ You have porphyria.
◆ You have previously had liver problems caused by medicines.
◆ You have previously had an allergic reaction to antifungal drugs.
◆ You have Addison's disease.
◆ You are taking other medicines.

Pregnancy Not usually prescribed. May cause defects in the developing baby. Discuss with your doctor.

Breast-feeding The drug passes into the breast milk and may affect the baby. Discuss with your doctor.

Infants and children Reduced dose necessary.

Over 60 No special problems.

Driving and hazardous work Not special problems.

Alcohol Avoid. Alcohol may interact with this drug to cause flushing and nausea.

PROLONGED USE

The risk of liver damage increases with use of oral ketoconazole for more than 14 days.
Monitoring Periodic blood tests are usually performed to check the drug's effect on the liver.

Ketoprofen

Brand names Ketocid, Ketovail, Ketozip, Orudis, Oruvail, Powergel, and many others
Used in the following combined preparations None

QUICK REFERENCE

Drug group Non-steroidal anti-inflammatory drug (p.50)
Overdose danger rating Medium
Dependence rating Low
Prescription needed Yes (except for some topical preparations)
Available as generic Yes

GENERAL INFORMATION

Ketoprofen is a non-steroidal anti-inflammatory (NSAID) which, like other NSAIDs, relieves pain and reduces inflammation and stiffness in rheumatoid arthritis, osteoarthritis, and ankylosing spondylitis. It does not cure the underlying disease, however.

Ketoprofen is also given to relieve mild to moderate pain of menstruation and soft tissue injuries, and pain following operations.

The most common adverse reactions to ketoprofen, as with all NSAIDs, are gastrointestinal disturbances such as nausea and indigestion. Switching to another NSAID may be recommended by your doctor if unwanted effects are persistent or troublesome.

INFORMATION FOR USERS

Follow instructions on the label. Call your doctor if symptoms worsen.
How taken/used Capsules, SR-capsules, injection, suppositories, gel.
Frequency and timing of doses Once daily (SR-capsules) or 2–4 x daily (capsules) with food; 4 x daily for up to 3 days (injection); 2 x daily (suppositories).
Adult dosage range 100–200mg daily.

Onset of effect Pain relief may be felt in 30 minutes to 2 hours. Full anti-inflammatory effect may not be felt for up to 2 weeks.
Duration of action Up to 8–12 hours.
Diet advice None.
Storage Keep in original container at room temperature out of the reach of children.
Missed dose Take as soon as you remember. If your next dose is due within 4 hours, take a single dose now and skip the next.
Stopping the drug Seek medical advice before stopping the drug.
Exceeding the dose An occasional unintentional extra dose is unlikely to be a cause for concern. Large overdoses may cause vomiting, confusion, or irritability. Notify your doctor.

POSSIBLE ADVERSE EFFECTS

Gastrointestinal disturbances, such as nausea, vomiting, abdominal pain, and heartburn are common with oral forms. Suppositories may cause rectal irritation. Dizziness, drowsiness, headache, and fluid retention (causing swollen feet or legs and weight gain) may also occur. If a rash or itching occur, stop taking the drug. If wheezing, breathlessness, or black or bloodstained faeces occur, stop taking the drug and get urgent medical attention.

INTERACTIONS

General note Ketoprofen interacts with a wide range of drugs, such as aspirin and other NSAIDs, oral anticoagulants, and corticosteroids, to increase the risk of bleeding and/or stomach ulcers.
Lithium, digoxin, and methotrexate Ketoprofen may raise blood levels of these drugs.
Phenytoin Ketoprofen may enhance its effects.
Quinolone antibiotics Ketoprofen may increase the risk of seizures if taken with these drugs.
Antihypertensive drugs Ketoprofen may reduce the beneficial effects of these drugs.

SPECIAL PRECAUTIONS

Be sure to consult your doctor or pharmacist before taking this drug if:
◆ You have long-term liver or kidney problems.
◆ You have heart problems.
◆ You have high blood pressure.
◆ You have asthma.

◆ You have had a peptic ulcer, oesophagitis, or acid indigestion.
◆ You have bleeding problems.
◆ You are allergic to aspirin or other NSAIDs.
◆ You are taking other medicines.

Pregnancy Safety in pregnancy not established. Discuss with your doctor.

Breast-feeding The drug passes into the breast milk and may affect the baby. Discuss with your doctor.

Infants and children Not recommended for children under 12 years.

Over 60 Increased likelihood of adverse effects. Reduced dose may therefore be necessary.

Driving and hazardous work Avoid such activities until you have learned how ketoprofen affects you because the drug can cause dizziness and drowsiness.

Alcohol Avoid. Alcohol may increase the risk of stomach disorders with ketoprofen.

Surgery and general anaesthetics Ketoprofen may prolong bleeding. Discuss this with your doctor or dentist before having any surgery.

PROLONGED USE

There is an increased risk of bleeding from peptic ulcers and in the bowel with prolonged use of ketoprofen. The lowest effective dose is given for the shortest duration.

Lactulose

Brand names Duphalac, Lactugal, Regulose
Used in the following combined preparations None

QUICK REFERENCE

Drug group Laxative (p.45)
Overdose danger rating Low
Dependence rating Low
Prescription needed No
Available as generic Yes

GENERAL INFORMATION

Lactulose is an effective laxative that softens faeces by increasing the amount of water in the large intestine. It is used for the relief of constipation and faecal impaction, especially in the elderly. It is less likely than some other laxatives to disrupt normal bowel action Lactulose is also to prevent and treat brain

disturbance associated with liver failure, a condition known as hepatic encephalopathy.

Because lactulose acts locally in the large intestine and is not absorbed into the body, it is safer than many other laxatives.

INFORMATION FOR USERS

Follow instructions on the label. Call your doctor if symptoms worsen.

How taken/used Liquid.
Frequency and timing of doses 2 x daily (chronic constipation); 3–4 x daily (liver failure).
Adult dosage range 15–30ml daily (chronic constipation); 90–150ml daily (liver failure).
Onset of effect 24–48 hours.
Duration of action 6–18 hours.
Diet advice It is important to maintain an adequate intake of fluid – up to 8 glasses of water daily.
Storage Keep in original container at room temperature out of the reach of children. Do not store after diluting, refrigerate, or freeze.
Missed dose Take as soon as you remember. If your next dose is due within 3 hours, take a single dose now and skip the next.
Stopping the drug In the treatment of constipation, the drug can be safely stopped as soon as you no longer need it.
Exceeding the dose An occasional unintentional extra dose is unlikely to be a cause for concern. But if you notice any unusual symptoms, or if a large overdose has been taken, notify your doctor.

POSSIBLE ADVERSE EFFECTS

Adverse effects, including belching, flatulence, nausea, vomiting, and abdominal cramps and distension are rarely serious and often disappear when your body adjusts to the medicine. Diarrhoea may indicate too high a dosage, requiring adjustment. Consult your doctor.

INTERACTIONS

No known significant interactions.

SPECIAL PRECAUTIONS

Be sure to consult your doctor or pharmacist before taking this drug if:
◆ You have severe abdominal pain.
◆ You have diabetes.
◆ You suffer from lactose intolerance or galactosaemia.

◆ You are taking other medicines.
Pregnancy No evidence of risk. Discuss with your doctor.
Breast-feeding No evidence of risk.
Infants and children Reduced dose necessary.
Over 60 No special problems.
Driving and hazardous work No known problems.
Alcohol No known problems.

PROLONGED USE

In children, prolonged use may contribute to the development of dental caries.

Lamotrigine

Brand name Lamictal
Used in the following combined preparations None

QUICK REFERENCE

Drug group Anticonvulsant drug (p.16)
Overdose danger rating Medium
Dependence rating Low
Prescription needed Yes
Available as generic Yes

GENERAL INFORMATION

Introduced in 1993, lamotrigine is an anticonvulsant prescribed, either alone or in combination with other anticonvulsants, for the treatment of epilepsy. It acts by restoring the balance between excitatory and inhibitory neurotransmitters in the brain. The drug may be less sedating than older anticonvulsants, and there is no need for blood tests to determine the level of the drug in the blood.

Lamotrigine may cause a number of minor adverse effects (see right), most of which will respond to an adjustment in dosage. Lamotrigine is also occasionally used in specialist centres to treat bipolar affective disorder.

INFORMATION FOR USERS

Your drug prescription is tailored for you. Do not alter dosage without checking with your doctor.
How taken/used Tablets, chewable tablets, dispersible tablets.
Frequency and timing of doses 1–2 x daily.
Adult dosage range 100–500mg daily (mainte-

nance); (100–200mg with sodium valproate). Smaller doses are used at start of treatment. Dose may vary if other anticonvulsant drugs are being taken.
Onset of effect Approximately 5 days at a constant dose.
Duration of action Up to 24 hours.
Diet advice None.
Storage Keep in original container at room temperature out of the reach of children.
Missed dose Take as soon as you remember. If your next dose is due within 2 hours, take a single dose now and skip the next.
Stopping the drug Do not stop taking the drug without consulting your doctor, who will supervise a gradual reduction in dosage. Abrupt cessation increases the risk of rebound fits.
Exceeding the dose An occasional unintentional extra dose is unlikely to be a cause for concern. Large overdoses may cause sedation, double vision, loss of muscular coordination, nausea, and vomiting. Contact your doctor immediately.

POSSIBLE ADVERSE EFFECTS

Serious adverse effects are rare with lamotrigine treatment. Headaches commonly occur. Blurred or double vision, tremor, and poor muscle coordination are also common, and they should be discussed with your doctor. Although common, a rash may indicate a serious hypersensitivity reaction, and you should call your doctor immediately; a rash is less likely to occur if the treatment is started at a low dose. If you develop a sore throat, facial swelling, flu-like symptoms, or if persistent or unusual bruising occurs, call your doctor immediately.

INTERACTIONS

Sodium valproate increases and prolongs the effectiveness of lamotrigine. A reduced dose of lamotrigine will be used.
Antidepressants, antipsychotics, mefloquine, and chloroquine may counteract the anticonvulsant effect of lamotrigine.
Carbamazepine may reduce lamotrigine blood levels, but lamotrigine may increase the side effects of carbamazepine.
Phenytoin and phenobarbital may decrease blood levels of lamotrigine, so a higher dose of lamotrigine may be needed.

SPECIAL PRECAUTIONS

Be sure to tell your doctor if:

◆ You have long-term liver or kidney problems.

◆ You have any blood disorder.

◆ You are taking other medicines.

Pregnancy Safety in pregnancy not established. Discuss with your doctor.

Breast-feeding The drug passes into the breast milk and may affect the baby. Discuss with your doctor.

Infants and children Not recommended under 2 years. Not recommended as a single therapy under 12 years. Doses may be relatively higher than adult doses due to increased metabolism.

Over 60 No special problems.

Driving and hazardous work Your underlying condition, in addition to the possibility of sedation, dizziness, and vision disturbances while taking lamotrigine, may make such activities inadvisable. Discuss with your doctor.

Alcohol Alcohol may increase the adverse effects of this drug.

PROLONGED USE

No special problems.

Lansoprazole

Brand name Zoton
Used in the following combined preparations None

QUICK REFERENCE

Drug group Anti-ulcer drug (p.43)
Overdose danger rating Low
Dependence rating Low
Prescription needed Yes
Available as generic No

GENERAL INFORMATION

Lansoprazole belongs to a group of drugs called proton pump inhibitors (see p.43). It is used to treat gastro-oesophageal reflux (rising of stomach acid into the oesophagus), Zollinger-Ellison syndrome (production of large quantities of stomach acid, leading to ulceration), and to prevent or treat peptic ulcers. It works by reducing the amount of stomach acid produced.

Lansoprazole may be used alone, or in combination with antibiotics as a 7-day course to eradicate *Helicobacter pylori* bacteria, the main cause of peptic ulcers. Because it may mask the symptoms of stomach cancer, the drug is prescribed only when the possibility of this disease has been ruled out.

INFORMATION FOR USERS

Your drug prescription is tailored for you. Do not alter dosage without checking with your doctor.

How taken/used Capsules, dispersible tablets, liquid (suspension).

Frequency and timing of doses Usually once, sometimes twice, daily before food in the morning.

Dosage range *Peptic ulcer/gastro-oesophageal reflux* 30mg daily. *NSAID-induced ulcer* 15–30mg daily. *Acid-related dyspepsia* 15–30mg daily. *Zollinger-Ellison syndrome* 60mg daily initially, adjusted according to response. *H. pylori-associated ulcer* 60mg daily, half the dose in the morning and half in the evening.

Onset of effect 1–2 hours.

Duration of action 24 hours.

Diet advice None, although spicy foods and alcohol may exacerbate the condition that is being treated.

Storage Keep in original container at room temperature out of the reach of children. Do not refrigerate.

Missed dose Take as soon as you remember. If your next dose is due within 8 hours, take a single dose now and skip the next.

Stopping the drug Do not stop taking the drug without consulting your doctor; symptoms may recur.

Exceeding the dose An occasional unintentional extra dose is unlikely to be a cause for concern. But if you notice any unusual symptoms, or if a large overdose has been taken, notify your doctor.

POSSIBLE ADVERSE EFFECTS

Common side effects include a headache and dizziness, diarrhoea or constipation, and flatulence and abdominal pain. Fatigue, malaise, muscle or joint pain, and bruising or swollen extremities are rare. If a rash or itching or nausea and vomiting occur, stop taking the drug. If a sore throat, wheezing, or breathing difficulties occur, stop taking the drug and seek immediate medical attention.

INTERACTIONS

Oral contraceptives, phenytoin, warfarin, carbamazepine, and theophylline Lansoprazole may reduce their effect.

Antacids and sucralfate These drugs may reduce the absorption of, and should not be taken within an hour of, lansoprazole.

Digoxin Lansoprazole may increase blood levels of digoxin.

Cilostazol Lansoprazole may increase the effect of cilostazol; the two drugs should not be taken together.

SPECIAL PRECAUTIONS

Be sure to tell your doctor if:
◆ You have liver problems.
◆ You are taking other medicines.

Pregnancy Safety not established. Discuss with your doctor.

Breast-feeding Safety not established. Discuss with your doctor.

Infants and children Not recommended.

Over 60 No special problems.

Driving and hazardous work No special problems.

Alcohol Avoid. Alcohol irritates the stomach.

PROLONGED USE

No problems expected.

Latanoprost

Brand name Xalatan
Used in the following combined preparation
Xalacom

QUICK REFERENCE

Drug group Drug for glaucoma (p.114)
Overdose danger rating Medium
Dependence rating Low
Prescription needed Yes
Available as generic No

GENERAL INFORMATION

Latanoprost is a synthetic derivative of the prostaglandin dinoprost, which constricts the smooth muscle in the blood vessels and bronchi. Latanoprost is used as eye drops to reduce pressure inside the eye in open-angle (chronic) glaucoma (see p.114) and ocular hypertension by constricting the pupils. The drug is used when patients have not responded to or cannot tolerate the drug of first choice, usually a beta blocker (such as timolol, p.408). Sometimes, combined eye drops of latanoprost and timolol may be prescribed when timolol alone is not adequately controlling the pressure.

The eye drops can gradually increase the amount of brown pigment in the eye, darkening the iris (due to increased amounts of melanin). This will be particularly noticeable if only one eye needs treatment. Irises of mixed coloration are especially susceptible; pure blue eyes do not seem to be affected. Latanoprost has also been reported to cause eyelashes to darken, thicken, and lengthen.

INFORMATION FOR USERS

Your drug prescription is tailored for you. Do not alter dosage without checking with your doctor.

How taken/used Eye drops.

Frequency and timing of doses 1 x daily, in the evening.

Adult dosage range 1 drop per eye, daily.

Onset of effect 3–4 hours.

Duration of action 24 hours.

Diet advice None.

Storage Keep the eye drops in the outer cardboard package to protect from light. Store at room temperature, out of the reach of children. Discard any unused solution 4 weeks after opening.

Missed dose Use the next dose as normal.

Stopping the drug Do not stop taking the drug without consulting your doctor; Symptoms may recur.

Exceeding the dose An occasional unintentional extra application is unlikely to cause problems. Excessive use may irritate the eye and produce adverse effects in other parts of the body. Notify your doctor.

POSSIBLE ADVERSE EFFECTS

Darkening of the iris, eye irritation, and eyelash changes are common. Consult your doctor if these are severe, or if you have eye pain, bloodshot or swollen eyes, inflamed eyelids, or facial swelling. Stop taking the drug and seek medical advice if chest pains, wheezing, or breathing difficulties occur.

INTERACTIONS

Other eye drops should not be used within 5 minutes of using latanoprost.

SPECIAL PRECAUTIONS

Be sure to tell your doctor if:
◆ You wear contact lenses.
◆ You are allergic to latanoprost or any of the ingredients in the formulation.
◆ You have asthma.
◆ You are taking other medicines.
Pregnancy Safety not established. Prostaglandins may affect the fetus. Discuss with your doctor.
Breast-feeding The drug may pass into the breast milk and may affect the baby. Discuss with your doctor.
Infants and children Not recommended. Safety not established.
Over 60 No special problems.
Driving and hazardous work No known problems.
Alcohol No known problems.

PROLONGED USE

No known problems except iris pigment and eyelashes changes, which do not affect vision, but do not diminish once treatment is stopped.
Monitoring Although there should be no problems with long-term use, your doctor will continue to monitor eye pigmentation as well as control of the glaucoma.

Levodopa/Co-beneldopa/Co-careldopa

Brand names None
Used in the following combined preparations Duodopa, Madopar, Madopar CR, Sinemet, Sinemet CR, Stalevo, Tilolec

QUICK REFERENCE

Drug group Drug for parkinsonism (p.18)
Overdose danger rating Medium
Dependence rating Low
Prescription needed Yes
Available as generic Yes

GENERAL INFORMATION

The treatment of Parkinson's disease underwent dramatic change in the 1960s with the introduction of levodopa. Since the body can transform levodopa into dopamine, a chemical messenger in the brain the absence or shortage of which causes Parkinson's disease (see p.18), rapid improvements in control were obtained. These improvements were not a cure but a marked relief of symptoms.

It was found, however, that, while levodopa was effective, it produced severe side effects, such as nausea, dizziness, and palpitations. Even when treatment was initiated gradually, it was difficult to balance the benefits against the adverse reactions.

Today the drug is prescribed in combination form with carbidopa (as co-careldopa) or benserazide (as co-beneldopa), both of which enhance the effects of levodopa in the brain, in addition to helping to reduce the side effects of levodopa. The drug is taken by mouth and, in severe cases, can be administered in the form of intestinal gel.

INFORMATION FOR USERS

Your drug prescription is tailored for you. Do not alter dosage without checking with your doctor.
How taken/used Tablets, dispersible tablets, capsules, intestinal gel.
Frequency and timing of doses 2–6 x daily with food or milk.
Adult dosage range 125–500mg initially, increased until benefits and side effects are balanced.
Onset of effect Within 1 hour.
Duration of action 2–12 hours.
Diet advice None.
Storage Keep in original container at room temperature out of the reach of children. Store intestinal gel in a refrigerator. Protect from light.
Missed dose Take as soon as you remember. If your next dose is due within 2 hours, take a single dose now and skip the next.
Stopping the drug Do not stop taking the drug without consulting your doctor; stopping the drug may lead to severe worsening of the underlying condition.
Exceeding the dose An occasional unintentional extra dose is unlikely to cause

problems. Larger overdoses may cause vomiting or drowsiness. Notify your doctor.

POSSIBLE ADVERSE EFFECTS
Adverse effects are related to dosage levels. At the start of treatment, on a low dosage, unwanted effects, such as dark urine, digestive disturbances, abnormal movements, nervousness or agitation, are usually mild but may increase in severity as dosage is increased. Discuss dizziness, fainting, and fatigue or sudden sleep episodes with your doctor. If palpitations occur, stop taking the drug and consult your doctor promptly.

INTERACTIONS
Antidepressant drugs Levodopa may interact with monoamine oxidase inhibitors (MAOIs) to cause a dangerous rise in blood pressure. The drug may also interact with tricyclic antidepressants.
Iron Absorption of levodopa may be reduced by iron.
Antipsychotic drugs Some of these drugs may reduce the effect of levodopa.

SPECIAL PRECAUTIONS
Be sure to tell your doctor if:
◆ You have heart problems.
◆ You have long-term liver or kidney problems.
◆ You have a lung disorder, such as asthma or bronchitis.
◆ You have glaucoma.
◆ You have a peptic ulcer.
◆ You have diabetes.
◆ You have any serious mental illness.
◆ You are taking other medicines.
Pregnancy Unlikely to be required.
Breast-feeding Unlikely to be required.
Infants and children Not normally used in children (and rarely given to patients under 25 years).
Over 60 No special problems.
Driving and hazardous work Your underlying condition, as well as the possibility of levodopa causing fainting, dizziness, and sudden sleep episodes, may make such activities inadvisable. Discuss with your doctor.
Alcohol No known problems, although levodopa may enhance the sedative effects of alcohol.

PROLONGED USE
Effectiveness usually declines in time, necessitating increased dosage. The adverse effects may become so severe that ultimately the drug must be stopped.

Levofloxacin

Brand name Tavanic
Used in the following combined preparations None

QUICK REFERENCE
Drug group Antibacterial (p.66)
Overdose danger rating Medium
Dependence rating Low
Prescription needed Yes
Available as generic No

GENERAL INFORMATION
Levofloxacin is a quinolone antibacterial drug used for soft-tissue and respiratory and urinary tract infections that have not responded to other antibiotics.

The drug is usually prescribed in the form of tablets, but it is administered by intravenous infusion to people with serious systemic infections or to those who cannot take drugs by mouth. Like other quinolones, levofloxacin may occasionally cause tendon inflammation and damage, especially in the elderly or in people taking corticosteroids. You should, therefore, report tendon pain or inflammation to your doctor immediately and stop taking the drug. The affected limb or limbs should be rested until the symptoms have subsided.

INFORMATION FOR USERS
Your drug prescription is tailored for you. Do not alter dosage without checking with your doctor.
How taken/used Tablets, injection.
Frequency and timing of doses 1 x 2 times daily for 7–14 days depending on infection (tablets).
Adult dosage range 250–1,000mg daily.
Onset of effect 1 hour.
Duration of action 12–24 hours.
Diet advice None.
Storage Keep in original container at room temperature out of the reach of children.

Missed dose Take as soon as you remember, then take your next dose when it is due.

Stopping the drug Take the full course. Even if you feel better, the original infection may still be present, and symptoms may recur if treatment is stopped too soon.

Exceeding the dose An occasional unintentional extra dose is unlikely to cause problems. Larger overdoses may cause mental disturbances and fits. Notify your doctor.

POSSIBLE ADVERSE EFFECTS

Nausea and vomiting are common with oral forms. Diarrhoea and abdominal pain are also common. Headache, dizziness, and drowsiness or restlessness may also occur. Given by injection, levofloxacin may cause palpitations and a fall in blood pressure. If a rash, itching, jaundice, fever, or an allergic reaction occur, stop taking the drug. If you experience confusion or convulsions or painful or inflamed tendons, stop taking the drug and seek immediate medical attention.

INTERACTIONS

Non-steroidal anti-inflammatory drugs (NSAIDs) and theophylline There is an increased risk of convulsions when these drugs are taken with levofloxacin.

Anticoagulants The effect of these drugs may be increased by levofloxacin.

Antacids, sucralfate, iron, and zinc These drugs may reduce the absorption of levofloxacin.

Ciclosporin There is an increased risk of kidney damage if ciclosporin is taken with levofloxacin.

SPECIAL PRECAUTIONS

Be sure to tell your doctor if:
◆ You have kidney problems.
◆ You suffer from epilepsy.
◆ You have glucose-6-phosphate dehydrogenase (G6PD) deficiency.
◆ You have porphyria.
◆ You have a history of psychotic illness.
◆ You have had a previous allergic reaction to a quinolone antibacterial.
◆ You have had a previous tendon problem with a quinolone.
◆ You are taking other medicines.

Pregnancy Safety not established. Discuss with your doctor.

Breast-feeding Safety not established. Discuss with your doctor.

Infants and children Not recommended.

Over 60 No special problems, except that tendon damage is more likely over the age of 60.

Driving and hazardous work Avoid such activities until you have learned how levofloxacin affects you because the drug can cause dizziness, drowsiness, visual disturbances, and hallucinations.

Alcohol Avoid. Alcohol may increase the sedative effects of levofloxacin.

Sunlight Avoid exposure to strong sunlight or artificial ultraviolet rays because photosensitization may occur.

PROLONGED USE

Levofloxacin is not usually prescribed for long-term use.

Levonorgestrel

Brand names Levonelle 1500, Levonelle One Step, Mirena, Norgeston
Used in the following combined preparations
Cyclo-progynova, Logynin ED, Microgynon 30, Ovranette, and others

QUICK REFERENCE

Drug group Female sex hormone (p.88) and oral contraceptive (p.105)
Overdose danger rating Low
Dependence rating Low
Prescription needed Yes (most preparations)
Available as generic No

GENERAL INFORMATION

Levonorgestrel is a synthetic hormone similar to progesterone, a natural female sex hormone. Its primary use is in oral contraceptives. It performs this function by thickening the mucus at the neck of the uterus (cervix), thereby making it difficult for sperm to enter the uterus.

Levonorgestrel is available in combined oral contraceptives with an oestrogen drug. It is also prescribed as a progestogen-only preparation (POP) for emergency, postcoital contraception and can also be obtained over the counter, as a single tablet, by women over the age of 16. It is also combined with an oestrogen drug in hormone replacement therapy (HRT) for the short-term treatment of menopausal symptoms (see p.89).

The drug rarely causes serious adverse effects. When it is used alone, menstrual irregularities, especially mid-cycle, or "breakthrough", bleeding may occur.

INFORMATION FOR USERS

Your drug prescription is tailored for you. Do not alter dosage without checking with your doctor.

How taken/used Tablets, intrauterine device (IUD), patches.

Frequency and timing of doses Once daily, at the same time each day (tablets).

Adult dosage range *Progestogen-only contraceptive* 30mcg daily. *Postcoital contraceptive* 1.5mg as a single dose as soon as possible, within 12 hours, but no later than after 72 hours. *HRT and combined oral contraceptive* Dosage varies according to preparation used.

Onset of effect Within 4 hours, but contraceptive protection may not be fully effective for 14 days, depending on day of cycle tablets are started.

Duration of action 24 hours. Some effects, not including contraception, may persist for up to 3 months after levonorgestrel is stopped.

Diet advice None.

Storage Keep in original container at room temperature out of the reach of children.

Missed dose *Progestogen-only contraceptive* If a tablet is delayed by 3 hours or more, regard it as a missed dose. See What to do if you miss a pill (p.109). *Postcoital contraceptive* If vomiting occurs within 3 hours, take another tablet immediately. If problem persists speak to your doctor or pharmacist without delay. *Combined oral contraceptive* Depends on preparation used. See What to do if you miss a pill (p.109).

Stopping the drug The drug can be safely stopped as soon as contraceptive protection is no longer required. For treatment of menopausal symptoms, consult your doctor before stopping the drug.

Exceeding the dose An occasional unintentional extra dose is unlikely to be a cause for concern. But if you notice any unusual symptoms, or if a large overdose has been taken, notify your doctor.

POSSIBLE ADVERSE EFFECTS

Menstrual irregularities (blood spotting between periods or absence of menstruation) are the most common side effects of levonorgestrel used alone and should be discussed with your doctor. Fluid retention, leading to swollen feet or ankles, or weight gain may also occur. Nausea, vomiting, and breast tenderness, are less common effects. If headache or depression occur, consult your doctor.

INTERACTIONS

General note The beneficial effects of many drugs, including bromocriptine, oral anticoagulants, anticonvulsants, and antidiabetic and antihypertensive drugs, may be affected by levonorgestrel. Many, including anticonvulsants, antibiotics, antituberculous drugs, and St John's wort, may reduce contraceptive protection.

SPECIAL PRECAUTIONS

Be sure to tell your doctor if:
◆ You have a liver or kidney problem.
◆ You have heart failure or high blood pressure.
◆ You have diabetes.
◆ You have unexplained abnormal vaginal bleeding.
◆ You have had blood clots or a stroke.
◆ You have ever had migraines or severe headaches.
◆ You have porphyria.
◆ You have a history of depression.
◆ You have asthma.
◆ You have epilepsy.
◆ You are taking other medicines.

Pregnancy Not prescribed. May cause abnormalities in the developing baby. Discuss with your doctor.

Breast-feeding The drug passes into the breast milk, but at normal doses adverse effects on the baby are unlikely. Discuss with your doctor.

Infants and children Not prescribed.

Over 60 Not prescribed.

Driving and hazardous work No known problems.

Alcohol No known problems.

PROLONGED USE

When used as part of HRT, levonorgestrel is usually only advised for short-term use around the menopause and is not normally recommended for long-term use or for treatment of osteoporosis.

Levothyroxine

Brand name Eltroxin
Used in the following combined preparations None

QUICK REFERENCE

Drug group Thyroid hormone (p.84)
Overdose danger rating Medium
Dependence rating Low
Prescription needed Yes
Available as generic Yes

GENERAL INFORMATION

Levothyroxine is the major hormone produced by the thyroid gland. A deficiency of the natural hormone causes hypothyroidism and may sometimes lead to myxoedema, a condition characterized by slowing of body functions and facial puffiness. A synthetic preparation is used to replace the natural hormone when it is deficient.

Certain types of goitre (enlarged thyroid gland) are helped by levothyroxine, and it may be given to prevent a goitre from developing during antithyroid drug treatment. Levothyroxine is also used for some forms of thyroid cancer.

Adults who have a severe thyroid deficiency are sensitive to thyroid hormones, so treatment is introduced gradually, and increased slowly, to prevent adverse effects. Particular care is required in patients with heart problems such as angina.

INFORMATION FOR USERS

Your drug prescription is tailored for you. Do not alter dosage without checking with your doctor.
How taken/used Tablets.
Frequency and timing of doses Once daily.
Dosage range *Adults* Doses of 50–100mcg daily, increased at 3–4-week intervals as required. The maximum dose is 200mcg daily.
Onset of effect Within 48 hours. Full beneficial effects may not be felt for several weeks.
Duration of action 1–3 weeks.

Diet advice None.
Storage Keep in original container at room temperature out of the reach of children. Protect from light.
Missed dose Take as soon as you remember. If your next dose is due within 8 hours, take a single dose now and skip the next.
Stopping the drug Do not stop taking the drug without consulting your doctor; symptoms may recur.
Exceeding the dose An occasional unintentional extra dose is unlikely to cause problems. Large overdoses may cause palpitations in the next few days. Notify your doctor.

POSSIBLE ADVERSE EFFECTS

Adverse effects are rare and are usually due to overdosage, causing thyroid overactivity. They include anxiety, agitation, diarrhoea, weight loss, sweating, flushing, muscle cramps, insomnia, and tremors. These effects diminish as the dose is lowered, but if they occur, consult your doctor. If palpitations or chest pain occur, seek immediate medical advice. Too low a dose of levothyroxine may cause signs of thyroid underactivity.

INTERACTIONS

Oral anticoagulants Levothyroxine may increase the effect of these drugs.
Colestyramine This drug may reduce the absorption of levothyroxine.
Amiodarone may affect thyroid activity; levothyroxine dosage may need adjustment.
Antiepileptic drugs These drugs may reduce the effect of levothyroxine.
Antidiabetic agents The doses of these drugs may need increasing once levothyroxine treatment is started.
Sucralfate Absorption of levothyroxine may be reduced by sucralfate.
Antidepressants Levothyroxine may enhance the effects of tricyclic antidepressants.

SPECIAL PRECAUTIONS

Be sure to tell your doctor if:
◆ You have high blood pressure.
◆ You have heart problems.
◆ You have diabetes.
◆ You are taking other medicines.
Pregnancy No evidence of risk, but dosage adjustment may be necessary.

Breast-feeding The drug passes into the breast milk, but at normal doses adverse effects on the baby are unlikely. Discuss with your doctor.
Infants and children Dosage depends on age and weight.
Over 60 Reduced dose usually necessary.
Driving and hazardous work No known problems.
Alcohol No known problems.

PROLONGED USE
No special problems.
Monitoring Periodic tests of thyroid function are required.

Lisinopril

Brand names Carace, Caralpha, Zestril
Used in the following combined preparations
Carace Plus, Lisicostad, Zestoretic

QUICK REFERENCE
Drug group ACE inhibitor vasodilator (p.31)
Overdose danger rating Medium
Dependence rating Low
Prescription needed Yes
Available as generic Yes

GENERAL INFORMATION
Lisinopril is an ACE inhibitor drug used in the treatment of high blood pressure (including that caused by diabetic kidney problems), heart failure, and following a heart attack. It works by relaxing the muscles in blood vessel walls, allowing them to dilate (widen), thereby easing blood flow.

Lisinopril can initially cause a rapid fall in blood pressure, especially when taken with a diuretic drug. Therefore, treatment for heart failure is usually started under close medical supervision, in hospital in severe cases. The first dose is usually very small, and it should be taken while you are lying down, preferably at bedtime.

INFORMATION FOR USERS
Your drug prescription is tailored for you. Do not alter dosage without checking with your doctor.
How taken/used Tablets.
Frequency and timing of doses Once daily.

Adult dosage range *Hypertension* 2.5–10mg (starting dose) up to 80mg. *Heart failure/diabetic nephropathy* 2.5mg (starting dose) up to 20mg. *Prevention of further heart attacks* 2.5–5mg (starting dose) up to 10mg.
Onset of effect 1–2 hours; full beneficial effect may take several weeks.
Duration of action 12–24 hours.
Diet advice None.
Storage Keep in original container at room temperature out of the reach of children.
Missed dose Take as soon as you remember. If your next dose is due within 8 hours, take a single dose now and skip the next.
Stopping the drug Do not stop taking the drug without consulting your doctor. Stopping the drug may lead to worsening of the underlying condition.
Exceeding the dose An occasional unintentional extra dose is unlikely to be a cause for concern. Larger overdoses may cause dizziness or fainting. Notify your doctor.

POSSIBLE ADVERSE EFFECTS
Common but unusual side effects of lisinopril are a persistent dry cough and altered sense of taste. A reduction of dosage may minimize these effects. Nausea, vomiting, and diarrhoea are also common. If dizziness, a rash or itching, runny nose, sore throat, confusion, mood changes, or jaundice occur, consult your doctor. If you experience chest pains, palpitations, fainting, or facial swelling, stop taking the drug and seek urgent medical advice.

INTERACTIONS
Potassium supplements, potassium-sparing diuretics, and ciclosporin Taken with lisinopril, these drugs increase the risk of high blood potassium levels.
Non-steroidal anti-inflammatory drugs (NSAIDs) Some of these drugs may reduce the effect of lisinopril, and the risk of kidney damage is increased.
Vasodilators, diuretics, and other drugs for hypertension These drugs may increase the effect of lisinopril.
Lithium Blood levels of lithium may be increased by lisinopril.
Insulin and antidiabetic drugs Lisinopril may increase the effect of these drugs.

SPECIAL PRECAUTIONS
Be sure to tell your doctor if:
◆ You are allergic to other ACE inhibitors.
◆ You have a history of angioedema.
◆ You have kidney problems or are on dialysis.
◆ You have peripheral vascular disease.
◆ You are taking a diuretic drug.
◆ You are on a low sodium diet.
◆ You are taking other medicines.

Pregnancy Not prescribed. May harm the developing baby.

Breast-feeding Safety not established. Discuss with your doctor.

Infants and children Not recommended.

Over 60 No special problems.

Driving and hazardous work Avoid such activities until you have learned how lisinopril affects you because the drug can cause dizziness and fainting.

Alcohol Avoid. Alcohol may increase the blood-pressure lowering and adverse effects of this drug.

PROLONGED USE
Rarely, prolonged use of lisinopril can lead to changes in blood count or kidney function.

Monitoring Periodic checks on potassium levels, white blood cell counts, and urine are usually performed.

Lithium

Brand names Camcolit, Li-liquid, Liskonum, Priadel
Used in the following combined preparations
None

QUICK REFERENCE
Drug group Antimanic drug (p.16)
Overdose danger rating High
Dependence rating Low
Prescription needed Yes
Available as generic No

GENERAL INFORMATION
Lithium, the lightest known metal, has been used since the 1940s in the treatment of manic depression (also known as bipolar affective disorder). Lithium decreases the intensity and frequency of the swings from extreme excitement to deep depression that characterize the disorder.

Lithium is sometimes used along with an antidepressant for depression that has not responded to an antidepressant alone. It is also sometimes used for aggressive or self-harming behaviour. Careful monitoring is required because high levels of lithium can cause serious adverse effects. Because any apparent benefit may take 2 to 3 weeks, an antipsychotic drug is often given with lithium until it becomes effective. Lithium cards, with details of side effects, etc., are available from pharmacy counters.

INFORMATION FOR USERS
Your drug prescription is tailored for you. Do not alter dosage without checking with your doctor.

How taken/used Tablets, SR-tablets, liquid.

Frequency and timing of doses 1–2 x daily with meals. Always take the same brand of lithium to ensure a consistent effect; change of brand must be closely supervised.

Adult dosage range 0.3–1.6g daily. Dosage may vary according to individual response and blood levels.

Onset of effect Some effects may be noticed in 3–5 days, but full benefits may not be felt for 4 weeks.

Duration of action 18–36 hours. Some effects may last for several days.

Diet advice Lithium levels in the blood are affected by the amount of salt in the body, so do not suddenly alter the amount of salt in your diet. Be sure to drink plenty of fluids, especially in hot weather.

Storage Keep in original container at room temperature out of the reach of children.

Missed dose Take as soon as you remember. If your next dose is due within 4 hours, take a single dose now and skip the next.

Stopping the drug Do not stop the drug without consulting your doctor; symptoms may recur.

OVERDOSE ACTION
Seek immediate medical advice in all cases. Take emergency action if convulsions or loss of consciousness occur.

POSSIBLE ADVERSE EFFECTS
Many effects are signs of high blood lithium levels. Increased urine production, thirst, nausea, vomiting, diarrhoea, and tremor are

common. Discuss these and any significant weight gain with your doctor. If drowsiness, lethargy, blurred vision, or unsteadiness occur, stop taking the drug and seek medical advice.

INTERACTIONS

General note Many drugs interact with lithium. Do not take any over-the-counter or prescription drugs without consulting your doctor or pharmacist. Paracetamol should be used in preference to other analgesics for everyday pain relief.

Diuretics, aspirin, and NSAIDs can increase lithium to a dangerous level. Blood levels of lithium should be monitored closely.

SPECIAL PRECAUTIONS

Be sure to tell your doctor if:
◆ You have long-term liver or kidney problems.
◆ You have heart or circulation problems.
◆ You have an overactive thyroid gland.
◆ You have Addison's disease.
◆ You are taking other medicines.

Pregnancy Not usually prescribed. May cause defects in the unborn baby. Discuss with your doctor.

Breast-feeding The drug passes into the breast milk and may affect the baby. Discuss with your doctor.

Infants and children Not recommended.

Over 60 Increased likelihood of adverse effects. Reduced dose may therefore be necessary.

Driving and hazardous work Avoid such activities until you have learned how lithium affects you because the drug can cause reduced alertness.

Alcohol Avoid. Alcohol may increase the sedative effects of this drug.

PROLONGED USE

Prolonged lithium use may lead to kidney problems. Treatment for periods of longer than 5 years is not normally advised unless the benefits are significant and tests show no sign of reduced kidney function.

Monitoring Once stabilized, lithium levels should be checked every 3 months. Thyroid function should be checked every 6–12 months. Kidney function should also be monitored regularly.

Lofepramine

Brand names Gamanil, Lomont
Used in the following combined preparations None

QUICK REFERENCE

Drug group Tricyclic antidepressant drug (p.14)
Overdose danger rating Medium
Dependence rating Low
Prescription needed Yes
Available as generic Yes

GENERAL INFORMATION

Lofepramine is a tricyclic antidepressant used primarily in the long-term treatment of depression. It serves to elevate mood, improve appetite, increase physical activity, and restore interest in everyday pursuits.

Less sedating than some of the other tricyclics, lofepramine is particularly useful when depression is accompanied by lethargy.

The main advantage of lofepramine over other similar drugs is that it seems to have a weaker anticholinergic action and therefore has milder side effects. In overdose, lofepramine is thought to be less harmful than other tricyclic antidepressant drugs.

INFORMATION FOR USERS

Your drug prescription is tailored for you. Do not alter dosage without checking with your doctor.

How taken/used Tablets, liquid.

Frequency and timing of doses 2–3 x daily.

Adult dosage range 140–210mg daily.

Onset of effect Sedation can occur within hours; full antidepressant effect may not be felt for 2–6 weeks.

Duration of action Antidepressant effect may last for 6 weeks; Common adverse effects, the first 1–2 weeks.

Diet advice None.

Storage Keep in original container at room temperature out of the reach of children. Protect from light.

Missed dose Take as soon as you remember. If your next dose is due within 3 hours, take a single dose now and skip the next.

Stopping the drug An abrupt stop can cause withdrawal symptoms and a recurrence of the original problem. Consult your doctor, who may supervise a gradual reduction in dosage over at least 4 weeks.

Exceeding the dose An occasional unintentional extra dose is unlikely to cause problems. If you notice any unusual symptoms or a large overdose has been taken, notify your doctor.

POSSIBLE ADVERSE EFFECTS

The possible adverse effects of this drug are mainly due to its mild anticholinergic action. Sweating, flushing, and drowsiness are common. Rarely, constipation or a dry mouth may also occur. If you experience blurred vision, or have difficulty in passing urine, consult your doctor. If dizziness, fainting, or palpitations occur, stop taking the drug and seek immediate medical attention.

INTERACTIONS

Sedatives All drugs that have sedative effects may intensify those of lofepramine.

Anti-arrhythmic drugs and sotalol may increase the risk of abnormal heart rhythms.

Antihypertensive drugs Lofepramine may reduce the effects of some of these drugs.

Warfarin Lofepramine may, rarely, increase the effects of warfarin.

Monoamine oxidase inhibitors (MAOIs) Serious interactions are possible. These drugs are prescribed together only under close specialist medical supervision.

Selective serotonin reuptake inhibitors (SSRIs) Some SSRIs can increase the amount of lofepramine in the body, leading to more marked adverse effects.

SPECIAL PRECAUTIONS

Be sure to tell your doctor if:
◆ You have heart problems.
◆ You have had epileptic fits.
◆ You have long-term liver or kidney problems.
◆ You have glaucoma.
◆ You have an overactive thyroid gland.
◆ You have prostate trouble.
◆ You have porphyria.
◆ You are taking other medicines.

Pregnancy Safety in pregnancy not established. Discuss with your doctor.

Breast-feeding The drug passes into the breast milk and may affect the baby. Discuss with your doctor.

Infants and children Not recommended.

Over 60 Reduced dose may be necessary as elderly patients are more sensitive to adverse reactions.

Driving and hazardous work Avoid such activities until you have learned how lofepramine affects you because the drug may cause blurred vision and reduced alertness.

Alcohol Avoid. Alcohol may increase the sedative effects of this drug.

Surgery and general anaesthetics Lofepramine may need to be stopped. Discuss with your doctor or dentist before you have any surgery.

PROLONGED USE

No problems expected.

Loperamide

Brand names Arret, Boots Diareze, Diasorb, Diocalm Ultra, Imodium, Norimode, Normaloe
Used in the following combined preparation
Diocalm Plus

QUICK REFERENCE

Drug group Antidiarrhoeal drug (p.44)
Overdose danger rating Medium
Dependence rating Low
Prescription needed No
(most preparations)
Available as generic Yes

GENERAL INFORMATION

Loperamide is an antidiarrhoeal drug available in tablet, capsule, or liquid form. It reduces the loss of water and salts from the bowel and slows bowel activity, resulting in the passage of firmer bowel movements at less frequent intervals.

A fast-acting drug, loperamide is widely used for both sudden and recurrent bouts of diarrhoea, but is not generally recommended for diarrhoea due to infection because it may delay expulsion of harmful substances from the bowel. It is often prescribed to people who have had a colostomy or ileostomy, to reduce fluid loss from the stoma (outlet).

Adverse effects are rare, and there is no risk of abuse, as there may be with opium-based antidiarrhoeals. Loperamide can be purchased over the pharmacy counter.

INFORMATION FOR USERS

Follow instructions on the label. Call your doctor if symptoms worsen.

How taken/used Tablets, capsules, liquid.

Frequency and timing of doses *Acute diarrhoea* Take a double dose at start of treatment, then a single dose after each loose faeces, to maximum daily dose. *Chronic diarrhoea* 2 x daily.

Adult dosage range *Acute diarrhoea* 4mg (starting dose), then 2mg after each loose bowel movement (12–16mg daily); usual dose 6–8mg daily. Use for up to 5 days only (3 days only for children 4–8 years), then consult your doctor. *Chronic diarrhoea* 4–8mg daily (up to 16mg daily).

Onset of effect Within 1–2 hours.

Duration of action 6–18 hours.

Diet advice Ensure adequate fluid, sugar, and salt intake during a diarrhoeal illness.

Storage Keep in original container at room temperature out of the reach of children.

Missed dose Do not take the missed dose. Take your next dose if needed.

Stopping the drug Can be safely stopped as soon as you no longer need it.

Exceeding the dose An occasional unintentional extra dose is unlikely to be a cause for concern. Large overdoses may cause constipation, vomiting, or drowsiness, and affect breathing. Notify your doctor.

POSSIBLE ADVERSE EFFECTS

Adverse effects are rare, but dry mouth, drowsiness, or dizziness may occur. Some effects are hard to distinguish from the effects of the diarrhoea that the drug is used to treat. If constipation occurs, stop taking the drug. If itching occurs, or bloating or abdominal pain or fever persist or worsen during treatment, consult your doctor. If a rash occurs, stop taking the drug and consult your doctor.

INTERACTIONS

None.

SPECIAL PRECAUTIONS

Be sure to consult your doctor or pharmacist before taking this drug if:

◆ You have long-term liver or kidney problems.

◆ You have had recent abdominal surgery.

◆ You have an infection or blockage in the intestine, pseudomembranous colitis, or ulcerative colitis.

◆ You are taking other medicines.

Pregnancy Safety in pregnancy not established. Discuss with your doctor.

Breast-feeding The drug passes into the breast milk and may affect the baby. Discuss with your doctor.

Infants and children Not to be given under 4 years. Reduced dose necessary in older children. Children can be very sensitive to the effects of this drug so care should be taken.

Over 60 No special problems.

Driving and hazardous work Avoid such activities until you have learned how loperamide affects you because the drug can cause dizziness or drowsiness.

Alcohol No known problems.

PROLONGED USE

Not usually taken for prolonged periods (except by persons with a medically diagnosed long-term gastrointestinal condition), but special problems are not expected.

Lopinavir/ritonavir

Brand name Kaletra
Used in the following combined preparations None

QUICK REFERENCE

Drug group Drug for HIV and immune deficiency (p.100)
Overdose danger rating Medium
Dependence rating Low
Prescription needed Yes
Available as generic No

GENERAL INFORMATION

Lopinavir and ritonavir are both antiretroviral drugs known as protease inhibitors. Combined as a single drug, they are used in the treatment of HIV infection. The drugs work by interfering with an enzyme that is used by the virus to produce genetic material.

The combination drug is prescribed with other antiretrovirals, usually two nucleoside analogues, which together slow down production of HIV. This therapy aims to reduce the damage the virus causes the immune system.

Combination antiretroviral therapy is not a cure for HIV. Taken regularly on a long-term basis, it can reduce the level of the virus in the body and improve the outlook. The patient will remain infectious, however, and will suffer a relapse if treatment is stopped.

INFORMATION FOR USERS

Your drug prescription is tailored for you. Do not alter dosage without checking with your doctor.

How taken/used Tablets, capsules, liquid.

Frequency and timing of doses Every 12 hours, with food.

Adult dosage range 2 tablets, 3 capsules, 5ml liquid.

Onset of effect Within 1 hour.

Duration of action 12 hours.

Diet advice None.

Storage Keep in original container at room temperature (tablets), or refrigerator (capsules and liquid) out of the reach of children.

Missed dose Take as soon as you remember. If your next dose is due within 2 hours, take a single dose now and skip the next. It is very important not to miss doses on a regular basis as this can lead to the development of drug-resistant HIV.

Stopping the drug Do not stop taking the drug without consulting your doctor.

Exceeding the dose An occasional unintentional extra dose is unlikely to cause problems. If you notice unusual symptoms, or if a large overdose has been taken, notify your doctor.

POSSIBLE ADVERSE EFFECTS

Fatigue and gastrointestinal upset, including nausea, vomiting, diarrhoea, and loss of appetite, are the most common effects. Changes in body shape, which are more likely to occur with prolonged use, should be discussed with your doctor. If severe abdominal pain occurs, seek immediate medical attention.

INTERACTIONS

General note Many drugs may interact with lopinavir and ritonavir, either increasing adverse effects or reducing the antiretrovirals' effect. Check with your doctor or pharmacist before taking any new drugs, including herbal medicines and those from the supermarket and dentist. Ritonavir is known to interact with some recreational drugs, including ecstasy, and it is essential to discuss the use of such drugs with your doctor or pharmacist.

SPECIAL PRECAUTIONS

Be sure to tell your doctor if:
◆ You have long-term liver or kidney problems.
◆ You take recreational drugs.
◆ You are taking other medicines.

Pregnancy Safety in pregnancy not established. Discuss with your doctor.

Breast-feeding Safety in breast-feeding not established. Breast-feeding is not recommended for HIV-positive mothers as the virus may be passed to the baby.

Infants and children Not recommended under 2 years. Reduced dose necessary over 2 years.

Over 60 Reduced dose may be necessary to minimize adverse effects.

Driving and hazardous work No known problems.

Alcohol Avoid excess. The liquid form of the drug contains a small amount of alcohol.

PROLONGED USE

Changes in body shape may occur.

Monitoring Your doctor will take regular blood samples to check the drugs' effect on the virus. Blood will also be checked for changes in lipids, cholesterol, and glucose levels.

Loratadine/desloratadine

Brand names [Loratadine] Boots Hayfever and Allergy Relief All Day, Clarityn, Clarityn Allergy, [Desloratadine] NeoClarityn

Used in the following combined preparations None

QUICK REFERENCE

Drug group Antihistamine (p.58)

Overdose danger rating Low

Dependence rating Low

Prescription needed No (loratadine); yes (desloratadine)

Available as generic Yes

GENERAL INFORMATION

Loratadine is a long-acting antihistamine for the relief of symptoms associated with allergic rhinitis, such as sneezing, nasal discharge, and itching and burning eyes. These are normally relieved within an hour with oral forms. It is also used to treat allergic skin conditions such as chronic urticaria (itching). An advantage of loratadine over older antihistamines, such as chlorphenamine, is that it has fewer sedative and anticholinergic effects, and is less likely to cause drowsiness.

Desloratadine is an active breakdown product of loratadine. It is available as a separate product (NeoClarityn).

Loratadine and desloratadine should be discontinued about 4 days prior to skin testing for allergy because they may decrease or prevent the detection of positive results.

INFORMATION FOR USERS

Follow instructions on the label. Call your doctor if symptoms worsen.

How taken/used Tablets, liquid.
Frequency and timing of doses Once daily.
Adult dosage range 10mg daily (loratadine); 5mg daily (desloratadine).
Onset of effect Usually within 1 hour.
Duration of action Up to 24 hours.
Diet advice None.
Storage Keep in original container at room temperature out of the reach of children.
Missed dose Take as soon as you remember. If your next dose is due within 6 hours, take a single dose now and skip the next.
Stopping the drug Can be safely stopped as soon as you no longer need it.
Exceeding the dose An occasional unintentional extra dose is unlikely to be a cause for concern. But if you notice any unusual symptoms, or if a large overdose has been taken, notify your doctor.

POSSIBLE ADVERSE EFFECTS

Adverse effects are rare, but fatigue, nausea, headache, and dry mouth may occur. If palpitations or fainting occur, consult your doctor.

INTERACTIONS

Cimetidine, clarithromycin, erythromycin, quinidine, ketoconazole, fluoxetine, and fluconazole may increase the blood levels and effects of loratadine and desloratadine, but this has not been found to cause problems.

SPECIAL PRECAUTIONS

Be sure to consult your doctor or pharmacist before taking this drug if:
◆ You are taking other medicines.
Pregnancy Safety in pregnancy not established. Discuss with your doctor.
Breast-feeding The drug passes into the breast milk. Discuss with your doctor.
Infants and children Not recommended under 2 years (loratadine) or 12 years (desloratadine).
Over 60 No problems expected.
Driving and hazardous work Problems are unlikely, but be aware of how the drug affects you before undertaking these activities.
Alcohol No known problems, but avoid excessive amounts.

PROLONGED USE

No problems expected.

Losartan

Brand name Cozaar
Used in the following combined preparation Cozaar-Comp

QUICK REFERENCE

Drug group Vasodilator (p.31) and antihypertensive drug (p.36)
Overdose danger rating Medium
Dependence rating Low
Prescription needed Yes
Available as generic No

GENERAL INFORMATION

Losartan is a member of a group of vasodilator drugs called angiotensin-II blockers. Used to treat hypertension, it works by blocking the action of angiotensin-II (a naturally occurring substance that constricts blood vessels). This action causes the blood vessel walls to relax, thereby easing blood pressure.

Unlike ACE inhibitors, losartan does not cause a persistent dry cough, and its use is now being evaluated in conditions such as heart failure, for which ACE inhibitors are currently being used.

Losartan is prescribed with caution to people with stenosis (narrowing) of the arteries to the kidneys because the initial dose causes a sudden drop in blood pressure.

Adverse effects include diarrhoea, dizziness, and fatigue, but they do not commonly occur.

INFORMATION FOR USERS

Your drug prescription is tailored for you. Do not alter dosage without checking with your doctor.

How taken/used Tablets.

Frequency and timing of doses Once daily.

Adult dosage range 50–100mg. People over 75 years, and other groups that are especially sensitive to the drug's effects, may start on 25mg.

Onset of effect *Blood pressure* 1–2 weeks, with maximum effect in 3–6 weeks from start of treatment. *Other conditions* Within 1 hour.

Duration of action 12–24 hours.

Diet advice None.

Storage Keep in original container at room temperature out of the reach of children.

Missed dose Take as soon as you remember. If your next dose is due within 8 hours, take a single dose now and skip the next.

Stopping the drug Do not stop the drug without consulting your doctor. Stopping the drug may lead to worsening of the underlying condition.

Exceeding the dose An occasional unintentional extra dose is unlikely to cause problems. Large overdoses may cause dizziness and fainting. Notify your doctor.

POSSIBLE ADVERSE EFFECTS

Side effects, of which dizziness and fatigue are the most common, are usually mild. Rarely, migraine, diarrhoea, and taste disturbance may also occur. If a rash, itching, or jaundice occur, consult your doctor. If wheezing occurs, or you develop facial swelling, stop taking the drug and seek immediate medical advice.

INTERACTIONS

Diuretics There is a risk of a sudden fall in blood pressure when these drugs are taken with losartan.

Potassium supplements, potassium-sparing diuretics, and ciclosporin Losartan increases the effect of these drugs, leading to raised levels of potassium in the blood.

Lithium Losartan may increase the levels and toxicity of lithium.

Non-steroidal anti-inflammatory drugs (NSAIDs) Certain NSAIDs may reduce the blood pressure lowering effect of losartan.

SPECIAL PRECAUTIONS

Be sure to tell your doctor if:
◆ You have stenosis of the kidney arteries.
◆ You have liver or kidney problems.
◆ You have congestive heart failure.
◆ You have primary aldosteronism.
◆ You have experienced angioedema.
◆ You are taking other medicines.

Pregnancy Not prescribed. May cause abnormalities in the fetus.

Breast-feeding Not prescribed. Safety not established.

Infants and children Not prescribed. Safety not established.

Over 60 Reduced dose may be necessary over 75 years.

Driving and hazardous work Do not undertake such activities until you have learned how losartan affects you because the drug can cause dizziness and fatigue.

Alcohol Avoid. Alcohol may raise blood pressure, reducing the drug's effectiveness. It also causes blood vessels to dilate, increasing the likelihood of an excessive fall in blood pressure.

PROLONGED USE

No special problems.

Monitoring Periodic checks on blood potassium levels may be performed.

Magnesium hydroxide

Brand names Cream of Magnesia, Milk of Magnesia
Used in the following combined preparations
Carbellon, Maalox, Mucogel, and others

QUICK REFERENCE

Drug group Antacid (p.42) and laxative (p.45)
Overdose danger rating Low
Dependence rating Low
Prescription needed No
Available as generic Yes

GENERAL INFORMATION

Magnesium hydroxide is a fast-acting antacid given to neutralize stomach acid. It is available in many over-the-counter preparations for the treatment of indigestion and heartburn. The drug also prevents the pain of stomach and duodenal ulcers, gastritis, and reflux oesophagitis, but other drugs are now normally used for these problems. Magnesium hydroxide also acts as a laxative by drawing water into the intestine from the surrounding blood vessels to soften the faeces.

Magnesium hydroxide is rarely used alone as an antacid due to its laxative effect; but this is countered when it is combined with aluminium hydroxide, which can cause constipation.

INFORMATION FOR USERS

Follow instructions on the label. Call your doctor if symptoms worsen.

How taken/used Tablets, liquid, powder.

Frequency and timing of doses 1–4 x daily as needed with water, preferably an hour after food and at bedtime.

Adult dosage range *Antacid* 1–2g per dose (tablets); 5–20ml per dose (liquid). *Laxative* 5–20ml per dose (liquid).

Onset of effect *Antacid* within 15 minutes. *Laxative* 2–8 hours.

Duration of action 2–4 hours.

Diet advice None.

Storage Keep in original container at room temperature out of the reach of children.

Missed dose Take as soon as you remember.

Stopping the drug When used as an antacid, can be safely stopped as soon as you no longer need it. When given as ulcer treatment, follow your doctor's advice.

Exceeding the dose An occasional unintentional extra dose is unlikely to be a cause for concern. But if you notice any unusual symptoms or if a large overdose has been taken, notify your doctor.

POSSIBLE ADVERSE EFFECTS

Diarrhoea is the only common adverse effect. Dizziness and muscle weakness due to absorption of excess magnesium may occur in people with poor kidney function.

INTERACTIONS

General note Magnesium hydroxide interferes with the absorption of a wide range of drugs taken by mouth including tetracycline antibiotics, iron supplements, diflunisal, phenytoin, gabapentin, and penicillamine.

Enteric-coated tablets As with other antacids, magnesium hydroxide may allow break-up of the enteric coating of tablets, sometimes leading to stomach irritation.

SPECIAL PRECAUTIONS

Be sure to consult your doctor or pharmacist before taking this drug if:
◆ You have a long-term kidney problem.
◆ You have a bowel disorder.
◆ You are taking other medicines.

Pregnancy No evidence of risk, but discuss the most appropriate treatment with your doctor.

Breast-feeding No evidence of risk, but discuss the most appropriate treatment with your doctor.

Infants and children Not recommended under 1 year except on the advice of a doctor. Reduced dose necessary for older children.

Over 60 No special problems.

Driving and hazardous work No known problems.

Alcohol Avoid excess. Alcohol irritates the stomach and may reduce the drug's benefits.

PROLONGED USE

Magnesium hydroxide should not be used long term without consulting your doctor. If you are over 40 years of age and are experiencing long-term indigestion or heartburn, your doctor will probably refer you to a specialist. Prolonged use in people with kidney damage may cause drowsiness, dizziness, and weakness due to accumulation of magnesium.

Malathion

Brand names Derbac-M, Prioderm, Quellada M
Used in the following combined preparations
None

QUICK REFERENCE

Drug group Drug to treat skin parasites (p.122)
Overdose danger rating Low (medium if swallowed)
Dependence rating Low
Prescription needed No
Available as generic No

GENERAL INFORMATION

Malathion is an insecticide used in the treatment of lice and mite infestations. The drug kills parasites by interfering with their nervous system function, causing paralysis and death.

Malathion is applied topically, either as a shampoo or a lotion. Lotion is more convenient to use than shampoo, requiring only a single application. It is also more effective because shampoo is diluted in use. Lotions with a high alcohol content are unsuitable for small children or asthmatics, who may be affected by the solvent, or for treating crab lice in the genital area. However, the water-based liquid is suitable. Care should be taken to avoid contact of the drug with the eyes or broken skin.

If resistance occurs during a course of treatment, your pharmacist will recommend an alternative insecticide. Treatment with malathion will not prevent infestation.

INFORMATION FOR USERS

Follow instructions on the label. Call your doctor if symptoms worsen.

How taken/used Topical liquid, lotion, shampoo.
Frequency and timing of doses *Scabies* Once only (lotion or topical liquid). *Lice* 3 applications 3 days apart (shampoo); 2 doses, 7 days apart (lotion or topical liquid).
Adult dosage range As directed. Family members and close contacts should also be treated.
Onset of effect *Lotion or topical liquid* leave on for 12 hours (lice), or 24 hours (scabies), before washing off. *Shampoo* leave on for 5 minutes, rinse off, repeat, then use fine-toothed comb.
Duration of action Until washed off.
Diet advice None.
Storage Keep in original container at room temperature out of the reach of children. Protect from light.
Missed dose When a repeat application of the shampoo has been missed, it should be carried out as soon as is practicable.
Stopping the drug Malathion should be applied as a single application or as a short course of treatment.
Exceeding the dose An extra application is unlikely to cause problems. Take emergency action if the insecticide has been swallowed.

POSSIBLE ADVERSE EFFECTS

Used correctly, malathion preparations are unlikely to produce adverse effects, but the alcoholic fumes given off by some lotions may cause wheezing in asthmatics. Skin irritation is rare; consult your doctor if this occurs.

INTERACTIONS
None.

SPECIAL PRECAUTIONS
Be sure to consult your doctor or pharmacist before using this drug if:
◆ You have asthma.
Pregnancy No evidence of risk. It is unlikely that enough malathion would be absorbed after occasional application to affect the developing fetus.
Breast-feeding No evidence of risk. It is unlikely that enough malathion would be absorbed after occasional application to affect the baby.
Infants and children No special problems; seek medical advice for infants under 6 months.
Over 60 No special problems.
Driving and hazardous work No special problems.
Alcohol No special problems.

PROLONGED USE
Malathion is intended for intermittent use only. The lotions should not be used more than once a week for 3 weeks at a time. If there is a need to use malathion more frequently, it is possible that resistance has built up; seek your doctor's advice.

Mebeverine

Brand names Colofac, Colofac IBS, Colofac MR, Equilon
Used in the following combined preparation Fybogel Mebeverine

QUICK REFERENCE
Drug group Drug for irritable bowel syndrome (p.45)
Overdose danger rating Low
Dependence rating Low
Prescription needed No (some preparations)
Available as generic Yes

GENERAL INFORMATION
Mebeverine is an antispasmodic drug used to relieve painful spasms of the intestine (known as colic), such as those that occur as

a result of irritable bowel syndrome and other intestinal disorders such as diverticular disease. It has a direct relaxing effect on the muscle in the bowel wall, and may also have an anticholinergic action, which reduces the transmission of nerve signals to the smooth muscle of the bowel wall and thereby prevents spasm. Mebeverine does not have serious side effects.

In addition to being available on its own, mebeverine is also produced in a combined form with ispaghula husk to provide roughage in an easily assimilable formulation. Both the drug on its own and the combined form are commonly used to control symptoms of irritable bowel syndrome.

INFORMATION FOR USERS
Follow instructions on the label. Call your doctor if symptoms worsen.
How taken/used Tablets, SR-capsules, liquid, granules.
Frequency and timing of doses 2–3 x daily, 20 minutes before meals.
Adult dosage range 300–450mg daily.
Onset of effect 30–60 minutes.
Duration of action 6–8 hours.
Diet advice None.
Storage Keep in original container at room temperature out of the reach of children. Protect from light.
Missed dose Take as soon as you remember, then return to your normal dosing schedule.
Stopping the drug The drug can be stopped as soon as you no longer need it.
Exceeding the dose An occasional unintentional extra dose is unlikely to be a cause for concern. Larger overdoses will probably cause constipation, and may cause central nervous system excitability.

POSSIBLE ADVERSE EFFECTS
Any side effects are likely to be recognized. Constipation is a common adverse effect of this drug. Rarer effects are agitation, confusion, blotchy skin, and breathlessness. If these occur, stop taking the drug and consult your doctor immediately.

INTERACTIONS
None.

SPECIAL PRECAUTIONS
Be sure to consult your doctor or pharmacist before taking this drug if:
◆ You have cystic fibrosis.
◆ You have porphyria.
Pregnancy Safety in pregnancy not established. Discuss with your doctor.
Breast-feeding Safety in breast-feeding not established. Discuss with your doctor.
Infants and children Not used in infants and children under 10 years.
Over 60 No special problems.
Driving and hazardous work No special problems.
Alcohol No special problems.

PROLONGED USE
No problems expected.

Medroxyprogesterone

Brand names Adgyn Medro, Depo-Provera, Farlutal, Provera
Used in the following combined preparations
Indivina, Premique, Tridestra

QUICK REFERENCE
Drug group Female sex hormone (p.88)
Overdose danger rating Low
Dependence rating Low
Prescription needed Yes
Available as generic No

GENERAL INFORMATION
Medroxyprogesterone is a progestogen, a synthetic female sex hormone similar to the natural hormone progesterone. This drug is used to treat a variety of menstrual disorders such as mid-cycle bleeding and amenorrhoea (absence of periods).

Medroxyprogesterone is also often used to treat endometriosis, a condition in which there is abnormal growth of the uterine-lining tissue in the pelvic cavity. Depot injections of the drug are used as a contraceptive. However, since they may cause serious side effects, such as persistent bleeding from the uterus, amenorrhoea, and prolonged infertility, their use remains controversial, and they are recommended only under special circumstances in Britain.

Medroxyprogesterone may be used to treat some types of cancer, such as cancer of the breast, uterus, or kidney.

INFORMATION FOR USERS

Your drug prescription is tailored for you. Do not alter dosage without checking with your doctor.

How taken/used Tablets, depot injection.

Frequency and timing of doses 1–3 x daily with plenty of water (by mouth); tablets may need to be taken at certain times during your cycle; follow the instructions you have been given. Every 3 months (depot injection).

Adult dosage range *Menstrual disorders* 2.5–10mg daily. *Endometriosis* 30mg daily. *Cancer* 100–1,500mg daily. *Contraception* 150mg.

Onset of effect 1–2 months (cancer); 1–2 weeks (other conditions).

Duration of action 1–2 days (by mouth); up to some months (depot injection).

Diet advice None.

Storage Keep in original container at room temperature out of the reach of children.

Missed dose Take as soon as you remember. If your next dose is due within 3 hours, take a single dose now and skip the next.

Stopping the drug Do not stop the drug without consulting your doctor because symptoms may recur.

Exceeding the dose An occasional unintentional extra dose is unlikely to be a cause for concern. But if you notice any unusual symptoms, or if a large overdose has been taken, notify your doctor.

POSSIBLE ADVERSE EFFECTS

Serious adverse effects are rare. Fluid retention may lead to weight gain, swollen feet or ankles, and, rarely, breast tenderness. Nausea, fatigue, depression, and irregular menstruation may also occur. If a rash, itching, or acne occur, stop taking the drug.

INTERACTIONS

Ciclosporin The effects of this drug may be increased by medroxyprogesterone.

Anticoagulants Medroxyprogesterone may reduce the effects of these drugs.

Rifamycin antibiotics, St John's wort, antiepileptics, griseofulvin, terbinafine, and barbiturates may reduce the effects of medroxyprogesterone.

SPECIAL PRECAUTIONS

Be sure to tell your doctor if:

◆ You have high blood pressure.

◆ You have diabetes.

◆ You have had blood clots or a stroke.

◆ You have long-term liver or kidney problems.

◆ You have porphyria.

◆ You have epilepsy.

◆ You are taking other medicines.

Pregnancy Not prescribed. May cause abnormalities in the unborn baby. Discuss with your doctor.

Breast-feeding The drug passes into the breast milk, but at normal doses adverse effects on the baby are unlikely. Discuss with your doctor.

Infants and children Not usually prescribed.

Over 60 No special problems.

Driving and hazardous work No known problems.

Alcohol No known problems.

PROLONGED USE

Long-term use may slightly increase the risk of blood clots in the leg veins. Irregular menstrual bleeding or spotting between periods may also occur during long-term use.

Monitoring Periodic checks on blood pressure, yearly cervical smear tests, and breast examinations are usually required.

Mefenamic acid

Brand names Dysman, Ponstan
Used in the following combined preparations None

QUICK REFERENCE

Drug group Non-steroidal anti-inflammatory drug (p.50)
Overdose danger rating Medium
Dependence rating Low
Prescription needed Yes
Available as generic Yes

GENERAL INFORMATION

Mefenamic acid, introduced in 1963, is a non-steroidal anti-inflammatory drug (NSAID). Like other NSAIDs, it relieves pain and inflammation. The drug is an effective analgesic, and is used to treat headache, toothache, and menstrual pains (dysmenorrhoea), as well as to reduce excessive menstrual bleeding (menorrhagia). Mefenamic acid is also prescribed for long-term relief of pain and stiffness in rheumatoid arthritis and osteoarthritis.

The most common side effects of mefenamic acid are gastrointestinal: abdominal pain, nausea and vomiting, and indigestion. Other, more serious effects include kidney problems and blood disorders.

INFORMATION FOR USERS

Your drug prescription is tailored for you. Do not alter dosage without checking with your doctor.

How taken/used Tablets, capsules, liquid.

Frequency and timing of doses 3 x daily with or after food.

Adult dosage range 1,500mg daily.

Onset of effect 1–2 hours.

Duration of action Up to 8 hours.

Diet advice None.

Storage Keep in original container at room temperature out of the reach of children.

Missed dose Take as soon as you remember. If your next dose is due within 2 hours, take a single dose now and skip the next.

Stopping the drug Can be safely stopped as soon as you no longer need it.

Exceeding the dose An occasional unintentional extra dose is unlikely to be a cause for concern. Large overdoses may cause poor coordination, muscle twitching, or fits. Notify your doctor.

POSSIBLE ADVERSE EFFECTS

Gastrointestinal disturbances such as indigestion and diarrhoea are common, but if diarrhoea occurs, stop taking the drug and consult your doctor. Rarely, dizziness, drowsiness, nausea, and vomiting occur; if abdominal pain occurs, consult your doctor. If you have a rash, wheezing or breathlessness, or black or bloodstained faeces, stop taking the drug and consult your doctor immediately.

INTERACTIONS

General note Mefenamic acid interacts with a wide range of drugs to increase the risk of bleeding and/or peptic ulcers. These drugs include other non-steroidal anti-inflammatory drugs (NSAIDs) such as aspirin, and also oral anticoagulant drugs, certain antidepressants, and corticosteroids.

Lithium, digoxin, phenytoin, and methotrexate Mefenamic acid may raise blood levels of these drugs to an undesirable extent.

Antihypertensive drugs and diuretics The beneficial effects of these drugs may be reduced by mefenamic acid.

Oral antidiabetics Mefenamic acid may increase their blood glucose-lowering effect.

Ciprofloxacin The risk of seizures with this drug and related antibiotics may be increased by mefenamic acid.

SPECIAL PRECAUTIONS

Be sure to tell your doctor if:
◆ You have liver or kidney problems.
◆ You have had a peptic ulcer, oesophagitis, or acid indigestion.
◆ You have inflammatory bowel disease.
◆ You have asthma.
◆ You have high blood pressure.
◆ You are allergic to aspirin.
◆ You have porphyria.
◆ You have any heart problems.
◆ You are taking other medicines.

Pregnancy Not usually prescribed. May cause defects in the unborn baby and, taken in late pregnancy, may affect the baby's cardiovascular system. Discuss with your doctor.

Breast-feeding The drug passes into the breast milk, but at normal doses adverse effects on the baby are unlikely. Discuss with your doctor.

Infants and children Reduced dose necessary.

Over 60 Increased likelihood of adverse effects.

Driving and hazardous work Avoid such activities until you have learned how mefenamic acid affects you because the drug can cause drowsiness and dizziness.

Alcohol Avoid. Alcohol may increase the risk of stomach irritation with mefenamic acid.

Surgery and general anaesthetics Mefenamic acid may prolong bleeding. Discuss the possibility of stopping treatment with your doctor or dentist before any surgery.

PROLONGED USE

Prolonged use of mefenamic acid increases the risk of bleeding from peptic ulcers and in the bowel. Rarely, the drug may affect the liver, kidney, and blood. Blood tests may be carried out. The lowest effective dose of any NSAID is given for the shortest duration.

Mefloquine

Brand name Lariam
Used in the following combined preparations None

QUICK REFERENCE

Drug group Antimalarial drug (p.75)
Overdose danger rating High
Dependence rating Low
Prescription needed Yes
Available as generic No

GENERAL INFORMATION

Mefloquine is used for the prevention and treatment of malaria. It is recommended for use in areas where malaria is resistant to other drugs. However, mefloquine's use is limited by the fact that it can cause, in some patients, serious side effects that include depression, suicidal tendencies, anxiety, panic, confusion, hallucinations, paranoid delusions, and convulsions. For most people, the benefits of mefloquine outweigh the risks, but this should be discussed with your doctor.

INFORMATION FOR USERS

Your drug prescription is tailored for you. Do not alter dosage without checking with your doctor.
How taken/used Tablets.
Frequency and timing of doses *Prevention* Once weekly. *Treatment* Up to 3 x daily every 6–8 hours, after food and with plenty of water.
Adult dosage range *Prevention* 250mg once weekly, starting 2–3 weeks before entering endemic area, and continuing until 4 weeks after leaving. *Treatment* 20–25mg/kg body weight up to a maximum dose of 1.5g.
Onset of effect 2–3 days.
Duration of action Over 1 week. Low levels of the drug may persist for several months.
Diet advice None.
Storage Keep in original container at room temperature out of the reach of children.
Missed dose Take as soon as you remember. If your next dose is due within 48 hours (if taken once weekly for prevention), take a single dose now and skip the next. If vomit-

ing occurs within 30 minutes of taking a dose, take another.
Stopping the drug If you feel it necessary to stop the drug, consult your doctor about alternative treatment before the next dose is due.

OVERDOSE ACTION

Seek immediate medical advice in all cases. Take emergency action if collapse or loss of consciousness occurs.

POSSIBLE ADVERSE EFFECTS

Dizziness, vertigo, nausea, vomiting, headache, and abdominal pain are common. Rarely, serious adverse effects on the nervous system can occur, including anxiety or panic attacks, depression, hallucinations, and paranoid delusions. If these or hearing disorders or palpitations occur, stop taking the drug and consult your doctor immediately.

INTERACTIONS

General note Mefloquine may increase the effects on the heart of drugs such as beta blockers, calcium channel blockers, and digitalis drugs. It may also affect live-vaccine immunization, which should be completed at least 3 days before the first dose of mefloquine.
Anticonvulsant drugs Mefloquine may decrease the effect of these drugs.
Other antimalarial drugs Mefloquine may increase the risk of adverse effects when taken with these drugs.

SPECIAL PRECAUTIONS

Be sure to tell your doctor if:
◆ You have long-term liver or kidney problems.
◆ You have had epileptic fits.
◆ You have had depression or other psychiatric illness.
◆ You have had a previous allergic reaction to mefloquine or quinine.
◆ You have heart problems.
◆ You are taking other medicines.
Pregnancy Not usually prescribed. If unavoidable, the drug is given only after the first trimester. Pregnancy must be avoided during and for 3 months after mefloquine use.
Breast-feeding Not prescribed. The drug passes into the breast milk.
Infants and children Not used under 3 months.

Reduced dose necessary in older children.

Over 60 Careful monitoring needed if liver or kidney problems or heart disease are present.

Driving and hazardous work Avoid such activities until you know how the drug affects you (prevention). Avoid during, and for 3 weeks after, treatment because the drug can cause dizziness or disturb balance.

Alcohol Keep consumption low.

PROLONGED USE
May be taken for prevention for up to a year.

Meloxicam

Brand name Mobic
Used in the following combined preparations None

QUICK REFERENCE
Drug group Non-steroidal anti-inflammatory drug (p.50)
Overdose danger rating Medium
Dependence rating Low
Prescription needed Yes
Available as generic No

GENERAL INFORMATION
Meloxicam is a non-steroidal anti-inflammatory (NSAID) drug that reduces pain, stiffness, and inflammation. It is used to relieve the symptoms of rheumatoid arthritis, ankylosing spondylitis, and acute episodes of osteoarthritis. It does not cure the underlying condition, however.

Meloxicam does not affect the stomach as severely as some other NSAIDs and is therefore less likely to cause gastrointestinal bleeding, ulceration, and perforation. Because elderly people are more sensitive to the drug's effects, they are usually prescribed only half the normal adult dose.

INFORMATION FOR USERS
Your drug prescription is tailored for you. Do not alter dosage without checking with your doctor.

How taken/used Tablets, suppositories.
Frequency and timing of doses Once daily with food.
Adult dosage range 7.5–15mg.
Onset of effect 1 hour. Full anti-inflamma-

tory effect may not be felt for up to 2 weeks.

Duration of action 24 hours.
Diet advice None.
Storage Keep in original container at room temperature out of the reach of children.
Missed dose Take as soon as you remember. If your next dose is due within 8 hours, take a single dose now and skip the next.
Stopping the drug The drug can be safely stopped as soon as you no longer need it (short term). Do not stop taking the drug without consulting your doctor (long term).
Exceeding the dose An occasional unintentional extra dose is unlikely to cause problems. Large overdoses can cause stomach and intestinal pain and damage. Notify your doctor.

POSSIBLE ADVERSE EFFECTS
Abdominal pain, indigestion, diarrhoea or constipation, lightheadedness, and drowsiness are common. A rash and itching are also common; if they occur, stop taking the drug. Rarely, vertigo, ringing in the ears, or a persistent sore throat may occur. If you have palpitations, wheezing or breathing difficulties, or black or bloodstained faeces, stop taking the drug and seek immediate medical attention.

INTERACTIONS
General note Meloxicam interacts with a wide range of drugs to increase the risk of bleeding and/or peptic ulcers. Such drugs include other NSAIDs, aspirin, and also oral anticoagulants, and corticosteroids.
Ciclosporin and tacrolimus increase the risk of kidney damage with meloxicam.
Lithium, digoxin, and methotrexate Meloxicam may increase the blood levels of these drugs to an undesirable extent.
Antibacterials Meloxicam may increase the risk of convulsions with ciprofloxacin and similar drugs.

SPECIAL PRECAUTIONS
Be sure to tell your doctor if:
◆ You have asthma.
◆ You are allergic to aspirin or other NSAIDs.
◆ You have had a peptic ulcer, oesophagitis, or acid indigestion.

◆ You have liver or kidney problems.
◆ You have a bleeding disorder, proctitis, or haemorrhoids.
◆ You have a heart problem or high blood pressure.
◆ You are taking other medicines.

Pregnancy Safety not established. May affect the developing fetus. Discuss with your doctor.
Breast-feeding Safety not established. Discuss with your doctor.
Infants and children Not recommended.
Over 60 Increased likelihood of adverse effects. Reduced doses necessary.
Driving and hazardous work Avoid such activities until you have learned how meloxicam affects you because the drug can cause vertigo and drowsiness.
Alcohol Keep consumption low. Alcohol may increase the risk of stomach irritation with meloxicam.
Surgery and general anaesthetics Meloxicam may prolong bleeding. Discuss with your doctor or dentist.

PROLONGED USE
Increased risk of bleeding from peptic ulcers and in the bowel. The lowest effective dose is given for the shortest duration.
Monitoring Periodic tests on kidney function may be performed.

Mercaptopurine

Brand name Puri-Nethol
Used in the following combined preparations None

QUICK REFERENCE
Drug group Anticancer drug (p.96)
Overdose danger rating Medium
Dependence rating Low
Prescription needed Yes
Available as generic No

GENERAL INFORMATION
Mercaptopurine is an anticancer drug that is widely used in the treatment of certain forms of leukaemia. It is usually given in combination with other anticancer drugs.

Common side effects of mercaptopurine (see Possible adverse effects, below) tend to be milder than those of other cytotoxic drugs,

and often disappear as the body adjusts. More seriously, the drug can interfere with blood cell production, resulting in blood clotting disorders and anaemia; it can also cause liver damage and increase the likelihood of infections.

INFORMATION FOR USERS
Your drug prescription is tailored for you. Do not alter dosage without checking with your doctor.
How taken/used Tablets.
Frequency and timing of doses Once daily.
Dosage range Dosage is determined individually according to body weight and response.
Onset of effect 1–2 weeks.
Duration of action Side effects may persist for several weeks after stopping treatment.
Diet advice None.
Storage Keep in original container at room temperature out of the reach of children. Protect from light.
Missed dose If your next dose is due within 6 hours, take a single dose now and skip the next. Tell your doctor that you missed a dose.
Stopping the drug Do not stop the drug without consulting your doctor; stopping the drug may worsen the underlying condition.
Exceeding the dose An occasional unintentional extra dose is unlikely to cause problems. Large overdoses may cause nausea and vomiting. Notify your doctor.

POSSIBLE ADVERSE EFFECTS
Nausea, vomiting, appetite loss, and mouth ulcers are common. Jaundice may also occur, but is reversible on stopping the drug. Because mercaptopurine interferes with blood-cell production, it may cause anaemia and blood clotting disorders; and infections are more likely. If, rarely, jaundice, black faeces, and bloodstained vomit occur, stop taking the drug and consult your doctor immediately.

INTERACTIONS
Co-trimoxazole, trimethoprim, mesalazine, olsalazine, and sulfasalazine These drugs increase the risk of blood problems with mercaptopurine.
Allopurinol This drug increases blood levels of mercaptopurine.
Warfarin The effects of warfarin may be decreased by mercaptopurine.

SPECIAL PRECAUTIONS

Be sure to tell your doctor if:

◆ You have long-term liver or kidney problems.

◆ You suffer from gout.

◆ You have recently had any infection.

◆ You have porphyria.

◆ You are taking other medicines.

Pregnancy Not usually prescribed. Discuss with your doctor.

Breast-feeding Not advised. The drug passes into the breast milk and may affect the baby adversely. Discuss with your doctor.

Infants and children Reduced dose necessary.

Over 60 Reduced dose may be necessary. Increased risk of adverse effects.

Driving and hazardous work No known problems.

Alcohol Avoid. Alcohol may increase the adverse effects of this drug.

PROLONGED USE

Prolonged use of this drug may reduce bone marrow activity, leading to a reduction of all types of blood cells.

Monitoring Regular blood checks and tests on liver function are required.

Mesalazine

Brand names Asacol, Pentasa, Salofalk
Used in the following combined preparations None

QUICK REFERENCE

Drug group Drug for inflammatory bowel disease (p.46)

Overdose danger rating Low

Dependence rating Low

Prescription needed Yes

Available as generic Yes

GENERAL INFORMATION

Mesalazine is prescribed for patients with ulcerative colitis and is sometimes used for Crohn's disease, which affects the large intestine. The drug is given to relieve symptoms in an acute attack and is also taken as a preventative measure. When mesalazine is used to treat severe cases, it is often taken with other drugs such as corticosteroids.

When the drug is taken as tablets, the active component is released in the large intestine, where its local effect relieves the inflamed mucosa. Always use the same brand of tablet. Enemas and suppositories are also available and are particularly useful when the disease affects the rectum and lower colon.

This drug produces fewer side effects than some older treatments, such as sulfasalazine. Patients unable to tolerate sulfasalazine may be able to take mesalazine with no problem. Anyone hypersensitive to salicylates, such as aspirin, should not take mesalazine.

INFORMATION FOR USERS

Your drug prescription is tailored for you. Do not alter dosage without checking with your doctor.

How taken/used Tablets, SR-tablets, granules, suppositories, enema (foam or liquid).

Frequency and timing of doses 3 x daily, swallowed whole and not chewed (tablets); 3 x daily (suppositories); once daily at bedtime (enema).

Adult dosage range 1.5–2.4g daily (acute attack); 750mg–2.4g daily (maintenance dose).

Onset of effect Adverse effects may be noticed within a few days, but full beneficial effects may not be felt for a couple of weeks.

Duration of action Up to 12 hours.

Diet advice Your doctor may advise you, taking account of the condition affecting you.

Storage Keep in original container at room temperature out of the reach of children. Protect from light. Keep aerosol container out of direct sunlight.

Missed dose Take as soon as you remember. If your next dose is due within 2 hours, take a single dose now and skip the next.

Stopping the drug Do not stop taking the drug without consulting your doctor; symptoms may recur.

Exceeding the dose An occasional unintentional extra dose is unlikely to be a cause for concern. But if you notice any unusual symptoms, or if a large overdose has been taken, notify your doctor.

POSSIBLE ADVERSE EFFECTS

Gastrointestinal problems such as nausea, abdominal pain, and diarrhoea are common. If your colitis worsens or you develop a rash, stop taking the drug. If unexplained bleeding, bruising, sore throat, fever, or malaise occur, stop taking the drug and consult your doctor, who will carry out a blood test to eliminate blood disorders.

INTERACTIONS

Lactulose The release of mesalazine at its site of action may be reduced by lactulose.

Warfarin Mesalazine may reduce the effect of warfarin.

Azathioprine and mercaptopurine may increase the risk of blood problems with mesalazine.

SPECIAL PRECAUTIONS

Be sure to tell your doctor if:
◆ You have long-term liver or kidney problems.
◆ You are allergic to aspirin.
◆ You are taking other medicines.

Pregnancy Negligible amounts of the drug cross the placenta. However, safety in pregnancy is not established. Discuss with your doctor.

Breast-feeding Negligible amounts of the drug pass into the breast milk, but safety is not established. Discuss with your doctor.

Infants and children Not recommended under 15 years.

Over 60 Dosage reduction not normally necessary unless there is kidney impairment.

Driving and hazardous work No special problems.

Alcohol No special problems.

PROLONGED USE

No problems expected.

Monitoring Regular blood tests and checks on kidney function are usually required.

Metformin

Brand name Glucophage
Used in the following combined preparations Avandamet, Competact

QUICK REFERENCE

Drug group Antidiabetic drug (p.82)
Overdose danger rating High
Dependence rating Low
Prescription needed Yes
Available as generic Yes

GENERAL INFORMATION

Metformin is an antidiabetic drug used to treat Type 2 diabetes in which some insulin-secreting cells are still active in the pancreas. It is usually prescribed for obese patients.

Metformin lowers blood glucose by reducing the absorption of glucose from the digestive tract into the bloodstream, by reducing the glucose production by cells in the liver and kidneys, and by increasing the sensitivity of cells to insulin so that they take up glucose more effectively from the blood.

The drug is given in conjunction with a diabetic diet that limits sugar and fat intake. It may be given with another antidiabetic drug that stimulates insulin secretion by the pancreas, or with insulin for maturity-onset diabetes, especially to obese patients.

INFORMATION FOR USERS

Your drug prescription is tailored for you. Do not alter dosage without checking with your doctor.

How taken/used Tablets.

Frequency and timing of doses 2–3 x daily with food.

Adult dosage range 1.5–3g daily, with a low dose at the start of treatment.

Onset of effect Within 2 hours. It may take 2 weeks to achieve control of diabetes.

Duration of action 8–12 hours.

Diet advice An individualized low-fat, low-sugar diet must be maintained for the drug to be fully effective. Follow your doctor's advice.

Storage Keep in original container at room temperature out of the reach of children.

Missed dose Take as soon as you remember. If your next dose is due within 2 hours, take a single dose now and skip the next.

Stopping the drug Do not stop taking the drug without consulting your doctor; stopping the drug may lead to worsening of the underlying condition.

OVERDOSE ACTION

Seek immediate medical advice in all cases. Take emergency action if fits or loss of consciousness occur.

POSSIBLE ADVERSE EFFECTS

A metallic taste in the mouth and minor gastrointestinal symptoms such as nausea, vomiting, and appetite loss are common and are often helped by taking the drug with food. Rarely, diarrhoea, dizziness, confusion, weakness, sweating, and a rash occur and should be discussed with your doctor.

INTERACTIONS

General note A number of drugs reduce the effects of metformin. These include corticosteroids, oestrogens, and diuretics. Other drugs, notably beta blockers and monoamine oxidase inhibitors (MAOIs), increase its effects.

Warfarin Metformin may increase the effect of this anticoagulant drug. The dosage of warfarin may need to be adjusted accordingly.

SPECIAL PRECAUTIONS

Be sure to tell your doctor if:
◆ You have long-term liver or kidney problems.
◆ You have heart failure.
◆ You are a heavy drinker.
◆ You are taking other medicines.

Pregnancy Not usually prescribed. Insulin is usually substituted because it provides better diabetic control during pregnancy. Discuss with your doctor.

Breast-feeding Safety not established. Discuss with your doctor.

Infants and children Not recommended under 10 years.

Over 60 Increased likelihood of adverse effects. Reduced dose may therefore be necessary.

Driving and hazardous work Usually no problems. Avoid such activities if you have warning signs of low blood glucose.

Alcohol Avoid. Alcohol increases the risk of low blood glucose, and can cause coma by increasing the acidity of the blood.

Surgery and general anaesthetics Surgery may reduce the response to this drug. Notify your doctor or dentist that you have diabetes before any surgery; insulin treatment may need to be substituted. Tell your doctor if you are to have a contrast X-ray; metformin should be stopped before the procedure.

PROLONGED USE

Prolonged treatment can deplete vitamin B_{12} reserves, and this may rarely cause anaemia.

Monitoring Regular checks on kidney function and on levels of sugar in the urine and/ or blood are usually required. Vitamin B_{12} levels may also be checked annually.

Methadone

Brand names Methadose, Metharose, Physeptone, Synastone
Used in the following combined preparations None

QUICK REFERENCE

Drug group Opioid analgesic (p.9)
Overdose danger rating High
Dependence rating High
Prescription needed Yes
Available as generic Yes

GENERAL INFORMATION

Methadone is a synthetic opioid analgesic drug used in the control of severe pain, and as a cough suppressant in terminal illness, but it is more widely used to replace morphine or heroin in the treatment of dependence. For this, methadone can be given once daily to prevent withdrawal symptoms. In some cases, dosage can be reduced until the drug is no longer needed.

Tolerance to methadone is marked. Although the initial dose for a person unused to opioids is very low, the dose needed by a dependent person could be fatal for a non-user.

INFORMATION FOR USERS

Your drug prescription is tailored for you. Do not alter dosage without checking with your doctor.

How taken/used Tablets, liquid, injection.
Frequency and timing of doses *Pain* 3–4 x daily; 2 x daily (prolonged use). *Cough* 4–6 x daily (starting dose); 2 x daily (prolonged use). *Opioid addiction* Once daily.
Adult dosage range *Pain* 5–10mg per dose initially, adjusted according to response. *Cough* 1–2mg per dose. *Opioid addiction* 10–20mg (starting dose); 40–60mg daily (maintenance).
Onset of effect 15–60 minutes.
Duration of action 36–48 hours.
Diet advice None.
Storage Keep in original container at room temperature out of the reach of children. Protect injections and liquids from light.

Missed dose Take as soon as you remember and return to your normal dosing schedule as soon as possible. If you missed the dose because it caused you to vomit, or if you cannot swallow, consult your doctor.

Stopping the drug If the reason for taking the drug no longer exists, it can be slowly reduced and safely stopped. Discuss with your doctor.

OVERDOSE ACTION

Seek immediate medical advice in all cases. Take emergency action if symptoms such as slow or irregular breathing, severe drowsiness, or loss of consciousness occur.

POSSIBLE ADVERSE EFFECTS

Nausea, vomiting, and drowsiness are common but diminish as the body adapts. Constipation is also common and may be longer lasting. Dizziness and confusion, although common, should be reported to your doctor. If, rarely, loss of consciousness or breathing difficulties occur, stop taking the drug and seek immediate medical attention.

INTERACTIONS

Phenytoin, carbamazepine, rifampicin, and ritonavir These drugs may reduce the effects of methadone.

Monoamine oxidase inhibitors (MAOIs) and selegiline may produce a dangerous rise or fall in blood pressure when taken with methadone.

Erythromycin, clarithromycin, and fluconazole These drugs may increase the effects of methadone.

Sedatives The effects of all drugs that have a sedative effect on the central nervous system are likely to be increased by methadone.

SPECIAL PRECAUTIONS

Be sure to tell your doctor if:
◆ You have heart or circulatory problems.
◆ You have liver or kidney problems.
◆ You have lung problems such as asthma or bronchitis.
◆ You have thyroid disease.
◆ You have a history of epileptic fits.
◆ You have problems with alcohol abuse.
◆ You are taking other medicines.

Pregnancy Not prescribed in late pregnancy if possible. May cause breathing difficulties in the newborn baby. Discuss with your doctor.

Breast-feeding Safety not established. The drug passes into breast milk and may affect the baby adversely. Discuss with your doctor.

Infants and children Not recommended.

Over 60 Reduced dose necessary.

Driving and hazardous work Your underlying condition may make such activities inadvisable. Discuss with your doctor.

Alcohol Avoid. Alcohol increases the drug's sedative effects and may depress breathing.

PROLONGED USE

Treatment with methadone is always closely monitored. If the drug is being taken long term, the dose must be carefully reduced before the drug is stopped.

Methotrexate

Brand name Maxtrex
Used in the following combined preparations None

QUICK REFERENCE

Drug group Anticancer drug (p.96), disease-modifying antirheumatic (p.52), and drug for psoriasis, (p.124)
Overdose danger rating Medium
Dependence rating Low
Prescription needed Yes
Available as generic Yes

GENERAL INFORMATION

Methotrexate is an anticancer drug used, together with other anticancer drugs, in the treatment of leukaemia, lymphoma, and solid cancers such as those of the breast, bladder, head, and neck. It is also used to treat severe uncontrolled psoriasis until less potent drugs can be re-introduced. It is also used to modify, halt, or slow the underlying disease process in severe acute rheumatoid arthritis that has not responded to other treatment. Once the condition is under control, the dose of methotrexate is reduced to a minimum.

As with most anticancer drugs, methotrexate affects both healthy and cancerous cells, so that its usefulness is limited by its adverse effects and toxicity. When it is given in high doses, methotrexate is usually given with folinic acid to prevent it from destroying bone marrow cells.

INFORMATION FOR USERS

Your drug prescription is tailored for you. Do not alter dosage without checking with your doctor.

How taken/used Tablets, injection.

Frequency and timing of doses *Cancer* Single dose once weekly or every 3 weeks. *Other conditions* Usually, single dose once weekly.

Adult dosage range *Cancer* Dosage is determined individually according to the nature of the condition, body weight, and response. *Rheumatoid arthritis* 7.5–20mg weekly. *Psoriasis* 10–25mg weekly.

Onset of effect 30–60 minutes.

Duration of action Short-term effects last 10–15 hours.

Diet advice None.

Storage Keep in original container at room temperature out of the reach of children. Wash your hands after handling the tablets.

Missed dose Take as soon as you remember and consult your doctor.

Stopping the drug Do not stop the drug without consulting your doctor; stopping may lead to worsening of the underlying condition.

Exceeding the dose Tell your doctor if you accidentally take an extra tablet. Large overdoses damage the bone marrow and cause nausea and abdominal pain. Notify your doctor immediately.

POSSIBLE ADVERSE EFFECTS

Nausea and vomiting commonly occur within a few hours of taking methotrexate. Diarrhoea and mouth ulcers/inflammation are also common, occurring a few days after treatment starts. A dry cough and chest pain are also common, but contact your doctor at once if they occur. Rarely, jaundice, mood changes, and confusion may occur. If mouth ulcers/inflammation or, rarely, sore throat, rash, or fever, occur, stop taking the drug and consult your doctor at once.

INTERACTIONS

General note Many drugs, including NSAIDs, diuretics, ciclosporin, phenytoin, and probenecid, may increase blood levels and toxicity of methotrexate.

Co-trimoxazole, trimethoprim, and certain antimalarial drugs These drugs may enhance the effects of methotrexate.

SPECIAL PRECAUTIONS

Be sure to tell your doctor if:
◆ You have liver or kidney problems.
◆ You have porphyria.
◆ You have a problem with alcohol abuse.
◆ You have a peptic or other digestive-tract ulcer.
◆ You are taking other medicines.

Pregnancy Not prescribed. Methotrexate may cause birth defects in the unborn baby.

Breast-feeding Not advised. The drug passes into the breast milk and may affect the baby adversely.

Infants and children For cancer treatment only. Reduced dose necessary.

Over 60 Increased likelihood of adverse effects. Reduced dose necessary.

Driving and hazardous work No special problems.

Alcohol Avoid. Alcohol may increase the adverse effects of methotrexate.

PROLONGED USE

Long-term treatment with methotrexate may be needed for rheumatoid arthritis. Once the condition is controlled, the drug is reduced as much as possible to the lowest effective dose.

Monitoring Full blood counts and kidney and liver function tests will be performed before treatment starts and at intervals during treatment. Blood concentrations of methotrexate may also be measured periodically.

Methylcellulose

Brand name Celevac
Used in the following combined preparations None

QUICK REFERENCE

Drug group Laxative (p.45) and antidiarrhoeal drug (p.44)
Overdose danger rating Low
Dependence rating Low
Prescription needed No
Available as generic Yes

GENERAL INFORMATION

Methylcellulose is a laxative used for the treatment of constipation, diverticular disease, and irritable bowel syndrome. Taken by mouth, it is not absorbed into the bloodstream but remains in the intestine, where it absorbs up to 25 times its volume of water, thereby softening and increasing the volume of faeces. Methylcellulose is also used to reduce the frequency and increase the firmness of faeces in chronic watery diarrhoea, and to control the consistency of faeces after colostomies and ileostomies.

Methylcellulose preparations are also used with appropriate dieting in some cases of obesity. The bulking agent swells to give a feeling of fullness, thereby encouraging adherence to a reducing diet.

INFORMATION FOR USERS

Follow instructions on the label. Call your doctor if symptoms worsen.

How taken/used Tablets.

Frequency and timing of doses 1–2 x daily. If used as laxative, unless otherwise instructed, break in mouth and swallow with full glass of water; do not take at bedtime.

Adult dosage range 1.5–6g daily.

Onset of effect Within 24 hours.

Duration of action Up to 3 days.

Diet advice If taken as a laxative, drink plenty of fluids, at least 6–8 glasses daily.

Storage Keep in original container at room temperature out of the reach of children.

Missed dose Take as soon as you remember. Take the next dose as scheduled.

Stopping the drug Can be safely stopped as soon as you no longer need it.

Exceeding the dose An occasional unintentional extra dose is unlikely to be a cause for concern. But if you notice any unusual symptoms, or if a large overdose has been taken, notify your doctor.

POSSIBLE ADVERSE EFFECTS

Adverse effects are rare, but when methylcellulose is taken by mouth it may cause bloating and excess wind. Insufficient fluid intake may cause blockage of the oesophagus (gullet) or intestine. Consult your doctor if you experience severe abdominal pain or if you have no bowel movement within 2 days of taking methylcellulose.

INTERACTIONS

None.

SPECIAL PRECAUTIONS

Be sure to consult your doctor or pharmacist before taking this drug if:

◆ You have severe constipation and/or abdominal pain.

◆ You have unexplained rectal bleeding.

◆ You have difficulty in swallowing.

◆ You vomit readily.

◆ You are taking other medicines.

Pregnancy No evidence of risk to developing baby, but discuss with your doctor.

Breast-feeding No evidence of risk.

Infants and children Reduced dose necessary, but discuss with your doctor.

Over 60 No special problems.

Driving and hazardous work No known problems.

Alcohol No known problems.

PROLONGED USE

No problems expected.

Metoclopramide

Brand names Maxolon, Maxolon High Dose, Maxolon SR, Primperan

Used in the following combined preparations MigraMax, Paramax

QUICK REFERENCE

Drug group Gastrointestinal motility regulator and anti-emetic drug (p.21)

Overdose danger rating Medium

Dependence rating Low

Prescription needed Yes

Available as generic Yes

GENERAL INFORMATION

Metoclopramide has a direct action on the gastrointestinal tract. It is used for conditions in which there is a need to encourage normal propulsion of food through the stomach and intestine.

Metoclopramide has powerful anti-emetic properties, and its most common use is in the prevention and treatment of nausea and vomiting. The drug is particularly effective for the relief of the nausea that sometimes accompanies migraine headaches and for the nausea resulting from treatment with anticancer drugs. Metoclopramide is also prescribed to alleviate symptoms of heartburn caused by acid reflux into the oesophagus.

One side effect of metoclopramide is muscle spasm of the face and neck, which is more likely to occur in children and young adults under the age of 20 years. Other side effects are not usually troublesome.

INFORMATION FOR USERS

Your drug prescription is tailored for you. Do not alter dosage without checking with your doctor.

How taken/used Tablets, SR-tablets/capsules, liquid, powder, injection.

Frequency and timing of doses Usually 3 x daily; 2 x daily (SR-preparations).

Adult dosage range Usually 15–30mg daily; may be higher for nausea caused by anticancer drugs.

Onset of effect Within 1 hour.

Duration of action 6–8 hours.

Diet advice Fatty and spicy foods and alcohol are best avoided if nausea is a problem.

Storage Keep in original container at room temperature out of the reach of children.

Missed dose Take as soon as you remember. If your next dose is due within 3 hours, take a single dose now and skip the next.

Stopping the drug Can be safely stopped as soon as you no longer need it.

Exceeding the dose An occasional unintentional extra dose is unlikely to be a cause for concern. However, large overdoses may cause drowsiness and muscle spasms. Notify your doctor.

POSSIBLE ADVERSE EFFECTS

Adverse effects are rare with metoclopramide. The main adverse effects of the drug are drowsiness and, even less commonly, uncontrolled muscle spasm. Other symptoms include restlessness, diarrhoea, muscle tremors and rigidity, and a rash. Consult your doctor if drowsiness becomes severe, and for all other effects. If you experience muscle spasms of the face, or you develop a rash, stop taking the drug and consult your doctor urgently.

INTERACTIONS

Sedatives The sedative properties of metoclopramide are increased by all drugs that have a sedative effect on the central nervous system. Such drugs include anti-anxiety and sleeping drugs, antihistamines, antidepressants, opioid analgesics, and antipsychotics.

Lithium Metoclopramide increases the risk of central nervous system side effects.

Ciclosporin Metoclopramide may increase the blood levels of this drug.

Drugs for parkinsonism There is an increased risk of adverse effects if these drugs are taken with metoclopramide.

Phenothiazine antipsychotics The likelihood of adverse effects from these drugs is increased by metoclopramide.

Opioid analgesics and anticholinergic drugs These drugs oppose the gastrointestinal effects of metoclopramide.

SPECIAL PRECAUTIONS

Be sure to tell your doctor if:

◆ You have long-term liver or kidney problems.

◆ You have epilepsy.

◆ You have Parkinson's disease.

◆ You have acute porphyria.

◆ You have a history of depression.

◆ You have phaeochromocytoma.

◆ You have stomach pains or cramps.

◆ You are taking other medicines.

Pregnancy Safety in pregnancy not established. Discuss with your doctor.

Breast-feeding The drug passes into the breast milk but at normal doses adverse effects on the baby are unlikely. Discuss with your doctor.

Infants and children Reduced dose necessary. Restricted use in patients younger than 20 years.

Over 60 Reduced dose may be necessary.

Driving and hazardous work Avoid such activities until you have learned how metoclopramide affects you because the drug can cause drowsiness.

Alcohol Avoid. Alcohol may oppose the beneficial effects and increase the sedative effects of this drug.

PROLONGED USE

Metoclopramide is not normally prescribed for long-term use, except for certain gastrointestinal disorders, and only under specialist supervision.

Metoprolol

Brand names Betaloc, Betaloc-SA, Lopresor, Lopresor SR
Used in the following combined preparation
Co-Betaloc

QUICK REFERENCE
Drug group Beta blocker (p.30)
Overdose danger rating High
Dependence rating Low
Prescription needed Yes
Available as generic Yes

GENERAL INFORMATION
Metoprolol is a beta blocker that is used to prevent the heart from beating too quickly in conditions such as angina, arrhythmias (abnormal heart rhythms), and hyperthyroidism (an overactive thyroid gland). The drug is also used to prevent migraine attacks and to protect the heart from further damage following a heart attack. Metoprolol is also used to treat hypertension (high blood pressure), but it is not usually used to initiate treatment.

Because metoprolol is cardioselective, it is less likely than other, non-cardioselective, beta blockers to provoke breathing difficulties. However, is not usually given to people with respiratory diseases.

INFORMATION FOR USERS
Your drug prescription is tailored for you. Do not alter dosage without checking with your doctor.
How taken/used Tablets, SR-tablets, injection.
Frequency and timing of doses 1–2 x daily (hypertension); 2–3 x daily (angina/arrhythmias); 4 x daily for 2 days, then 2 x daily (prevention of heart attack); 2 x daily (prevention of migraine); 4 x daily (hyperthyroidism).
Adult dosage range 100–400mg daily.
Onset of effect 1–2 hours.
Duration of action 3–7 hours.
Diet advice None.
Storage Keep in original container at room temperature out of the reach of children.
Missed dose Take as soon as you remember. If your next dose is due within 2 hours, take a single dose now and skip the next.

Stopping the drug Do not stop taking the drug without consulting your doctor. Stopping suddenly may lead to worsening of the underlying condition.

OVERDOSE ACTION
Seek immediate medical advice in all cases. Take emergency action if breathing difficulties, collapse, or loss of consciousness occur.

POSSIBLE ADVERSE EFFECTS
Like all beta blockers, treatment with metoprolol is commonly associated with nightmares and cold fingers and toes. Drowsiness, fatigue, dizziness, and headache are also common adverse effects. Rarely, nausea, vomiting, and abdominal pain may occur. If, rarely, you develop breathing difficulties or wheezing, or fainting occurs, seek immediate medical attention.

INTERACTIONS
Verapamil When first taken with metoprolol, this drug may seriously slow or stop the heart beat and lower blood pressure.
Decongestants may increase blood pressure and heart rate with metoprolol.
Alpha blockers, antidepressants, calcium channel blockers, sympathomimetics, and some diuretics may increase the blood pressure lowering effect of metoprolol.
Ergotamine Taken with metoprolol, this drug increases the constriction of blood vessels in the extremities.
Antidiabetic drugs Taken with metoprolol, these drugs may increase the risk of low blood glucose or mask its symptoms.
Non-steroidal anti-inflammatory drugs (NSAIDs) may oppose the blood pressure lowering effects of metoprolol.

SPECIAL PRECAUTIONS
Be sure to tell your doctor if:
◆ You have liver or kidney problems.
◆ You have asthma, bronchitis, or emphysema.
◆ You have heart failure.
◆ You have diabetes.
◆ You have hyperthyroidism.
◆ You have phaeochromocytoma.
◆ You have psoriasis.
◆ You have poor circulation in the legs.
◆ You are taking other medicines.

Pregnancy Not usually prescribed. May affect the baby, but the drug may be given under close supervision. Discuss with your doctor.

Breast-feeding The drug passes into the breast milk, but at normal doses adverse effects on the baby are unlikely. Discuss with your doctor.

Infants and children Not recommended.

Over 60 Reduced doses necessary. There may be an increased risk of adverse effects.

Driving and hazardous work Avoid such activities until you have learned how metoprolol affects you because the drug can cause fatigue, dizziness, and drowsiness.

Alcohol No special problems.

PROLONGED USE

No special problems.

Metronidazole

Brand names Anabact, Elyzol, Flagyl, Metrogel, Metrolyl, Metrotop, Metrozol, Noritate, Rozex, Vaginyl, Zidoval, Zyomet

Used in the following combined preparations None

QUICK REFERENCE

Drug group Antibacterial (p.66) and antiprotozoal drug (p.73)

Overdose danger rating Low

Dependence rating Low

Prescription needed Yes

Available as generic Yes

GENERAL INFORMATION

Metronidazole is prescribed to fight both protozoal infections and a variety of bacterial infections.

It is widely used in the treatment of trichomonas infection of the vagina. Because the organism responsible for this disorder is sexually transmitted and may not cause any symptoms, a simultaneous course of treatment is usually advised for the sexual partner.

Certain infections of the abdomen, pelvis, and gums also respond well to metronidazole treatment. The drug is used to treat septicaemia and infected leg ulcers and pressure sores. Metronidazole may be given to prevent or treat infections following surgery. Because the drug in high doses can penetrate the brain, it is prescribed to treat abscesses occurring there.

Metronidazole is also prescribed for the treatment of amoebic dysentery and giardiasis, a rare protozoal infection.

Metronidazole may be applied topically in the form of a gel to treat some forms of acne, rosacea, infected tumours, and gum disease.

INFORMATION FOR USERS

Your drug prescription is tailored for you. Do not alter dosage without checking with your doctor.

How taken/used Tablets, liquid, injection, suppositories, gel, cream.

Frequency and timing of doses 3 x daily for 5–10 days, depending on condition being treated. Sometimes a single large dose is prescribed. Tablets should be taken after meals and swallowed whole with plenty of water. 1–2 x daily (topical preparations).

Adult dosage range 600–2,000mg daily (by mouth); 3g daily (suppositories); 1.5g daily (injection).

Onset of effect The drug starts to work within an hour or so, but beneficial effects may not be felt for 1–2 days.

Duration of action 6–12 hours.

Diet advice None.

Storage Keep in original container at room temperature out of the reach of children. Protect from light.

Missed dose Take as soon as you remember. If your next dose is due within 2 hours, take a single dose now and skip the next.

Stopping the drug Take the full course. Even if you feel better the infection may still be present and symptoms may recur if treatment is stopped too soon.

Exceeding the dose An occasional unintentional extra dose is unlikely to be a cause for concern. However, if you notice unusual symptoms, especially numbness or tingling, or if a large overdose has been taken, notify your doctor.

POSSIBLE ADVERSE EFFECTS

Various minor gastrointestinal disturbances are common but tend to diminish with time. The drug may commonly cause a darkening of the urine, which is no cause for concern.

Nausea and loss of appetite are also common. A dry mouth, metallic taste in the mouth, headache, and dizziness are rare. More serious adverse effects on the nervous system, causing numbness and tingling, are extremely rare with metronidazole, but, if they occur, consult your doctor immediately.

INTERACTIONS

Oral anticoagulants, ciclosporin, phenytoin, and fluorouracil Metronidazole may increase the effects of these drugs.

Lithium Metronidazole increases the risk of adverse effects on the kidneys.

Cimetidine This drug may increase the levels of metronidazole in the body.

Phenobarbital This drug may reduce the effects of metronidazole.

SPECIAL PRECAUTIONS

Be sure to tell your doctor if:
◆ You have long-term liver or kidney problems.
◆ You have a blood disorder.
◆ You have a disorder of the central nervous system, such as epilepsy.
◆ You have porphyria.
◆ You have a history of angioedema.
◆ You are taking other medicines.

Pregnancy Safety in pregnancy not established. Discuss with your doctor.

Breast-feeding The drug passes into the breast milk, but at normal doses adverse effects on the baby are unlikely. However, metronidazole may give the milk a bitter taste. Discuss with your doctor.

Infants and children Reduced dose necessary.

Over 60 No special problems.

Driving and hazardous work Avoid such activities until you have learned how metronidazole affects you because the drug can cause drowsiness.

Alcohol Avoid. Taken with metronidazole, alcohol may cause flushing, nausea, vomiting, abdominal pain, and headache.

PROLONGED USE

Not usually prescribed for longer than 10 days. Prolonged treatment may cause loss of sensation in the hands and feet (usually temporary), and may also reduce production of white blood cells.

Miconazole

Brand names Daktarin, Gyno-Daktarin
Used in the following combined preparation Daktacort

QUICK REFERENCE

Drug group Antifungal drug (p.76)
Overdose danger rating Low
Dependence rating Low
Prescription needed No (cream, powder) Yes (other preparations)
Available as generic Yes

GENERAL INFORMATION

Miconazole is an antifungal drug used to treat candida (yeast) infections of the mouth, candida and bacterial infections of the vagina, and a range of other fungal infections affecting the skin. It is available as a treatment for oral infections in the form of a gel to be used on dentures. Cream, dusting powder, or ointment are used for skin infections, and a variety of vaginal preparations is available.

Side effects usually occur only with oral preparations because miconazole is absorbed in only very small quantities following topical or vaginal application.

The pessaries, vaginal capsules, and vaginal cream damage latex condoms and diaphragms.

INFORMATION FOR USERS

Follow instructions on the label. Call your doctor if symptoms worsen.

How taken/used Pessaries, vaginal cream, vaginal capsules, cream, ointment, oral gel, spray powder.

Frequency and timing of doses 4 x daily after food (oral gel); 1–2 x daily (vaginal/skin preparations).

Adult dosage range *Vaginal infections* 1 x 5g applicatorful (cream); 1 x 100mg pessary; 1 x 1.2g vaginal capsule. *Oral/skin infections* As directed.

Onset of effect 2–3 days.

Duration of action Up to 12 hours.

Diet advice None.

Storage Keep in original container at room temperature out of the reach of children.

Missed dose No cause for concern, but apply missed dose or application as soon as you remember.

Stopping the drug Apply the full course. Even if you feel better, the original infection may still be present and may recur if treatment is stopped too soon.

Exceeding the dose An occasional unintentional extra dose is unlikely to cause problems. But if you notice any unusual symptoms or if a large amount has been swallowed, notify your doctor.

POSSIBLE ADVERSE EFFECTS

Adverse effects are rare with miconazole and usually occur only with oral use. The effects include skin irritation, nausea, vomiting, and vaginal irritation, which should be reported to your doctor. If you experience wheezing or a blotchy rash, stop the drug and consult your doctor promptly.

INTERACTIONS

Oral anticoagulants, ciclosporin, phenytoin, antidiabetics, terfenadine, quinidine, and pimozide Miconazole oral gel may increase the effects and toxicity of these drugs.

Carbamazepine, phenytoin, calcium channel blockers, sirolimus, and tacrolimus Miconazole oral gel may increase the effects and toxicity of these drugs.

Simvastatin There is an increased risk of muscle damage if this drug is taken with miconazole.

SPECIAL PRECAUTIONS

Be sure to consult your doctor or pharmacist before taking this drug if:
◆ You have porphyria.
◆ You have liver problems.
◆ You are taking other medicines.

Pregnancy Safety not established. Discuss with your doctor.

Breast-feeding Safety not established. Discuss with your doctor.

Infants and children Reduced dose necessary (oral gel).

Over 60 No special problems.

Driving and hazardous work No special problems.

Alcohol No special problems.

PROLONGED USE

No problems expected. Most types of miconazole are not usually prescribed in the long term. However, the oral gel may cause diarrhoea if it is used for a long time.

Minocycline

Brand names Aknemin, Blemix, Dentomycin, Minocin, Minocin MR
Used in the following combined preparations None

QUICK REFERENCE

Drug group Tetracycline antibiotic (p.62)
Overdose danger rating Low
Dependence rating Low
Prescription needed Yes
Available as generic Yes

GENERAL INFORMATION

Minocycline is a member of the tetracycline group of antibiotics, but it has a substantially longer duration of action than tetracycline itself. Minocycline is most commonly used to treat acne.

Minocycline may be given to treat pneumonia or to prevent infection in people who have chronic bronchitis. The drug is also used for the treatment of gonorrhoea and non-gonococcal urethritis and may be used to treat other sexually transmitted diseases. Minocycline is also used to treat chronic gum disease in adults.

The drug's most frequent side effects are nausea, vomiting, and diarrhoea. It also interferes with the functioning of the balance mechanism in the inner ear, with resultant nausea, dizziness, and unsteadiness, but these symptoms generally disappear after the drug is stopped. Minocycline is not prescribed for people with poor kidney function.

INFORMATION FOR USERS

Your drug prescription is tailored for you. Do not alter dosage without checking with your doctor.

How taken/used Tablets, capsules, MR-capsules, gel.

Frequency and timing of doses 1–2 x daily.

Dosage range *Adults* 100–200mg daily. *Children* Reduced dose according to age and weight.

Onset of effect 4–12 hours.

Duration of action Up to 24 hours.

Diet advice Milk products may impair absorption; avoid from 1 hour before to 2 hours after dosage.

Storage Keep in original container at room temperature out of the reach of children.

Missed dose Take as soon as you remember. If your next dose is due within 4 hours, take a single dose now and skip the next.

Stopping the drug Use the full course. Even if you feel better, the original infection may still be present and symptoms may recur if treatment is stopped too soon.

Exceeding the dose An occasional unintentional extra dose is unlikely to be a cause for concern. But if you notice any unusual symptoms, or if a large overdose has been taken, notify your doctor.

POSSIBLE ADVERSE EFFECTS

Minocycline may occasionally cause nausea, vomiting, or diarrhoea. Other less common adverse effects include dizziness and loss of balance (vertigo), a rash, itching, increased sensitivity of the skin to sunlight, headache, or blurred vision. If any of these effects occur, stop taking the drug and consult your doctor promptly.

INTERACTIONS

Oral anticoagulants Minocycline may increase the anticoagulant action of these drugs.

Retinoids Taken with minocycline these drugs may increase the risk of benign intracranial hypertension (high pressure in the skull) leading to headaches, nausea, and vomiting.

Oral contraceptives Minocycline can reduce the effectiveness of these drugs.

Penicillin antibiotics Minocycline interferes with the antibacterial action of these drugs.

Iron may interfere with the absorption of minocycline and may reduce its effectiveness.

Antacids, zinc preparations, and milk interfere with absorption of minocycline and may reduce its effectiveness. Doses should be separated by 1–2 hours.

SPECIAL PRECAUTIONS

Be sure to tell your doctor if:
◆ You have liver or kidney problems.
◆ You have previously suffered an allergic reaction to a tetracycline antibiotic.
◆ You have myasthenia gravis.
◆ You are taking other medicines.

Pregnancy Not prescribed. May damage the teeth and bones of the developing baby, as well as the mother's liver. Discuss with your doctor.

Breast-feeding The drug passes into the breast milk and may lead to discoloration of the baby's teeth. Discuss with your doctor.

Infants and children Not recommended under 13 years. Reduced dose necessary in older children.

Over 60 No special problems.

Driving and hazardous work Avoid such activities until you have learned how minocycline affects you because the drug can cause dizziness.

Alcohol No known problems.

How to take your tablets To prevent minocycline from sticking in your throat, take a small amount of water before, and a full glass of water after, each dose. Take this medication while sitting or standing and do not lie down immediately afterwards.

PROLONGED USE

Prolonged use of minocycline may occasionally cause skin darkening and discoloration of the teeth.

Monitoring Regular blood tests should be carried out to assess liver function.

Minoxidil

Brand names Loniten, Regaine
Used in the following combined preparations None

QUICK REFERENCE

Drug group Antihypertensive drug (p.36) and treatment for hair loss (p.127)
Overdose danger rating Medium
Dependence rating Low
Prescription needed Yes (except for scalp lotions)
Available as generic No

GENERAL INFORMATION

Minoxidil is a vasodilator drug (see p.31) that works by relaxing the muscles of artery walls and dilating blood vessels. It is effective in controlling dangerously high blood pressure that is rising very rapidly. Because minoxidil is stronger acting than many other antihypertensive drugs, it is particularly useful for people whose blood pressure is not controlled by other treatment.

Because minoxidil can cause fluid retention and increase the heart rate, it should be prescribed with a diuretic and a beta blocker to increase effectiveness and to counteract its side effects. Unlike many other drugs in the antihypertensive group, minoxidil rarely causes dizziness and fainting. The major drawback of minoxidil is that, if it is taken for more than 2 months, it increases hair growth, especially on the face. Although this effect can be controlled by shaving or depilatories, some people find the abnormal growth distressing. This effect is put to use, however, to treat baldness in men and women, and for this purpose minoxidil is applied locally as a solution.

INFORMATION FOR USERS

Your drug prescription is tailored for you. Do not alter dosage without checking with your doctor.

How taken/used Tablets, topical solution.
Frequency and timing of doses Once or twice daily.
Adult dosage range 5mg daily initially, increasing gradually to a maximum of 50mg daily.
Onset of effect *Blood pressure* Within 1 hour (tablets). *Hair growth* Up to 1 year (solution).
Duration of action Up to 24 hours. Some effect may last for 2–5 days after stopping the drug.
Diet advice None.
Storage Keep in original container at room temperature out of the reach of children.
Missed dose Take as soon as you remember (tablets). If your next dose is due within 5 hours, take a single dose now and skip the next.
Stopping the drug Do not stop the drug without consulting your doctor; stopping the drug may lead to worsening of the underlying condition.
Exceeding the dose An occasional unintentional extra dose is unlikely to cause problems. Large overdoses may cause nausea, vomiting, palpitations, or dizziness. Notify your doctor.

POSSIBLE ADVERSE EFFECTS

Fluid retention is a common adverse effect of minoxidil, which may lead to an increase in weight; diuretics are often prescribed to control this effect. Another common adverse effect is increased hair growth. Nausea may also occur. If you experience breast tenderness, dizziness, or lightheadedness, or you develop a rash, consult your doctor. If you have palpitations, stop taking the drug and consult your doctor immediately. Allergic and irritant dermatitis may occur with minoxidil topical solution.

INTERACTIONS

Antidepressant drugs The hypotensive effects of minoxidil may be enhanced by antidepressant drugs.
Other antihypertensives These drugs may increase the effects of minoxidil.
Oestrogens and progestogens (including those in some contraceptive pills) may reduce the effects of minoxidil.

SPECIAL PRECAUTIONS

Be sure to tell your doctor if:
◆ You have a long-term kidney problem.
◆ You have heart problems.
◆ You retain fluid.
◆ You are taking other medicines.
Pregnancy Safety in pregnancy not established. Discuss with your doctor.
Breast-feeding The drug passes into the breast milk, but at normal doses adverse effects on the baby are unlikely. Discuss with your doctor.
Infants and children Reduced dose necessary.
Over 60 Reduced dose may be necessary.
Driving and hazardous work Avoid such activities until you have learned how minoxidil affects you because the drug can cause dizziness and lightheadedness.
Alcohol Avoid. Alcohol may further reduce blood pressure.
Surgery and general anaesthetics Minoxidil treatment may need to be stopped before you have a general anaesthetic. Discuss this with your doctor or dentist before any surgery.

PROLONGED USE

Prolonged use of this drug may lead to swelling of the ankles and increased hair growth.

Mirtazepine

Brand names SolTab, Zispin
Used in the following combined preparations
None

QUICK REFERENCE

Drug group Antidepressant drug (p.14)
Overdose danger rating Medium
Dependence rating Low
Prescription needed Yes
Available as generic Yes

GENERAL INFORMATION

Mirtazepine is an antidepressant drug that works by increasing the naturally occurring chemicals in the brain, serotonin and noradrenaline. It is used in the treatment of major depression, the symptoms of which may include feelings of worthlessness, anxiety, and increased or decreased appetite.

Mirtazepine may be given at a low dose initially and increased gradually according to the response of the individual. If there is no response to mirtazepine at the maximum dose within 2 to 4 weeks, the treatment may be discontinued.

Mirtazepine is available as tablets, orosoluble tablets (which are placed on the tongue and allowed to dissolve), and an oral solution.

INFORMATION FOR USERS

Your drug prescription is tailored for you. Do not alter dosage without checking with your doctor.
How taken/used Tablets, orosoluble tablets, liquid (oral solution).
Frequency and timing of doses Usually 1 x 3 daily at bedtime or 2 divided doses.
Adult dosage range 15mg (initial dose), increased gradually to 45mg, according to response.
Onset of effect Within 1–2 weeks, but full beneficial effect may not be felt for 2–4 weeks.
Duration of action At least 24 hours.
Diet advice None.
Storage Keep in original container at room temperature out of the reach of children.
Missed dose Take as soon as you remember, then return to your normal dosing schedule. Do not take an extra dose to make up.

Stopping the drug Do not stop taking the drug without consulting your doctor, who will supervise gradual dosage reduction. Stopping abruptly can lead to withdrawal symptoms.
Exceeding the dose An occasional unintentional extra dose is unlikely to cause problems. Larger overdoses may cause drowsiness and disorientation. Notify your doctor.

POSSIBLE ADVERSE EFFECTS

A number of mirtazepine's effects are similar to symptoms of the illness. The drug has few anticholinergic effects, but causes sedation at the start of treatment. Increased appetite, weight gain, drowsiness, sedation, and fatigue are common; discuss swollen ankles and feet (oedema) with your doctor. Rarely, dizziness, headache, nightmares, and vivid dreams may occur. If jaundice, fever, or sore throat occur, stop taking the drug and consult your doctor immediately.

INTERACTIONS

Monoamine oxidase inhibitors (MAOIs) should not be taken with, or within 2 weeks of stopping, mirtazepine and vice versa.
Warfarin Mirtazepine increases the anticoagulant effect of warfarin.
Antimalarials (artemether with lumefantrine) should not be taken with mirtazepine.
Sibutramine may have increased side effects if taken with mirtazepine.

SPECIAL PRECAUTIONS

Be sure to tell your doctor if:
◆ You have epilepsy.
◆ You have liver or kidney problems.
◆ You have angina or have had a recent heart attack.
◆ You have hypertension.
◆ You have diabetes.
◆ You have a psychiatric disease or bipolar disorder.
◆ You have any eye diseases such as glaucoma.
◆ You have had a previous allergic reaction to mirtazepine.
◆ You are taking other medicines.
Pregnancy Not recommended. Safety not established. Discuss with your doctor.
Breast-feeding Small amounts of the drug pass into the breast milk, but safety not established. Discuss with your doctor.

Infants and children Not recommended.
Over 60 Not recommended.
Driving and hazardous work Do not undertake such activities until you have learned how mirtazepine affects you because the drug can cause initial sedation and impaired alertness and concentration.
Alcohol Avoid. Mirtazepine may increase the sedative effects of alcohol.

PROLONGED USE
No known problems.
Monitoring Periodic tests of liver function are usually carried out.

Misoprostol

Brand name Cytotec
Used in the following combined preparations
Arthrotec, Napratec

QUICK REFERENCE
Drug group Anti-ulcer drug (p.43)
Overdose danger rating Low
Dependence rating Low
Prescription needed Yes
Available as generic No

GENERAL INFORMATION
Misoprostol reduces the amount of acid that is secreted in the stomach and promotes healing of gastric and duodenal ulcers. The drug is related to naturally occurring chemicals known as prostaglandins. Gastric and duodenal ulcers may be caused by aspirin (see p.146) and non-steroidal anti-inflammatory drugs (see p.50), which block certain prostaglandins, and misoprostol can be used to prevent or cure these ulcers. The ulcers usually heal after a few weeks' treatment with misoprostol. In some cases, misoprostol is given during treatment with these drugs as a preventative measure, and combined preparations are available that reduce the likelihood of the ulcers occurring. The most likely adverse effects of treatment with misoprostol are diarrhoea and indigestion; if these are severe it may be necessary to stop treatment with the drug. Diarrhoea can be made worse by antacids containing magnesium; these should therefore be avoided.

INFORMATION FOR USERS
Your drug prescription is tailored for you. Do not alter dosage without checking with your doctor.
How taken/used Tablets.
Frequency and timing of doses 2–4 x daily, with or after food.
Adult dosage range 400–800mcg daily.
Onset of effect Within 24 hours.
Duration of action Up to 24 hours; some effects may be longer lasting.
Diet advice None.
Storage Keep in original container at room temperature out of the reach of children.
Missed dose Take as soon as you remember. If your next dose is due within 3 hours, take a single dose now and skip the next.
Stopping the drug Do not stop the drug without consulting your doctor; symptoms may recur.
Exceeding the dose An occasional unintentional extra dose is unlikely to be a cause for concern. But if you notice any unusual symptoms, or if a large overdose has been taken, notify your doctor.

POSSIBLE ADVERSE EFFECTS
Adverse effects on the gastrointestinal tract, such as diarrhoea and indigestion, can occur. These effects may be reduced by spacing the doses out during the day. Taking the drug with food may be recommended. Rarely, nausea and vomiting may occur. Vaginal and intermenstrual bleeding, abdominal pain, dizziness, and a skin rash are also rare and should be discussed with your doctor; if you develop a skin rash, stop taking the drug.

INTERACTIONS
Magnesium-containing antacids These may increase the severity of any diarrhoea caused by misoprostol.

SPECIAL PRECAUTIONS
Be sure to tell your doctor if:
◆ You are, or are intending to become, pregnant.
◆ You have had a stroke.
◆ You have heart or circulation problems.
◆ You have high blood pressure.
◆ You have bowel problems.
◆ You are taking other medicines.

Pregnancy Misoprostol should not be taken by women of childbearing age. In exceptional cases, it may be prescribed on the condition that effective contraception is used. If taken during pregnancy, the drug can cause the uterus to contract before the baby is due.

Breast-feeding Safety not established. Discuss with your doctor.

Infants and children Not recommended.

Over 60 No special problems.

Driving and hazardous work Avoid such activities until you have learned how the drug affects you; it can cause dizziness.

Alcohol No problems expected, but excess may undermine the drug's desired effect.

PROLONGED USE

No problems expected.

Mometasone

Brand names Asmanex, Elocon, Nasonex
Used in the following combined preparations None

QUICK REFERENCE

Drug group Corticosteroid (p.78)
Overdose danger rating Low
Dependence rating Low
Prescription needed Yes
Available as generic No

GENERAL INFORMATION

Mometasone is a corticosteroid drug used as an inhaler to prevent asthma attacks and as a nasal spray to relieve the symptoms of allergic rhinitis. It is also used topically for the treatment of severe inflammatory skin disorders and in conditions such as eczema that have not responded to other corticosteroids (see Topical corticosteroids, p.120).

Serious adverse effects are rare if the drug is used for short periods or in small amounts, but prolonged or excessive topical use may cause local side effects such as thin skin and systemic side effects such as weak bones, muscle weakness, and peptic ulcers.

Fungal infections causing irritation of the mouth and throat are a possible side effect of taking mometasone by inhaler. These can be avoided to some degree by rinsing the mouth and gargling with water after each inhalation, however.

INFORMATION FOR USERS

Your drug prescription is tailored for you. Do not alter dosage without checking with your doctor.

How taken/used cream, ointment, scalp lotion, inhaler, powder for inhalation, nasal spray.

Frequency and timing of doses 1 x 2 times daily (inhaler); once daily (other forms).

Dosage range *Inhaler* 200–800mcg. *Nasal spray* 100mcg (2 puffs) into each nostril. *Topical preparations* As directed, applied thinly.

Onset of effect 12 hours. Full beneficial effect after 48 hours.

Duration of action 24 hours. Effects can last for several days after the drug is stopped.

Diet advice None.

Storage Keep in original container at room temperature out of the reach of children.

Missed dose Take as soon as you remember. If your next dose/application is due within 8 hours, take a single dose or apply the usual amount now and skip the next.

Stopping the drug Do not stop the drug without consulting your doctor; symptoms may recur.

Exceeding the dose An occasional unintentional extra dose/application may not be a cause for concern, but if you notice any unusual symptoms, notify your doctor.

POSSIBLE ADVERSE EFFECTS

Irritation of, and sometimes bleeding from, the nose are the most common adverse effects; loss of skin pigmentation, headache, a sore throat and mouth, hoarseness, thinning skin, increased capillary size in the skin, and acne or dermatitis around the mouth, are also common; discuss with your doctor. Rarely, weight gain and mood changes may occur; discuss these with your doctor. If breathing difficulties, a rash, or facial swelling occur, consult your doctor immediately.

INTERACTIONS

Ketoconazole and itraconazole These may increase the systemic effect of mometasone.

SPECIAL PRECAUTIONS

Be sure to tell your doctor if:

◆ You have a cold sore, measles, chickenpox, or tuberculosis.
◆ You have any other nasal or skin infection.
◆ You have rosacea or acne.
◆ You have had nasal ulcers or surgery.

Pregnancy Safety not established. Discuss with your doctor.

Breast-feeding No evidence of risk. Discuss with your doctor.

Infants and children Used only for very short courses in children.

Over 60 No special problems.

Driving and hazardous work No special problems.

Alcohol No special problems.

Infection Avoid exposure to chickenpox, measles, or shingles while using mometasone.

PROLONGED USE

Asthma prevention is the condition for which prolonged use may be required. High doses inhaled for a prolonged period can lead to peptic ulcers, fragile bones, glaucoma, muscle weakness, and growth retardation in children. Patients taking the drug long term are advised to carry a "steroid card" or wear a MedicAlert bracelet.

Monitoring If large doses are being taken, periodic checks may be needed to ensure that the adrenal glands are working properly. Children using inhalers should have their growth (height) monitored regularly.

Montelukast

Brand name Singulair
Used in the following combined preparations None

QUICK REFERENCE

Drug group Anti-allergy drug (p.24)
Overdose danger rating Low
Dependence rating Low
Prescription needed Yes
Available as generic No

GENERAL INFORMATION

Montelukast belongs to the leukotriene receptor antagonist (blocker) group of anti-allergy drugs and is used in the prevention of asthma. It is thought that stimulation of leu-kotriene receptors by naturally occurring leukotrienes from the mast cells plays a part in causing asthma. Montelukast works by blocking these receptors.

Montelukast is given as an additional medication when combined treatment with corticosteroids and bronchodilators does not give adequate control. The drug is usually given by mouth as tablets, and a chewable form is available for children. Montelukast is not a bronchodilator, and it cannot, therefore, be used to treat an acute asthma attack.

INFORMATION FOR USERS

Your drug prescription is tailored for you. Do not alter dosage without checking with your doctor.

How taken/used Tablets, chewable tablets.
Frequency and timing of doses Once daily at bedtime.
Adult dosage range 10mg.
Onset of effect 2 hours.
Duration of action 24 hours.
Diet advice None.
Storage Keep in original container at room temperature out of the reach of children. Protect from light.
Missed dose Take as soon as you remember. If your next dose is due within 8 hours, take a single dose now and skip the next.
Stopping the drug Do not stop the drug without consulting your doctor, symptoms may recur.
Exceeding the dose An occasional unintentional extra dose is unlikely to be a cause for concern. But if you notice any unusual symptoms, or if a large overdose has been taken, notify your doctor.

POSSIBLE ADVERSE EFFECTS

Severe adverse effects are rare. There seems to be an increase in the incidence of chest infections among people taking montelukast. Abdominal pain and headache are common. Rarely, diarrhoea, dizziness, drowsiness, and weakness may occur. If a fever, a productive cough, a rash, worsening chest symptoms, or numbness, or tingling occur, consult your doctor.

INTERACTIONS

None.

SPECIAL PRECAUTIONS

Be sure to tell your doctor if:
◆ You have phenylketonuria.
◆ You have galactose intolerance.
◆ You have lactase deficiency.
◆ You are taking other medicines.

Pregnancy Safety not established. Discuss with your doctor.

Breast-feeding Safety not established. Discuss with your doctor.

Infants and children Reduced dose necessary.

Over 60 No special problems.

Driving and hazardous work Avoid such activities until you have learned how the drug affects you; it can cause dizziness and drowsiness.

Alcohol No special problems.

PROLONGED USE

No special problems.

Morphine/diamorphine

Brand names Morphgesic SR, MST Continus, MXL, Oramorph, Oramorph SR, Sevredol, Zomorph
Used in the following combined preparation Cyclimorph

QUICK REFERENCE

Drug group Opioid analgesic (p.9)
Overdose danger rating High
Dependence rating High
Prescription needed Yes
Available as generic Yes

GENERAL INFORMATION

In use since the 19th century, morphine and diamorphine are opioid analgesics (see p.11), which are derived from opium, obtained from the unripe seed capsules of the opium poppy.

Morphine and diamorphine are used to relieve severe pain that can be caused by heart attack, injury, surgery, or chronic diseases such as cancer. They are also sometimes given as premedication before surgery.

Morphine and diamorphine's painkilling effect wears off quickly, in contrast to some other opioid analgesics, and the drugs may be given in a special slow-release (long-acting) form to relieve continuous severe pain.

These drugs are habit-forming, and dependence and addiction can occur. However, most patients who take them for pain relief over brief periods do not become dependent and are able to stop taking them without difficulty.

INFORMATION FOR USERS

Your drug prescription is tailored for you. Do not alter your dosage without checking with your doctor.

How taken/used Tablets, SR-tablets, capsules, SR-capsules, liquid, SR-granules, injection, suppositories, SR-suppositories.

Frequency and timing of doses Every 4 hours; every 12–24 hours (SR-preparations).

Adult dosage range 5–25mg per dose; however, some patients may need 75mg or more per dose. Doses vary considerably for each individual.

Onset of effect Within 1 hour; within 4 hours (SR-preparations).

Duration of action 4 hours; up to 24 hours (SR-preparations).

Diet advice None.

Storage Keep in original container at room temperature out of the reach of children.

Missed dose Take as soon as you remember. Return to your normal dosing schedule as soon as possible.

Stopping the drug If the reason for taking the drug no longer exists, you may stop the drug and notify your doctor.

OVERDOSE ACTION

Seek immediate medical advice in all cases. Take emergency action if symptoms such as slow or irregular breathing, severe drowsiness, or loss of consciousness occur.

POSSIBLE ADVERSE EFFECTS

Nausea, vomiting, constipation, and drowsiness are common, especially with high doses. Anti-nausea drugs or laxatives may be needed to counteract these effects. Dizziness is also common; consult your doctor. Confusion and breathing difficulties are rare; if you experience breathing difficulties, stop taking the drug and consult your doctor promptly.

INTERACTIONS

Monoamine oxidase inhibitors (MAOIs) These drugs may produce a severe rise in blood pressure when taken with morphine and diamorphine.

Esmolol The effects of this beta blocker may be increased by morphine and diamorphine.

Sedatives Morphine and diamorphine increase the sedative effects of other sedating drugs including antidepressants, antipsychotics, sleeping drugs, and antihistamines.

SPECIAL PRECAUTIONS

Be sure to tell your doctor if:
◆ You have long-term liver or kidney problems.
◆ You have heart or circulatory problems.
◆ You have a lung disorder such as asthma or bronchitis.
◆ You have thyroid disease.
◆ You have a history of epileptic fits.
◆ You are taking other medicines.

Pregnancy Not usually prescribed. May cause breathing difficulties in the newborn baby. Discuss with your doctor.

Breast-feeding The drug passes into the breast milk, but at low doses adverse effects on the baby are unlikely. Discuss with your doctor.

Infants and children Reduced dose necessary.

Over 60 Increased likelihood of adverse effects. Reduced dose may be necessary.

Driving and hazardous work People on morphine treatment are unlikely to be well enough to undertake such activities.

Alcohol Avoid. Alcohol may increase the sedative effects of these drugs.

PROLONGED USE

The effects of these drugs usually become weaker as the body adapts. Dependence may occur if they are taken for extended periods although this is unusual in patients taking the correct dose for pain relief.

Moxonidine

Brand name Physiotens
Used in the following combined preparations None

QUICK REFERENCE

Drug group Antihypertensive drug (p.36)
Overdose danger rating Medium
Dependence rating Low
Prescription needed Yes
Available as generic Yes

GENERAL INFORMATION

Moxonidine is an antihypertensive drug that is related to clonidine but is more selective and may therefore have fewer side effects. It works by stimulating alpha-receptors within the central nervous system, reducing the signals that constrict the blood vessels. Moxonidine also reduces resistance to blood flow in the peripheral blood vessels. It also seems to have actions on the kidneys that result in more sodium and water being excreted.

The drug is less likely than clonidine to cause dry mouth, and, unlike clonidine, has no effect on blood fat levels or glucose. However, other side effects, such as headache and dizziness, may still occur.

INFORMATION FOR USERS

Your drug prescription is tailored for you. Do not alter dosage without checking with your doctor.

How taken/used Tablets.

Frequency and timing of doses Once daily in the morning (initially); 1–2 x daily.

Adult dosage range 200mcg daily initially; increasing after 3 weeks to 400mcg daily, if necessary; increasing again after a further 3 weeks to maximum of 600mcg daily in 2 divided doses if necessary.

Onset of effect 30–180 minutes.

Duration of action 12 hours.

Diet advice None.

Storage Keep in original container at room temperature out of the reach of children.

Missed dose Take as soon as you remember. If your next dose is due within 4 hours, take a single dose now and skip the next.

Stopping the drug Do not stop taking the drug without consulting your doctor, who will supervise a gradual reduction in dosage over a period of 2 weeks.

Exceeding the dose An occasional unintentional extra dose is unlikely to cause problems. Large overdoses may cause drowsiness and a fall in blood pressure.

POSSIBLE ADVERSE EFFECTS

Side effects often decrease in frequency and intensity during treatment. Dry mouth, headache, weakness, and fatigue are common. Rarely, dizziness, nausea, sleep disturbance, sedation, and a rash occur.

INTERACTIONS

Other antihypertensives, thymoxamine, moxisy-lyte, and muscle relaxants may increase moxonidine's blood pressure lowering effect.

Sedatives and hypnotics The effect of these drugs may be increased by moxonidine.

SPECIAL PRECAUTIONS

Be sure to tell your doctor if:
◆ You have heart, liver, or kidney problems.
◆ You have a history of angioedema.
◆ You have Raynaud's syndrome.
◆ You have epilepsy.
◆ You suffer from depression.
◆ You have Parkinson's disease.
◆ You have glaucoma.
◆ You are taking other medicines.

Pregnancy Safety not established. Discuss with your doctor.

Breast-feeding Safety in breast-feeding not established. Discuss with your doctor.

Infants and children Not recommended.

Over 60 No special problems.

Driving and hazardous work Avoid such activities until you have learned how the drug affects you; it can cause drowsiness and dizziness.

Alcohol Avoid. Alcohol may increase the sedative effects of this drug.

PROLONGED USE

No special problems.

Naftidrofuryl

Brand name Praxilene
Used in the following combined preparations None

QUICK REFERENCE

Drug group Vasodilator (p.31)
Overdose danger rating Medium
Dependence rating Low
Prescription needed Yes
Available as generic Yes

GENERAL INFORMATION

Naftidrofuryl is a vasodilator used in the treatment of peripheral circulatory disorders such as Raynaud's syndrome or intermittent claudication (cramplike pain). Most of these are caused by blocked blood vessels due to spasms or sclerosis (hardening) of the vessel walls.

Naftidrofuryl may improve symptoms and mobility in these conditions, but its influence on their progress is unknown. Lifestyle changes such as exercise and giving up smoking (and keeping warm in the case of Raynaud's) are often helpful. The drug has also been used to treat night cramps, but how it works to reduce them is not known. It has also been tried for circulatory disorders in the brain.

INFORMATION FOR USERS

Your drug prescription is tailored for you. Do not alter dosage without checking with your doctor.

How taken/used Capsules.

Frequency and timing of doses 3 x daily with meals, swallowed whole with at least one glass of water.

Adult dosage range 300–600mg daily.

Onset of effect 1 hour.

Duration of action 8 hours.

Diet advice Drink plenty of water during treatment.

Storage Keep in original container at room temperature out of the reach of children.

Missed dose Take when you remember. If your next dose is due within 2 hours, take a single dose now and skip the next.

Stopping the drug Do not stop taking the drug without consulting your doctor; symptoms may recur.

Exceeding the dose An occasional unintentional extra dose is unlikely to cause problems. Large overdoses may cause heart problems and convulsions. Notify your doctor immediately.

POSSIBLE ADVERSE EFFECTS

Naftidrofuryl is generally well tolerated. Nausea is common. Rarely, chest pain, a rash, jaundice, or convulsions may occur; consult your doctor and, if jaundice or convulsions occur, stop taking the drug.

INTERACTIONS

None known.

SPECIAL PRECAUTIONS

Be sure to tell your doctor if:
◆ You have liver or kidney problems.
◆ You are taking other medicines.

Pregnancy Safety not established. Discuss with your doctor.
Breast-feeding Safety not established. Discuss with your doctor.
Infants and children Not recommended.
Over 60 No special problems.
Driving and hazardous work No special problems.
Alcohol No special problems.

PROLONGED USE
Treatment should be reviewed after 3 months to see if the condition is improving, or if the drug should be stopped.

Naproxen

Brand names Arthrocin, Arthroxen, Naprosyn, Nycopren, Synflex, Timpron, and others
Used in the following combined preparation Napratec

QUICK REFERENCE
Drug group Non-steroidal anti-inflammatory drug (p.50) and drug for gout (p.53)
Overdose danger rating Medium
Dependence rating Low
Prescription needed Yes
Available as generic Yes

GENERAL INFORMATION
Naproxen is a non-steroidal anti-inflammatory (NSAID) used to reduce pain, stiffness, and inflammation. It relieves the symptoms of adult and juvenile rheumatoid arthritis, ankylosing spondylitis, and osteoarthritis, but it does not cure the underlying disease.

It is also used to treat acute gout attacks, and may sometimes be given for relief of migraine and pain after orthopaedic surgery, dental treatment, strains, and sprains. It is also effective for treating menstrual cramps.

Gastrointestinal side effects are fairly common, and there is increased risk of bleeding, but naproxen is safer than aspirin, and long term, it needs to be taken only twice daily.

INFORMATION FOR USERS
Your drug prescription is tailored for you. Do not alter dosage without checking with your doctor.

How taken/used Tablets.
Frequency and timing of doses Every 6–8 hours as required (general pain relief); 1–2 x daily (arthritis); every 6–8 hours (gout). All doses should be taken with food.
Adult dosage range *Mild to moderate pain, menstrual cramps* 500mg (starting dose), then 250mg every 6–8 hours as required. *Arthritis* 500–1,000mg daily. *Gout* 750mg (starting dose), then 250mg every 8 hours until attack has subsided.
Onset of effect Pain relief begins within 1 hour. Full anti-inflammatory effect may take 2 weeks.
Duration of action Up to 12 hours.
Diet advice None.
Storage Keep in original container at room temperature out of the reach of children. Protect from light.
Missed dose Take as soon as you remember. If your next dose is due within 4 hours, take a single dose now and skip the next.
Stopping the drug When taken for short-term pain relief, naproxen can be safely stopped as soon as you no longer need it. If prescribed for long-term treatment, however, you should seek medical advice before stopping the drug.
Exceeding the dose An occasional unintentional extra dose is unlikely to cause problems. If you notice unusual symptoms or a large overdose has been taken, notify your doctor.

POSSIBLE ADVERSE EFFECTS
Most adverse effects are not serious and may diminish with time. Gastrointestinal disorders are common, but a headache and the inability to concentrate may also occur. If you have ringing in the ears or swollen feet and ankles, consult your doctor. If a rash or itching occur, stop taking the drug. If you have black or bloodstained faeces, or wheezing or breathlessness, stop taking the drug and consult your doctor urgently.

INTERACTIONS
General note Naproxen interacts with a wide range of drugs to increase the risk of bleeding and/or peptic ulcers. It may also increase the blood levels of lithium, methotrexate, and digoxin to an undesirable extent.
Antihypertensive drugs and diuretics Their beneficial effects may be reduced by naproxen.

SPECIAL PRECAUTIONS

Be sure to tell your doctor if:
◆ You have long-term liver or kidney problems.
◆ You have heart problems, high blood pressure, or a bleeding disorder.
◆ You have had a peptic ulcer, oesophagitis, or acid indigestion.
◆ You are allergic to aspirin or other NSAIDs.
◆ You suffer from asthma.
◆ You are taking other medicines.

Pregnancy Not usually prescribed. When taken in the last 3 months of pregnancy, may increase the risk of adverse effects on the baby's heart and may prolong labour. Discuss with your doctor.

Breast-feeding The drug passes into the breast milk, but at normal doses adverse effects on the baby are unlikely. Discuss with your doctor.

Infants and children Prescribed only to treat juvenile arthritis. Reduced dose necessary.

Over 60 Increased likelihood of adverse effects. Reduced dose may therefore be necessary.

Driving and hazardous work Avoid such activities until you have learned how naproxen affects you because the drug may reduce your ability to concentrate.

Alcohol Keep consumption low. Alcohol may increase the risk of stomach irritation.

Surgery and general anaesthetics Naproxen may prolong bleeding. Discuss with your doctor or dentist before surgery.

PROLONGED USE

Increased risk of bleeding from peptic ulcers and in the bowel. The lowest effective dose is given for the shortest duration.

Nicorandil

Brand name Ikorel
Used in the following combined preparations None

QUICK REFERENCE

Drug group Anti-angina drug (p.35)
Overdose danger rating Medium
Dependence rating Low
Prescription needed Yes
Available as generic No

GENERAL INFORMATION

Nicorandil is the only generally available member of a group of drugs known as potassium channel openers. It is used to treat angina pectoris.

The symptoms of angina result from the failure of narrowed coronary blood vessels to deliver sufficient oxygen to the heart. Nicorandil acts by widening blood vessels by a different mechanism from other anti-angina drugs, and is notable because it widens both veins and arteries. As a result, more oxygen-carrying blood reaches the heart muscle, and the heart's work load is reduced as the resistance against which it has to pump is decreased.

Nicorandil is as effective as other drugs used to treat angina, and when used in combination with others may add to their effects.

INFORMATION FOR USERS

Your drug prescription is tailored for you. Do not alter dosage without checking with your doctor.

How taken/used Tablets.
Frequency and timing of doses 2 x daily.
Adult dosage range 10–60mg daily.
Onset of effect Within 1 hour.
Duration of action Approximately 12 hours.
Diet advice None.
Storage Keep in original container at room temperature out of the reach of children.
Missed dose Take as soon as you remember. If your next dose is due within 4 hours, take a single dose now and skip the next.
Stopping the drug Do not stop taking the drug without consulting your doctor; stopping the drug may lead to worsening of the underlying condition.
Exceeding the dose An occasional unintentional extra dose is unlikely to cause problems. Large overdoses may cause unusual dizziness and dangerously low blood pressure. Notify your doctor.

POSSIBLE ADVERSE EFFECTS

Adverse effects are usually minor, and wear off with continued treatment, but may necessitate dosage reduction in some cases. Headache, flushing, nausea, and vomiting are common. Discuss mouth ulcers, dizziness, weakness, jaundice, and facial swelling with your doctor. If a rash or palpitations occur, stop taking the drug and consult your doctor immediately.

INTERACTIONS

Antihypertensive drugs Nicorandil may increase the effects of these drugs.

Sildenafil greatly increases the effects of nicorandil on blood pressure.

Tricyclic antidepressant drugs may increase the effects of nicorandil on blood pressure, resulting in dizziness.

SPECIAL PRECAUTIONS

Be sure to tell your doctor if:
◆ You have low blood pressure.
◆ You have other heart problems.
◆ You have a history of angioedema.
◆ You are taking other medicines.

Pregnancy Safety in pregnancy not established. Discuss with your doctor.

Breast-feeding Safety not established. Discuss with your doctor.

Infants and children Not recommended.

Over 60 No special problems.

Driving and hazardous work Avoid such activities until you have learned how nicorandil affects you because the drug can cause dizziness as a result of lowered blood pressure.

Alcohol Avoid until you are accustomed to the effect of nicorandil. Alcohol may further reduce blood pressure, causing dizziness or other symptoms.

PROLONGED USE

No problems expected.

Nicotine

Brand names Nicorette, Nicotinell, NiQuitin CQ
Used in the following combined preparations None

QUICK REFERENCE

Overdose danger rating Medium
Dependence rating Low
Prescription needed No
Available as generic Yes

GENERAL INFORMATION

Smoking is a difficult habit to stop due to the addiction to nicotine and the psychological attachment to cigarettes or a pipe. Taking nicotine in a different form can help the smoker deal with the two aspects of the habit separately. Nicotine comes as chewing gum, nasal spray, sublingual tablets, skin patches, lozenges, and inhalator for the relief of withdrawal symptoms.

The patches should be applied every 24 hours to unbroken, dry, and non-hairy skin on the trunk or the upper arm. Replacement patches should be placed on a different area, and the same area of application avoided for several days. The strength of the patch is gradually reduced, and abstinence is generally achieved within three months.

The lozenges, chewing gum, nasal spray, and inhalator are used whenever the urge to smoke occurs. Gum is chewed slowly for up to 30 minutes, by which time all available nicotine has been released.

INFORMATION FOR USERS

Follow instructions on the label.

How taken/used Sublingual tablets, lozenges, chewing gum, skin patches, nasal spray, inhalator.

Frequency and timing of doses Hourly (tablets and lozenges); every 24 hours, removing the patch after 16 hours (patches); when the urge to smoke is felt (gum, inhalator, or spray).

Adult dosage range Will depend on your previous smoking habits. 7–22mg per day (patches); 1 x 2mg piece to 15 x 4mg pieces per day (gum); up to 64 x 0.5mg puffs (spray).

Onset of effect A few hours (patches); within minutes (other forms).

Duration of action Up to 24 hours (patches); 30 minutes (other forms).

Diet advice None.

Storage Keep in original container at room temperature out of the reach of children.

Missed dose Change your patch as soon as you remember, and keep the new patch on for the required amount of time before removing it.

Stopping the drug The dose of nicotine is normally reduced gradually.

Exceeding the dose Application of several nicotine patches at the same time could result in serious overdosage. Remove the patches and seek immediate medical help.

Overdosage with the tablets, lozenges, gum, or spray can occur only if tablets or lozenges are taken more often than every hour, if many pieces of gum are chewed simultaneously, or if the spray is used more than 4 times an hour. Seek immediate medical help.

POSSIBLE ADVERSE EFFECTS

Any skin reaction to patches will usually disappear in a couple of days. The chewing gum and nasal spray may cause local irritation of the throat or nose and increased salivation. The most common effects are local irritation, headache, dizziness, and nausea. Rarely, indigestion, cold and flu-like symptoms, and insomnia may occur.

INTERACTIONS

General note Stopping smoking may increase the blood levels of some drugs (such as warfarin, theophylline/aminophylline, and antipsychotics). Discuss this with your doctor or pharmacist.

Nicotine patches, chewing gum, and nasal spray should not be used with other nicotine-containing products, including cigarettes.

SPECIAL PRECAUTIONS

Be sure to consult your doctor or pharmacist before taking this drug if:
◆ You have long-term liver or kidney problems.
◆ You have diabetes mellitus.
◆ You have thyroid disease.
◆ You have circulation problems.
◆ You have heart problems.
◆ You have a peptic ulcer.
◆ You have phaeochromocytoma.
◆ You have any skin disorders.
◆ You are taking other medicines.
Pregnancy Nicotine should not be used (in any form) during pregnancy. Nicotine replacement is recommended for pregnant smokers unable to quit.
Breast-feeding Nicotine should not be used (in any form) during breast-feeding.
Infants and children Nicotine products should not be administered to children.
Over 60 No special problems.
Driving and hazardous work Usually no problems.
Alcohol No special problems.

PROLONGED USE

Nicotine replacement therapy should not normally be used for more than 3–6 months.

Nifedipine

Brand names Adalat, Adipine MR, Angiopine, Cardilate MR, Coracten, Coroday MR, Fortipine LA, Tensipine MR, and others
Used in the following combined preparations Beta-Adalat, Tenif

QUICK REFERENCE

Drug group Anti-angina drug (p.35) and antihypertensive drug (p.36)
Overdose danger rating Medium
Dependence rating Low
Prescription needed Yes
Available as generic Yes

GENERAL INFORMATION

Nifedipine belongs to a group of drugs called calcium channel blockers (see p.37), which interfere with conduction of signals in the muscles of the heart and blood vessels.

Nifedipine is given as a regular medication to help prevent angina attacks. The drug can be used safely by asthmatics, unlike some other anti-angina drugs (such as beta blockers).

Nifedipine is also widely used to reduce high blood pressure and is often helpful in improving circulation to the limbs in disorders such as Raynaud's disease.

Like other drugs of its class, nifedipine may cause the blood pressure to fall too low, and it occasionally causes disturbances of heart rhythm. In rare cases, angina worsens as a result of taking nifedipine, and another drug must be substituted.

INFORMATION FOR USERS

Your drug prescription is tailored for you. Do not alter dosage without checking with your doctor.
How taken/used Tablets, capsules, SR-tablets, SR-capsules.
Frequency and timing of doses 3 x daily; 1–2 x daily (SR-preparations).
Adult dosage range 15–90mg daily.
Onset of effect 30–60 minutes.

Duration of action 6–24 hours.

Diet advice Nifedipine should not be taken with grapefruit juice.

Storage Keep in original container at room temperature out of the reach of children. Protect from light.

Missed dose Take as soon as you remember, or when needed. If your next dose is due within 3 hours, take a single dose now and skip the next.

Stopping the drug Do not stop taking the drug without consulting your doctor; sudden withdrawal may make angina worse.

Exceeding the dose An occasional unintentional extra dose is unlikely to cause problems. Large overdoses may cause dizziness. Notify your doctor.

POSSIBLE ADVERSE EFFECTS

Nifedipine can cause a variety of minor adverse effects. Dizziness, especially on rising, may be caused by reduced blood pressure. Patients with angina may notice an increase in severity or frequency of attacks after starting nifedipine treatment. This should always be reported to your doctor. Sometimes an adjustment in dosage or a change of drug may be necessary. The more common effects are headache, dizziness, fatigue, flushing, ankle swelling, and palpitations. Frequency in passing urine, and a rash, are less common, and should be reported to your doctor if they occur. If you experience an increase in your angina, stop taking the drug and consult your doctor immediately.

INTERACTIONS

General note Nifedipine may interfere with the beneficial effects of drugs such as carbamazepine, ciclosporin, magnesium (by injection), tacrolimus, and theophylline. Consult your doctor or pharmacist.

Antihypertensive drugs Nifedipine may increase the effects of these drugs.

Phenytoin This drug may reduce the effects of nifedipine.

Digoxin Nifedipine may increase the effects and toxicity of digoxin.

Rifampicin This drug may decrease the effects of nifedipine.

Grapefruit juice may block breakdown of nifedipine, increasing its effects.

SPECIAL PRECAUTIONS

Be sure to tell your doctor if:
◆ You have liver or kidney problems.
◆ You have heart failure.
◆ You have had a recent heart attack.
◆ You have aortic stenosis.
◆ You have diabetes.
◆ You have porphyria.
◆ You are taking other medicines.

Pregnancy Not usually prescribed. The drug may cause abnormalities in the developing fetus and delay labour. Discuss with your doctor.

Breast-feeding The drug passes into the breast milk and may affect the baby. Discuss with your doctor.

Infants and children Not recommended.

Over 60 Increased likelihood of adverse effects. Reduced dose may therefore be necessary.

Driving and hazardous work Avoid such activities until you have learned how nifedipine affects you because the drug can cause dizziness as a result of lowered blood pressure.

Alcohol Avoid. Alcohol may further reduce blood pressure, causing dizziness or other symptoms.

Surgery and general anaesthetics Nifedipine may interact with some general anaesthetics causing a fall in blood pressure. Discuss this with your doctor or dentist before any surgery.

PROLONGED USE

No problems expected.

Nitrazepam

Brand names Mogadon, Remnos, Somnite
Used in the following combined preparations
None

QUICK REFERENCE

Drug group Benzodiazepine sleeping drug (p.11)
Overdose danger rating Medium
Dependence rating High
Prescription needed Yes
Available as generic Yes

GENERAL INFORMATION

Nitrazepam is a long-acting benzodiazepine used for the short-term treatment of insomnia. Benzodiazepines relieve tension and nervousness, relax muscles, and encourage sleep. When nitrazepam is taken at night, there are often effects the next day. Taken every night, its effects gradually accumulate. Therefore, short courses of 1 or 2 weeks are usually prescribed. Long-term use of the drug leads to daytime sedation, tolerance, and dependence.

Stopping treatment with nitrazepam after prolonged use results in rebound insomnia, anxiety, and a withdrawal syndrome that may include confusion, toxic psychosis, and convulsions. In these patients a tapering off period will be needed. The actual time that is needed for withdrawal can vary from weeks to many months.

It is recommended that benzodiazepines should be used to treat insomnia only when the problem is severe, disabling, or very distressing.

INFORMATION FOR USERS

Your drug prescription is tailored for you. Do not alter dosage without checking with your doctor.

How taken/used Tablets, liquid.

Frequency and timing of doses Once daily, at bedtime.

Adult dosage range 5–10mg daily.

Onset of effect 1–2 hours.

Duration of action 24 hours or more.

Diet advice None.

Storage Keep in original container at room temperature out of the reach of children.

Missed dose If you fall asleep without having taken a dose and wake some hours later, do not take the missed dose. If necessary, return to your normal dose schedule the following night.

Stopping the drug If you have taken the drug for 2 weeks or less, it can be safely stopped. If you have been taking the drug for longer, consult your doctor, who may supervise a gradual reduction in dosage. Stopping abruptly may lead to withdrawal symptoms.

Exceeding the dose An occasional unintentional extra dose is unlikely to be a cause for concern. Large overdoses may cause unusual drowsiness. Notify your doctor.

POSSIBLE ADVERSE EFFECTS

The main adverse effects of nitrazepam are related primarily to its sedative and tranquil-lizing properties. These effects include drowsiness the following day, confusion and forgetfulness, uncoordinated walking, dizziness, and double vision. Rarely, you may experience a headache and vertigo. If you experience mood changes or restlessness, consult your doctor.

INTERACTIONS

Sedatives All drugs that have a sedative effect on the central nervous system are likely to increase the sedative properties of nitrazepam. Such drugs include other sleeping drugs, anti-anxiety drugs, antihistamines, opioid analgesics, antidepressants, and antipsychotics.

Rifampicin This drug reduces the effect of nitrazepam.

Antiepileptic drugs The side effects and toxicity of these drugs may be increased by nitrazepam.

SPECIAL PRECAUTIONS

Be sure to tell your doctor if:
♦ You have severe respiratory disease.
♦ You have kidney or liver problems.
♦ You have myasthenia gravis.
♦ You suffer from sleep apnoea.
♦ You have had problems with alcohol or drug abuse.
♦ You are taking other medicines.

Pregnancy Safety not established. The drug is known to affect the baby in the womb. The baby may be born with dependence and have withdrawal symptoms. Discuss with your doctor.

Breast-feeding Avoid. Nitrazepam passes into the breast milk.

Infants and children Not recommended

Over 60 The elderly are more likely to suffer adverse effects. Reduced dose necessary.

Driving and hazardous work Do not drive. Nitrazepam's effects are still present during the day after taking a dose. The drug reduces alertness, slows reactions, impairs concentration, and causes drowsiness.

Alcohol Avoid. Alcohol will add to the sedative effects.

PROLONGED USE

Not recommended. Produces tolerance and dependence.

Norethisterone

Brand names Micronor, Noriday, Noristerat, Primolut N, Utovlan
Used in the following combined preparations Brevinor, Climagest, Loestrin, Norinyl, Synphase, TriNovum, and others

QUICK REFERENCE

Drug group Female sex hormone (p.88)
Overdose danger rating Low
Dependence rating Low
Prescription needed Yes
Available as generic Yes

GENERAL INFORMATION

Norethisterone is a progestogen, a synthetic hormone similar to the natural female sex hormone progesterone. It has a wide variety of uses including the postponement of menstruation and the treatment of menstrual disorders such as endometriosis (see p.105). When used for these disorders, it is taken only on certain days during the menstrual cycle. The drug is also prescribed as hormone replacement therapy (HRT), but this is usually only advised for short-term use around the menopause, and in the treatment of certain breast cancers.

One of norethisterone's major uses is as an oral contraceptive. It may be used on its own or with an oestrogen. It is also available, in special circumstances, in an injectable contraceptive preparation.

Adverse effects are rare, but oral contraceptives may cause "breakthrough" bleeding (see p.107).

INFORMATION FOR USERS

Your drug prescription is tailored for you. Do not alter dosage without checking with your doctor.
How taken/used Tablets, injection, skin patch.
Frequency and timing of doses 1–3 x daily (tablets); once every 8 weeks (injection); 2 x weekly (skin patch).
Adult dosage range 10–15mg daily (menstrual disorders); 15mg daily (postponement of menstruation); 350mcg daily (progestogen-only contraceptives); 700mcg–1mg daily (HRT); 30–60mg daily (cancer).

Onset of effect Within a few hours.
Duration of action 24 hours.
Diet advice None.
Storage Keep in original container at room temperature out of the reach of children. Protect from light.
Missed dose Take as soon as you remember. If you are taking the drug for contraception, see What to do if you miss a pill (p.109).
Stopping the drug The drug can be safely stopped as soon as contraceptive protection is no longer required. If it is prescribed for an underlying disorder, do not stop taking the drug without consulting your doctor. When the drug is used to treat menstrual disorders, a normal period should occur 2 to 3 days after it is stopped.
Exceeding the dose An occasional unintentional extra dose is unlikely to be a cause for concern. But if you notice any unusual symptoms, or if a large overdose has been taken, notify your doctor.

POSSIBLE ADVERSE EFFECTS

Adverse effects are rarely troublesome and are generally typical of drugs of this type. Prolonged treatment may cause jaundice due to liver damage. Breakthrough bleeding is common and should be discussed with your doctor. Rarely, swollen feet and ankles or weight gain may occur. Depression, headache, and jaundice are also rare and should be discussed with your doctor; stop taking the drug if jaundice occurs. If pain or tightness in the chest or visual or hearing disturbances occur, stop taking the drug and consult your doctor urgently.

INTERACTIONS

General note Norethisterone may interfere with the beneficial effects of many drugs, including oral anticoagulants, anticonvulsants, antihypertensives, and antidiabetic drugs. Many other drugs may reduce the contraceptive effect of norethisterone-containing pills. These include anticonvulsants, antituberculous drugs, certain antivirals, and antibiotics. Be sure to inform your doctor that you are taking norethisterone before taking additional prescribed medication.
Ciclosporin Levels of ciclosporin may be raised by norethisterone.

SPECIAL PRECAUTIONS

Be sure to tell your doctor if:
◆ You have liver or kidney problems.
◆ You have diabetes.
◆ You have had epileptic fits.
◆ You suffer from migraine.
◆ You have acute porphyria.
◆ You have heart or circulatory problems.
◆ You are taking other medicines.

Pregnancy Not usually prescribed. May cause defects in the baby. Discuss with your doctor.

Breast-feeding The drug passes into the breast milk, but at normal doses adverse effects on the baby are unlikely. Discuss with your doctor.

Infants and children Not prescribed.

Over 60 Not usually prescribed.

Driving and hazardous work No special problems.

Alcohol No special problems.

Surgery and general anaesthetics Inform your doctor or dentist that you are taking norethisterone. He or she will tell you when to stop taking it prior to any surgery.

PROLONGED USE

No special problems but, as part of HRT, norethisterone is usually advised only for short-term use around the menopause; it is not normally recommended long term or for treatment of osteoporosis. Prolonged use may in rare cases cause liver damage.

Monitoring Blood tests to check liver function may be carried out.

Nystatin

Brand names Nystamont, Nystan
Used in the following combined preparations
Dermovate-NN, Nystaform, Timodine, Tinaderm-M, and others

QUICK REFERENCE

Drug group Antifungal drug (p.76)
Overdose danger rating Low
Dependence rating Low
Prescription needed Yes
Available as generic Yes

GENERAL INFORMATION

Nystatin is an antifungal drug named after the New York State Institute of Health, where it was developed in the early 1950s. The drug has been used effectively against candidiasis (thrush), an infection caused by the *Candida* yeast. Available in a variety of dosage forms, it is used to treat infections of the skin, mouth, throat, intestinal tract, oesophagus, and vagina. As the drug is poorly absorbed into the bloodstream from the digestive tract, it is of little use against systemic infections. It is not given by injection.

Nystatin rarely causes adverse effects and can be used during pregnancy to treat vaginal candidiasis.

INFORMATION FOR USERS

Your drug prescription is tailored for you. Do not alter dosage without checking with your doctor.

How taken/used Tablets, pastilles, liquid, pessaries, cream, ointment.

Frequency and timing of doses *Mouth or throat infections* 4 x daily. Take after food and hold in the mouth for several minutes before swallowing (liquid); do not eat or drink 5 minutes before or for 1 hour after (pastilles). *Intestinal infections* 4 x daily. *Skin infections* 2–4 x daily. *Vaginal infections* Once daily for 2 weeks.

Adult dosage range 2–4 million units daily (by mouth); 100,000–200,000 units at night (pessaries); 1–2 applicatorfuls (vaginal cream); as directed (skin preparations).

Onset of effect Full beneficial effect may not be felt for 7–14 days.

Duration of action Up to 6 hours.

Diet advice None.

Storage Keep in original container at room temperature out of the reach of children. Protect from light.

Missed dose Take as soon as you remember. Take your next dose as usual.

Stopping the drug Take the full course, and continue with the treatment for at least 48 hours after symptoms have disappeared. Even if the affected area seems to be cured, the original infection may still be present, and symptoms may recur if treatment is stopped too soon.

Exceeding the dose An occasional unintentional extra dose is unlikely to be a cause for concern. But if you notice any unusual symptoms, or if a large overdose has been taken, notify your doctor.

POSSIBLE ADVERSE EFFECTS

Adverse effects are uncommon with nystatin and are usually mild and transient. Nausea and vomiting may occur when high doses of the drug are taken by mouth. Diarrhoea and a rash are other rare side effects of this drug; consult your doctor if you develop a rash.

INTERACTIONS

None.

SPECIAL PRECAUTIONS

Be sure to tell your doctor if:
◆ You are taking other medicines.
Pregnancy No evidence of risk to developing fetus.
Breast-feeding No evidence of risk.
Infants and children Reduced dose necessary.
Over 60 No special problems.
Driving and hazardous work No known problems.
Alcohol No known problems.

PROLONGED USE

No problems expected. Usually given as a course of treatment until infection is cured.

Olanzapine

Brand names Zyprexa, Zyprexa Velotab
Used in the following combined preparations None

QUICK REFERENCE

Drug group Antipsychotic drug (p.15)
Overdose danger rating Medium
Dependence rating Low
Prescription needed Yes
Available as generic No

GENERAL INFORMATION

Olanzapine is an atypical antipsychotic drug prescribed for the treatment of schizophrenia and mania and for long-term treatment of bipolar disorder. It works by blocking several different receptors, including dopamine, histamine, and serotonin receptors.

In schizophrenia, the drug can be used to treat both "positive" symptoms (delusions, hallucinations, and thought disorders) and "negative" symptoms (blunted affect, emotional and social withdrawal). In mania, olanzapine can be used alone or in combination with other drugs.

Olanzapine injection is used short term for its calming effects in agitation associated with schizophrenia or mania.

INFORMATION FOR USERS

Your drug prescription is tailored for you. Do not alter dosage without checking with your doctor.
How taken/used Tablets, dispersible tablets, injection.
Frequency and timing of doses Once daily (tablets); 1–2 x daily (injection).
Adult dosage range *Schizophrenia* 10mg (starting dose). *Mania* 15mg if used alone or 10mg if used in combination with other drugs (starting dose). For all conditions, the dose can be adjusted between 5mg and 20mg daily (tablets) and 5mg and 10mg daily (injection).
Onset of effect 4–8 hours (tablets); 15–45 minutes (injection).
Duration of action 30–38 hours.
Diet advice None.
Storage Keep in original container at room temperature out of the reach of children. Protect from light.
Missed dose Take as soon as you remember. If your next dose is due within 8 hours take a single dose now and skip the next.
Stopping the drug Do not stop taking the drug without consulting your doctor; symptoms may recur.
Exceeding the dose An occasional unintentional extra dose is unlikely to cause problems. Large overdoses may cause unusual drowsiness, depressed breathing, and low blood pressure. Notify your doctor.

POSSIBLE ADVERSE EFFECTS

Unusual drowsiness and increased appetite and weight gain are common. Dizziness and fainting are also common but should be discussed with your doctor. Rarely, you may experience frequency in passing urine, which should also be discussed with your doctor.

INTERACTIONS

Sedatives All drugs that have a sedative effect may increase olanzapine's sedative effects.

Carbamazepine and smoking These can reduce the effects of olanzapine.

Diabetic medication Olanzapine can affect diabetic control. Dosage of diabetic medications may need to be adjusted.

SPECIAL PRECAUTIONS

Be sure to tell your doctor if:
◆ You have kidney or liver problems.
◆ You have diabetes.
◆ You have glaucoma.
◆ You have epilepsy.
◆ You have had, or are at risk of having, a stroke.
◆ You are taking other medicines.

Pregnancy Safety not established. Discuss with your doctor.

Breast-feeding Safety not established. Discuss with your doctor.

Infants and children Not recommended.

Over 60 Reduced dose may be necessary.

Driving and hazardous work Avoid such activities until you have learned how the drug affects you; it can cause unusual drowsiness.

Alcohol Avoid. Alcohol increases the sedative effects of this drug.

PROLONGED USE

Prolonged use of olanzapine may, rarely, cause tardive dyskinesia, in which there are involuntary movements of the tongue and face.

Omeprazole

Brand names Losec, Mepradec
Used in the following combined preparations None

QUICK REFERENCE

Drug group Anti-ulcer drug (p.43)
Overdose danger rating Low
Dependence rating Low
Prescription needed Yes
Available as generic Yes

GENERAL INFORMATION

Omeprazole is used to treat stomach and duodenal ulcers as well as reflux oesophagitis, a condition in which stomach acid rises into the oesophagus. It reduces (by about 70 per cent) the amount of acid the stomach produces, and works in a different way from other anti-ulcer drugs that reduce acid secretion. It is also used for acid reflux disease and Zollinger–Ellison syndrome.

Treatment for an ulcer is usually given for 4–8 weeks, depending on where the ulcer is situated. Omeprazole may also be given with antibiotics to eradicate the *Helicobacter pylori* bacteria that cause many gastric ulcers. Reflux oesophagitis may be treated for 4–12 weeks.

Omeprazole causes few serious side effects. However, because it may affect the actions of enzymes in the liver, where many drugs are broken down, it may increase the effects of ciclosporin, warfarin, and phenytoin, and these drugs require more careful monitoring when used with omeprazole. As with other anti-ulcer drugs, it may mask signs of stomach cancer, so it is used only when the possibility of this disease has been ruled out.

INFORMATION FOR USERS

Your drug prescription is tailored for you. Do not alter dosage without checking with your doctor.

How taken/used Tablets, capsules, injection, intravenous infusion.

Frequency and timing of doses 1–2 x daily; (2 x daily for doses above 80mg).

Adult dosage range 10–40mg daily and sometimes up to 120mg daily.

Onset of effect 2–5 hours.

Duration of action 24 hours.

Diet advice None, but spicy foods and alcohol may exacerbate the underlying condition.

Storage Keep in original container at room temperature out of the reach of children. The drug is very sensitive to moisture. It must not be transferred to another container and must be used within 3 months of opening.

Missed dose Take as soon as you remember. If your next dose is due within 8 hours, take a single dose now and skip the next.

Stopping the drug Do not stop the drug without consulting your doctor; symptoms may recur.

Exceeding the dose An occasional unintentional extra dose is unlikely to be a cause for concern. But if you notice any unusual symptoms, or if a large overdose has been taken, notify your doctor.

POSSIBLE ADVERSE EFFECTS

Adverse effects such as headache and diar-rhoea are common but are usually mild and often diminish with continued use of the drug. Rarely, nausea and constipation may occur. If a rash occurs, stop taking the drug and consult your doctor.

INTERACTIONS

Warfarin The effects of warfarin may be increased by omeprazole.

Phenytoin The effects of phenytoin may be increased by omeprazole.

Ciclosporin Blood levels of ciclosporin are raised by omeprazole.

Atazanavir The effects of this drug are reduced by omeprazole.

SPECIAL PRECAUTIONS

Be sure to tell your doctor if:
◆ You have a long-term liver problem.
◆ You are taking other medicines.

Pregnancy No evidence of risk, but discuss with your doctor.

Breast-feeding The drug may pass into the breast milk. Safety in breast-feeding not established. Discuss with your doctor.

Infants and children Not usually recommended under 1 year. Reduced dose necessary in older children.

Over 60 No special problems.

Driving and hazardous work No special problems.

Alcohol Avoid. Alcohol irritates the stomach.

PROLONGED USE

No problems expected.

Ondansetron

Brand name Zofran
Used in the following combined preparations None

QUICK REFERENCE

Drug group Anti-emetic (p.21)
Overdose danger rating Low
Dependence rating Low
Prescription needed Yes (except for low-dose oral forms)
Available as generic No

GENERAL INFORMATION

Ondansetron, an anti-emetic, is used especially for treating the nausea and vomiting associated with radiotherapy and anticancer drugs such as cisplatin. It may also be prescribed for the nausea and vomiting that occur after surgery.

The dose given and the frequency will depend on which anti cancer drug you are having and its dose. In most instances, you will receive a dose of ondansetron, either by mouth or injection, before infusion of the anti cancer agent, then tablets for up to 5 days after treatment has finished. The drug is less effective against the delayed nausea and vomiting that occur several days after chemotherapy than against symptoms that occur soon after anticancer treatment. For nausea and vomiting after surgery, one dose is usually given before the surgery, and two doses after.

To enhance the effectiveness of ondansetron, it is usually taken with other drugs such as dexamethasone. Serious adverse effects are unlikely to occur.

INFORMATION FOR USERS

Your drug prescription is tailored for you. Do not alter dosage without checking with your doctor.

How taken/used Tablets, liquid, injection, suppositories.

Frequency and timing of doses Normally 2 x daily but the frequency will depend on the reason for which the drug is being used.

Adult dosage range 4–32mg daily depending on the reason for which it is being used.

Onset of effect Within 1 hour.

Duration of action Approximately 12 hours.

Diet advice None.

Storage Keep in original container at room temperature out of the reach of children. Protect from light.

Missed dose Take as soon as you remember. If your next dose is due within 2 hours, take a single dose now and skip the next.

Stopping the drug Can be safely stopped as soon as you no longer need it.

Exceeding the dose An occasional unintentional extra dose is unlikely to be a cause for concern. But if you notice any unusual symptoms, or if a large overdose has been taken, notify your doctor.

POSSIBLE ADVERSE EFFECTS

Ondansetron is considered safe, is generally well tolerated, and does not cause sedation and movement disorders. Constipation and headache are common. Rarely, a warm feeling in the head or stomach, palpitations, fits, and muscle stiffness may occur; consult your doctor. If wheezing, chest pain, dizziness, rash, or swollen eyelids, face, or lips occur, stop the drug and consult your doctor urgently.

INTERACTIONS
None.

SPECIAL PRECAUTIONS

Be sure to tell your doctor if:
◆ You have a long-term liver problem.
◆ You have bowel problems.
◆ You are taking other medicines.
Pregnancy Safety in pregnancy not established. Discuss with your doctor.
Breast-feeding The drug may pass into the breast milk. Discuss with your doctor.
Infants and children Reduced dose necessary.
Over 60 No special problems.
Driving and hazardous work No problems expected.
Alcohol No known problems.

PROLONGED USE
Not generally prescribed long term.

Orlistat

Brand name Xenical
Used in the following combined preparations None

QUICK REFERENCE
Overdose danger rating Low
Dependence rating Low
Prescription needed Yes
Available as generic No

GENERAL INFORMATION

Orlistat blocks the action of stomach and pancreatic enzymes (lipases) that digest fats: the fats are not absorbed and are passed out in faeces. As a result, the body must burn stored fat for energy, which should gradually reduce the fat stores and produce weight loss. The effectiveness of orlistat varies from person to person.

Because of the way orlistat works, the faeces become oily, and this can cause flatulence. Part of the drug's effect may be due to people reducing fat intake to avoid these side effects.

As fat absorption is greatly reduced, there is a danger of fat soluble vitamins being lost to the body, and vitamin supplements may be prescribed to compensate. The vitamins should be taken at a different time from the orlistat; bedtime might be best, or at least 2 hours apart from any orlistat dose.

INFORMATION FOR USERS

Your drug prescription is tailored for you. Do not alter dosage without checking with your doctor.
How taken/used Capsules.
Frequency and timing of doses Just before, during, or up to 1 hour after each main meal (up to 3 x daily). If a meal is omitted or contains no fat, do not take the dose of orlistat.
Adult dosage range 120–360mg daily.
Onset of effect 30 minutes; excretion of excess faecal fat begins about 24–48 hours after the first dose.
Duration of action Orlistat is not absorbed from the gut, and potentially continues to work as it passes through the intestines. If you stop taking the drug, faecal fat returns to normal in 48–72 hours.
Diet advice Eat a nutritionally balanced diet that does not contain quite enough calories, and that provides about 30 per cent of the calories as fat. Eat lots of fruit and vegetables. The intake of fat, carbohydrate, and protein should be distributed over the 3 main meals.
Storage Keep in original container at room temperature out of the reach of children.
Missed dose No cause for concern. Take the next dose with the next meal.
Stopping the drug The drug can be safely stopped as soon as it is no longer needed, but notify your doctor.
Exceeding the dose An occasional unintentional extra dose is unlikely to cause be a cause for concern. But if you notice any unusual symptoms, or if a large overdose has been taken, notify your doctor

POSSIBLE ADVERSE EFFECTS

Most side effects depend on how much fat is eaten and the dose of orlistat. Liquid and oily stools, faecal urgency, flatulence, abdominal or rectal pain, headache, menstrual irregularities, anxiety, fatigue, nausea, infections (such as influenza), and hypoglycaemia are common.

INTERACTIONS

General note Orlistat may lower the effect of ciclosporin, acarbose, oral anticoagulants, and amiodarone.

Lipid-lowering drugs Orlistat increases blood levels and toxicity of pravastatin.

SPECIAL PRECAUTIONS

Be sure to tell your doctor if:
◆ You have diabetes.
◆ You have chronic malabsorption syndrome.
◆ You have gallbladder or liver problems.
◆ You are taking lipid-lowering drugs.
◆ You are taking other medicines.

Pregnancy Safety not established. Discuss with your doctor.

Breast-feeding Safety not established. Discuss with your doctor.

Infants and children Not prescribed.

Over 60 No special problems.

Driving and hazardous work No special problems.

Alcohol No special problems.

PROLONGED USE

Treatment should be stopped after 12 weeks if you have not lost 5 per cent of your body weight since the start of treatment. It should also be stopped if you have lost less than 10 per cent of your body weight over the first 6 months. If you have, the drug may be continued for a maximum of 2 years until your target weight is approached. When treatment is stopped, there may be gradual weight gain.

Orphenadrine

Brand names Biorphen, Disipal
Used in the following combined preparations None

QUICK REFERENCE

Drug group Drug for parkinsonism (p.54)
Overdose danger rating High
Dependence rating Low
Prescription needed Yes
Available as generic Yes

GENERAL INFORMATION

Orphenadrine is an anticholinergic drug used to treat all forms of Parkinson's disease. It is less effective than other drugs used in the treatment of this disorder, but is often preferred because its adverse effects tend to be less severe. Orphenadrine is particularly valuable for relieving the muscle rigidity that often occurs with Parkinson's disease; it is less helpful for improving the slowing of movement that also commonly occurs. The effects of the drug may become less noticeable after it has been taken for a long time.

Orphenadrine also possesses muscle-relaxant properties and is occasionally used to treat muscle pain and restless leg syndrome.

INFORMATION FOR USERS

Your drug prescription is tailored for you. Do not alter dosage without checking with your doctor.

How taken/used Tablets, liquid.

Frequency and timing of doses 2–3 x daily.

Adult dosage range 150–400mg daily.

Onset of effect Within 60 minutes.

Duration of action 8–12 hours.

Diet advice None.

Storage Keep in original container at room temperature out of the reach of children. Protect from light.

Missed dose Take as soon as you remember. If your next dose is due within 2 hours, take a single dose now and skip the next.

Stopping the drug Do not stop taking the drug without consulting your doctor; symptoms may recur.

OVERDOSE ACTION

Seek immediate medical advice in all cases. Take emergency action if palpitations, fits, or loss of consciousness occur.

POSSIBLE ADVERSE EFFECTS

Adverse effects are similar to those of other anticholinergic drugs; common symptoms such as a dry mouth and blurred vision can often be overcome by dosage reduction. Difficulty in passing urine, constipation, and dizziness are also common. Rarely, confusion and agitation occur and should be discussed with your doctor. If palpitations occur, stop taking the drug and consult your doctor promptly.

INTERACTIONS

Anticholinergic drugs The anticholinergic effects of orphenadrine are likely to be increased by these drugs.

SPECIAL PRECAUTIONS

Be sure to tell your doctor if:
◆ You have long-term liver or kidney problems.
◆ You have heart problems.
◆ You have glaucoma.
◆ You have difficulty in passing urine and have an enlarged prostate.
◆ You have myasthenia gravis.
◆ You are taking other medicines.

Pregnancy Safety in pregnancy not established. Discuss with your doctor.

Breast-feeding Safety in breast feeding not established. Discuss with your doctor.

Infants and children Not usually prescribed.

Over 60 Increased likelihood of adverse effects. Reduced dose may therefore be necessary.

Driving and hazardous work Avoid such activities until you have learned how orphenadrine affects you because the drug can cause dizziness, lightheadedness, and blurred vision.

Alcohol Avoid. Alcohol can worsen some of the adverse effects of orphenadrine.

PROLONGED USE

No problems expected. Effectiveness in treating Parkinson's disease may diminish with time.

Oseltamivir

Brand name Tamiflu
Used in the following combined preparations None

QUICK REFERENCE

Drug group Antiviral drug (p.69)
Overdose danger rating Low
Dependence rating Low
Prescription needed Yes
Available as generic No

GENERAL INFORMATION

Oseltamivir is a type of antiviral drug that is used to prevent or treat influenza (flu), a virus that infects, and multiplies within, the lungs. Oseltamivir works by attacking the virus, preventing it from multiplying and spreading within the body, thereby relieving or preventing the symptoms of flu. These symptoms include the sudden onset of fever, sweating and shivering, cough, runny or stuffy nose, headache, aching muscles, and extreme fatigue. The drug should be taken within 48 hours of the onset of symptoms.

Oseltamivir is not a substitute for flu vaccination, but, because it does not alter the vaccine's effectiveness, it can be taken even if you have been vaccinated.

INFORMATION FOR USERS

Your drug prescription is tailored for you. Do not alter dosage without checking with your doctor.

How taken/used Tablets, liquid (suspension).

Frequency and timing of doses Once daily (prevention); 2 x daily (treatment).

Dosage range *Adults and adolescents over 13 years* 75mg daily (prevention); 150mg daily (treatment).
Children up to 12 years 60–120mg, according to bodyweight (treatment).

Onset of effect Within 24 hours.

Duration of action 12–24 hours.

Diet advice None.

Storage Keep in original container at room temperature out of the reach of children.

Missed dose Take as soon as you remember. If your next dose is due within 2 hours, take a single dose now and skip the next.

Stopping the drug Do not stop taking the drug without consulting your doctor; symptoms may recur.

Exceeding the dose An occasional unintentional extra dose is unlikely to cause problems. However, if you notice any unusual symptoms, or if a large overdose has been taken, notify your doctor.

POSSIBLE ADVERSE EFFECTS

The most common side effects usually occur following the first dose and generally subside as treatment continues. Taking oseltamivir with food helps to reduce these effects, but you should consult your doctor if they persist. Nausea, vomiting, and abdominal pain are common. If a rash occurs, stop taking the drug and consult your doctor.

INTERACTIONS
None known.

SPECIAL PRECAUTIONS
Be sure to tell your doctor if:
◆ You have kidney problems.
◆ You have ever had an allergic reaction to oseltamivir.
◆ You are taking other medicines.
Pregnancy Safety in pregnancy not established. Discuss with your doctor.
Breast-feeding Safety in breast-feeding not established. Discuss with your doctor.
Infants and children No problems expected; not usually given under 1 year.
Over 60 No special problems.
Driving and hazardous work No known problems.
Alcohol No known problems.

PROLONGED USE
No problems expected. The drug is not usually prescribed for longer than 5 days (children), 7 days (adults), or 6 weeks (adults, during an epidemic).

Oxybutynin

Brand names Contimin, Cystrin, Kentera, Lyrinel XL
Used in the following combined preparations None

QUICK REFERENCE
Drug group Drug for urinary disorders (p.112)
Overdose danger rating Medium
Dependence rating Low
Prescription needed Yes
Available as generic Yes

GENERAL INFORMATION
Oxybutynin is an anticholinergic and antispasmodic drug used, in adults, to treat urinary incontinence and, in children, frequency and bedwetting. It works by reducing bladder contraction, allowing the bladder to hold more urine. The drug stops bladder spasms and delays the desire to empty the bladder. It also has some local anaesthetic effect.

The drug's usefulness is limited to some extent by its side effects, especially in children and the elderly. It can aggravate conditions such as an enlarged prostate or coronary heart disease in the elderly. Children are more susceptible to effects on the central nervous system (CNS), such as restlessness, disorientation, hallucinations, and convulsions.

INFORMATION FOR USERS
Your drug prescription is tailored for you. Do not alter dosage without checking with your doctor.
How taken/used Tablets, liquid, patches.
Frequency and timing of doses 2–4 x daily (tablets, liquid); 1–2 x weekly (patch).
Adult dosage range 10–20mg daily (tablets, liquid); 36mg twice weekly (patch).
Onset of effect 1 hour (tablets, liquid); 24–48 hours (patch).
Duration of action Up to 10 hours (tablets, liquid); 96 hours (patch).
Diet advice None.
Storage Keep in original container at room temperature out of the reach of children. Protect liquid from light.
Missed dose Take as soon as you remember. If your next dose is due within 2 hours, take a single dose now and skip the next (tablets, liquid). Apply when you remember (patches).
Stopping the drug Do not stop taking the drug without consulting your doctor; symptoms may recur.
Exceeding the dose An occasional unintentional extra dose is unlikely to cause problems. Larger overdoses may cause restlessness or psychotic behaviour, fall in blood pressure, breathing difficulties, paralysis, or coma. Notify your doctor immediately.

POSSIBLE ADVERSE EFFECTS
Dosage adjustment is necessary in children and the elderly to minimize adverse effects. The drug can also precipitate glaucoma. Dry mouth, constipation, nausea, facial flushing, and difficulty in passing urine are common. Rarely, blurred vision, eye pain, headache, and confusion may occur. Discuss dry skin with your doctor. If you develop a rash, stop taking the drug and consult your doctor urgently.

INTERACTIONS
General note If oxybutynin is taken with other drugs with anticholinergic effects, the risk of anticholinergic side effects is increased.

SPECIAL PRECAUTIONS

Be sure to tell your doctor if:

◆ You have liver or kidney problems.
◆ You have hyperthyroidism.
◆ You have heart problems.
◆ You have an enlarged prostate.
◆ You have hiatus hernia.
◆ You have ulcerative colitis.
◆ You have glaucoma.
◆ You have myasthenia gravis.
◆ You are taking other medicines.

Pregnancy Safety not established. May harm the unborn baby. Discuss with your doctor.

Breast-feeding Safety not established. Discuss with your doctor.

Infants and children Not recommended under 5 years. Reduced dose necessary in older children.

Over 60 Reduced dose necessary.

Driving and hazardous work Avoid such activities until you have learned how oxybutynin affects you because the drug can cause drowsiness, disorientation, and blurred vision.

Alcohol Avoid. Alcohol increases the sedative effects of oxybutynin.

PROLONGED USE

No special problems. The need for continued treatment may be reviewed after 6 months.

Monitoring Periodic eye tests for glaucoma may be performed.

Paracetamol

Brand names Alvedon, Calpol, Disprol, Hedex, Panadol, Panaleve, and many others

Used in the following combined preparations
Anadin Extra, Migraleve, Panadeine, Paradote, Tylex, and others

QUICK REFERENCE

Drug group Non-opioid analgesic (p.9)
Overdose danger rating High
Dependence rating Low
Prescription needed No
Available as generic Yes

GENERAL INFORMATION

Although paracetamol has been known since the early 1900s, it was not widely used as an analgesic until the 1950s. One of a group of drugs known as the non-opioid analgesics, it is kept in the home to relieve occasional bouts of mild pain and to reduce fever. It is suitable for children as well as adults.

One of the primary advantages of paracetamol is that it does not cause stomach upset or bleeding problems. This makes it a particularly useful alternative for people who suffer from peptic ulcers or those who cannot tolerate aspirin. The drug is also safe for occasional use by those who are being treated with anticoagulants.

Paracetamol is safe when used as directed, but is dangerous in overdose; it is capable of causing serious liver and kidney damage. Large doses may also be toxic if you regularly drink even moderate amounts of alcohol.

INFORMATION FOR USERS

Follow instructions on the label. Call your doctor if symptoms worsen.

How taken/used Tablets, capsules, liquid, suppositories.

Frequency and timing of doses Every 4–6 hours as necessary, but not more than 4 doses per 24 hours in children.

Dosage range *Adults* 500mg–1g per dose up to 4g daily. *Children* 60mg (2 months, for fever following immunization; 2 doses only); 60–120mg per dose (3 months–1 year); 120–250mg per dose (1–5 years); 250–500mg per dose (6–12 years).

Onset of effect Within 15–60 minutes.

Duration of action Up to 6 hours.

Diet advice None.

Storage Keep in original container at room temperature out of the reach of children.

Missed dose Take as soon as you remember if required to relieve pain. Otherwise do not take the missed dose, and take a further dose only when you are in pain.

Stopping the drug Can be safely stopped as soon as you no longer need it.

OVERDOSE ACTION

Seek immediate medical advice in all cases. Take emergency action if nausea, vomiting, or stomach pain occur.

POSSIBLE ADVERSE EFFECTS

Paracetamol has rarely been found to produce side effects when taken as recommended, although nausea may occur. If you develop a rash, stop taking the drug and consult your doctor promptly.

INTERACTIONS

Anticoagulants such as warfarin may need dosage adjustment if paracetamol is taken regularly in high doses.

Colestyramine reduces the absorption of paracetamol and may reduce its effectiveness.

SPECIAL PRECAUTIONS

Be sure to consult your doctor or pharmacist before using this drug if:
◆ You have long-term liver or kidney problems.
◆ You are taking other medicines.

Pregnancy No evidence of risk with occasional use.

Breast-feeding No evidence of risk.

Infants and children Usually only given to infants under 3 months on doctor's advice except for relief of fever following vaccination at 2 months. Reduced dose necessary up to 12 years.

Over 60 No special problems.

Driving and hazardous work No special problems.

Alcohol Prolonged heavy intake of alcohol in combination with excess paracetamol may substantially increase the risk of injury to the liver.

PROLONGED USE

You should not normally take this drug for longer than 48 hours except on the advice of your doctor. However, there is no evidence of harm from long-term use.

Paroxetine

Brand name Seroxat
Used in the following combined preparations None

QUICK REFERENCE

Drug group Antidepressant drug (p.14)
Overdose danger rating Low
Dependence rating Low
Prescription needed Yes
Available as generic Yes

GENERAL INFORMATION

Paroxetine is one of a group of antidepressants known as selective serotonin re-uptake inhibitors (SSRIs). It is used in the treatment of depression, and helps to control the anxiety that often accompanies it. It is also used to treat generalized anxiety disorder, social phobia, panic disorder, obsessive-compulsive disorders, and post-traumatic stress disorder. Like other SSRIs, paroxetine is sometimes given to treat severe premenstrual syndrome.

It is less likely than the older tricyclic antidepressants to cause anticholinergic side effects such as dry mouth, blurred vision, and difficulty in passing urine, and is much less dangerous in overdose.

The most common adverse effects include nausea, diarrhoea, insomnia, and sexual problems, such as lack of orgasm and ejaculation difficulties. Withdrawal symptoms can occur if the drug is not stopped gradually over at least 4 weeks.

INFORMATION FOR USERS

Your drug prescription is tailored for you. Do not alter dosage without checking with your doctor.

How taken/used Tablets, liquid.

Frequency and timing of doses Once daily, in the morning.

Dosage range 10–60mg daily.

Onset of effect Onset of therapeutic response, usually within 14 days; full antidepressant effect may not be felt for 6 weeks (or longer for anxiety disorders).

Duration of action Antidepressant effect may last for some time following prolonged use.

Diet advice None.

Storage Keep in original container at room temperature out of the reach of children.

Missed dose Take as soon as you remember.

Stopping the drug Do not stop the drug without consulting your doctor. Stopping abruptly can cause withdrawal symptoms.

Exceeding the dose An occasional unintentional extra dose is unlikely to be a cause for concern. Large doses may cause unusual drowsiness. Notify your doctor immediately.

POSSIBLE ADVERSE EFFECTS

Common adverse effects include nausea, diarrhoea, drowsiness, dizziness, sweating, tremor, weakness, insomnia, and sexual dysfunction in both sexes (lack of orgasm, male ejaculation problems). Rarely, nervousness, anxiety, and agitation occur. If there are suicidal thoughts (or suicide attempts), stop taking the drug and seek urgent medical help.

INTERACTIONS

General note Any drug that affects the breakdown of others in the liver may alter blood levels of paroxetine or vice versa.

Anticoagulants Paroxetine may increase the effects of these drugs.

Antipsychotics Paroxetine may increase levels and effects of some antipsychotics.

Monoamine oxidase inhibitors (MAOIs) Paroxetine should not be taken during or within 14 days of MAOI treatment because serious reactions may occur.

Tricyclic antidepressants Paroxetine may increase the toxicity of these drugs.

SPECIAL PRECAUTIONS

Be sure to tell your doctor if:
◆ You have long-term liver or kidney problems.
◆ You have a history of mania.
◆ You have a history or a family history of epilepsy.
◆ You have had problems withdrawing from other antidepressants.
◆ You are taking other medicines.

Pregnancy Safety in pregnancy not established. Discuss with your doctor.

Breast-feeding The drug passes into the breast milk. Discuss with your doctor.

Infants and children Not recommended under 18 years.

Over 60 Increased likelihood of adverse effects. Reduced dose may be necessary.

Driving and hazardous work Avoid such activities until you have learned how paroxetine affects you; the drug can cause drowsiness.

Alcohol Avoid. Alcohol may increase the sedative effects of this drug.

PROLONGED USE

Withdrawal symptoms may occur if the drug is not stopped gradually over at least 4 weeks. Such symptoms include dizziness, electric shock sensations, anxiety, nausea, and insomnia. These rarely last for more than 1–2 weeks.

Monitoring Any person experiencing drowsiness, confusion, muscle cramps, or convulsions should be monitored for low sodium levels in the blood.

Perindopril

Brand name Coversyl
Used in the following combined preparation
Coversyl Plus

QUICK REFERENCE

Drug group ACE inhibitor (p.31)
Overdose danger rating Medium
Dependence rating Low
Prescription needed Yes
Available as generic No

GENERAL INFORMATION

Perindopril is an ACE inhibitor, a group of drugs used to treat high blood pressure, heart failure, and to reduce the risk of cardiac events such as a heart attack in patients with certain heart conditions. The drug relaxes the muscles in the blood-vessel walls, allowing the vessels to dilate, thereby easing blood flow. Perindopril lowers blood pressure promptly, but may need to be taken for several weeks to achieve maximum effect. For heart failure, it is usually combined with a diuretic. This can give dramatic improvement, relaxing the muscle in blood vessel walls and reducing the heart's workload.

At the start of treatment, ACE inhibitors can cause a very rapid fall in blood pressure. Therefore, the first dose is usually low and taken at bedtime so that the patient can stay lying down.

The most characteristic adverse effect of perindopril is a persistent dry cough, which may occur in up to 20 per cent of patients. The throat may become irritated, and the voice husky or hoarse.

INFORMATION FOR USERS

Your drug prescription is tailored for you. Do not alter dosage without checking with your doctor.

How taken/used Tablets.
Frequency and timing of doses Once daily, 30 minutes before food, usually in the morning.

Adult dosage range 2mg initially, then 4–8mg daily.

Onset of effect 30–60 minutes.

Duration of action 24 hours.

Diet advice None.

Storage Keep in original container at room temperature out of the reach of children.

Missed dose Take as soon as you remember. If your next dose is due within the next 8 hours, take a single dose now, and skip the next.

Stopping the drug Do not stop the drug without consulting your doctor; stopping the drug may lead to worsening of the underlying condition.

Exceeding the dose An occasional unintentional extra dose is unlikely to cause problems. Large overdoses may cause dizziness or fainting. Notify your doctor.

POSSIBLE ADVERSE EFFECTS

Perindopril may cause kidney impairment and a drastic fall in blood pressure. Loss of taste, a rash and itching, and nausea and abdominal pain are common. If you have a persistent dry cough, consult your doctor. If, rarely, fatigue, sore throat, fever, dizziness, and fainting occur consult your doctor.

INTERACTIONS

Lithium Blood levels and toxicity of this drug may be raised by perindopril.

Diuretics cause a very rapid fall in blood pressure with perindopril; you may be advised to stop the diuretic for 2–3 days before the start of treatment.

Vasodilators (e.g. nitrates) may reduce blood pressure even further with perindopril.

Ciclosporin, potassium salts, and potassium-sparing diuretics increase the risk of high blood potassium levels with perindopril and should be avoided.

Non-steroidal anti-inflammatory drugs (NSAIDs) may reduce the effects of perindopril. There is also a risk of kidney damage when they are taken together.

SPECIAL PRECAUTIONS

Be sure to tell your doctor if:

◆ You have long-term liver or kidney problems.

◆ You have a history of allergy to any ACE inhibitor.

◆ You are on a low sodium diet.

◆ You have blood problems.

◆ You are taking other medicines.

Pregnancy Not prescribed. May expose the fetus to toxicity.

Breast-feeding Safety in breast-feeding not established. Discuss with your doctor.

Infants and children Not recommended.

Over 60 Elderly people may be more sensitive to the drug. Reduced dose necessary.

Driving and hazardous work Avoid such activities until you have learned how perindopril affects you because the drug can cause dizziness and fainting.

Alcohol Avoid. Alcohol may increase the blood pressure lowering and adverse effects of the drug.

Surgery and general anaesthetics Perindopril may need to be stopped before you have a general anaesthetic. Discuss with your doctor or dentist before any operation.

PROLONGED USE

Rarely, long-term use of perindopril can lead to changes in the blood count or in kidney function.

Monitoring Periodic checks on potassium levels, white blood cell count, kidney function, and urine contents are usually performed.

Permethrin

Brand name Lyclear
Used in the following combined preparations None

QUICK REFERENCE

Drug group Drug to treat skin parasites (p.122)
Overdose danger rating Low
Dependence rating Low
Prescription needed No
Available as generic Yes

GENERAL INFORMATION

Permethrin is an insecticide used to treat pubic lice and scabies infestations. The drug works by interfering with the nervous system function of the parasites, causing paralysis and death. Permethrin has the advantage of being less toxic than some of the other types of insecticide.

Permethrin is applied topically as a cream to treat pubic lice and scabies infestations. In children and elderly people, the entire body surface, including the face, scalp, neck, and ears, may have to be covered; adults are treated from the neck downwards. For pubic lice, the entire body should be treated and the permethrin left on overnight. A second treatment 7 days later is needed.

For both pubic lice and scabies, all family members should be treated at the same time, to prevent recontamination, and the process repeated after a week.

There are signs that the parasites are developing resistance to permethrin. If the drug does not work for you, your pharmacist should be able to suggest an alternative treatment.

INFORMATION FOR USERS

Follow instructions on the label. Call your doctor if symptoms worsen.

How taken/used Cream.

Frequency and timing of doses Once only, repeating after 7 days (2 years and over); under specialist supervision only (infants and children under 2 years). Avoid contact with eyes and broken or infected skin.

Adult dosage range As directed.

Onset of effect *Public lice* Wash off after 12–24 hours. *Scabies* Wash off after 8–12 hours.

Duration of action Until washed off.

Diet advice None.

Storage Keep in original container at room temperature out of the reach of children. Protect from light.

Missed dose Timing of the second application is not rigid; use as soon as you remember.

Stopping the drug Not applicable.

Exceeding the dose An occasional extra application is unlikely to cause problems. If permethrin is accidentally swallowed, take emergency action.

POSSIBLE ADVERSE EFFECTS

In general, permethrin is well tolerated on the skin, although mild skin irritation is common; the skin may become itchy or reddened. Rarely, a rash may occur.

INTERACTIONS

Corticosteroids Treatment of eczema-like reactions to permethrin with corticosteroids may lower the immune response to the mites. These drugs should not be given at the same time as treatment with permethrin.

SPECIAL PRECAUTIONS

Be sure to consult your doctor or pharmacist before taking this drug if:

◆ You are taking other medicines.

Pregnancy Safety not established. Discuss with your doctor.

Breast-feeding Safety not established. Discuss with your doctor.

Infants and children Under specialist supervision only under 2 years. No special problems in older children.

Over 60 No special problems, but consult your doctor or a health professional.

Driving and hazardous work No special problems.

Alcohol No special problems.

PROLONGED USE

Permethrin should not be used for prolonged periods, The drug is intended for intermittent use only.

Phenobarbital

Brand names None
Used in the following combined preparations None

QUICK REFERENCE

Drug group Barbiturate anticonvulsant drug (p.16)
Overdose danger rating High
Dependence rating High
Prescription needed Yes
Available as generic Yes

GENERAL INFORMATION

Phenobarbital, which was introduced more than 70 years ago, belongs to the group of drugs known as barbiturates. The drug is used mainly in the treatment of epilepsy, but it was also used as a sleeping drug and sedative before the development of safer drugs.

In the treatment of epilepsy, the drug is usually given together with another anticonvulsant drug such as phenytoin. The main disadvantage of the drug is that it often causes unwanted sedation. However, tolerance develops within a week or two, and most patients have no problem in long-term use. In children and the elderly, it may occasionally cause excessive excitement.

Because of their sedative effects, phenobarbital and other barbiturates are sometimes abused.

INFORMATION FOR USERS

Your drug prescription is tailored for you. Do not alter dosage without checking with your doctor.

How taken/used Tablets, liquid, injection.
Frequency and timing of doses Once daily, usually at night.
Dosage range Adults 60–180mg daily.
Onset of effect 30–60 minutes (by mouth).
Duration of action 24–48 hours (some effect may persist for up to 6 days).
Diet advice None.
Storage Keep in original container at room temperature out of the reach of children.
Missed dose Take as soon as you remember. If the next dose is due within 10 hours, take a single dose now and skip the next.
Stopping the drug Do not stop taking the drug without consulting your doctor, who may supervise a gradual reduction in dosage. Abrupt cessation may cause fits or lead to restlessness, trembling, and insomnia.

OVERDOSE ACTION

Seek immediate medical advice in all cases. Take emergency action if unsteadiness, severe weakness, confusion, or loss of consciousness occur.

POSSIBLE ADVERSE EFFECTS

Most adverse effects of phenobarbital are the result of its sedative effect. These can sometimes be minimized by a medically supervised reduction in dosage. Drowsiness, clumsiness, unsteadiness, dizziness, and fainting are common. If, rarely, confusion, mood changes, or impaired memory occur, consult your doctor. If a rash or localized swellings occur stop taking the drug and consult your doctor urgently.

INTERACTIONS

General note Phenobarbital interacts with a wide range of other drugs. Consult your doctor or pharmacist before taking any new drugs, including herbal remedies.

Anticoagulants, corticosteroids, oral contraceptives, and protease inhibitor antiretroviral drugs Phenobarbital may decrease the effect of these drugs.

Antipsychotic drugs, antidepressants, St John's wort, mefloquine, and chloroquine These may reduce the anticonvulsant effect of phenobarbital.

Sedatives All drugs that have a sedative effect on the central nervous system are likely to increase the sedative properties of phenobarbital.

SPECIAL PRECAUTIONS

Be sure to tell your doctor if:

◆ You have long-term liver or kidney problems.

◆ You have heart problems.

◆ You have poor circulation.

◆ You have porphyria.

◆ You have breathing problems.

◆ You have depression.

◆ You are taking other medicines.

Pregnancy The drug may affect the fetus and increase the tendency of bleeding in the newborn. Discuss with your doctor.

Breast-feeding The drug passes into the breast milk and could cause drowsiness in the baby. Discuss with your doctor.

Infants and children Reduced dose necessary.

Over 60 Increased likelihood of confusion. Reduced dose may therefore be necessary.

Driving and hazardous work Your underlying condition, in addition to the possibility of reduced alertness while taking phenobarbital, may make such activities inadvisable. Discuss with your doctor.

Alcohol Never drink alcohol while undergoing treatment with phenobarbital. Alcohol may interact dangerously with this drug.

PROLONGED USE

The sedative effect of phenobarbital can build up, causing excessive drowsiness and lethargy. However, tolerance may develop, thereby reducing these effects. Dependence may also result. Withdrawal symptoms may occur if phenobarbital is stopped suddenly.

Monitoring Blood samples may be taken periodically to test blood levels of the drug.

Phenoxymethylpenicillin

Brand names None
Used in the following combined preparations None

QUICK REFERENCE
Drug group Penicillin antibiotic (p.62)
Overdose danger rating Low
Dependence rating Low
Prescription needed Yes
Available as generic Yes

GENERAL INFORMATION
Phenoxymethylpenicillin, also known as penicillin V, is a synthetic penicillin-type antibiotic that is prescribed for a wide range of infections.

Various commonly occurring respiratory tract infections, such as some types of tonsillitis and pharyngitis, as well as ear infections, often respond well to this drug. It is also effective for the treatment of the gum disease, Vincent's gingivitis.

Phenoxymethylpenicillin is also used to treat less common infections caused by the *Streptococcus* bacterium, such as scarlet fever and erysipelas (a skin infection). It is also prescribed long term to prevent the recurrence of rheumatic fever, a rare, although potentially serious condition. It is also used long term to prevent infections following removal of the spleen or in sickle cell disease.

As with other penicillin antibiotics, the most serious adverse effect that may rarely occur is an allergic reaction that may cause collapse, wheezing, and a rash in susceptible people.

INFORMATION FOR USERS
Your drug prescription is tailored for you. Do not alter dosage without checking with your doctor.
How taken/used Tablets, liquid.
Frequency and timing of doses 4 x daily, at least 30 minutes before food.
Dosage range *Adults* 2–4g daily. *Children* Reduced dose according to age.
Onset of effect 1–2 days.
Duration of action Up to 12 hours.
Diet advice None.
Storage Keep in original container at room temperature out of the reach of children.

Missed dose Take as soon as you remember. If your next dose is due within 2 hours, take a single dose now and skip the next.
Stopping the drug Take the full course. Even if you feel better, the original infection may still be present and may recur if the treatment is stopped too soon.
Exceeding the dose An occasional unintentional extra dose is unlikely to be a cause for concern. But if you notice any unusual symptoms, or if a large overdose has been taken, notify your doctor.

POSSIBLE ADVERSE EFFECTS
Most people do not experience any serious adverse effects, but the drug may provoke an allergic reaction in susceptible people. Nausea and vomiting are common, and diarrhoea may occur. If a rash, itching, or breathing difficulties occur, stop taking the drug and seek immediate medical attention.

INTERACTIONS
Oral contraceptives Phenoxymethylpenicillin may reduce the contraceptive effect of these drugs. Discuss with your doctor.
Probenecid increases the level of phenoxymethylpenicillin in the blood.
Neomycin reduces the level of phenoxymetylpenicillin in the blood.
Methotrexate Excretion of this drug may be greatly reduced by phenoxymethylpenicillin, leading to toxicity.

SPECIAL PRECAUTIONS
Be sure to tell your doctor if:
◆ You have a long-term kidney problem.
◆ You have had a previous allergic reaction to a penicillin or cephalosporin antibiotic.
◆ You have an allergic disorder such as asthma or urticaria.
◆ You are taking other medicines.
Pregnancy No evidence of risk.
Breast-feeding The drug passes into the breast milk, but at normal doses adverse effects on the baby are unlikely. Discuss with your doctor.
Infants and children Reduced dose necessary.
Over 60 No special problems.
Driving and hazardous work No known problems.
Alcohol No known problems.

PROLONGED USE

Prolonged use may increase the risk of *Candida* infections and diarrhoea.

Phenytoin/Fosphenytoin

Brand names [Phenytoin] Epanutin, [Fosphenytoin] Pro-Epanutin
Used in the following combined preparations None

QUICK REFERENCE

Drug group Anticonvulsant drug (p.16)
Overdose danger rating Medium
Dependence rating Low
Prescription needed Yes
Available as generic Yes

GENERAL INFORMATION

Phenytoin decreases the likelihood of convulsions by reducing abnormal electrical discharges within the brain. Introduced in the 1930s, it is prescribed for the treatment of epilepsy, including tonic/clonic and temporal lobe epilepsy. Fosphenytoin is a new type of phenytoin given by injection for severe fits.

The drug has also been used for other disorders, such as migraine, trigeminal neuralgia, and the correction of certain abnormal heart rhythms.

Because some adverse effects are more pronounced in children, the drug is prescribed for them only when other drugs are unsuitable. The dose may be adjusted according to blood levels of the drug. Patients are advised to remain on the same brand of phenytoin.

INFORMATION FOR USERS

Your drug prescription is tailored for you. Do not alter dosage without checking with your doctor.
How taken/used Tablets, chewable tablets, capsules, liquid, injection.
Frequency and timing of doses 1–2 x daily with food or plenty of water.
Dosage range *Adults* 200–500mg daily (usually as a single dose). *Children* According to age and weight.
Onset of effect Full anticonvulsant effect may not be felt for 7–10 days.
Duration of action 24 hours.

Diet advice Folic acid and vitamin D deficiency may occasionally occur while taking this drug. Make sure you eat a balanced diet containing fresh, green vegetables.
Storage Keep in original container at room temperature out of the reach of children.
Missed dose Take as soon as you remember.
Stopping the drug Do not stop the drug without consulting your doctor; seizures may recur.
Exceeding the dose An occasional, unintentional extra dose is unlikely to cause problems but if you notice vision problems, drowsiness, slurred speech, or confusion, notify your doctor immediately.

POSSIBLE ADVERSE EFFECTS

Phenytoin has a number of adverse effects, many of which appear only after prolonged use. If they become severe, your doctor may prescribe a different anticonvulsant. Dizziness, headache, confusion, nausea, vomiting, and insomnia are common. If, rarely, you have increased body hair, overgrowth of gums, a rash, fever, sore throat, or mouth ulcers, consult your doctor at once.

INTERACTIONS

General note Many drugs may interact with phenytoin, causing either an increase or a reduction in the phenytoin blood level. The dosage of phenytoin may need to be adjusted. Consult your doctor or pharmacist.
Oral contraceptives Phenytoin may reduce their effectiveness.
Antidepressants, antipsychotics, mefloquine, chloroquine, and St John's wort These preparations may reduce the effect of phenytoin.
Warfarin The anticoagulant effect of this drug may be altered. An adjustment in its dosage may be necessary.

SPECIAL PRECAUTIONS

Be sure to tell your doctor if:
◆ You have long-term liver or kidney problems.
◆ You have diabetes.
◆ You have porphyria.
◆ You are taking other medicines.
Pregnancy The drug may be associated with malformation and a tendency to bleeding in the newborn baby. Folic acid supplements should be taken by the mother. Discuss with your doctor.

Breast-feeding The drug passes into the breast milk, but at normal doses adverse effects on the baby are unlikely. Discuss with your doctor.

Infants and children Reduced dose necessary. Increased likelihood of overgrowth of the gums and excessive growth of body hair.

Over 60 Reduced dose may be necessary.

Driving and hazardous work Your underlying condition, as well as the effects of phenytoin, may make such activities inadvisable. Discuss with your doctor.

Alcohol Avoid. Alcohol increases the sedative effects of this drug.

PROLONGED USE

There is a slight risk that blood abnormalities may occur. Prolonged use may also lead to adverse effects on skin, gums, and bones. It may also disrupt control of diabetes.

Monitoring Periodic blood tests may be performed to monitor levels of the drug in the body and composition of the blood cells and blood chemistry.

Pilocarpine

Brand names Isopto, Minims Pilocarpine, Pilogel, Salagen
Used in the following combined preparations None

QUICK REFERENCE

Drug group Miotic drug for glaucoma (p.114)
Overdose danger rating Medium
Dependence rating Low
Prescription needed Yes
Available as generic Yes

GENERAL INFORMATION

Pilocarpine is a miotic drug used to treat chronic and severe glaucoma prior to surgery.

The eye drops are quick-acting, but they have to be re-applied every 4–8 hours. Eye gel is longer acting and needs to be applied only once a day. Pilocarpine frequently causes blurred vision; and spasm of the eye muscles may cause headaches, particularly at the start of treatment. However, serious adverse effects are rare.

As tablets it is used to treat dry mouth following radiotherapy to the head and neck.

INFORMATION FOR USERS

Your drug prescription is tailored for you. Do not alter dosage without checking with your doctor.

How taken/used Tablets, eye gel, eye drops.

Frequency and timing of doses *Eye drops* 4 x daily (chronic glaucoma); 5-minute intervals until condition is controlled (acute glaucoma). *Eye gel* Once daily. *Tablets* 3–4 x daily after food with plenty of water.

Dosage range According to formulation and condition. In general, 1–2 eye drops are used per application. *Tablets* 15–30mg daily.

Onset of effect 15–30 minutes.

Duration of action 4–8 weeks for maximum effect (tablets); 3–8 hours (eye drops); up to 24 hours (eye gel).

Diet advice None.

Storage Keep in original container at room temperature out of the reach of children (tablets/eye drops). Discard eye drops 1 month after opening.

Missed dose Use as soon as you remember. If not remembered until 2 hours before next dose, skip missed dose and take next dose now.

Stopping the drug Do not stop the drug without consulting your doctor; symptoms may recur.

Exceeding the dose An occasional unintentional extra application is unlikely to cause problems. Excessive use may cause flushing, increased saliva, and sweating. If the drops or gel are accidentally swallowed, seek immediate medical attention.

POSSIBLE ADVERSE EFFECTS

Eye drops/gel Blurred vision or poor night vision, sweating, and chills are common. Headache or browache and eye pain or irritation are also common and usually wear off in a few days; if they do not, or they become severe, consult your doctor. If, rarely, red, watery eyes or twitching eyelids occur, consult your doctor. *Tablets* nausea, diarrhoea, dizziness, headache, and urinary frequency are common.

INTERACTIONS

General note A wide range of drugs (including aminoglycoside antibiotics, clindamycin, colistin, chloroquine, quinine, quinidine, lithium, and procainamide) may antagonize pilocarpine.

Beta blockers may reduce pilocarpine's effects.
Calcium channel blockers These drugs may increase pilocarpine's systemic effect.

SPECIAL PRECAUTIONS

Be sure to tell your doctor if:
◆ You have asthma.
◆ You have inflamed eyes.
◆ You wear contact lenses.
◆ You have heart, liver, or gastrointestinal problems.
◆ You are taking other medicines.

Pregnancy No evidence of risk with eye drops at doses used for chronic glaucoma. Safety of tablets in pregnancy not established. Discuss with your doctor.
Breast-feeding The drug passes into the breast milk, but at normal doses adverse effects on the baby are unlikely. Discuss with your doctor.
Infants and children Not usually prescribed.
Over 60 Reduced night vision is particularly noticeable; no dosage adjustment required.
Driving and hazardous work Avoid such activities, especially in poor light, until you have learned how pilocarpine affects you because it may cause short sight and poor night vision.
Alcohol No known problems.

PROLONGED USE

The drug's effect may occasionally wear off as the body adapts but may be restored by changing temporarily to a similar drug.

Piroxicam

Brand names Brexidol, Feldene, Pirozip
Used in the following combined preparations None

QUICK REFERENCE

Drug group Non-steroidal anti-inflammatory drug (p.50) and drug for gout (p.53)
Overdose danger rating Medium
Dependence rating Low
Prescription needed Yes
Available as generic Yes

GENERAL INFORMATION

Piroxicam, introduced in 1980, is a non-steroidal anti-inflammatory drug (NSAID) that, like others in this group, reduces pain, stiffness, and inflammation. Blood levels of the drug remain high for many hours after a dose, so it needs to be taken only once daily.

Piroxicam is used for osteoarthritis, rheumatoid arthritis, acute attacks of gout, and ankylosing spondylitis. It gives relief of the symptoms of arthritis, although it does not cure the disease. It is sometimes prescribed in conjunction with slow-acting drugs in rheumatoid arthritis to relieve pain and inflammation while these drugs take effect. The drug may also be given for pain relief after sports injuries, for conditions such as tendinitis and bursitis, and following minor surgery.

This drug is less likely than aspirin to cause stomach ulcers.

INFORMATION FOR USERS

Your drug prescription is tailored for you. Do not alter dosage without checking with your doctor.
How taken/used Tablets, capsules, melts, injection, gel.
Frequency and timing of doses 1–3 x daily with food or plenty of water.
Adult dosage range 10–40mg daily.
Onset of effect 3–4 hours (pain relief); full effect develops over 2–4 weeks (arthritis) or 4–5 days (gout).
Duration of action Up to 2 days. Some effect may last for 7–10 days after treatment has been stopped.
Diet advice None.
Storage Keep in original container at room temperature out of the reach of children. Protect from light.
Missed dose Take as soon as you remember. If your next dose is due within 4 hours, take a single dose now and skip the next.
Stopping the drug When taken for short-term pain relief, the drug can be safely stopped as soon as you no longer need it. If it is prescribed for long-term treatment of arthritis, seek medical advice before stopping the drug.
Exceeding the dose An occasional unintentional extra dose is unlikely to be a cause for concern. Large overdoses may cause nausea and vomiting. Notify your doctor.

POSSIBLE ADVERSE EFFECTS

Dizziness, headache, and gastrointestinal effects such as nausea, indigestion, and abdominal pain are not usually serious. Swollen feet and ankles are less common; discuss with your doctor. If you have a rash or itching, stop taking the drug and consult your doctor immediately. If wheezing, breathlessness, bruising or bleeding, or black or bloodstained faeces occur, stop taking the drug and seek immediate medical attention.

INTERACTIONS

General note Piroxicam interacts with many drugs, including other NSAIDs, corticosteroids, and oral anticoagulants, to increase the risk of bleeding and/or peptic ulcers.

Lithium, digoxin, and methotrexate Piroxicam may raise blood levels of these drugs to an undesirable extent.

Antihypertensive drugs and diuretics Their beneficial effects may be reduced by piroxicam.

Ciprofloxacin, norfloxacin, and ofloxacin Piroxicam may increase the risk of convulsions when taken with these drugs.

SPECIAL PRECAUTIONS

Be sure to tell your doctor if:
◆ You have liver or kidney problems.
◆ You have heart problems or high blood pressure.
◆ You have had a peptic ulcer, oesophagitis, or acid indigestion.
◆ You have porphyria.
◆ You have asthma.
◆ You are allergic to aspirin or other NSAIDs.
◆ You are taking other medicines.

Pregnancy Not usually prescribed. When taken in the last 3 months of pregnancy, the drug increases the risk of adverse effects on the baby's heart and may prolong labour. Discuss with your doctor.

Breast-feeding The drug passes into the breast milk but at normal doses adverse effects are unlikely. Discuss with your doctor.

Infants and children Not recommended under 6 years. Reduced dose necessary.

Over 60 Increased likelihood of adverse effects. Reduced dose may therefore be necessary.

Driving and hazardous work Avoid such activities until you have learned how piroxicam affects you; the drug can cause dizziness.

Alcohol Avoid. Alcohol may increase the risk of stomach disorders with piroxicam.

Surgery and general anaesthetics Piroxicam may prolong bleeding. Discuss with your doctor or dentist before any surgery.

PROLONGED USE

Increased risk of bleeding from peptic ulcers and in the bowel. The lowest effective dose is given for the shortest duration.

Monitoring Periodic blood counts and liver function tests may be performed.

Pizotifen

Brand name Sanomigran
Used in the following combined preparations None

QUICK REFERENCE

Drug group Drug for migraine (p.20)
Overdose danger rating Medium
Dependence rating Low
Prescription needed Yes
Available as generic Yes

GENERAL INFORMATION

Pizotifen is an antihistamine drug with a chemical structure similar to that of tricyclic antidepressants (see p.14); it also has similar anticholinergic effects. This drug is prescribed for the prevention of migraine headaches in people who suffer frequent, disabling attacks. The drug is thought to work by blocking the chemicals (histamine and serotonin) that act on blood vessels in the brain.

The main disadvantage of prolonged use of pizotifen is that it stimulates the appetite and, as a result, often causes weight gain. It is usually prescribed only for people in whom other measures for migraine prevention, such as avoidance of trigger factors, have failed.

The sweetener used in the liquid medication is hydrogenated glucose syrup, and this may affect levels of blood glucose.

INFORMATION FOR USERS

Your drug prescription is tailored for you. Do not alter dosage without checking with your doctor.

How taken/used Tablets, liquid.

Frequency and timing of doses Once a day (at night) or 3 x daily.

Adult dosage range 1.5–4.5mg daily.

Maximum single dose 3mg.

Onset of effect Full beneficial effects may not be felt for several days.

Duration of action Effects of this drug may last for several weeks.

Diet advice You may be advised to avoid foods that trigger headaches in your case.

Storage Keep in original container at room temperature out of the reach of children. Protect from light.

Missed dose Take as soon as you remember. If your next dose is due within 4 hours, take a single dose now and skip the next.

Stopping the drug Do not stop the drug without consulting your doctor; symptoms may recur.

Exceeding the dose An occasional unintentional extra dose is unlikely to cause problems. Large overdoses may cause drowsiness, nausea, palpitations, fits, and coma. Notify your doctor.

POSSIBLE ADVERSE EFFECTS

Drowsiness is common, but it can often be minimized by starting with a low dose that is gradually increased. Increased appetite and weight gain are also common. Nausea, dizziness, muscle pains, dry mouth, and blurred vision occur less commonly. If you have depression or anxiety, consult your doctor.

INTERACTIONS

Anticholinergic drugs including tricyclic antidepressants, may increase the weak anticholinergic effects of pizotifen.

Antihypertensive drugs The blood pressure lowering effects of guanethidine and debrisoquine are reduced by pizotifen.

Sedatives All drugs that have a sedative effect on the central nervous system are likely to increase the sedative properties of pizotifen. These include sleeping drugs, anti-anxiety drugs, opioid analgesics, and antihistamines.

SPECIAL PRECAUTIONS

Be sure to tell your doctor if:
◆ You have a long-term kidney problem.
◆ You have glaucoma.
◆ You have urinary retention.
◆ You have prostate trouble.
◆ You are taking other medicines.

Pregnancy Safety in pregnancy not established. Discuss with your doctor.

Breast-feeding The drug passes into the breast milk, but at normal doses adverse effects on the baby are unlikely. Discuss with your doctor.

Infants and children Reduced dose usually necessary.

Over 60 No special problems.

Driving and hazardous work Avoid such activities until you have learned how pizotifen affects you because the drug can cause drowsiness and blurred vision.

Alcohol Avoid. Alcohol may increase the sedative effects of this drug.

PROLONGED USE

Long term, pizotifen often causes weight gain. Treatment is usually reviewed every 6 months.

Pravastatin

Brand name Lipostat
Used in the following combined preparations None

QUICK REFERENCE

Drug group Lipid-lowering drug (p.37)
Overdose danger rating Medium
Dependence rating Low
Prescription needed Yes
Available as generic Yes

GENERAL INFORMATION

Pravastatin belongs to the statin group of lipid-lowering drugs. It is prescribed for people with hypercholesterolaemia (high levels of cholesterol in the blood) who have not responded to other treatments, such as a special diet, and who are at risk of developing heart disease. The drug works by blocking the action of an enzyme that is needed for the manufacture of cholesterol, mainly in the liver. As a result, blood levels of cholesterol are lowered, which can help to prevent heart disease.

Like most other statins, pravastatin is taken at night because that is when most cholesterol is produced.

Rarely, statins can cause muscle pain, inflammation, and damage. This seems to be more likely if another kind of lipid-lowering drug called a fibrate is given with the statin.

INFORMATION FOR USERS

Your drug prescription is tailored for you. Do not alter dosage without checking with your doctor.

How taken/used Tablets.

Frequency and timing of doses Once daily at night.

Adult dosage range 10–40mg daily, changed after intervals of at least 4 weeks.

Onset of effect Within 2 weeks. Full beneficial effect may be felt within 4 weeks.

Duration of action 24 hours.

Diet advice A low-fat diet is usually advised.

Storage Keep in original container at room temperature out of the reach of children. Protect from light.

Missed dose Take as soon as you remember. If your next dose is due within 8 hours, do not take the missed dose, but take the next dose as usual.

Stopping the drug Do not stop taking the drug without consulting your doctor; stopping the drug may lead to worsening of the underlying condition.

Exceeding the dose An occasional unintentional extra dose is unlikely to cause problems. Large overdoses may cause liver problems. Notify your doctor.

POSSIBLE ADVERSE EFFECTS

Most adverse effects are mild and usually disappear with time. Headache and nausea are common. Rarely, fatigue and chest pain may occur. If jaundice or abdominal pain occur, consult your doctor. If a rash or muscle pain or weakness occur, stop taking the drug and seek immediate medical advice.

INTERACTIONS

Anticoagulants Pravastatin may increase the effect of these drugs.

Antifungal drugs Taken with pravastatin, itraconazole, ketoconazole, and possibly other antifungal drugs, may increase the risk of muscle damage.

Orlistat This drug increases blood levels and toxicity of pravastatin.

Other lipid-lowering drugs (fibrates) Taken with pravastatin, these drugs may increase the risk of muscle damage.

Ciclosporin and other immunosuppressant drugs There is an increased risk of muscle damage if pravastatin is taken with these drugs. They are not usually prescribed together.

SPECIAL PRECAUTIONS

Be sure to tell your doctor if:
◆ You have had liver problems.
◆ You have had side effects on your muscles from any other lipid-lowering drugs.
◆ You are taking other medicines.

Pregnancy Not prescribed. Discuss with your doctor.

Breast-feeding Not recommended. The drug passes into the breast milk. Discuss with your doctor.

Infants and children Not recommended under 8 years.

Over 60 No special problems.

Driving and hazardous work No special problems.

Alcohol Avoid excessive amounts. Alcohol may increase the risk of developing liver problems with this drug.

PROLONGED USE

Long-term use of pravastatin can affect liver function.

Monitoring Regular blood tests to check liver and muscle function are usually required.

Prednisolone

Brand names Deltacortril, Deltastab, Minims prednisolone, Predenema, Predfoam, Pred Forte, Predsol, and others

Used in the following combined preparations Predsol-N, Scheriproct

QUICK REFERENCE

Drug group Corticosteroid (p.80)
Overdose danger rating Low
Dependence rating Low
Prescription needed Yes
Available as generic Yes

GENERAL INFORMATION

Prednisolone, a powerful corticosteroid, is used for a wide range of conditions, including some skin diseases, rheumatic disorders, allergic states, and certain blood disorders. It is used as eye drops to reduce inflammation in conjunctivitis or iritis and may be given as an enema to treat inflammatory bowel disease. It is also prescribed with fludrocortisone for pituitary or adrenal gland disorders.

Prednisolone taken short term either by mouth or topically rarely causes serious side effects. However, long-term treatment with high doses can cause fluid retention, indigestion, diabetes, hypertension, and acne. Enteric-coated tablets reduce the local effects of the drug on the stomach but not the systemic effects.

INFORMATION FOR USERS

Your drug prescription is tailored for you. Do not alter dosage without checking with your doctor.

How taken/used Tablets, suppositories, enema, foam, injection, eye and ear drops.

Frequency and timing of doses Usually once daily or on alternate days with food (tablets); 2–4 x daily, more frequently initially (eye/ear drops).

Adult dosage range Considerable variation. Follow your doctor's instructions.

Onset of effect 2–4 days.

Duration of action 12–72 hours.

Diet advice A low-sodium and high-potassium diet is recommended when the oral or injected form of the drug is used for extended periods. Follow the advice of your doctor.

Storage Keep in original container at room temperature out of the reach of children. Protect from light.

Missed dose Take as soon as you remember. If your next dose is due within 6 hours, take a single dose now and skip the next.

Stopping the drug Do not stop the drug without consulting your doctor. Abrupt cessation of long-term treatment by mouth may be dangerous.

Exceeding the dose An occasional unintentional extra dose is unlikely to be a cause for concern. But if you notice any unusual symptoms, or if a large overdose has been taken, notify your doctor.

POSSIBLE ADVERSE EFFECTS

The rare but more serious adverse effects occur only with high doses taken by mouth or injection or for long periods. If taking oral forms, you should avoid close personal contact with chickenpox or herpes zoster, and seek urgent medical attention if exposed. In-digestion and acne are common; discuss with your doctor. Rarely, muscle weakness, mood changes, and depression occur, and should also be discussed with your doctor. If you have black or bloodstained faeces, stop taking the drug and consult your doctor urgently.

INTERACTIONS

Anticonvulsant drugs Carbamazepine, phenytoin, and phenobarbital can reduce the effects of prednisolone.

Vaccines Serious reactions can occur when vaccinations are given with this drug. Discuss with your doctor.

Anticoagulant drugs Prednisolone may affect the response to these drugs.

Diuretics Prednisolone may increase the adverse effects of these drugs.

Antihypertensive and antidiabetic drugs and insulin Prednisolone may reduce their effects, requiring larger doses of them.

Ciclosporin and tacrolimus may reduce daily or alternate-day dose of prednisolone required.

SPECIAL PRECAUTIONS

Be sure to tell your doctor if:
◆ You have had a peptic ulcer.
◆ You have glaucoma.
◆ You have had tuberculosis.
◆ You suffer from depression.
◆ You have any infection.
◆ You have diabetes.
◆ You have osteoporosis.
◆ You are taking other medicines.

Pregnancy No evidence of risk with eye or ear drops. Harm to the fetus is unlikely when the drug is taken as tablets in low doses. Discuss with your doctor.

Breast-feeding No evidence of risk with drops or injections. Taken by mouth, the drug passes into the breast milk, but at low doses adverse effects on the baby are unlikely. Discuss with your doctor.

Infants and children Only given when essential. Alternate-day dosing preferred to prevent growth retardation.

Over 60 Increased likelihood of adverse effects. Reduced dose may therefore be necessary.

Driving and hazardous work No known problems.

Alcohol Keep consumption low. Increased risk of peptic ulcers (by mouth or injection).

Infection Avoid exposure to chickenpox, shingles, or measles if having systemic treatment.

PROLONGED USE
Prolonged use by mouth can lead to peptic ulcers, glaucoma, muscle weakness, fragile bones, and growth retardation in children. Prolonged use of topical forms may also lead to skin thinning. People having long-term treatment should carry a "steroid" card.

Prochlorperazine

Brand names Buccastem, Proziére, Stemetil
Used in the following combined preparations None

QUICK REFERENCE
Drug group Phenothiazine antipsychotic drug (p.15) and anti-emetic (p.21)
Overdose danger rating Medium
Dependence rating Low
Prescription needed Yes (most preparations)
Available as generic Yes

GENERAL INFORMATION
Introduced in the late 1950s, prochlorperazine belongs to a group of drugs called phenothiazines, which act on the central nervous system.

In small doses, prochlorperazine controls nausea and vomiting, especially when they are side effects of medical treatment by drugs or radiation, or of anaesthesia. It is available over the counter for nausea and vomiting associated with migraine. It is also used to treat the nausea that occurs with inner-ear disorders such as vertigo. In large doses, it is sometimes used as an antipsychotic to reduce aggressiveness and suppress abnormal behaviour. It thus minimizes and controls the abnormal behaviour of schizophrenia, mania, and other mental disorders. Prochlorperazine does not cure any of these diseases, but helps to relieve symptoms.

INFORMATION FOR USERS
Your drug prescription is tailored for you. Do not alter the dosage without checking with your doctor.
How taken/used Tablets, buccal tablets, effervescent granules, liquid, injection.
Frequency and timing of doses 2–3 x daily.

Adult dosage range *Nausea and vomiting* 20mg initially, then 5–10mg per dose (tablets); 5–25mg per dose (suppositories). *Mental illness* 25–100mg daily. Larger doses may be given.
Onset of effect Within 60 minutes (by mouth or suppository); 10–20 minutes (injection).
Duration of action 3–6 hours.
Diet advice None.
Storage Keep in original container at room temperature out of the reach of children. Protect from light.
Missed dose Take as soon as you remember. If your next dose is due within 2 hours, take a single dose now and skip the next.
Stopping the drug Do not stop the drug without consulting your doctor; symptoms may recur.
Exceeding the dose An occasional unintentional extra dose is unlikely to cause problems. Large overdoses may cause unusual drowsiness and may affect the heart. Notify your doctor.

POSSIBLE ADVERSE EFFECTS
Prochlorperazine has a strong anticholinergic effect (see Autonomic nervous system, p.8), which can cause a variety of minor symptoms that often become less marked with time. The most significant effect with high doses is abnormal movements of the face and limbs (parkinsonism) caused by changes in the balance of brain chemicals. Drowsiness, lethargy, dry mouth, and constipation are common, as are dizziness, fainting, and parkinsonism, which should be discussed with your doctor. If tensing of muscles occurs, consult your doctor. If a rash occurs, stop taking the drug and consult your doctor urgently.

INTERACTIONS
Sedatives All drugs with a sedative effect are likely to increase the sedative effects of prochlorperazine.
Drugs for parkinsonism Prochlorperazine may block the beneficial effect of these.
Anticholinergic drugs Prochlorperazine may increase the side effects of these drugs.

SPECIAL PRECAUTIONS
Be sure to tell your doctor if:
◆ You have heart, liver, or kidney problems.
◆ You have had epileptic fits.
◆ You have Parkinson's disease.

◆ You have prostate problems.
◆ You have glaucoma.
◆ You are taking other medicines.

Pregnancy Safety in pregnancy not established. Discuss with your doctor.

Breast-feeding The drug passes into the breast milk and may affect the baby. Discuss with your doctor.

Infants and children Not recommended in infants weighing less than 10kg and young children. Reduced dose necessary in older children due to increased risk of adverse effects.

Over 60 Increased likelihood of adverse effects. Reduced dose may be necessary.

Driving and hazardous work Avoid such activities until you have learned how prochlorperazine affects you because it can cause drowsiness and reduced alertness.

Alcohol Avoid. Alcohol may increase and prolong the sedative effects of this drug.

PROLONGED USE

Use of this drug for more than a few months may lead to the development of involuntary, potentially irreversible movements of the eye, mouth, and tongue (tardive dyskinesia). Occasionally, jaundice may occur.

Monitoring Periodic blood tests may be performed.

Procyclidine

Brand names Arpicolin, Kemadrin
Used in the following combined preparations None

QUICK REFERENCE

Drug group Anticholinergic drug for parkinsonism (p.18)
Overdose danger rating High
Dependence rating Low
Prescription needed Yes
Available as generic Yes

GENERAL INFORMATION

Introduced in the 1950s, procyclidine is an anticholinergic drug (see Autonomic nervous system, p.8) used to treat Parkinson's disease. The drug is especially helpful in the early stages for treating muscle rigidity. It also helps to reduce excess salivation. However, it has little effect on the characteristic shuffling gait and slow muscular movements of the disease.

Procyclidine is also often used to treat parkinsonism resulting from treatment with antipsychotics. It may cause various adverse effects (see below), but these are rarely serious enough to warrant stopping treatment.

INFORMATION FOR USERS

Your drug prescription is tailored for you. Do not alter dosage without checking with your doctor.

How taken/used Tablets, liquid, injection.
Frequency and timing of doses 2–3 x daily.
Adult dosage range 7.5–30mg daily, exceptionally up to 60mg daily. Dosage is determined individually in order to find the best balance between effective relief of symptoms and the occurrence of adverse effects.
Onset of effect Within 30 minutes.
Duration of action 8–12 hours.
Diet advice None.
Storage Keep in original container at room temperature out of the reach of children.
Missed dose Take as soon as you remember. If your next dose is due within 2 hours, take a single dose now and skip the next.
Stopping the drug Do not stop the drug without consulting your doctor; symptoms may recur.

OVERDOSE ACTION

Seek immediate medical advice in all cases. Take emergency action if palpitations, fits, or unconsciousness occur.

POSSIBLE ADVERSE EFFECTS

Procyclidine's possible adverse effects are mainly due to its anticholinergic action. Dry mouth, constipation, drowsiness, dizziness, and blurred vision may be overcome by dosage adjustment. If you have blurred vision or difficulty in passing urine, consult your doctor. Nausea, vomiting, nervousness, confusion, and a rash have occasionally been reported and should be discussed with your doctor.

INTERACTIONS

Anticholinergic and antihistamine drugs These may increase procyclidine's adverse effects.
Tricyclic antidepressants and antipsychotic drugs may increase the side effects of procyclidine.

SPECIAL PRECAUTIONS

Be sure to tell your doctor if:
◆ You have long-term liver or kidney problems.
◆ You suffer from or have a family history of glaucoma.
◆ You have high blood pressure.
◆ You suffer from constipation.
◆ You have prostate trouble.
◆ You are taking other medicines.

Pregnancy Safety in pregnancy not established. Discuss with your doctor.

Breast-feeding The drug passes into the breast milk and may affect the baby. Discuss with your doctor.

Infants and children Not recommended.

Over 60 Reduced dose may be necessary.

Driving and hazardous work Avoid such activities until you have learned how procyclidine affects you because the drug can cause drowsiness, blurred vision, and mild confusion.

Alcohol Avoid. Alcohol may increase the sedative effect of this drug.

PROLONGED USE

This may provoke the onset of glaucoma.

Monitoring Periodic eye examinations are usually advised.

Proguanil with Atovaquone

Brand name Malarone
Used in the following combined preparations None

QUICK REFERENCE

Drug group Antimalarial drug (p.75)
Overdose danger rating Medium
Dependence rating Low
Prescription needed Yes
Available as generic No

GENERAL INFORMATION

Proguanil is an antimalarial used to prevent the development of malaria. Microbial resistance to its effects can occur, which has led to it being used in combination with other drugs.

Atovaquone is an antiprotozoal that is also active against the fungus *Pneumocystis carinii* (a cause of pneumonia in people with poor immunity). Alone, it is less useful for malaria, but combined with proguanil it rapidly treats the infection. The combination is also used for prevention of malaria, especially in areas where there is resistance to other drugs.

For prevention, you should start taking the tablets a day or two before travelling. Continue taking them during your stay, and for 7 days after your return. It is important to take other precautions, such as using insect repellent at all times and a mosquito net at night. If you develop an illness after your return from a malarial zone, and especially in the first 3 months, go to your doctor immediately and tell him or her where you have been.

INFORMATION FOR USERS

Your drug prescription is tailored for you. Do not alter dosage without checking with your doctor.

How taken/used Tablets.

Frequency and timing of doses *Prevention* Once daily with food or a milky drink, at the same time each day. Start 1–2 days before travel and continue for period of stay (which should not exceed 28 days) and for 7 days after return. *Treatment* Once daily for 3 days, with food or a milky drink.

Adult dosage range *Prevention* 1 tablet. *Treatment* 4 tablets.

Onset of effect After 24 hours.

Duration of action 24–48 hours.

Diet advice None.

Storage Keep in original container at room temperature out of the reach of children.

Missed dose Take as soon as you remember. If next dose is due now, take both doses together.

Stopping the drug Do not stop the drug for 1 week after leaving a malaria-infected area; there is a risk of developing the disease.

Exceeding the dose An occasional unintentional extra dose is unlikely to cause problems. Large overdoses may cause abdominal pain and vomiting. Notify your doctor.

POSSIBLE ADVERSE EFFECTS

Adverse effects are generally fairly mild. Diarrhoea is common. Rarely, nausea, vomiting, abdominal pain, indigestion, and mouth ulcers occur. Discuss hair loss, jaundice, or a rash with your doctor. If you develop a sore throat or fever, consult your doctor urgently.

INTERACTIONS

Warfarin The effects of warfarin may be enhanced by proguanil with atovaquone.

Antacids may reduce the absorption of proguanil with atovaquone.

Rifampicin, metoclopramide, and tetracycline antibiotics These drugs reduce the effect of proguanil with atovaquone.

SPECIAL PRECAUTIONS

Be sure to tell your doctor if:
◆ You have a long-term kidney problem.
◆ You have a liver problem.
◆ You are suffering from diarrhoea and vomiting.
◆ You are taking other medicines.

Pregnancy Safety in pregnancy not established, but benefits are generally considered to outweigh risks. Folic acid supplements must be taken. Discuss with your doctor.

Breast-feeding The drug passes into breast milk and may affect the baby. Breast-feeding is not recommended; the drug will not protect your baby from malaria. Discuss with your doctor.

Infants and children Reduced dose necessary.

Over 60 No known problems.

Driving and hazardous work Avoid until you know how the drug affects you because it may cause dizziness.

Alcohol No special problems.

PROLONGED USE

No known problems.

Promazine

Brand names None
Used in the following combined preparations None

QUICK REFERENCE

Drug group Anti-anxiety drug (p.13) and antipsychotic drug (p.15)
Overdose danger rating Medium
Dependence rating Low
Prescription needed Yes
Available as generic Yes

GENERAL INFORMATION

Promazine, introduced in the late 1950s, is a member of a group of drugs called phenothiazines, which act on the brain to regulate abnormal behaviour.

The main use of promazine is to calm agitated and restless behaviour. It is also given as a sedative for the short-term treatment of severe anxiety, especially that which occurs in the elderly and during terminal illness.

Promazine is less likely to cause parkinsonism (abnormal movements and shaking of the arms and legs) and other side effects experienced with other phenothiazines.

INFORMATION FOR USERS

Your drug prescription is tailored for you. Do not alter dosage without checking with your doctor.

How taken/used Tablets, liquid.
Frequency and timing of doses 4 x daily.
Adult dosage range 100–800mg daily (tablets).
Onset of effect 30 minutes–1 hour.
Duration of action 4–6 hours.
Diet advice None.
Storage Keep in original container at room temperature out of the reach of children. Protect from light.
Missed dose Take as soon as you remember. If your next dose is due within 2 hours, take a single dose now and skip the next.
Stopping the drug Do not stop the drug without consulting your doctor; symptoms may recur.
Exceeding the dose An occasional unintentional extra dose is unlikely to be a cause for concern. Large overdoses may cause drowsiness, dizziness, unsteadiness, fits, and coma. Notify your doctor.

POSSIBLE ADVERSE EFFECTS

Drowsiness, lethargy, dry mouth, constipation, and blurred vision are common and may be helped by dosage reduction. Rarely, the drug may affect the body's ability to regulate temperature (especially in the elderly). Parkinsonism is less common; discuss this with your doctor. If jaundice occurs, stop taking the drug and consult your doctor at once.

INTERACTIONS

Sedatives All drugs that have a sedative effect are likely to increase the sedative properties of promazine.

Drugs for parkinsonism Promazine may reduce the effectiveness of these drugs.

SPECIAL PRECAUTIONS
Be sure to tell your doctor if:
◆ You have heart problems.
◆ You have long-term liver or kidney problems.
◆ You have had epileptic fits.
◆ You have prostate problems.
◆ You have glaucoma.
◆ You have Parkinson's disease.
◆ You are taking other medicines.

Pregnancy Safety in pregnancy not established. Discuss with your doctor.
Breast-feeding Safety in breast-feeding not established. Discuss with your doctor.
Infants and children Not recommended.
Over 60 Increased likelihood of adverse effects. Reduced dose may therefore be necessary.
Driving and hazardous work Avoid such activities until you have learned how promazine affects you because the drug can cause drowsiness and reduced alertness.
Alcohol Avoid. Alcohol may increase the sedative effect of this drug.

PROLONGED USE
Use of this drug for more than a few months may be associated with jaundice and abnormal movements. Sometimes a reduction in dose may be recommended.
Monitoring Periodic blood tests and eye examinations should be performed.

Promethazine

Brand names Avomine, Phenergan, Sominex
Used in the following combined preparations
Night Nurse, Tixylix Night-time

QUICK REFERENCE
Drug group Antihistamine (p.58) and anti-emetic (p.21)
Overdose danger rating Medium
Dependence rating Low
Prescription needed No (most preparations) Yes (injection)
Available as generic No

GENERAL INFORMATION
Promethazine is one of a class of drugs known as the phenothiazines, which were developed in the 1950s for their beneficial effect on abnormal behaviour arising from mental illnesses (see Antipsychotics, p.15). Promethazine was found, however, to have effects more like the antihistamines used to treat allergies (see p.58) and some types of nausea and vomiting (see Anti-emetics, p.21). The drug is widely used to reduce itching in a variety of skin conditions, including urticaria (hives), chickenpox, and eczema. It can also relieve the nausea and vomiting caused by inner ear disturbances such as Ménière's disease and motion sickness. Because of its sedative effect, promethazine is sometimes used for short periods as a sleeping medicine, and is also given as premedication before surgery.

Promethazine is used in combined preparations together with opioid cough suppressants for the relief of coughs and nasal congestion, and it is given at night for its sedative effect.

INFORMATION FOR USERS
Follow instructions on the label. Call your doctor if symptoms worsen.
How taken/used Tablets, liquid, injection.
Frequency and timing of doses *Allergic symptoms* 1–3 x daily or as a single dose at night. *Motion sickness* Bedtime on night before travelling, repeating following morning if necessary, then every 6–8 hours as necessary. *Nausea and vomiting* Every 4–6 hours as necessary.
Dosage range *Adults* 25–100mg per dose, depending on preparation and use. *Children* Reduced dose according to age.
Onset of effect Within 1 hour. If dose is taken after nausea has started, the onset of effect is delayed.
Duration of action 8–16 hours.
Diet advice None.
Storage Keep in original container at room temperature out of the reach of children. Protect from light.
Missed dose No cause for concern, but take as soon as you remember. Adjust the timing of your next dose accordingly.
Stopping the drug Can be safely stopped as soon as symptoms disappear.
Exceeding the dose An occasional unintentional extra dose is unlikely to cause problems. Large overdoses may cause drowsiness or agitation, fits, unsteadiness, and coma. Notify your doctor.

POSSIBLE ADVERSE EFFECTS

Promethazine usually causes only minor anticholinergic effects. More serious adverse effects generally occur only during long-term use or with abnormally high doses. Common adverse effects are drowsiness, lethargy, dry mouth, blurred vision, and urinary retention, which should be discussed with your doctor. Palpitations are less common, and, if they occur, you should consult your doctor. If you develop a light-sensitive rash, stop taking the drug and consult your doctor promptly.

INTERACTIONS

Sedatives All drugs that have a sedative effect are likely to increase the sedative properties of promethazine. Such drugs include other antihistamines, sleeping drugs, and antipsychotics.

Pregnancy urine test Promethazine may interfere with this test, giving a false result.

SPECIAL PRECAUTIONS

Be sure to consult your doctor or pharmacist before taking this drug if:
◆ You have liver or kidney problems.
◆ You have had epileptic fits.
◆ You have heart disease.
◆ You suffer from asthma or bronchitis.
◆ You are taking other medicines.

Pregnancy Occasionally used by specialist services. Discuss with your doctor.

Breast-feeding The drug passes into the breast milk, but at normal doses adverse effects on the baby are unlikely. Discuss with your doctor.

Infants and children Not recommended for infants under 2 years. Reduced dose necessary for older children.

Over 60 Reduced dose may be necessary.

Driving and hazardous work Avoid such activities until you have learned how promethazine affects you because the drug can cause drowsiness.

Alcohol Avoid. Alcohol may increase the sedative effects of this drug.

Sunlight Avoid exposure to strong sunlight because, rarely, skin reactions may occur.

PROLONGED USE

Use of this drug for long periods is rarely necessary.

Propranolol

Brand names Angilol, Bedranol, Beta-Prograne, Half Inderal, Inderal, Slo-Pro, Syprol, and others
Used in the following combined preparations None

QUICK REFERENCE

Drug group Beta blocker (p.30) and anti-anxiety drug (p.13)
Overdose danger rating High
Dependence rating Low
Prescription needed Yes
Available as generic Yes

GENERAL INFORMATION

Propranolol, introduced in 1965, was the first widely available beta blocker in the United Kingdom. It is mainly used to treat angina and abnormal heart rhythms and is helpful in controlling the fast heart rate and other symptoms of an overactive thyroid gland. It also helps to reduce the palpitations, sweating, and tremor of severe anxiety and to prevent migraine. The drug is also used to treat hypertension (high blood pressure) but is not usually used to initiate treatment.

Propranolol is not given to people with respiratory diseases because it can cause breathing difficulties. It should be used with caution by people with diabetes because, like all beta blockers, it affects the body's response to low blood glucose.

INFORMATION FOR USERS

Your drug prescription is tailored for you. Do not alter dosage without checking with your doctor.

How taken/used Tablets, SR-capsules, liquid, injection.

Frequency and timing of doses 2–4 x daily. Once daily (SR-capsules).

Adult dosage range *Abnormal heart rhythms* 30–160mg daily. *Angina* 80–240mg daily. *Hypertension* 160–320mg daily. *Migraine prevention and anxiety* 40–160mg daily.

Onset of effect 1–2 hours (tablets); after 4 hours (SR-capsules). In hypertension and migraine, it may be several weeks before full benefits of this drug are felt.

Duration of action 6–12 hours (tablets); 24–30 hours (SR-capsules).

Diet advice None.

Storage Keep in original container at room temperature out of the reach of children. Protect from light.

Missed dose Take as soon as you remember. If your next dose is due within 2 hours (tablets) or 12 hours (SR-capsules), take a single dose now and skip the next.

Stopping the drug Do not stop the drug without consulting your doctor. Abrupt cessation may lead to worsening of the underlying condition.

OVERDOSE ACTION

Seek immediate medical advice in all cases. Take emergency action if breathing difficulties, collapse, or loss of consciousness occur.

POSSIBLE ADVERSE EFFECTS

Propranolol has adverse effects, such as cold hands and feet, that are common to most beta blockers. Symptoms such as fatigue and nausea are usually temporary and diminish with long-term use. Fainting (which may be a sign that the drug has slowed the heart beat excessively), nightmares, vivid dreams, dry eyes, and visual disturbances are rare; if they occur, stop taking the drug and consult your doctor immediately.

INTERACTIONS

Antihypertensive drugs Propranolol may enhance the blood pressure lowering effect.

Diltiazem and verapamil Combining either of these drugs with propranolol may have adverse effects on heart function.

Cimetidine and hydralazine These drugs may increase the effects of propranolol.

Non-steroidal anti-inflammatory drugs (NSAIDs) (e.g. indometacin) may reduce the antihypertensive effect of propranolol.

SPECIAL PRECAUTIONS

Be sure to tell your doctor if:
◆ You have long-term liver or kidney problems.
◆ You have a breathing disorder such as asthma, bronchitis, or emphysema.
◆ You have heart failure.
◆ You have diabetes.
◆ You have poor circulation in the legs.

◆ You are taking other medicines.

Pregnancy May affect the baby. Discuss with your doctor.

Breast-feeding The drug passes into the breast milk, but at normal doses adverse effects on the baby are unlikely. Discuss with your doctor.

Infants and children Reduced dose necessary.

Over 60 Increased risk of adverse effects. Reduced starting dose will therefore be necessary.

Driving and hazardous work No special problems.

Alcohol No special problems.

Surgery and general anaesthetics Propranolol may need to be stopped before you have a general anaesthetic. Discuss this with your doctor or dentist before any surgery.

PROLONGED USE

No problems expected.

Propylthiouracil

Brand names None
Used in the following combined preparations None

QUICK REFERENCE

Drug group Drug for thyroid disorders (p.84)
Overdose danger rating Medium
Dependence rating Low
Prescription needed Yes
Available as generic Yes

GENERAL INFORMATION

Propylthiouracil is an antithyroid drug used to manage an overactive thyroid gland (hyperthyroidism). In some people, particularly those with Graves' disease (the most common form of the disorder), drug treatment alone may bring on a remission. Propylthiouracil may also be prescribed for long-term treatment of the disease in people who may be at special risk from surgery, such as children and pregnant women.

The drug is also used to restore the normal functioning of the thyroid gland before its partial removal by surgery. It is sometimes given with thyroxine in order to prevent the development of hypothyroidism (low thyroid hormone levels). Propylthiouracil is preferred to other antithyroid drugs when treatment is essential during pregnancy.

The most important adverse effect that sometimes occurs is a reduction in white blood cells, leading to the risk of infection. If you develop a sore throat or mouth ulceration, see your doctor immediately; this might be a sign that your blood is being affected.

INFORMATION FOR USERS

Your drug prescription is tailored for you. Do not alter dosage without consulting your doctor.

How taken/used Tablets.

Frequency and timing of doses 1–3 x daily.

Dosage range Initially 200–400mg daily. Usually the dose can be reduced to 50–150mg daily.

Onset of effect 10–20 days. Full beneficial effects may not be felt for 6–10 weeks.

Duration of action 24–36 hours.

Diet advice Your doctor may advise you to avoid foods high in iodine (see Minerals, p.93).

Storage Keep in original container at room temperature out of the reach of children. Protect from light.

Missed dose Take as soon as you remember. If your next dose is due within 3 hours, take a single dose now and skip the next.

Stopping the drug Do not stop the drug without consulting your doctor; stopping the drug may lead to a recurrence of hyperthyroidism.

Exceeding the dose An occasional unintentional extra dose is unlikely to cause problems. Large overdoses may cause nausea, vomiting, and headache. Notify your doctor.

POSSIBLE ADVERSE EFFECTS

Serious side effects are rare. Rash, itching, headache, nausea, and joint pain are fairly common. A sore throat, fever, or jaundice may indicate adverse effects on the blood. If these occur, stop taking the drug and inform your doctor immediately.

INTERACTIONS

Anticoagulants Propylthiouracil may reduce the effects of oral anticoagulants.

SPECIAL PRECAUTIONS

Be sure to tell your doctor if:
◆ You have long-term liver or kidney problems.

◆ You are pregnant.
◆ You are taking other medicines.

Pregnancy Prescribed with caution. Risk of goitre and thyroid hormone deficiency (hypothyroidism) in the newborn infant if too high a dose is used. Discuss with your doctor.

Breast-feeding The drug passes into the breast milk and may affect the baby. Discuss with your doctor.

Infants and children Not recommended under 6 years. Reduced dose necessary in older children.

Over 60 No special problems.

Driving and hazardous work No problems expected.

Alcohol No known problems.

PROLONGED USE

High doses of propylthiouracil over a prolonged period may reduce the number of white blood cells.

Monitoring Periodic tests of thyroid function are usually required, and blood cell counts may also be carried out.

Pyridostigmine

Brand name Mestinon
Used in the following combined preparations None

QUICK REFERENCE

Drug group Drug for myasthenia gravis (p.55)
Overdose danger rating High
Dependence rating Low
Prescription needed Yes
Available as generic No

GENERAL INFORMATION

Pyridostigmine is used to treat a rare auto immune condition, known as myasthenia gravis, which involves the faulty transmission of nerve impulses to the muscles. Pyridostigmine improves muscle strength by prolonging nerve signals, although it does not cure the underlying disease. In severe cases, the drug may be prescribed with corticosteroids or other drugs. Pyridostigmine may also be given to reverse temporary paralysis of the bowel and urinary retention following an operation.

Side effects, including abdominal cramps, nausea, and diarrhoea, usually disappear on reduction of the dosage of pyridostigmine.

INFORMATION FOR USERS

Your drug prescription is tailored for you. Do not alter dosage without checking with your doctor.

How taken/used Tablets.

Frequency and timing of doses Every 3–4 hours initially. Thereafter, according to the needs of the individual.

Dosage range *Adults* 300mg–1.2g daily (by mouth) according to response and side effects. *Children* Reduced dose necessary according to age and weight.

Onset of effect 30–60 minutes.

Duration of action 3–6 hours.

Diet advice None.

Storage Keep in original container at room temperature out of the reach of children. Protect from light.

Missed dose Take as soon as you remember. If your next dose is due within 2 hours, take a single dose now and skip the next.

Stopping the drug Do not stop taking the drug without consulting your doctor; symptoms may recur.

OVERDOSE ACTION

Seek immediate medical advice in all cases. You may experience severe abdominal cramps, vomiting, weakness, and tremor. Take emergency action if troubled breathing, unusually slow heart beat, fits, or loss of consciousness occur.

POSSIBLE ADVERSE EFFECTS

Adverse effects of pyridostigmine are usually dose-related and can be avoided by adjusting the dose. Nausea, vomiting, increased salivation, and sweating are common, as are abdominal cramps and diarrhoea, which should be discussed with your doctor. Watering eyes and small pupils, and hypersensitivity (leading to an allergic rash), are rare; consult your doctor.

INTERACTIONS

General note Drugs that suppress the transmission of nerve signals may oppose the effect of pyridostigmine. Such drugs include aminoglycoside antibiotics, digoxin, procainamide, quinidine, lithium, and chloroquine. **Hydrocortisone and prednisolone** may decrease pyridostigmine's effectiveness.

SPECIAL PRECAUTIONS

Be sure to tell your doctor if:
◆ You have a long-term kidney problem.
◆ You have heart problems.
◆ You have had epileptic fits.
◆ You have asthma.
◆ You have difficulty in passing urine.
◆ You have a peptic ulcer.
◆ You have Parkinson's disease.
◆ You are taking other medicines.

Pregnancy No evidence of risk to the developing fetus in the first 6 months. Large doses near the time of delivery may cause premature labour and temporary muscle weakness in the baby. Discuss with your doctor.

Breast-feeding No evidence of risk, but the baby should be monitored for signs of muscle weakness.

Infants and children Reduced dose necessary, calculated according to age and weight.

Over 60 Reduced dose may need to be given. Increased likelihood of adverse effects.

Driving and hazardous work Your underlying condition may make such activities inadvisable. Discuss with your doctor.

Alcohol No special problems.

Surgery and general anaesthetics Pyridostigmine interacts with some anaesthetic agents. Notify your doctor or dentist that you are taking it before any surgery.

PROLONGED USE

No problems expected.

Pyrimethamine

Brand name Daraprim
Used in the following combined preparation Fansidar

QUICK REFERENCE

Drug group Antimalarial drug (p.75)
Overdose danger rating Medium
Dependence rating Low
Prescription needed Yes
Available as generic No

GENERAL INFORMATION

Pyrimethamine is an antimalarial drug. Because malaria parasites can readily develop resistance to pyrimethamine, the drug is now always given combined with the antibacterial drug sulfadoxine (Fansidar) for the treatment of malaria. The activity of the combination greatly exceeds that of either drug alone. Fansidar is used with quinine in the treatment of malaria. Pyrimethamine is not used for the prevention of malaria. Pyrimethamine is sometimes given with another drug, sulfadiazine, to treat toxoplasmosis in people with lowered immunity. Such treatment must be supervised by an expert.

Blood disorders can sometimes arise during prolonged treatment, and, because of this, blood counts are monitored regularly and vitamin supplements are given.

INFORMATION FOR USERS

Your drug prescription is tailored for you. Do not alter dosage without checking with your doctor.

How taken/used Tablets.

Frequency and timing of doses Once only, daily, or weekly, depending on condition treated.

Dosage range *Adults* Depends on condition being treated. *Children* Reduced dose necessary according to age.

Onset of effect 24 hours.

Duration of action Up to 1 week.

Diet advice None.

Storage Keep in original container at room temperature out of the reach of children. Protect from light.

Missed dose If you are being treated for toxoplasmosis, take as soon as you remember. If your next dose is due within 24 hours, take a single dose now and alter the dosing day so that your next dose is one week later.

Stopping the drug Do not stop taking the drug without discussing it with your doctor.

Exceeding the dose An occasional unintentional extra dose is unlikely to cause problems. Large overdoses may cause trembling, breathing difficulty, fits, blood disorders, and vomiting. Notify your doctor.

POSSIBLE ADVERSE EFFECTS

Loss of appetite, insomnia, gastric irritation, and a rash may occur and should be discussed with your doctor. Unusual tiredness, weakness, bleeding, bruising, and a sore throat may be signs of a blood disorder; notify your doctor immediately if they occur. Breathing difficulties or signs of a chest infection should also be reported to your doctor immediately.

INTERACTIONS

General note Drugs that suppress the bone marrow or cause folic acid deficiency may increase the risk of serious blood disorders when they are taken with pyrimethamine. Such drugs include anticancer drugs, antirheumatic drugs, sulfasalazine, co-trimoxazole, trimethoprim, phenytoin, and phenylbutazone.

SPECIAL PRECAUTIONS

Be sure to tell your doctor if:
◆ You have long-term liver or kidney problems.
◆ You have had epileptic fits.
◆ You have anaemia.
◆ You are allergic to sulphonamides.
◆ You have glucose-6-phosphate dehydrogenase (G6PD) deficiency.
◆ You are taking other medicines.

Pregnancy Pyrimethamine may cause deficiency of folic acid in the unborn baby. Pregnant women receiving this drug should take a folic acid supplement. Discuss this with your doctor.

Breast-feeding The drug passes into the breast milk, but at normal doses adverse effects on the baby are unlikely. Discuss with your doctor.

Infants and children Reduced dose necessary.

Over 60 No special problems.

Driving and hazardous work No special problems.

Alcohol No known problems.

Sunlight Avoid excessive exposure to sunlight.

PROLONGED USE

Prolonged use of pyrimethamine may cause folic acid deficiency, leading to serious blood disorders. Folic acid supplements may be recommended (in the form of folinic acid).

Monitoring Regular blood cell counts are required during high-dose or long-term treatment with pyrimethamine.

Quetiapine

Brand name Seroquel
Used in the following combined preparations None

QUICK REFERENCE

Drug group Antipsychotic drug (p.15)
Overdose danger rating Medium
Dependence rating Low
Prescription needed Yes
Available as generic No

GENERAL INFORMATION

Quetiapine is an atypical antipsychotic drug that is prescribed for the treatment of schizophrenia and mania. It can be used to treat "positive" symptoms (thought disorders, delusions, and hallucinations) and "negative" symptoms (blunted affect and emotional and social withdrawal in schizophrenia).

Elderly people excrete quetiapine up to 50 per cent more slowly than the usual adult rate. They therefore need to be prescribed much lower doses in order for them to avoid adverse effects.

INFORMATION FOR USERS

Your drug prescription is tailored for you. Do not alter dosage without checking with your doctor.

How taken/used Tablets.
Frequency and timing of doses 2 x daily.
Adult dosage range *Schizophrenia* 50mg daily (starting dose). *Mania* 100mg daily (starting dose). The dose is increased over several days (both). Usual range is 300–450mg daily, maximum 750mg daily (schizophrenia); 800mg (mania).
Onset of effect 1 hour.
Duration of action Up to 12 hours.
Diet advice None.
Storage Keep in original container at room temperature out of the reach of children.
Missed dose Take as soon as you remember. If your next dose is due within 4 hours take a single dose now and skip the next.
Stopping the drug Do not stop the drug without consulting your doctor; symptoms may recur.
Exceeding the dose An occasional unintentional extra dose is unlikely to cause problems. Large overdoses may cause unusual drowsiness, palpitations, and low blood pressure. Notify your doctor.

POSSIBLE ADVERSE EFFECTS

Unusual drowsiness, weight gain, and digestive disturbance are common adverse effects of treatment with quetiapine. Dizziness and fainting, which are also common, should be discussed with your doctor. A persistent sore throat is a less common adverse effect, and, if it occurs, you should notify your doctor. If you experience palpitations, consult your doctor promptly.

INTERACTIONS

Antiepileptics Quetiapine may oppose the effect of these drugs. However, phenytoin and carbamazepine may also reduce the effects of quetiapine.
Sedatives All drugs that have a sedative effect on the central nervous system are likely to increase the sedative properties of quetiapine.

SPECIAL PRECAUTIONS

Be sure to tell your doctor if:
◆ You have epilepsy.
◆ You have diabetes.
◆ You have liver or kidney problems.
◆ You have heart problems.
◆ You are taking other medicines.
Pregnancy Safety not established. Discuss with your doctor.
Breast-feeding Safety not established. Discuss with your doctor.
Infants and children Not recommended.
Over 60 Reduced doses necessary. The elderly eliminate quetiapine more slowly than younger adults.
Driving and hazardous work Avoid such activities until you have learned how quetiapine affects you because the drug can cause drowsiness.
Alcohol Avoid. Alcohol increases the sedative effects of this drug.

PROLONGED USE

Prolonged use of quetiapine has been reported to produce tardive dyskinesia (in which there are involuntary movements of the tongue and face).

Quinine

Brand names None
Used in the following combined preparations None

QUICK REFERENCE

Drug group Antimalarial drug (p.75) and muscle relaxant (p.54)
Overdose danger rating High
Dependence rating Low
Prescription needed Yes
Available as generic Yes

GENERAL INFORMATION

Quinine, obtained from the bark of the cinchona tree, is the earliest antimalarial drug. It often causes side effects, but is still given for cases of malaria that are resistant to safer treatments. Owing to the resistance of malaria parasites to chloroquine and some of the more modern antimalarials, quinine remains the mainstay of treatment, but it is not used as a preventative.

At the high doses used to treat malaria, quinine may cause ringing in the ears, headaches, nausea, hearing loss, and blurred vision: a group of symptoms known as cinchonism. In rare cases, the drug may cause bleeding into the skin as a result of reduced blood platelets.

In many countries quinine is often used, in small doses, to prevent painful night-time leg cramps.

INFORMATION FOR USERS

Your drug prescription is tailored for you. Do not alter dosage without checking with your doctor.
How taken/used Tablets, injection.
Frequency and timing of doses *Malaria* Every 8 hours. *Muscle cramps* Once daily at bedtime.
Adult dosage range 1.8g daily (malaria); 200–300mg daily (cramps).
Onset of effect 1–2 days (malaria); up to 4 weeks (cramps).
Duration of action Up to 24 hours.
Diet advice None.
Storage Keep in original container at room temperature out of the reach of children. Protect from light.
Missed dose Take as soon as you remember.

If your next dose is due within 4 hours, skip the missed one and return to your normal dosing schedule thereafter.
Stopping the drug If the drug is prescribed for malaria, take the full course. Even if you feel better, the original infection may still be present and may recur if treatment is stopped too soon. If taken for muscle cramps, the drug can safely be stopped as soon as you no longer need it.

OVERDOSE ACTION

Seek immediate medical advice in all cases. Take emergency action if breathing problems, fits, or loss of consciousness occur.

POSSIBLE ADVERSE EFFECTS

Adverse effects are unlikely with low doses. At antimalarial doses, hearing disturbances, headache, and blurred vision are more common. Nausea and diarrhoea may also occur. If you develop a rash, itching, hearing loss, or blurred vision, stop taking the drug and consult your doctor immediately.

INTERACTIONS

Digoxin Quinine increases blood levels of digoxin; the dose of digoxin should be reduced. Discuss with your doctor.
Cimetidine This drug increases the blood levels of quinine.

SPECIAL PRECAUTIONS

Be sure to consult your doctor if:
◆ You have a long-term kidney problem.
◆ You have tinnitus (ringing in the ears).
◆ You have optic neuritis.
◆ You have myasthenia gravis.
◆ You have glucose-6-phosphate dehydrogenase (G6PD) deficiency.
◆ You have heart problems.
◆ You have diabetes.
◆ You are taking other medicines.
Pregnancy Not usually prescribed. May cause defects in the unborn baby. Discuss with your doctor.
Breast-feeding The drug passes into the breast milk, but at normal doses adverse effects on the baby are unlikely. Discuss with your doctor.
Infants and children Reduced dose necessary.
Over 60 No special problems.

Driving and hazardous work Avoid these activities until you know how quinine affects you; the drug's side effects may distract you.
Alcohol No known problems.

PROLONGED USE

No problems expected with low doses used to control night-time leg cramps. Treatment may be stopped after 3 months to assess the need to continue.

Rabeprazole

Brand name Pariet
Used in the following combined preparations
None

QUICK REFERENCE

Drug group Anti-ulcer drug (p.43)
Overdose danger rating Low
Dependence rating Low
Prescription needed Yes
Available as generic No

GENERAL INFORMATION

Rabeprazole belongs to a class of anti-ulcer drugs known as proton pump inhibitors (see p.43). Because the drug inhibits the secretion of gastric acid, it is used to treat gastro-oesophageal reflux disease (GORD), also called heartburn, and to help prevent it from recurring. It may also be used in the treatment of Zollinger–Ellison syndrome (a condition in which the stomach produces extremely high amounts of acid).

Rabeprazole may also be used to treat active duodenal and peptic ulcers by protecting them from the action of stomach acid, allowing them to heal. It is also used in combination with antibiotics to eradicate *Helicobacter pylori* bacteria in patients with peptic ulcer disease. Rabeprazole is also occasionally prescribed to people who have the gastrointestinal adverse effects associated with non-steroidal anti-inflammatory drugs (NSAIDs) but need to continue NSAID treatment.

INFORMATION FOR USERS

Your drug prescription is tailored for you. Do not alter dosage without checking with your doctor.

How taken/used Tablets.
Frequency and timing of doses Once daily, generally in the morning, before food. Swallow whole; do not crush or chew.
Adult dosage range 10–20mg. Zollinger–Ellison syndrome 60–120mg.
Onset of effect 2–3 hours. Pain should improve in 2–3 days.
Duration of action 12–24 hours.
Diet advice None, but spicy foods and alcohol may exacerbate the condition being treated.
Storage Keep in original container at room temperature out of the reach of children.
Missed dose Take as soon as you remember, then return to your normal dosing schedule. Do not take an extra dose to make up.
Stopping the drug The drug can be safely stopped as soon as you no longer need it.
Exceeding the dose An occasional unintentional extra dose is unlikely to cause problems. If you notice unusual symptoms or a large overdose has been taken, notify your doctor.

POSSIBLE ADVERSE EFFECTS

Most common adverse effects of rabeprazole are mild and usually resolve without the need to discontinue treatment. They include headache, diarrhoea, abdominal pain, flatulence, and insomnia. A cough, bronchitis, and sinusitis are also common but should be discussed with your doctor. Jaundice is rare, but if it occurs, stop taking the drug and seek prompt medical attention.

INTERACTIONS

Itraconazole and ketoconazole Rabeprazole reduces the effects of these drugs.
Digoxin Rabeprazole may increase the effects of digoxin.
Warfarin Rabeprazole increases the anticoagulant effect of warfarin.
Atazanavir Rabeprazole can reduce the blood levels of this drug.

SPECIAL PRECAUTIONS

Be sure to tell your doctor if:
◆ You are allergic to other proton pump inhibitors.
◆ You think you might be pregnant, or you are breast-feeding.
◆ You have a history of liver disease.
◆ You are taking other medicines.

Pregnancy Not prescribed. Safety not established.

Breast-feeding Not recommended. It is not known whether the drug passes into the breast milk. Discuss with your doctor.

Infants and children Not recommended.

Over 60 No special problems.

Driving and hazardous work Do not undertake such activities until you have learned how rabeprazole affects you because the drug can cause drowsiness.

Alcohol Avoid. Alcohol irritates the stomach.

PROLONGED USE

No problems expected.

Raloxifene

Brand name Evista
Used in the following combined preparations None

QUICK REFERENCE

Drug group Drug for bone disorders (p.56)
Overdose danger rating Low
Dependence rating Low
Prescription needed Yes
Available as generic No

GENERAL INFORMATION

Raloxifene is a non-steroidal anti-oestrogen drug (oestrogen is a naturally occurring female sex hormone, see p.88) that is related to clomifene and tamoxifen. It is prescribed to prevent vertebral fractures in postmenopausal women who are at increased risk of osteoporosis. There is some evidence that the drug would also be useful for preventing fractures of the hip, but its use in the prevention of other bone fractures is uncertain.

Raloxifene has no beneficial effect on other menopausal problems such as hot flushes. It is not prescribed to women who might become pregnant because it may harm the unborn baby, and it is not prescribed to men.

There is an increased risk of a thrombosis (blood clot) developing in a vein in the leg, but the risk is similar to that due to HRT (see p.89). However, because of this risk, raloxifene is usually stopped if the woman taking it becomes immobile or bedbound, when clots are more likely to form. Treatment is restarted when full activity is resumed.

INFORMATION FOR USERS

Your drug prescription is tailored for you. Do not alter dosage without checking with your doctor.

How taken/used Tablets.

Frequency and timing of doses Once daily.

Adult dosage range 60mg daily.

Onset of effect 1–4 hours.

Duration of action 24–48 hours.

Diet advice Calcium supplements are recommended if dietary calcium is low.

Storage Keep in original container at room temperature out of the reach of children. Protect from light.

Missed dose Take as soon as you remember. If your next dose is due within 8 hours, take a single dose now and skip the next.

Stopping the drug Do not stop the drug without consulting your doctor except under conditions specified in advance, such as immobility, which increases the risk of blood clots forming.

Exceeding the dose An occasional unintentional extra dose is unlikely to be a cause for concern. But if you notice any unusual symptoms, or if a large overdose has been taken, notify your doctor.

POSSIBLE ADVERSE EFFECTS

Hot flushes, leg cramps, swollen ankles or feet, and flu-like symptoms are common adverse effects. Headache is rare and should be discussed with your doctor. A rash is also rare; and if you develop a rash, you should stop taking the drug. Some adverse effects of raloxifene are indications of a thrombosis (blood clot) in a vein in the leg. If a clot develops somewhere else in the body, there might not be any obvious symptoms. Rarely, you may experience pain, tenderness, swelling, discoloration, or ulceration of the leg, or inflammation of the capillaries. If any of these occur, stop taking the drug and seek immediate medical attention.

INTERACTIONS

Anticoagulants Raloxifene reduces the effect of warfarin and acenocoumarol (nicoumalone).

Colestyramine This drug reduces the absorption of raloxifene by the body.

SPECIAL PRECAUTIONS

Be sure to tell your doctor if:
◆ You have had a blood clot in a vein.
◆ You have uterine bleeding.
◆ You have liver or kidney problems.
◆ You are taking other medicines.

Pregnancy Not prescribed to premenopausal women.

Breast-feeding Not prescribed to premenopausal women.

Infants and children Not prescribed.

Over 60 No special problems.

Driving and hazardous work No special problems.

Alcohol No special problems.

PROLONGED USE

No special problems. Raloxifene is normally used long term.

Monitoring Liver function tests may be performed periodically.

Ramipril

Brand names Lopace, Tritace
Used in the following combined preparations
Triapin, Triapin mite

QUICK REFERENCE

Drug group ACE inhibitor vasodilator (p.31) and antihypertensive drug (p.36)
Overdose danger rating Medium
Dependence rating Low
Prescription needed Yes
Available as generic Yes

GENERAL INFORMATION

Ramipril belongs to a group of drugs known as ACE (angiotensin converting enzyme) inhibitors. It works by dilating the blood vessels, which enables the blood to circulate more easily. The drug is used to treat high blood pressure (see p.31) and to reduce the strain on the heart in patients with heart failure after a heart attack. The first dose of an ACE inhibitor can cause the blood pressure to drop very suddenly, so a few hours' bed rest afterwards may be advised. You may need to stay in hospital until you are stabilized on the treatment.

Side effects of ramipril, such as headache, nausea, and dizziness are usually mild. Like all ACE inhibitors, however, ramipril causes the body to retain potassium, an excess of which can cause a number of adverse effects (see Possible adverse effects, below).

INFORMATION FOR USERS

Your drug prescription is tailored for you. Do not alter dosage without checking with your doctor.

How taken/used Tablets, capsules.

Frequency and timing of doses *High blood pressure* Usually once daily. *Heart failure or after a heart attack* 1–2 x daily.

Adult dosage range *High blood pressure* 1.25–10mg daily. *Heart failure or after heart attack* 5–10mg daily.

Onset of effect Within 2 hours.

Duration of action Up to 24 hours.

Diet advice Your doctor may advise you to decrease your salt intake to help control your blood pressure.

Storage Keep in original container at room temperature out of the reach of children.

Missed dose Take as soon as you remember. If your next dose is due within 6 hours, take a single dose now and skip the next. Subsequently, continue with your usual routine.

Stopping the drug Do not stop taking the drug without consulting your doctor. Treatment of hypertension and heart failure is normally lifelong, it may be necessary to substitute alternative therapy.

Exceeding the dose If you notice any unusual symptoms or if a large overdose has been taken, notify your doctor.

POSSIBLE ADVERSE EFFECTS

Nausea, dizziness, and headache are common adverse effects of treatment with ramipril, but they are usually mild and transient. Also common are taste disturbance and an irritating dry cough (which can be minimized with smaller, more frequent doses, but it may be necessary for some people to stop taking the drug). Jaundice, a rash, and itching are rare but should be reported to your doctor. If you experience swelling of the face or mouth, breathing difficulties, chest pain, or unconsciousness, stop taking the drug and seek immediate medical attention.

INTERACTIONS

Non-steroidal anti-inflammatory drugs (NSAIDs) (e.g. ibuprofen) may reduce the antihypertensive effect of ramipril and increase the risk of kidney damage.

Ciclosporin increases the risk of high potassium levels in the blood.

Potassium supplements and potassium-sparing diuretics may cause excess levels of potassium in the body.

Lithium Like other ACE inhibitors, ramipril may raise blood lithium levels and toxicity.

SPECIAL PRECAUTIONS

Be sure to tell your doctor if:
◆ You have long-term liver or kidney problems.
◆ You have ever suffered from severe allergies or angioedema.
◆ You have had heart-valve problems.
◆ You have peripheral vascular disease or atherosclerosis.
◆ You suffer from systemic lupus erythematosus or scleroderma.
◆ You are taking other medicines.

Pregnancy Not usually prescribed. May cause defects in the unborn baby. Discuss with your doctor.

Breast-feeding The drug passes into the breast milk and may affect the baby adversely. Discuss with your doctor.

Infants and children Not recommended.

Over 60 Reduced dose may be necessary.

Driving and hazardous work Avoid such activities until you have learned how ramipril affects you because the drug may cause dizziness due to low blood pressure.

Alcohol Avoid. Alcohol may lower blood pressure further at first dose or dosage adjustment.

Surgery and general anaesthetics Notify your doctor or dentist that you are taking ramipril as anaesthetics can increase its effects.

PROLONGED USE

No problems expected.

Monitoring If you have other medical conditions, blood counts and kidney function tests may be performed at intervals.

Ranitidine

Brand names Gavilast, Ranitic, Ranitil, Rantec, Ranzac, Zantac
Used in the following combined preparations None

QUICK REFERENCE

Drug group Anti-ulcer drug (p.43)
Overdose danger rating Low
Dependence rating Low
Prescription needed No (tablets in limited quantities); Yes (other preparations)
Available as generic Yes

GENERAL INFORMATION

Ranitidine is prescribed in the treatment of stomach and duodenal ulcers. In combination with antibiotics, the drug is used for ulcers caused by *Helicobacter pylori* infection. It is also used to protect against duodenal (but not stomach) ulcers in people taking NSAIDs (see p.50), who may be prone to ulcers. This drug reduces the discomfort and ulceration of reflux oesophagitis, and may prevent stress ulceration and gastric bleeding in severely ill patients. Ranitidine reduces the amount of stomach acid produced, allowing ulcers to heal. It is usually given in courses lasting 4–8 weeks, with further courses if symptoms recur.

Ranitidine does not affect the actions of enzymes in the liver, where many drugs are broken down. Consequently, unlike the similar drug cimetidine, ranitidine does not increase blood levels of other drugs such as anticoagulants and anticonvulsants, which might reduce the effectiveness of treatment.

Most people experience no serious effects during ranitidine treatment. As it promotes healing of the stomach lining, there is a risk that ranitidine may mask stomach cancer, delaying diagnosis. It is therefore usually prescribed only when the possibility of stomach cancer has been ruled out.

INFORMATION FOR USERS

Your drug prescription is tailored for you. Do not alter dosage without checking with your doctor.

How taken/used Tablets, effervescent tablets, liquid, injection.

Frequency and timing of doses Once daily at bedtime or 2–3 x daily.

Adult dosage range 150mg–6g daily, depending on the condition being treated. Usual dose is 150mg twice daily.

Onset of effect Within 1 hour.

Duration of action 12 hours.

Diet advice None.

Storage Keep in original container at room temperature out of the reach of children. Protect from light.

Missed dose Take as soon as you remember. If your next dose is due within 3 hours, take a single dose now and skip the next.

Stopping the drug Do not stop taking the drug without consulting your doctor; symptoms may recur.

Exceeding the dose An occasional unintentional extra dose is unlikely to be a cause for concern. But if you notice any unusual symptoms, or if a large overdose has been taken, notify your doctor.

POSSIBLE ADVERSE EFFECTS

Adverse effects of ranitidine, of which headache and dizziness are the most common, are usually related to the dosage level and almost always disappear when treatment has finished. Nausea, vomiting, constipation, diarrhoea, jaundice, and mental problems may occur rarely; jaundice and mental problems should be discussed with your doctor. If you develop a sore throat or fever, contact your doctor immediately.

INTERACTIONS

Ketoconazole Ranitidine may reduce the absorption of ketoconazole. Ranitidine should be taken at least 2 hours after ketoconazole.

Sucralfate High doses (2g) of sucralfate may reduce the absorption of ranitidine. Sucralfate should be taken at least 2 hours after ranitidine.

SPECIAL PRECAUTIONS

Be sure to tell your doctor if:
◆ You have long-term liver or kidney problems.
◆ You have porphyria.
◆ You are taking other medicines.

Pregnancy Safety in pregnancy not established. Discuss with your doctor.

Breast-feeding The drug passes into the breast milk and may affect the baby. Discuss with your doctor.

Infants and children Reduced dose necessary.

Over 60 No special problems.

Driving and hazardous work No known problems. Dizziness can occur in a very small proportion of patients.

Alcohol Avoid. Alcohol may aggravate your underlying condition and reduce the beneficial effects of this drug.

PROLONGED USE

No problems expected.

Repaglinide

Brand name NovoNorm
Used in the following combined preparations None

QUICK REFERENCE

Drug group Oral antidiabetic drug (p.82)
Overdose danger rating Medium
Dependence rating Low
Prescription needed Yes
Available as generic No

GENERAL INFORMATION

Repaglinide is a drug used to treat non-insulin dependent diabetes that cannot be adequately controlled by diet and exercise alone. It acts in a similar manner to sulphonylurea drugs by stimulating the release of insulin from the pancreas. Therefore, some of the pancreatic cells need to be functioning in order for it to be effective.

Repaglinide is quick acting, but its effects last for only about 4 hours. The drug is sometimes given together with metformin if the metformin is not providing adequate diabetic control.

It is best to take repaglinide just before a meal in order for the insulin that is released to cope with the food. If a meal is likely to be missed, then the dose of repaglinide should not be taken. If a tablet has been taken and a meal is not forthcoming, some carbohydrate (as specified by your doctor or dietitian) should be eaten as soon as possible.

INFORMATION FOR USERS

Your drug prescription is tailored for you. Do not alter dosage without checking with your doctor.

How taken/used Tablets.

Frequency and timing of doses 1–4 x daily (up to 30 minutes before a meal, and up to 4 meals a day). If you are going to miss a meal, do not take the tablet.

Adult dosage range 500mcg (starting dose), increased at intervals of 1–2 weeks according to response; 4–16mg daily (maintenance dose).

Onset of effect 30 minutes.

Duration of action 4 hours.

Diet advice Follow the diet advised by your doctor or dietitian.

Storage Keep in original container at room temperature out of the reach of children.

Missed dose Do not take tablets between meals. Discuss with your doctor.

Stopping the drug Do not stop taking the drug without consulting your doctor.

Exceeding the dose An overdose will cause hypoglycaemia with dizziness, sweating, trembling, confusion, and headache. Notify your doctor.

POSSIBLE ADVERSE EFFECTS

Intestinal problems are common at the start of treatment with repaglinide. However, such adverse effects tend to become less troublesome as treatment continues. Nausea, vomiting, abdominal pain, diarrhoea, or constipation are common. If, rarely, a rash or itching occur, consult your doctor.

INTERACTIONS

Clarithromycin, itraconazole, ketoconazole, monoamine oxidase inhibitors (MAOIs), trimethoprim, beta blockers, ACE inhibitors, salicylates, and non-steroidal anti-inflammatory drugs (NSAIDs) These may enhance and/or prolong the hypoglycaemic effect of repaglinide.

Oral contraceptives, thiazide diuretics, corticosteroids, thyroid hormones, danazol, sympathomimetics, rifampicin, barbiturates and carbamazepine These drugs may decrease the effect of repaglinide.

SPECIAL PRECAUTIONS

Be sure to tell your doctor if:

◆ You have liver or kidney problems.

◆ You are taking other medicines.

Pregnancy Safety not established. Discuss with your doctor.

Breast-feeding Safety not established. Discuss with your doctor.

Infants and children Not recommended.

Over 60 No special problems, but safety not established over 75 years.

Driving and hazardous work Avoid such activities until you have learned how repaglinide affects you, as you are likely to experience low blood glucose without warning signs.

Alcohol Avoid. Alcohol may upset diabetic control and may increase and prolong the effects of repaglinide.

PROLONGED USE

No special problems. Repaglinide is usually prescribed indefinitely.

Rifampicin

Brand names Rifadin, Rimactane
Used in the following combined preparations Rifater, Rifinah, Rimactazid

QUICK REFERENCE

Drug group Antituberculous drug (p.67)
Overdose danger rating Medium
Dependence rating Low
Prescription needed Yes
Available as generic Yes

GENERAL INFORMATION

Rifampicin is an antibacterial drug that is highly effective in the treatment of tuberculosis. Taken by mouth, the drug is well absorbed in the intestine and widely distributed throughout the body, including the brain. As a result, it is particularly useful in the treatment of tuberculous meningitis.

Rifampicin is also used to treat leprosy (see Drug treatment for Hansen's disease, p.67) and other serious infections, including Legionnaires' disease and infections of the bone (osteomyelitis). Additionally, the drug is given to anyone who comes into close contact with a person with meningococcal meningitis to prevent infection. Rifampicin is always prescribed together with other antibiotics or antituberculous drugs because of rapid resistance in some bacteria.

A red-orange coloration may be imparted to the urine, saliva, and tears, and soft contact lenses may become permanently stained. This is harmless, however.

INFORMATION FOR USERS

Your drug prescription is tailored for you. Do not alter dosage without checking with your doctor.

How taken/used Tablets, capsules, liquid, injection.

Frequency and timing of doses 1 x daily, 30 minutes before breakfast (leprosy, tuberculosis) or once a month (leprosy); 2 x daily (prevention of meningococcal meningitis); 2–4 x daily, 30 minutes before or 2 hours after meals (other serious infections).

Adult dosage range According to weight; usually 450–600mg daily (for tuberculosis and leprosy) or 600mg once a month (for leprosy); 600mg–1.2g daily (for other serious infections); 1.2g daily for 2 days (for meningococcal meningitis).

Onset of effect Over several days.

Duration of action Up to 24 hours.

Diet advice None.

Storage Keep in original container at room temperature out of the reach of children. Protect from light.

Missed dose Take as soon as you remember. If your next dose is due within 6 hours, take a single dose now, then return to normal dosing schedule.

Stopping the drug Take the full course. Even if you feel better, the original infection may still be present and symptoms may recur if the treatment is stopped too soon. In rare cases stopping the drug suddenly after treatment with high doses can lead to a severe flu-like illness.

Exceeding the dose An occasional unintentional extra dose is unlikely to cause problems. Large overdoses may cause liver damage, nausea, vomiting, and lethargy. Notify your doctor immediately.

POSSIBLE ADVERSE EFFECTS

Serious adverse effects are rare with rifampicin. A red-orange discoloration of body fluids normally occurs, but this is harmless. Headache and breathing difficulties may occur after treatment with high doses is stopped. Rarely, you may experience nausea, vomiting, or diarrhoea. Muscle cramps or aches, a rash, and itching are also rare; and if any of these occur, you should consult your doctor. Rarely, you may develop jaundice, which usually improves during treatment; but you should report it to your doctor if it occurs. If, rarely, you develop any flu-like symptoms, stop taking the drug and consult your doctor immediately.

INTERACTIONS

General note Rifampicin may reduce the effectiveness of a wide variety of drugs, such as oral contraceptives (in which case alternative contraceptive methods may be necessary), phenytoin, corticosteroids, oral antidiabetics, disopyramide, and oral anticoagulants. Dosage adjustment of these drugs may be necessary at the start or end of treatment with rifampicin. Consult your doctor or pharmacist for advice.

SPECIAL PRECAUTIONS

Be sure to tell your doctor if:
◆ You have a long-term liver or kidney problem.
◆ You have porphyria.
◆ You wear contact lenses.
◆ You are taking other medicines.

Pregnancy Safety in pregnancy not established. Discuss with your doctor.

Breast-feeding The drug passes into the breast milk, but at normal doses adverse effects on the baby are unlikely. Discuss with your doctor.

Infants and children Reduced dose necessary.

Over 60 Increased risk of adverse effects. Reduced dose may therefore be necessary.

Driving and hazardous work No problems expected.

Alcohol Avoid excessive amounts. Heavy consumption of alcohol may increase the risk of liver damage.

PROLONGED USE

Prolonged use of rifampicin may cause liver damage.

Monitoring Periodic blood tests may be performed to monitor liver function.

Rimonabant

Brand name Acomplia
Used in the following combined preparations
None

QUICK REFERENCE
Drug group Cannabinoid blocker for obesity
Overdose danger rating Low
Dependence rating Low
Prescription needed Yes
Available as generic No

GENERAL INFORMATION

Rimonabant is prescribed, in combination with diet and exercise, for the treatment of obesity. It is centrally acting, and reduces appetite by blocking receptors in the brain known as cannabinoid-1 (CB1) receptors.

Rimonabant has particular advantages for people with diabetes mellitus. Apart from reducing weight, it may also reduce key risk factors, including certain cholesterol markers and HbA1c (an important reference for determining the severity of diabetes and effective management of disease).

Rimonabant is prescribed to people with a body mass index (BMI) above 30kg/m^2, or those with a BMI above 27kg/m^2 with associated risk factors, such as Type 2 diabetes or dyslipidaemia (cholesterol abnormalities).

Because the presence of food reduces rimonabant's effectiveness, the drug should be taken first thing in the morning on an empty stomach.

INFORMATION FOR USERS

Your drug prescription is tailored for you. Do not alter dosage without checking with your doctor.
How taken/used Tablets.
Frequency and timing of doses Once daily in the morning, before food.
Adult dosage range 20mg.
Onset of effect 2–4 weeks.
Duration of action 24 hours.
Diet advice It is important that you adhere to a reduced-calorie diet; your doctor will advise you on a diet that is specific to your condition.
Storage Keep in original container at room temperature out of the reach of children.

Missed dose Take as soon as you remember, then return to your normal dosing schedule. Do not take an extra dose to make up.
Stopping the drug The drug can be safely stopped as soon as you no longer need it.
Exceeding the dose An occasional unintentional extra dose is unlikely to be a cause for concern. However, if you notice any unusual symptoms, or if a large overdose has been taken, notify your doctor.

POSSIBLE ADVERSE EFFECTS

Adverse effects of rimonabant are generally mild and transient. Nausea, digestive disturbance, vomiting, upper respiratory tract infection, sleep disturbances, back or muscle pain, and memory loss are common. Depression, irritability, and anxiety are also common but should be discussed with your doctor. If, rarely, excessive sweating, altered sensation to the hands or feet, anger, and restlessness occur, consult your doctor. If itching occurs, stop taking the drug and consult your doctor immediately.

INTERACTIONS

Erythromycin, clarithromycin, itraconazole, keto-conazole, atazanavir, and ritonavir may increase the effects of rimonabant.
Antiepileptics (e.g. carbamazepine, phenytoin, and primidone) may reduce the effects of rimonabant.

SPECIAL PRECAUTIONS

Be sure to tell your doctor if:
◆ You are allergic to rimonabant.
◆ You have liver or kidney problems.
◆ You have epilepsy.
◆ You have depression or a psychotic illness.
◆ You are breast-feeding.
◆ You are taking other medicines.
Pregnancy Not prescribed.
Breast-feeding Not prescribed. Consult your doctor before starting treatment if you are breast-feeding.
Infants and children Not recommended.
Over 60 No special problems.
Driving and hazardous work Do not undertake such activities until you have learned how rimonabant affects you because the drug can cause fatigue.
Alcohol No special problems.

PROLONGED USE

Safety not established for long-term use.
Monitoring Periodic BMI measurements are usually carried out, and periodic liver-function tests may be performed.

Risedronate

Brand name Actonel
Used in the following combined preparations
None

QUICK REFERENCE

Drug group Drug for bone disorders (p.56)
Overdose danger rating Low
Dependence rating Low
Prescription needed Yes
Available as generic No

GENERAL INFORMATION

Risedronate belongs to a group of drugs known as bisphosphonates. Used in the treatment of bone disorders such as Paget's disease, the drug works directly on the bones by increasing the amount of calcium they absorb, thereby making them stronger.

Risedronate is also used in the prevention and treatment of osteoporosis in postmenopausal women. Taken as either a daily or a weekly dose, it reduces the risk of fractures of the hip or vertebrae. The drug is also used to treat steroid-induced osteoporosis.

To reduce the risk of gastrointestinal adverse effects, you should take risedronate first thing in the morning, on an empty stomach and in a standing position, and remain upright for at least 30 minutes afterwards. Risedronate should not be taken at bedtime.

INFORMATION FOR USERS

Your drug prescription is tailored for you. Do not alter dosage without checking with your doctor.
How taken/used Tablets.
Frequency and timing of doses *Paget's disease* Once daily (30mg dose). *Osteoporosis* Once daily (5mg dose); once weekly, on the same day (35mg dose). Swallow whole with water, on rising and before food; or avoid food or drink for at least 2 hours before and after the dose.

Adult dosage range *Paget's disease* 30mg daily. *Osteoporosis* 5mg daily; 35mg weekly.
Onset of effect Within 1 month.
Duration of action 24 hours for 5mg tablet, 1 week for 35mg tablet.
Diet advice Avoid products that contain calcium (for example, milk or cheese), vitamin and mineral supplements, and antacids for at least 2 hours before and after the dose of risedronate.
Storage Keep in original container at room temperature out of the reach of children.
Missed dose Take as soon as you remember. Then return to your original dosing schedule. Do not make up for the missed dose (weekly).
Stopping the drug The drug can be safely stopped as soon as you no longer need it.
Exceeding the dose An occasional unintentional dose is unlikely to cause problems. However, if you notice any unusual symptoms, or if a large overdose has been taken, drink a large glass of milk and notify your doctor.

POSSIBLE ADVERSE EFFECTS

Most adverse effects of risedronate are mild to moderate and do not usually require the treatment to be stopped. Common effects of the drug include dyspepsia, nausea, diarrhoea or constipation, muscle pain, and headache. Abdominal pain is also common but should be discussed with your doctor. If you have pain or difficulty in swallowing, jaundice, an allergic rash, itching, or facial swelling, stop taking the drug and seek immediate medical attention.

INTERACTIONS

Mineral supplements and antacids reduce the absorption of risedronate and should be taken at a different time of day.

SPECIAL PRECAUTIONS

Be sure to tell your doctor if:
◆ You are allergic to risedronate.
◆ You have kidney problems.
◆ You are/may be pregnant or are planning pregnancy.
◆ You are breast-feeding.
◆ You are unable to sit or stand upright for at least 30 minutes.

◆ You have had pain or difficulty in swallowing.

◆ You are taking other medicines.

Pregnancy Not recommended. Safety in pregnancy not established. Discuss with your doctor.

Breast-feeding Not recommended. Safety in breast-feeding not established. Discuss with your doctor.

Infants and children Not recommended.

Over 60 No special problems.

Driving and hazardous work No special problems.

Alcohol Keep consumption low. Alcohol may increase the gastrointestinal adverse effects of risedronate.

PROLONGED USE

Monitoring Your doctor may monitor your bone mineral density. Blood and urine tests may be carried out.

Risperidone

Brand names Risperdal, Risperdal Consta, Risperdal Quicklet

Used in the following combined preparations None

QUICK REFERENCE

Drug group Antipsychotic drug (p.15)
Overdose danger rating Medium
Dependence rating Low
Prescription needed Yes
Available as generic No

GENERAL INFORMATION

Risperidone is an antipsychotic drug that is used to treat patients who have acute psychiatric disorders and long-term psychotic illnesses such as schizophrenia and mania. Although it does not cure the disorder, risperidone helps to alleviate distressing symptoms. It is effective for relieving "positive" symptoms (such as hallucinations, thought disturbances, and hostility) and "negative" symptoms (such as emotional and social withdrawal). The drug may also help to alleviate various other symptoms, such as depression and anxiety, that are often associated with schizophrenia. Risperidone is an atypi-

cal antipsychotic, and it has less of a sedative effect and is less likely to cause movement disorders as a side effect than some of the other antipsychotics.

INFORMATION FOR USERS

Your drug prescription is tailored for you. Do not alter dosage without checking with your doctor.

How taken/used Tablets, dispersible tablets, liquid, injection.

Frequency and timing of doses 1–2 x daily (tablets, liquid).

Adult dosage range *Tablets* 2mg daily (starting dose) increasing to 4–6mg daily (usual maintenance dose); maximum 16mg daily. *Injection* 25mg every 2 weeks (starting dose) increasing to 50mg every 2 weeks (maximum maintenance dose).

Onset of effect *Tablets* Within 2–3 days, but may take up to 6 weeks before maximum effect is seen. *Injection* Up to 3 weeks before onset of effect.

Duration of action Approximately 2 days.

Diet advice None.

Storage Keep in original container at room temperature (tablets) or refrigerate (injection) out of reach of children. Protect from light.

Missed dose Take as soon as you remember. If your next dose is due within 3 hours, take a single dose now and skip the next.

Stopping the drug Do not stop taking the drug without consulting your doctor; symptoms may recur.

Exceeding the dose An occasional unintentional extra dose is unlikely to cause problems. If larger doses have been taken, notify your doctor.

POSSIBLE ADVERSE EFFECTS

Risperidone is generally well tolerated and has a low incidence of movement disorders. It is less sedating than some other antipsychotic drugs. Insomnia, anxiety, agitation, headache, difficulty in concentrating, and weight gain are common. Shakiness and tremors, which are also common, and sexual dysfunction, dizziness, and drowsiness, which are rare, should be discussed with your doctor. If you develop a high fever, or you have rigid muscles, stop taking the drug and seek immediate medical attention.

INTERACTIONS

Sedatives All drugs that have a sedative effect on the central nervous system are likely to increase any sedative effect of risperidone.

Fluoxetine and paroxetine These drugs increase the blood levels of risperidone and the risk of side effects.

Carbamazepine reduces the effects of risperidone. Other liver-enzyme inducing drugs (e.g. phenytoin) may have the same effect.

Drugs for parkinsonism Risperidone may reduce the effect of these drugs.

SPECIAL PRECAUTIONS

Be sure to tell your doctor if:
◆ You have liver or kidney problems.
◆ You have heart or circulation problems.
◆ You have, or are at risk of having, diabetes.
◆ You have had epileptic fits.
◆ You have Parkinson's disease.
◆ You have had, or are at risk of having, a stroke.
◆ You are taking other medicines.

Pregnancy Safety in pregnancy not established. Discuss with your doctor.

Breast-feeding The drug probably passes into breast milk. Discuss with your doctor.

Infants and children Not recommended under 15 years.

Over 60 Reduced dose may be necessary.

Driving and hazardous work Avoid such activities until you have learned how risperidone affects you because the drug may cause difficulty in concentration and slowed reactions.

Alcohol Avoid. Alcohol may increase the sedative effects of this drug.

PROLONGED USE

If used long term, permanent movement disorders (tardive dyskinesia) may occur, although they are less likely than with many other antipsychotic drugs.

Rivastigmine

Brand name Exelon
Used in the following combined preparations None

QUICK REFERENCE

Drug group Drug for dementia (p.19)

Overdose danger rating Medium
Dependence rating Low
Prescription needed Yes
Available as generic No

GENERAL INFORMATION

Rivastigmine is an inhibitor of an enzyme called anticholinesterase. This enzyme breaks down a naturally occurring neurotransmitter called acetylcholine to limit its effects. Blocking anticholinesterase raises the levels of acetylcholine which, in the brain, increases alertness, awareness and memory. Rivastigmine has been found to improve the symptoms of dementia in Alzheimer's disease, and is used to slow the rate of deterioration in that disease. The drug is not currently recommended for dementia due to other causes. Treatment is initiated under specialist supervision. It is usual to assess those being treated at 6 monthly intervals to decide whether the drug is helping. As the disease progresses, the benefit obtained may diminish.

Side effects of rivastigmine may include agitation, confusion, and depression, which could be thought due to Alzheimer's disease. Weight loss should be monitored.

INFORMATION FOR USERS

Your drug prescription is tailored for you. Do not alter dosage without checking with your doctor.

How taken/used Capsules, liquid.

Frequency and timing of doses 2 x daily.

Adult dosage range 3mg daily (starting dose); 6–12mg daily (maintenance dose).

Onset of effect 30–60 minutes. Full effect may take up to 3 months.

Duration of action 9–12 hours.

Diet advice None.

Storage Keep in original container at room temperature out of the reach of children.

Missed dose Take as soon as you remember. If your next dose is due within 4 hours, take a single dose now and skip the next. A carer should be overseeing the taking of tablets.

Stopping the drug Do not stop the drug without consulting your doctor; symptoms may recur.

Exceeding the dose An occasional unintentional extra dose is unlikely to be a problem.

Large overdoses may cause nausea, vomiting, and diarrhoea. Notify your doctor.

POSSIBLE ADVERSE EFFECTS

Common adverse effects of rivastigmine include drowsiness, dizziness, weakness, sweating, and malaise. Reduced appetite, weight loss, nausea, abdominal pain, agitation, confusion, urinary incontinence, and infection are also common, but these should be discussed with your doctor. Mental changes and intestinal problems, although common, are usually quite mild. Women may be more susceptible to nausea, vomiting, and weight loss.

INTERACTIONS

Muscle relaxants used in surgery Rivastigmine may increase the effects of some muscle relaxants, but it may also block the effects of some others.

SPECIAL PRECAUTIONS

Be sure to tell your doctor if:
◆ You have a heart problem.
◆ You have liver or kidney problems.
◆ You have asthma or respiratory problems.
◆ You have had a gastric or duodenal ulcer.
◆ You are taking other medicines.
Pregnancy Not recommended. Safety in pregnancy not established.
Breast-feeding Not recommended.
Infants and children Not recommended.
Over 60 No special problems.
Driving and hazardous work Your underlying condition may make such activities inadvisable. Discuss with your doctor.
Alcohol Avoid. Alcohol increases the sedative effects of rivastigmine.
Surgery and general anaesthetics Treatment with rivastigmine may need to be stopped before you have a general anaesthetic. Discuss this with your doctor or dentist before any operation.

PROLONGED USE

May be continued for as long as there is benefit. Stopping the drug leads to a gradual loss of the improvements.
Monitoring Periodic checks may be performed to test whether the drug is still providing some benefit.

Rosiglitazone

Brand name Avandia
Used in the following combined preparation Avandamet

QUICK REFERENCE

Drug group Antidiabetic drug (p.82)
Overdose danger rating High
Dependence rating Low
Prescription needed Yes
Available as generic No

GENERAL INFORMATION

Rosiglitazone is used to treat Type 2 diabetes. It works by reducing insulin resistance in fatty tissue, skeletal muscle, and in the liver, which leads to a reduction of blood glucose levels. The effects appear gradually and reach their full extent in about 8 weeks. For some patients, rosiglitazone may be used alone. Often, however, it is used in addition to metformin and/or a sulphonylurea; it is available as a combined preparation with metformin. Rosiglitazone works better in obese diabetics, although it often causes weight gain. Anaemia is another adverse effect.

Rosiglitazone is not used with insulin because this combination may increase the risk of heart failure.

INFORMATION FOR USERS

Your drug prescription is tailored for you. Do not alter dosage without checking with your doctor.
How taken/used Tablets.
Frequency and timing of doses 1–2 x daily.
Adult dosage range 4–8mg daily.
Onset of effect 60 minutes; it can take 8 weeks for full effects to appear.
Duration of action 12–24 hours.
Diet advice An individualized low-fat, low-sugar diet must be maintained in order for the drug to be fully effective. Follow your doctor's advice.
Storage Keep in original container at room temperature out of the reach of children.
Missed dose Take as soon as you remember. If your next dose is due within 2 hours, take a single dose now and skip the next.
Stopping the drug Do not stop taking the drug without consulting your doctor; stopping

the drug may lead to worsening of the underlying condition.

OVERDOSE ACTION

Seek immediate medical advice in all cases. Take emergency action if loss of consciousness occurs.

POSSIBLE ADVERSE EFFECTS

Fatigue and weakness (as a result of anaemia) and weight gain (even in those people on a strict diabetic diet) are common side effects, and they should be discussed with your doctor. Less commonly, rosiglitazone has been associated with heart failure. Other common side effects of the drug include nausea, abdominal pain, indigestion, flatulence, and headache; you should discuss headaches with your doctor. Dark urine, dizziness, sleepiness, swollen ankles, painful breathing, or a cough at night are rare, but should also be discussed with your doctor.

INTERACTIONS

Paclitaxel may reduce the metabolism and increase the effects of rosiglitazone.

Non-steroidal anti-inflammatory drugs (NSAIDs) may increase the risk of fluid retention.

ACE inhibitors may increase the effects of rosiglitazone.

Diazoxide, corticosteroids, and diuretics reduce the effects of rosiglitazone.

SPECIAL PRECAUTIONS

Be sure to tell your doctor if:

◆ You have liver problems.

◆ You are anaemic.

◆ You have heart failure.

◆ You have severe kidney failure.

◆ You are taking other medicines.

Pregnancy Safety not established. Discuss with your doctor.

Breast-feeding Safety not established. Discuss with your doctor.

Infants and children Not recommended.

Over 60 No special problems, but the elderly may be more susceptible to side effects.

Driving and hazardous work No known problems.

Alcohol Avoid excessive intake. Alcohol can increase rosiglitazone's effect.

PROLONGED USE

Rosiglitazone, like other antidiabetic drugs, is used indefinitely.

Monitoring Initial and periodic blood tests of liver function will be performed. Weight will be measured at intervals. Blood glucose levels should be monitored regularly.

Rosuvastatin

Brand name Crestor
Used in the following combined preparations None

QUICK REFERENCE

Drug group Lipid-lowering drug (p.37)
Overdose danger rating Low
Dependence rating Low
Prescription needed Yes
Available as generic No

GENERAL INFORMATION

Rosuvastatin is a "statin" lipid-lowering drug that is used in the treatment of hypercholesterolaemia (high levels of cholesterol in the blood). It is prescribed to people who have not responded to other forms of therapy, such as a special diet, and are at risk of developing, or have existing, coronary heart disease.

Cholesterol is a lipid (fat) that is necessary for production of many chemicals and hormones in the body. Raised cholesterol levels may result in fatty deposits on artery walls, a common cause of heart disease. Rosuvastatin works by inhibiting an enzyme involved in the manufacture of cholesterol in the liver.

Adverse effects of rosuvastatin are usually mild and wear off with time. However, any unexplained aches or pains or muscle weakness should be reported to your doctor immediately. People of Asian origin are given lower starting doses because they are at increased risk of muscle damage.

INFORMATION FOR USERS

Your drug prescription is tailored for you. Do not alter dosage without checking with your doctor.

How taken/used Tablets.

Frequency and timing of doses Once daily at the same time each day.

Adult dosage range 5–40mg (5–20mg for patients of Asian origin); 10mg (initial dose), increased to 20mg after 4 weeks, if necessary; a maximum dose of 40mg may be given for severe hypercholesterolaemia.

Onset of effect 2–4 weeks.

Duration of action 24 hours.

Diet advice A low-fat diet is usually recommended.

Storage Keep in original container at room temperature, out of the reach of children.

Missed dose Do not take the missed dose. Take the next scheduled dose as usual.

Stopping the drug Do not stop taking the drug without consulting your doctor. Symptoms may recur.

Exceeding the dose An occasional unintentional extra dose is unlikely to be a cause for concern. However, if you notice any unusual symptoms, or if a large overdose has been taken, notify your doctor.

POSSIBLE ADVERSE EFFECTS

Common adverse effects of rosuvastatin include headache, constipation, stomach pain, and dizziness, but these are usually mild and transient. If, rarely, muscle pain, weakness, blood in the urine, an allergic rash, and facial swelling occur, stop taking the drug and seek immediate medical attention.

INTERACTIONS

Ciclosporin increases blood levels of rosuvastatin

Warfarin Rosuvastatin enhances the effects of warfarin.

Erythromycin reduces the effectiveness of rosuvastatin.

Gemfibrozil and other lipid-lowering drugs There is an increased risk of adverse effects when these drugs are taken with rosuvastatin.

Antacids may reduce the effectiveness of rosuvastatin.

SPECIAL PRECAUTIONS

Be sure to tell your doctor if:

◆ You have had a previous allergic reaction to rosuvastatin.

◆ You have liver or kidney problems.

◆ You have myopathy or a family history of myopathy.

◆ You have an underactive thyroid gland.

◆ You regularly drink larger-than-average amounts of alcohol per day.

◆ You are of Asian origin.

◆ You are taking other medicines, especially "fibrates".

Pregnancy Not usually prescribed. Safety not established. Discuss with your doctor.

Breast-feeding Not recommended. Safety not established. Discuss with your doctor.

Infants and children Not recommended.

Over 60 Reduced initial dose. Discuss with your doctor.

Driving and hazardous work Do not undertake such activities until you have learned how the drug affects you; it can cause dizziness.

Alcohol No special problems.

PROLONGED USE

No known problems.

Monitoring Regular blood tests to check the drug's effectiveness in reducing cholesterol levels may be performed. Blood tests of liver and muscle function may also be carried out.

Salbutamol

Brand names Airomir, Asmasal, Salamol, Ventmax, Ventodisks, Ventolin, Volmax, and others
Used in the following combined preparation Combivent

QUICK REFERENCE

Drug group Bronchodilator (p.23), drug to treat asthma (p.24), and drug used in premature labour (p.110)
Overdose danger rating Low
Dependence rating Low
Prescription needed Yes
Available as generic Yes

GENERAL INFORMATION

Salbutamol is a sympathomimetic bronchodilator that relaxes the muscle surrounding the bronchioles (the airways in the lungs).

This drug is used to relieve symptoms of asthma, chronic bronchitis, and emphysema. Although it can be taken by mouth, inhalation is considered more effective because the drug is delivered directly to the bronchioles, thus giving rapid relief, allowing smaller doses, and causing fewer side effects.

Compared to some similar drugs, salbutamol has little stimulant effect on the heart rate and blood pressure, making it safer for people with heart problems or high blood pressure. Because salbutamol relaxes the muscles of the uterus, it is also used to prevent premature labour.

The drug's most common side effect is fine tremor of the hands, which may interfere with precise manual work. Anxiety, tension, and restlessness may also occur.

INFORMATION FOR USERS

Your drug prescription is tailored for you. Do not alter dosage without checking with your doctor.

How taken/used Tablets, SR-tablets, SR-capsules, liquid, injection, inhaler, nebules for nebulizer, powder for inhalation.

Frequency and timing of doses 3–4 x daily (tablets/liquid); 2 x daily (SR-preparations); 1–2 inhalations 3–4 x daily (inhaler); up to 4 x daily (nebules).

Dosage range 8–16mg daily (by mouth); 400–800mcg daily (inhaler); 2.5–20mg daily (nebules).

Onset of effect Within 30–60 minutes (by mouth); within 5–15 minutes (inhaler/nebules).

Duration of action Up to 8 hours (tablets); up to 6 hours (inhaler); up to 12 hours (SR-preparations).

Diet advice None.

Storage Keep in original container at room temperature out of reach of children. Protect from light. Do not puncture or burn inhalers.

Missed dose Take as soon as you remember if you need it. If your next dose is due within 2 hours, take a single dose now and skip the next.

Stopping the drug Do not stop the drug without consulting your doctor; symptoms may recur.

Exceeding the dose An occasional unintentional extra dose is unlikely to be a cause for concern. But if you notice any unusual symptoms, or if a large overdose has been taken, notify your doctor.

POSSIBLE ADVERSE EFFECTS

Muscle tremor (which particularly affects the hands), anxiety, restlessness, and headache are common adverse effects. Muscle cramps may occur rarely, and should be discussed with your doctor. Palpitations are also rare, and if you experience them, stop taking the drug and consult your doctor promptly.

INTERACTIONS

Theophylline, corticosteroids, and diuretics There is a risk of low potassium levels in blood occurring if this drug is taken with salbutamol.

Other sympathomimetic drugs may increase the effects of salbutamol, thereby also increasing the risk of adverse effects.

Digoxin Salbutamol may cause low potassium levels, increasing the risk of digoxin toxicity. Salbutamol by mouth or injection can reduce digoxin levels.

Beta blockers Drugs in this group may reduce the action of salbutamol.

SPECIAL PRECAUTIONS

Be sure to tell your doctor if:
◆ You have heart problems.
◆ You have high blood pressure.
◆ You have an overactive thyroid gland.
◆ You have diabetes.
◆ You are taking other medicines.

Pregnancy No evidence of risk when used to treat asthma, or to treat or prevent premature labour. Discuss with your doctor.

Breast-feeding The drug passes into the breast milk, but at normal doses adverse effects on the baby are unlikely. Discuss with your doctor.

Infants and children Reduced dose necessary.

Over 60 Increased likelihood of adverse effects. Reduced dose may therefore be necessary.

Driving and hazardous work Avoid such activities until you have learned how salbutamol affects you because the drug can cause tremors.

Alcohol No known problems.

PROLONGED USE

No problems expected. However, you should contact your doctor if you find you are needing to use your salbutamol inhaler more than usual (more than 8 puffs in 24 hours). Failure to respond to salbutamol may be a result of worsening asthma that requires urgent medical attention.

Monitoring Periodic blood tests for potassium may be needed in people on high-dose treatment with salbutamol combined with other asthma drugs.

Salmeterol

Brand name Serevent
Used in the following combined preparation Seretide

QUICK REFERENCE

Drug group Bronchodilator (p.23), drug to treat asthma (p.24)
Overdose danger rating Low
Dependence rating Low
Prescription needed Yes
Available as generic No

GENERAL INFORMATION

Salmeterol is a sympathomimetic bronchodilator that is used to treat conditions, such as asthma, chronic obstructive pulmonary disease (COPD) and bronchospasm, in which the airways become constricted. The advantage of salmeterol over salbutamol (see p.379) is that is has a longer acting.

Salmeterol relaxes the muscle surrounding the airways in the lungs but, because of its slow onset of effect, it is not used for immediate relief of symptoms of asthma. It is prescribed to prevent attacks, however, and can be helpful in preventing night-time asthma.

Salmeterol should always be used in combination with inhaled or oral corticosteroids. Taken by inhalation, the drug is delivered directly to the airways. This allows smaller doses to be taken and reduces the risk of adverse effects.

INFORMATION FOR USERS

Your drug prescription is tailored for you. Do not alter dosage without checking with your doctor.
How taken/used Inhaler, powder for inhalation.
Frequency and timing of doses 2 x daily.
Dosage range 100–200mcg daily.
Onset of effect 10–20 minutes.
Duration of action 12 hours.
Diet advice None.
Storage Keep in original container at room temperature out of the reach of children.
Missed dose Take as soon as you remember. If your next dose is due within 4 hours, take a single dose now and skip the next.
Stopping the drug Do not stop the drug without consulting your doctor; symptoms may recur.
Exceeding the dose An occasional unintentional extra dose is unlikely to be a cause for concern. But if you notice any unusual symptoms, or if a large overdose has been taken, notify your doctor.

POSSIBLE ADVERSE EFFECTS

Side effects of salmeterol are usually mild, and tremor commonly occurs. Wheezing and sudden breathlessness (paradoxical bronchospasm) are rare; if you experience these, stop taking the drug and notify your doctor immediately. Palpitations, headache, and muscle cramps are also rare and should be discussed with your doctor.

INTERACTIONS

Corticosteroids, theophylline, and diuretics There is an increased risk of low blood potassium levels when high doses of salmeterol are taken with these drugs.
Other sympathomimetics may increase the effects of salmeterol, thereby also increasing the risk of adverse effects.
Digoxin Salmeterol may cause low potasssium levels in the blood, which increases the risk of digoxin toxicity.

SPECIAL PRECAUTIONS

Be sure to tell your doctor if:
◆ You have heart problems.
◆ You have high blood pressure.
◆ You have an overactive thyroid gland.
◆ You have diabetes.
◆ You are taking other medicines.
Pregnancy No evidence of risk when used to treat asthma. Benefits of treatment usually outweigh risk that mother's worsening asthma has on developing baby. Discuss with your doctor.
Breast-feeding The drug passes into the breast milk, but at normal doses adverse effects on the baby are unlikely. Discuss with your doctor.
Infants and children Reduced dose necessary. Not recommended for children under 4 years.

Over 60 No special problems.
Driving and hazardous work No special problems.
Alcohol No known problems.

PROLONGED USE
Salmeterol is intended to be used long term. The main problem comes from using combinations of anti-asthma drugs, leading to low blood potassium levels.

Monitoring Periodic blood tests are usually carried out to monitor potassium levels.

Sertraline

Brand name Lustral
Used in the following combined preparations None

QUICK REFERENCE
Drug group Antidepressant (p.14)
Overdose danger rating Low
Dependence rating Low
Prescription needed Yes
Available as generic Yes

GENERAL INFORMATION
Sertraline is a member of the group of antidepressant drugs called selective serotonin re-uptake inhibitors (SSRIs). These drugs tend to cause less sedation and have different side effects from older types of antidepressants. Sertraline elevates mood, increases physical activity, and restores interest in everyday activities. It is used to treat depression, including accompanying anxiety, and obsessive-compulsive disorder (OCD). Sertraline is also prescribed for post-traumatic stress disorder (PTSD) in women; it has not been shown to work in men with this condition.

Treatment with sertraline is usually stopped gradually over at least four weeks because symptoms such as headache, nausea, and dizziness may occur if the drug is withdrawn suddenly.

INFORMATION FOR USERS
Your drug prescription is tailored for you. Do not alter dosage without checking with your doctor.
How taken/used Tablets.
Frequency and timing of doses Once daily, usually in the morning.
Adult dosage range 50–200mg daily.
Onset of effect Some benefits may appear within 14 days; full effects may take another 6 weeks; anxiety disorders may take longer.
Duration of action Antidepressant effect may continue for some weeks following prolonged use.
Diet advice None.
Storage Keep in original container at room temperature out of the reach of children.
Missed dose Take as soon as you remember. If your next dose is due within 8 hours, take a single dose now and skip the next.
Stopping the drug Do not stop the drug without consulting your doctor, who may supervise a gradual reduction in dosage.
Exceeding the dose An occasional unintentional extra dose is unlikely to cause problems. Large overdoses may cause adverse effects. Notify your doctor.

POSSIBLE ADVERSE EFFECTS
Common adverse effects of sertraline include gastrointestinal problems (such as nausea, indigestion, diarrhoea/loose stools), restlessness, insomnia or sleepiness, anxiety, and sexual dysfunction. A rash, itching, skin eruptions, and suicidal thoughts (or suicidal attempts) occur rarely. If you experience any of these, stop taking the drug and seek immediate medical attention.

INTERACTIONS
St John's wort There is a danger of increasing the side effects of both substances.
Monoamine oxidase inhibitors (MAOIs) Sertraline's effects and toxicity are greatly increased by MAOIs.
Tramadol and $5HT_1$ agonists (e.g. sumatriptan) There is an increased risk of adverse effects if these drugs are taken with sertraline.
Antipsychotics Sertraline may increase the levels and effects of some antipsychotics.
Anticoagulants The effects of these may be increased by sertraline.

SPECIAL PRECAUTIONS
Be sure to tell your doctor if:
◆ You have long-term liver or kidney problems.
◆ You have had epileptic fits.
◆ You have heart problems.

◆ You have a history of bleeding disorders.

◆ You have a history of mania.

◆ You are taking other medicines.

Pregnancy Safety not established. Discuss with your doctor.

Breast-feeding Safety not established. Discuss with your doctor.

Infants and children Not generally recommended under 18 years.

Over 60 No special problems.

Driving and hazardous work Avoid such activities until you know how sertraline affects you because the drug can cause drowsiness and visual disturbances.

Alcohol Avoid excessive intake. SSRIs may increase the sedative effects of alcohol.

PROLONGED USE

No known problems.

Monitoring Any person experiencing drowsiness, confusion, muscle cramps, or convulsions should be monitored for low sodium levels in the blood.

Sibutramine

Brand name Reductil
Used in the following combined preparations None

QUICK REFERENCE

Drug group Appetite suppressant (see Nervous system stimulants, p.19)
Overdose danger rating Medium
Dependence rating Low
Prescription needed Yes
Available as generic No

GENERAL INFORMATION

Sibutramine is a drug that acts on brain neurotransmitters. It is used to suppress the appetite of people who are obese (those who have a body Mass Index (BMI) of 30kg/m^2 or more) or overweight (those who have a BMI of 27kg/m^2 or more) and who have a condition such as Type 2 diabetes (see p.82) or high blood lipid levels (see p.37). For these people, losing weight reduces the risk of stroke, improves the control of diabetes and gallstones, and reduces the load on joints in conditions such as osteoarthritis.

Treatment with sibutramine must be accompanied by a suitable diet. The drug is prescribed to patients in whom dieting alone has failed. They also need to make lifestyle changes in order to avoid weight being regained when the drug is withdrawn. Psychological help from a support group is beneficial for some people.

INFORMATION FOR USERS

Your drug prescription is tailored for you. Do not alter dosage without checking with your doctor.

How taken/used Capsules.

Frequency and timing of doses Once daily, in the morning.

Adult dosage range 10–15mg daily.

Onset of effect 30–60 minutes.

Duration of action 24 hours.

Diet advice Low fat, low calorie diet.

Storage Keep in original container at room temperature out of the reach of children.

Missed dose Take as soon as you remember. If your next dose is due within 12 hours, wait until you are due to take the next dose.

Stopping the drug Do not stop taking the drug without consulting your doctor. Stopping the drug may result in your gaining weight again.

Exceeding the dose An occasional unintentional extra dose is unlikely to cause problems. Large overdoses may cause adverse effects. Notify your doctor.

POSSIBLE ADVERSE EFFECTS

Sibutramine has a wide range of unwanted effects, which are usually mild; the most common of these are increased heart rate and mild mental stimulation. Other common adverse effects of sibutramine include constipation, haemorrhoids, a dry mouth, nausea, insomnia, anxiety, palpitations, lightheadedness, headache, hot flushes, sweating, and taste disturbances.

INTERACTIONS

Troleandomycin, erythromycin, clarithromycin, ciclosporin, ketoconazole, and itraconazole These drugs increase blood levels and the effects of sibutramine.

Dihydroergotamine, sumatriptan, SSRIs, St John's wort, and some opioid analgesics All of these drugs inhibit serotonin re-uptake and can increase the effects of sibutramine.

Monoamine oxidase inhibitors (MAOIs), some antidepressants, and some antipsychotics Adverse effects occur if these drugs are taken with sibutramine; concomitant use should be avoided.

Cough and cold remedies These preparations may add to the blood pressure-raising effect of sibutramine.

SPECIAL PRECAUTIONS

Be sure to tell your doctor if:
◆ You have liver or kidney problems.
◆ You have high blood pressure.
◆ You have a psychiatric illness.
◆ You have heart problems.
◆ You have an overactive thyroid.
◆ You have prostate problems.
◆ You have glaucoma.
◆ You have a history of drug abuse.
◆ You are taking other medicines.

Pregnancy Safety not established. Weight reducing drugs should not be used in pregnancy.

Breast-feeding It is not known whether sibutramine is secreted in breast milk. Do not use the drug during the period when you are breast-feeding.

Infants and children Not generally recommended under 18 years.

Over 60 Not recommended for people over 65 years.

Driving and hazardous work Avoid until you have learned how sibutramine affects you because the drug may cause lightheadedness, blurred vision, fits, and impaired thinking.

Alcohol Alcohol contains calories and should not be part of a diet supported by sibutramine.

PROLONGED USE

Sibutramine must be stopped after 1 year. On withdrawal, there is often an increase in appetite.

Monitoring The pulse rate and blood pressure will be checked regularly. Body weight will be checked at intervals. If the weight loss is insufficient (less than 5 per cent of starting body weight), the drug will be stopped.

Sildenafil

Brand name Viagra
Used in the following combined preparations None

QUICK REFERENCE

Drug group Drug for erectile dysfunction (p.110)
Overdose danger rating Medium
Dependence rating Low
Prescription needed Yes
Available as generic No

GENERAL INFORMATION

Sildenafil is a drug that is used to treat erectile dysfunction (commonly known as impotence). It does not cause an erection directly, but it produces a chemical change that prevents the muscle walls of the blood-filled chambers in the penis from relaxing.

Sildenafil does not need to be taken regularly; the drug is only used to produce an erection and only needs to be taken before sexual activity is undertaken.

Because it is a vasodilator (see p.31), sildenafil can cause a small fall in blood pressure while it is active, and it may increase the effect of antihypertensive drugs. It is not usually prescribed with nitrates (see p.35) because it greatly increases their effects.

INFORMATION FOR USERS

Your drug prescription is tailored for you. Do not alter dosage without checking with your doctor.

How taken/used Tablets.

Frequency and timing of doses Maximum once daily, 1 hour before sexual activity.

Adult dosage range 25–100mg daily.

Onset of effect 30 minutes.

Duration of action 4 hours.

Diet advice None, although sildenafil will take longer to work after a meal, especially a high fat meal. It is absorbed faster on an empty stomach.

Storage Keep in original container at room temperature out of the reach of children.

Missed dose Take the next dose when you need to. Do not use more than one dose in a 24-hour period.

Stopping the drug Can be safely stopped as soon as you no longer need it.

Exceeding the dose An occasional unintentional extra dose is unlikely to cause problems. Large overdoses may cause headache, dizziness, flushing, altered vision, and nasal congestion. Notify your doctor.

POSSIBLE ADVERSE EFFECTS

Most adverse effects are common and include headache, flushing, dizziness, indigestion, nasal congestion, blurred vision, and altered colour vision. Sildenafil has been reported to cause muscle aches when taken more frequently than recommended; it is not certain that this effect is due to the drug, however. Priapism (a persistent, painful erection) is rare and, if it occurs, stop taking the drug and consult your doctor. If chest pain, which is also rare, occurs, stop taking the drug and consult your doctor urgently.

INTERACTIONS

Nitrates The effects of these drugs are greatly increased by sildenafil, and they are therefore not prescribed with it.

Antihypertensive drugs Sildenafil may enhance their blood pressure-lowering effect.

Cimetidine, erythromycin, nicorandil, ketoconazole (oral), and antivirals These drugs increase the blood levels and toxicity of sildenafil.

SPECIAL PRECAUTIONS

Be sure to tell your doctor if:
◆ You have heart problems.
◆ You have had a stroke or heart attack.
◆ You have liver or kidney problems.
◆ You have an inherited eye problem.
◆ You have an abnormality of the penis.
◆ You are taking a nitrate drug.
◆ You are taking other medicines.

Pregnancy Not prescribed.

Breast-feeding Not prescribed.

Infants and children Not prescribed under 18 years.

Over 60 Reduced dose may be necessary.

Driving and hazardous work Avoid such activities until you have learned how sildenafil affects you because the drug can cause dizziness and altered vision.

Alcohol No special problems.

PROLONGED USE

No problems expected.

Simvastatin

Brand names Zocor, Zocor Heart-Pro
Used in the following combined preparation Inegy

QUICK REFERENCE

Drug group Lipid-lowering drug (p.37)
Overdose danger rating Medium
Dependence rating Low
Prescription needed Yes (except low-dose preparations)
Available as generic Yes

GENERAL INFORMATION

Simvastatin is a lipid-lowering drug that was introduced in 1989. It blocks the action of an enzyme that is needed for cholesterol to be manufactured in the liver, and as a result the blood levels of cholesterol are lowered. The drug is prescribed for people with hypercholesterolaemia (high levels of cholesterol in the blood) who have not responded to other forms of therapy, such as a special diet, and who are at risk of developing or have existing coronary heart disease. Low-dose simvastatin is available over the counter to help lower cholesterol levels in certain people.

Side effects are usually mild and often wear off with time. In the body, simvastatin is found mainly in the liver, and it may raise the levels of various liver enzymes. This does not usually indicate serious liver damage.

INFORMATION FOR USERS

Your drug prescription is tailored for you. Do not alter dosage without checking with your doctor.

How taken/used Tablets.

Frequency and timing of doses Once daily at night.

Adult dosage range 10–80mg daily.

Onset of effect Within 2 weeks; full beneficial effects may not be reached for 4–6 weeks.

Duration of action Up to 24 hours.

Diet advice A low-fat diet is usually recommended. Avoid grapefruit juice.

Storage Keep in original container at room temperature out of the reach of children. Protect from light.

Missed dose Take as soon as you remember. If your next dose is due within 8 hours, do not take the missed dose, but take the next dose on schedule.

Stopping the drug Do not stop taking the drug without consulting your doctor. Stopping the drug may lead to worsening of the underlying condition.

Exceeding the dose An occasional unintentional extra dose is unlikely to cause problems. Large overdoses may cause liver problems. Notify your doctor.

POSSIBLE ADVERSE EFFECTS

Adverse effects are usually mild and do not last long. The most common are those affecting the gastrointestinal system, such as nausea, abdominal pain, constipation, diarrhoea, and flatulence. Headache may also occur. If, also rarely, you develop a rash or jaundice, stop taking the drug and consult your doctor urgently. Simvastatin may very rarely cause muscle problems; stop taking the drug and consult your doctor immediately if muscle pain or weakness occur.

INTERACTIONS

Ciclosporin, danazol, fibrates, nicotinic acid, amiodarone, verapamil, diltiazem Itraconazole, ketoconazole, HIV protease inhibitors, macrolide antibiotics (e.g. erythromycin), and nefazodone Used with simvastatin, these drugs in-crease the risk of muscle toxicity. If they are required, simvastatin is withheld temporarily.

Anticoagulants Simvastatin may increase the effect of anticoagulants. The dose may need to be adjusted, and prothrombin time should be monitored regularly.

Grapefruit juice increases blood levels of simvastatin; regular consumption should be avoided.

SPECIAL PRECAUTIONS

Be sure to tell your doctor if:
◆ You have liver or kidney problems.
◆ You have eye or vision problems.
◆ You have muscle weakness or pain.
◆ You have a thyroid disorder.
◆ You have had problems with alcohol abuse.
◆ You have porphyria.
◆ You have angina.
◆ You have high blood pressure.
◆ You are taking other medicines.

Pregnancy Not used. The drug should be stopped during pregnancy. Discuss with your doctor.

Breast-feeding The drug passes into the breast milk and may affect the baby. Discuss with your doctor.

Infants and children No recommended under 5 years. Reduced dose necessary in older children, under specialist advice.

Over 60 No special problems.

Driving and hazardous work No special problems.

Alcohol Avoid excessive amounts. Alcohol may increase the risk of developing liver problems with this drug.

PROLONGED USE

Prolonged treatment can adversely affect liver function.

Monitoring Periodic blood tests to test for muscle toxicity and assess liver function are recommended.

Sodium cromoglicate

Brand names Cromogen, Hay-Crom, Intal, Nalcrom, Opticrom, Rynacrom, Vividrin and others
Used in the following combined preparations None

QUICK REFERENCE

Drug group Anti-allergy drug (p.24)
Overdose danger rating Low
Dependence rating Low
Prescription needed No (some preparations)
Available as generic Yes

GENERAL INFORMATION

Sodium cromoglicate, introduced in the 1970s, is used primarily to prevent asthma and allergic conditions.

When taken by inhaler as a powder (Spinhaler) or spray, sodium cromoglicate is commonly used to reduce the frequency and severity of asthma attacks, and is also effective in helping to prevent attacks induced by exercise or cold air. The drug has a slow onset of action, and it may take up to six weeks for its full anti-asthmatic effect to be felt. Sodium cromoglicate is not effective for the relief of an asthma attack.

Sodium cromoglicate is also given in the

form of eye drops to prevent or treat allergic conjunctivitis. Taken as a nasal spray, it is used to prevent or treat allergic rhinitis (hay fever). It is also given, in the form of capsules, for food allergy.

Side effects are mild. Coughing and wheezing occurring on inhalation of the drug may be prevented by using a sympathomimetic bronchodilator (see p.23) first. Hoarseness and throat irritation can be avoided by rinsing the mouth with water after inhalation.

INFORMATION FOR USERS

Follow instructions on the label. Call your doctor if symptoms worsen.

How taken/used Capsules, inhaler (various types), eye drops, nasal spray.

Frequency and timing of doses *Capsules* 4 x daily before meals, swallowed whole or dissolved in water. *Inhaler, nasal spray* 4–6 x daily. *Eye preparations* 4 x daily (drops).

Adult dosage range 800mg daily (capsules); as directed (inhaler); apply to each nostril as directed (nasal spray); 1–2 drops in each eye per dose (eye drops).

Onset of effect Varies with dosage, form, and condition being treated. Eye conditions and allergic rhinitis may respond after a few days' treatment with drops, while asthma and chronic allergic rhinitis may take 2–6 weeks to show improvement.

Duration of action 4–6 hours. Some effect persists for several days after treatment is stopped.

Diet advice Capsules: you may be advised to avoid certain foods. Follow your doctor's advice.

Storage Keep in original container at room temperature out of the reach of children. Protect from light.

Missed dose Take as soon as you remember. If your next dose is due within 2 hours, take a single dose now and skip the next.

Stopping the drug Do not stop the drug without consulting your doctor; symptoms may recur.

Exceeding the dose An occasional unintentional extra dose is unlikely to be a cause for concern. But if you notice any unusual symptoms, or if a large overdose has been taken, notify your doctor.

POSSIBLE ADVERSE EFFECTS

Coughing and hoarseness and local irritation are common with inhalation of sodium cromoglicate; and nasal spray may cause sneezing. These symptoms usually diminish with continued use. Headache and dizziness are rare, as are wheezing or breathlessness, which should be reported to your doctor. The capsules may, rarely, cause nausea, vomiting, joint pain, or a rash. If any of these occur, consult your doctor immediately.

INTERACTIONS
None.

SPECIAL PRECAUTIONS

Be sure to tell your doctor or pharmacist before taking this drug if:
◆ You are taking other medicines.

Pregnancy No evidence of risk.

Breast-feeding It is not known whether the drug passes into the breast milk. Discuss with your doctor.

Infants and children Reduced dose necessary.

Over 60 No special problems.

Driving and hazardous work No known problems.

Alcohol No known problems.

PROLONGED USE
No problems expected.

Sodium valproate (valproate)

Brand names Convulex (valproic acid), Epilim, Epilim Chrono, Depakote, Orlept
Used in the following combined preparations None

QUICK REFERENCE

Drug group Anticonvulsant drug (p.16)
Overdose danger rating Medium
Dependence rating Low
Prescription needed Yes
Available as generic Yes

GENERAL INFORMATION

Sodium valproate is an anticonvulsant drug that is often used for the treatment of different types of epilepsy. The action of sodium valproate is similar to that of other anticonvulsants, reducing electrical discharges in the brain to prevent the excessive build-up of discharges that can lead to epileptic fits.

Beneficial in long-term treatment, this drug does not usually have a sedative effect. This makes it particularly suitable for children who suffer either from atonic epilepsy (the sudden relaxing of the muscles throughout the body) or from absence seizures (during which the person appears to be daydreaming).

Care should be taken if changing between preparations.

Sodium valproate is also sometimes used for the treatment of manic episodes and, in the long term, for bipolar illness.

INFORMATION FOR USERS

Your drug prescription is tailored for you. Do not alter dosage without checking with your doctor.

How taken/used Tablets, MR-tablets, capsules, liquid, injection.

Frequency and timing of doses 1–2 x daily, after food.

Dosage range 600mg–2.5g daily, adjusted as necessary.

Onset of effect Within 60 minutes.

Duration of action 12 hours or more.

Diet advice None.

Storage Keep in original container at room temperature out of the reach of children. Protect from light.

Missed dose Take as soon as you remember. If your next dose is due within 2 hours, take a single dose now and skip the next.

Stopping the drug Do not stop the drug without consulting your doctor; symptoms may recur.

Exceeding the dose An occasional unintentional extra dose is unlikely to cause problems. Large overdoses may lead to coma. Notify your doctor.

POSSIBLE ADVERSE EFFECTS

Most adverse effects of sodium valproate are uncommon and the most serious ones are even rarer. They include liver failure, and platelet and bleeding abnormalities. Menstrual periods may become irregular or cease altogether. The drug may also cause temporary hair loss, weight gain, nausea, or indigestion. Report a rash, drowsiness, jaundice, or bruising or bleeding to your doctor at once.

INTERACTIONS

Other anticonvulsant drugs These drugs may reduce blood levels of sodium valproate.

Antidepressants, antipsychotics, mefloquine, and chloroquine These drugs may reduce the effectiveness of sodium valproate to prevent seizures.

Clarithromycin and erythromycin These drugs may increase the effects of sodium valproate.

Zidovudine When zidovudine and sodium valproate are taken together, the blood levels of zidovudine may increase, leading to increased adverse effects.

Lamotrigine Sodium valproate increases levels of lamotrigine and may lead to increased adverse effects.

SPECIAL PRECAUTIONS

Be sure to tell your doctor if:
◆ You have long-term liver or kidney problems.
◆ You have porphyria.
◆ You have any blood disorders.
◆ You are taking other medicines.

Pregnancy Not recommended. May cause abnormalities in the unborn baby. If sodium valproate is essential, extra folic acid supplements must also be taken. Discuss with your doctor.

Breast-feeding The drug passes into the breast milk, but at normal doses adverse effects on the baby are unlikely. Discuss with your doctor.

Infants and children Reduced dose necessary. The dose is often based on the weight of the child.

Over 60 Reduced dose may be necessary.

Driving and hazardous work Your underlying condition, as well as the possibility of reduced alertness while taking sodium valproate, may make such activities inadvisable. Discuss with your doctor.

Alcohol Avoid. Alcohol may increase the sedative effects of this drug.

PROLONGED USE

Use of this drug can, very rarely, cause liver damage, which is more likely in the first 6 months of use.

Monitoring Periodic blood tests of liver function and blood composition may be carried out.

Sotalol

Brand names Beta-Cardone, Sotacor
Used in the following combined preparations None

QUICK REFERENCE
Drug group Beta blocker (p.30)
Overdose danger rating Medium
Dependence rating Low
Prescription needed Yes
Available as generic Yes

GENERAL INFORMATION
Sotalol is a non-cardioselective beta blocker used in the prevention and treatment of ventricular and supraventricular arrhythmias (see p.34). It has an additional anti-arrhythmic action to other beta blockers.

Sotalol is no longer prescribed for the other conditions that beta blockers are prescribed for. This is due to the risk of a serious side effect called 'torsades de pointes', a kind of ventricular arrhythmia that is serious enough to produce symptoms that can be serious and, rarely, life-threatening. For this reason, anyone prescribed sotalol will be carefully monitored.

INFORMATION FOR USERS
Your drug prescription is tailored for you. Do not alter dosage without checking with your doctor.
How taken/used Tablets, injection.
Frequency and timing of doses 2 x daily (tablets); 6-hourly intervals when necessary (injections).
Adult dosage range 80mg daily initially, increased at 2–3-day intervals to 160–320mg daily. Higher doses of 480–640mg under specialist supervision.
Onset of effect 12 hours.
Duration of action 12 hours.
Diet advice None.
Storage Keep in original container at room temperature out of the reach of children. Protect from light.

Missed dose Take as soon as you remember. If your next dose is due within 3 hours, take a single dose now and skip the next.
Stopping the drug Do not stop the drug without consulting your doctor, who will supervise a gradual reduction in dosage. Sudden withdrawal may lead to worsening of your condition.
Exceeding the dose An occasional unintentional extra dose is unlikely to be a cause for concern. Large overdoses may cause low blood pressure, slow heart rate, heart block, bronchospasm, and heart arrhythmias. Notify your doctor immediately.

POSSIBLE ADVERSE EFFECTS
A very fast heart rate with palpitations could be a symptom of torsades de pointes, which should be reported to your doctor immediately. Lethargy, dizziness, and cold hands or feet are common. Nightmares or vivid dreams are also common; discuss these with your doctor. If, rarely, a rash, dry eyes, wheezing, breathlessness, palpitations, or fainting occur, contact your doctor urgently.

INTERACTIONS
Phenothiazines, antidepressants, astemizole, moxifloxacin, mizolastine, ivabradine, antipsychotics, terfenadine, and erythromycin (IV) These drugs increase the risk of torsades de pointes with sotalol.
Calcium channel blockers These may cause low blood pressure, slow heartbeats and heart failure if taken with sotalol.
Diuretics, amphotericin, corticosteroids, and some laxatives These drugs may lower blood potassium levels, increasing the risk of torsades de pointes.
Anti-arrhythmics such as amiodarone, disopyramide, quinidine, lidocaine, and procainamide Taking any of these drugs with sotalol may slow the heart rate and affect heart function.
Sympathomimetics such as epinephrine (adrenaline), norepinephrine (noradrenaline), and dobutamine There is a risk of severe high blood pressure if these drugs are taken with sotalol.

SPECIAL PRECAUTIONS
Be sure to tell your doctor if:
◆ You have liver or kidney problems.

◆ You have a breathing disorder such as asthma, bronchitis, or emphysema.
◆ You have heart failure.
◆ You have diabetes.
◆ You have psoriasis.
◆ You have hyperthyroidism.
◆ You have phaeochromocytoma.
◆ You have poor circulation in the legs.
◆ You are taking other medicines.

Pregnancy Not usually prescribed. May affect the unborn baby. Discuss with your doctor.

Breast-feeding The drug passes into the breast milk and may affect the baby. Discuss with your doctor.

Infants and children Not prescribed.

Over 60 Reduced dose may be necessary.

Driving and hazardous work Do not undertake such activities until you have learned how sotalol affects you because the drug can cause dizziness and fatigue.

Alcohol No special problems.

Surgery and general anaesthetics Sotalol may interact with some anaesthetics. Discuss with your doctor or dentist.

PROLONGED USE

Sotalol may be taken indefinitely for prevention of ventricular arrhythmias.

Monitoring Periodic blood tests are usually performed to monitor levels of potassium and magnesium. The heartbeat is usually monitored for signs of development of torsades de pointes.

Spironolactone

Brand names Aldactone, Laractone, Spiroctan, Spirolone, Spirospare
Used in the following combined preparations
Aldactide, Lasilactone, Spiro-Co

QUICK REFERENCE

Drug group Potassium-sparing diuretic (p.32)
Overdose danger rating Low
Dependence rating Low
Prescription needed Yes
Available as generic Yes

GENERAL INFORMATION

Spironolactone belongs to the class of drugs known as potassium-sparing diuretics. Combined with thiazide or loop diuretics, it is used in the treatment of oedema (fluid retention) resulting from congestive heart failure. On its own or, more commonly, in combination with a thiazide, spironolactone may be used to treat oedema associated with cirrhosis of the liver, nephrotic syndrome (a kidney disorder), and a rare disease called Conn's syndrome, which is caused by a benign tumour in one of the adrenal glands.

Spironolactone is relatively slow to act, and its effects may appear only after several days of treatment. As with other potassium-sparing diuretics, there is a risk of unusually high levels of potassium in the blood if the kidneys are functioning abnormally. For this reason, the drug is prescribed with caution to people with kidney failure.

It does not worsen gout or diabetes, as do some other diuretics. The major side effect is nausea, but abnormal breast enlargement may occur in men if high doses are given.

INFORMATION FOR USERS

Your drug prescription is tailored for you. Do not alter dosage without checking with your doctor.

How taken/used Tablets, capsules, liquid.

Frequency and timing of doses Once daily, usually in the morning.

Adult dosage range 25–400mg daily.

Onset of effect Within 1–3 days, but full effect may take up to 2 weeks.

Duration of action 2–3 days.

Diet advice Avoid foods that are high in potassium, for example, dried fruit and salt substitutes.

Storage Keep in original container at room temperature out of the reach of children. Protect from light.

Missed dose Take as soon as you remember.

Stopping the drug Do not stop the drug without consulting your doctor; symptoms may recur.

Exceeding the dose An occasional unintentional extra dose is unlikely to be a cause for concern. But if you notice any unusual symptoms, or if a large overdose has been taken, notify your doctor.

POSSIBLE ADVERSE EFFECTS

There are few common adverse effects; the main problem is the possibility that potassium may be retained by the body, causing muscle weakness and numbness. Nausea and vomiting are common. Headache, lethargy, drowsiness, and irregular menstruation may occur rarely. Breast enlargement or impotence may also occur rarely in men; consult your doctor. If a rash occurs, stop taking the drug and consult your doctor immediately.

INTERACTIONS

ACE inhibitors, NSAIDs, angiotensin II blockers, ciclosporin, tacrolimus, and potassium salts These drugs may increase the risk of raised blood levels of potassium, and can enhance the lowering of blood pressure caused by spironolactone.

Lithium Spironolactone may increase the blood levels of lithium, leading to an increased risk of lithium toxicity.

Digoxin Adverse effects may result from increased digoxin levels.

SPECIAL PRECAUTIONS

Be sure to tell your doctor if:
◆ You have long-term liver or kidney problems.
◆ You have porphyria.
◆ You have Addison's disease.
◆ You have a metabolic disorder.
◆ You are taking other medicines.

Pregnancy Not usually prescribed. May have adverse effects on the baby. Discuss with your doctor.

Breast-feeding The drug passes into the breast milk, but at normal doses adverse effects on the baby are unlikely. Discuss with your doctor.

Infants and children Reduced dose necessary.

Over 60 Increased likelihood of adverse effects. Reduced dose may be necessary.

Driving and hazardous work Avoid such activities until you have learned how spironolactone affects you because the drug may occasionally cause drowsiness.

Alcohol No known problems.

PROLONGED USE

Long-term use in the young is avoided if possible.

Monitoring Blood tests may be performed to check on kidney function and levels of body salts.

Streptokinase

Brand name Streptase
Used in the following combined preparation
Varidase

QUICK REFERENCE

Drug group Thrombolytic drug (p.40)
Overdose danger rating Medium
Dependence rating Low
Prescription needed Yes
Available as generic Yes

GENERAL INFORMATION

Streptokinase, an enzyme produced by the streptococcus bacteria, is used in hospitals to dissolve the fibrin of blood clots, especially those in the arteries of the heart and lungs. It is also used on the clots formed in shunts during kidney dialysis.

A fast-acting thrombolytic drug (see p.107), streptokinase is most effective in dissolving any newly formed clots, and it is often released at the site of the clot via a catheter inserted into an artery. Administered in the early stages of a heart attack to dissolve a clot (thrombosis) in the coronary arteries, it can reduce the amount of damage to heart muscle. Because excessive bleeding is a common side effect of streptokinase, treatment is closely supervised.

Streptokinase is also used to treat wounds and ulcers in combination with another enzyme called streptodornase. For this use, powder is applied locally.

Because streptokinase is a protein, it can cause allergic reactions. To reduce this risk, an antihistamine may be given at the start of treatment.

INFORMATION FOR USERS

The drug is given only under medical supervision and is not for self administration.

How taken/used Injection, topical powder.

Frequency and timing of doses By a single injection or continuously over a period of 24–72 hours. *Powder* 1–2 x daily.

Dosage range Dosages are determined individually by the condition and response of the patient.

Onset of effect As soon as streptokinase reaches the blood clot, the clot begins to

dissolve within minutes. Most of the blood clot will have dissolved within a few hours.
Duration of action Effect disappears within a few minutes of stopping the drug.
Diet advice None.
Storage Not applicable. This drug is not normally kept in the home.
Missed dose Not applicable. This drug is given only in hospital under close medical supervision.
Stopping the drug The drug is usually given for up to 3 days.
Exceeding the dose Overdose is unlikely since treatment is carefully monitored.

POSSIBLE ADVERSE EFFECTS

Because streptokinase is given only under strict medical supervision, all of its adverse effects will be closely monitored in order for them to be dealt with quickly. All of the adverse effects listed here should be reported to your doctor immediately. Nausea, vomiting, and excessive bleeding are common. Rarely, a fever, wheezing, or abnormal heart rhythms may occur. If a rash, itching, or collapse (signs of an allergic reaction) occur, the treatment should be stopped.

INTERACTIONS

Anticoagulant drugs There is an increased risk of bleeding when these are taken at the same time as streptokinase.
Antiplatelet drugs There is an increased risk of bleeding if these drugs are given with streptokinase.

SPECIAL PRECAUTIONS

Streptokinase is prescribed only under close medical supervision, usually only in life-threatening circumstances.
Pregnancy Not usually prescribed. If the drug is used during the first 18 weeks of pregnancy there is a risk that the placenta may separate from the wall of the uterus.
Breast-feeding It is not known whether the drug passes into breast milk or is harmful. Discard breast milk for first 24 hours after treatment.
Infants and children Reduced dose necessary.
Over 60 Increased likelihood of bleeding into the brain.
Driving and hazardous work Not applicable.

Alcohol Not applicable.

PROLONGED USE

Streptokinase is never used long term.
Further instructions Once you have had a dose of streptokinase, you will be given a card, which you must keep with you at all times and present to any doctor, in case further treatment is required. A second course of treatment would not normally be given within 12 months of the first.

Sucralfate

Brand name Antepsin
Used in the following combined preparations None

QUICK REFERENCE
Drug group Ulcer-healing drug (p.43)
Overdose danger rating Low
Dependence rating Low
Prescription needed Yes
Available as generic No

GENERAL INFORMATION

Sucralfate is a drug that is partly derived from aluminium. It is prescribed to treat gastric and duodenal ulcers. Sucralfate does not neutralize stomach acid, but it forms a protective barrier over the ulcer that protects it from attack by digestive juices, giving it time to heal.

If it is necessary, during treatment with sucralfate, to take antacids to relieve pain, they should be taken at least half an hour before or after taking sucralfate.

There have been a few reports of seriously ill patients developing bezoars (balls of indigestible material) in their stomachs while they are undergoing treatment with sucralfate. The safety of the drug for long-term use has not yet been confirmed. Therefore, courses of more than 12 weeks are not recommended.

INFORMATION FOR USERS

Your drug prescription is tailored for you. Do not alter dosage without checking with your doctor.
How taken/used Tablets, liquid.

Frequency and timing of doses 2–6 x daily, 1 hour before each meal and at bedtime, at least 2 hours after food. The tablets may be dispersed in a small glass of water before being swallowed.

Dosage range 4–8g daily.

Onset of effect Some improvement may be noted after one or two doses, but it takes a few weeks for an ulcer to heal.

Duration of action Up to 5 hours.

Diet advice Your doctor will advise if supplements are needed.

Storage Keep in original container at room temperature out of the reach of children.

Missed dose Do not make up the dose you missed. Take your next dose on your original schedule.

Stopping the drug Do not stop the drug without consulting your doctor; symptoms may recur.

Exceeding the dose An occasional unintentional extra dose is unlikely to be a cause for concern. But if you notice any unusual symptoms, or if a large overdose has been taken, notify your doctor.

POSSIBLE ADVERSE EFFECTS

Most people do not experience any adverse effects while they are taking sucralfate. The most common adverse effect is constipation, which will diminish as your body adjusts to the drug; indigestion is also common. Rarely, diarrhoea, a dry mouth, and headache may occur. Nausea, a rash, itching, dizziness, or vertigo are also rare and should be discussed with your doctor.

INTERACTIONS

General note Sucralfate may reduce the absorption and effect of a range of drugs, including ranitidine, digoxin, phenytoin, warfarin, levothyroxine, and antibacterials. Take these and other medications at least 30 minutes before or 2 hours after sucralfate.

Antacids and other indigestion remedies These reduce the effectiveness of sucralfate and should be taken at least 30 minutes before or after sucralfate.

SPECIAL PRECAUTIONS

Be sure to tell your doctor if:
♦ You have a long-term kidney problem.

♦ You are taking other medicines.

Pregnancy Safety in pregnancy not established. Discuss with your doctor.

Breast-feeding It is not known whether the drug passes into breast milk. Discuss with your doctor.

Infants and children Not usually prescribed.

Over 60 No special problems.

Driving and hazardous work Usually no problems, but sucralfate may cause dizziness in some people.

Alcohol Avoid. Alcohol may counteract the beneficial effect of this drug.

PROLONGED USE

Sucralfate is not usually prescribed for longer than 12 weeks at a time. Prolonged use of the drug may lead to deficiencies of vitamins A, D, E, and K.

Sulfasalazine

Brand names Salazopyrin, Sulazine EC
Used in the following combined preparations None

QUICK REFERENCE

Drug group Drug for inflammatory bowel disease (p.46) and disease-modifying antirheumatic drug (p.52)
Overdose danger rating Low
Dependence rating Low
Prescription needed Yes
Available as generic Yes

GENERAL INFORMATION

Sulfasalazine, a chemical combination of a sulphonamide and a salicylate, is used to treat 2 inflammatory disorders affecting the bowel: ulcerative colitis (which mainly affects the large intestine), and Crohn's disease (which usually affects the small intestine). Sulfasalazine is also used to modify, halt, or slow the underlying disease process in severe rheumatoid arthritis.

Adverse effects of sulfasalazine, such as nausea, loss of appetite, and general discomfort are more likely to occur when higher doses are taken. Side effects caused by stomach irritation may be avoided by changing to a specially coated tablet form of the drug. Allergic reactions to sulfasalazine, such as a fever and skin rash may be avoided or minimized by taking low initial doses of the drug, followed by gradual increases. Maintenance of adequate fluid intake is important while you are taking this drug. In rare cases among men, temporary sterility may occur.

INFORMATION FOR USERS

Your drug prescription is tailored for you. Do not alter dosage without checking with your doctor.

How taken/used Tablets, liquid, suppositories, enema.

Frequency and timing of doses 4 x daily after meals with a glass of water (tablets); 2 x daily (suppositories); once daily, usually at bedtime (enema).

Adult dosage range 4–8g daily (Crohn's disease/ulcerative colitis); 500mg–3g daily (rheumatoid arthritis).

Onset of effect Adverse effects may occur within a few days, but full beneficial effects may take 1–3 weeks, depending on the severity of the condition.

Duration of action Up to 24 hours.

Diet advice It is important to drink plenty of liquids (at least 1.5 litres a day) during treatment. Sulfasalazine may reduce the absorption of folic acid from the intestine, leading to a deficiency of this vitamin. Eat plenty of green vegetables.

Storage Keep in original container at room temperature out of the reach of children.

Missed dose Take as soon as you remember. If your next dose is due within 2 hours, take a single dose now and skip the next.

Stopping the drug Do not stop the drug without consulting your doctor; symptoms may recur.

Exceeding the dose An occasional unintentional extra dose is unlikely to be a cause for concern. But if you notice any unusual symptoms, or if a large overdose has been taken, notify your doctor.

POSSIBLE ADVERSE EFFECTS

Adverse effects are common with high doses of sulfasalazine, but they may disappear with a reduction in dosage. Symptoms such as nausea and vomiting are common and may

be helped if you take the drug with food. Orange or yellow discoloration of the urine is no cause for concern. Malaise, loss of appetite are also common side effects of the drug. Headache and joint pain, which are also common, should be discussed with your doctor. Ringing in the ears is rare, and you should consult your doctor if it occurs. If, rarely, you develop a fever or a rash, or you experience bleeding or bruising, seek immediate medical attention.

INTERACTIONS

General note 1 Sulfasalazine may increase the effects of some drugs, including mercaptopurine and azathioprine.

General note 2 Sulfasalazine reduces the absorption and effect of some drugs, including digoxin, folic acid, and iron.

SPECIAL PRECAUTIONS

Be sure to tell your doctor if:
◆ You have long-term liver or kidney problems.
◆ You have glucose-6-phosphate dehydrogenase (G6PD) deficiency.
◆ You have a blood disorder.
◆ You suffer from porphyria.
◆ You are allergic to sulphonamides or salicylates.
◆ You wear soft contact lenses.
◆ You are taking other medicines.

Pregnancy No evidence of risk to developing fetus. Folic acid supplements may be required. Discuss with your doctor.

Breast-feeding The drug passes into the breast milk and may affect the baby. Discuss with your doctor.

Infants and children Not recommended under 2 years. Reduced dose necessary for older children, according to body weight.

Over 60 No special problems.

Driving and hazardous work No special problems.

Alcohol No known problems.

PROLONGED USE

Blood disorders may occur with prolonged use of this drug. Maintenance dosage is usually continued indefinitely.

Monitoring Periodic tests of blood composition and liver function are usually required.

Sumatriptan

Brand name Imigran
**Used in the following combined
preparations** None

QUICK REFERENCE

Drug group Drug for migraine (p.20)
Overdose danger rating Medium
Dependence rating Low
Prescription needed Yes (injection and nasal spray)
No (others)
Available as generic Yes

GENERAL INFORMATION

Sumatriptan is a highly effective drug for migraine. It is usually given to people who fail
to respond to analgesics (such as aspirin and
paracetamol). Sumatriptan is of considerable
value in the treatment of acute attacks of
migraine, whether or not they are preceded
by an aura, but the drug is not meant to
be taken regularly to prevent attacks from
occurring. Sumatriptan is also used for the
acute treatment of cluster headache (a form
of migraine headache). It should be taken as
soon as possible after the onset of the attack,
although, unlike other drugs used in migraine, it will still be of benefit at whatever
stage of the attack it is taken.

Sumatriptan relieves the symptoms of migraine by preventing the dilation of blood
vessels in the brain, which causes the attack.

INFORMATION FOR USERS

Your drug prescription is tailored for you.
Do not alter dosage without checking with
your doctor.
How taken/used Tablets, injection, nasal spray.
Frequency and timing of doses Sumatriptan
should be taken as soon as possible after the
onset of an attack, but it is equally effective at
any stage. Do not take a second dose for the
same attack, or within 2 hours if migraine
recurs.
Adult dosage range *Tablets* 50–100mg per
attack, up to a maximum of 300mg in
24 hours if another attack occurs. Do not
take a second dose for the same attack, or
within 2 hours if migraine recurs. *Injection*
6mg per attack, up to a maximum of 12mg
(2 injections) in 24 hours if another attack

occurs. Do not take a second dose for the
same attack, or within 1 hour if migraine
recurs. *Nasal spray* Adults: 1 x 20mg puff
into one nostril per attack, to a maximum of
40mg (2 puffs) in 24 hours if another attack
occurs; Age 12 to 17 years: 1 x 10mg puff into
one nostril per attack, to a maximum of
20mg (2 puffs) in 24 hours if another attack
occurs.
Onset of effect 30–45 minutes (tablets);
10–15 minutes (injection); 15 minutes (nasal
spray).
Duration of action *Tablets* 2–4 hours. *Injection*
1½–2 hours. *Tablets* 2–4 hours. *Nasal spray*
1–3 hours.
Diet advice None, unless otherwise advised.
Storage Keep in original container at room
temperature out of the reach of children.
Protect from light.
Missed dose Not applicable, as it is taken only
to treat a migraine attack.
Stopping the drug Taken only to treat a migraine attack.
Exceeding the dose An occasional unintentional extra tablet or injection is unlikely to
cause problems. But if you notice any unusual symptoms, or if a large overdose has
been taken, notify your doctor.

POSSIBLE ADVERSE EFFECTS

Many of the adverse effects of sumatriptan
will disappear after about an hour as your
body becomes adjusted to the medicine. If
the symptoms persist or are severe, contact
your doctor. Commonly, there may be pain
at the injection site, flushing, a feeling of tingling or heat or a feeling of heaviness or
weakness. Rare side effects of the drug
include dizziness, fatigue, and drowsiness. If
you experience palpitations or chest pain,
stop taking the drug and seek immediate
medical attention.

INTERACTIONS

Antidepressants Monoamine oxidase inhibitors (MAOIs) and some other antidepressants, such as fluvoxamine, fluoxetine,
paroxetine, sertraline, and St John's wort
increase the risk of adverse effects with
sumatriptan.
Lithium High risk of adverse effects if these
drugs are taken with sumatriptan.

Ergotamine Must be taken at least 6 hours after you have taken sumatriptan, and sumatriptan must be taken at least 24 hours after ergotamine.

SPECIAL PRECAUTIONS

Be sure to tell your doctor if:
◆ You have liver or kidney problems.
◆ You have heart problems.
◆ You have high blood pressure.
◆ You have had a heart attack.
◆ You have had a stroke.
◆ You have angina.
◆ You are allergic to some medicines.
◆ You are taking other medicines.

Pregnancy Safety in pregnancy not established. Discuss with your doctor.

Breast-feeding Safety not established. Discuss with your doctor.

Infants and children Not recommended under 12 years.

Over 60 No recommended for patients over 65 years.

Driving and hazardous work Avoid such activities until you have learned how sumatriptan affects you because the drug can cause drowsiness.

Alcohol No special problems, but some drinks may provoke migraine in some people (see p.20).

Surgery and general anaesthetics Notify your doctor or dentist if you have used sumatriptan within 48 hours prior to surgery.

PROLONGED USE

Sumatriptan should not be used continuously to prevent migraine but only to treat migraine attacks.

Tamoxifen

Brand names Nolvadex, Soltamox
Used in the following combined preparations None

QUICK REFERENCE

Drug group Anticancer drug (p.96)
Overdose danger rating Low
Dependence rating Low
Prescription needed Yes
Available as generic Yes

GENERAL INFORMATION

Tamoxifen is an anti-oestrogen drug (oestrogen is a naturally occurring female sex hormone, see p.88). It is used for two conditions: infertility and breast cancer. When given as treatment of certain types of infertility, the drug is taken only on certain days of the menstrual cycle. Used as an anticancer drug for breast cancer, it works against oestrogens. By latching on to cells that recognize these hormones, it can slow the growth of the tumour and even shrink it. It is effective in reducing the recurrence of breast cancer after surgical removal of the tumour.

Because its effect is specific, tamoxifen has fewer adverse effects than most other drugs that are used for breast cancer. However, it may cause eye damage if high doses are taken for long periods.

INFORMATION FOR USERS

Your drug prescription is tailored for you. Do not alter dosage without checking with your doctor.

How taken/used Tablets, liquid.

Frequency and timing of doses 1–2 x daily.

Adult dosage range 20mg daily (breast cancer). 20–80mg daily (infertility).

Onset of effect Side effects may be felt within days, but beneficial effects may take 4–10 weeks.

Duration of action Effects may be felt for several weeks after stopping the drug.

Diet advice None.

Storage Keep in original container at room temperature out of the reach of children. Protect from light.

Missed dose Take as soon as you remember. If your next dose is due within 2 hours, take a single dose now and skip the next.

Stopping the drug Do not stop the drug without consulting your doctor; stopping the drug may lead to worsening of your underlying condition.

Exceeding the dose An occasional unintentional extra dose is unlikely to be a cause for concern. But if you notice any unusual symptoms, or if a large overdose has been taken, notify your doctor.

POSSIBLE ADVERSE EFFECTS

Adverse effects are rarely serious with tamoxifen and do not usually require the treatment to be stopped. Nausea, vomiting, and hot flushes are the most common reactions. There is a small risk of endometrial cancer (cancer of the lining of the uterus) developing; therefore, you should notify your doctor of any symptoms such as irregular vaginal bleeding or discharge as soon as possible. Rarely, bone and tumour pain, a rash, itching, blurred vision, and headache may occur and should be discussed with your doctor. If you experience calf pain or swelling, contact your doctor immediately.

INTERACTIONS

Anticoagulants People treated with anticoagulants such as warfarin usually need a lower dose of the anticoagulant.

Anticancer medicines Cytotoxic medicines taken with tamoxifen may increase the risk of side effects.

SPECIAL PRECAUTIONS

Be sure to tell your doctor if:
◆ You have cataracts or poor eyesight.
◆ You suffer from porphyria.
◆ You are taking other medicines.

Pregnancy Not usually prescribed. May have effects on the developing baby. Discuss with your doctor.

Breast-feeding Not usually prescribed. Discuss with your doctor.

Infants and children Not prescribed.

Over 60 No special problems.

Driving and hazardous work Do not drive until you have learned how tamoxifen affects you because the drug can cause dizziness and blurred vision.

Alcohol No known problems.

Surgery and general anaesthetics Tell your doctor or anaesthetist that you are taking tamoxifen before you have any surgery. You may be advised to stop taking the drug 6 weeks before.

PROLONGED USE

There is a risk of damage to the eye with long-term, high-dose treatment.

There is a small increased risk of endometrial cancer with long-term treatment but this is far outweighed by the benefits of treatment.

Monitoring Your eyesight may be tested periodically.

Tamsulosin

Brand names Flomaxtra XL, Omnic MR, Stronazon MR
Used in the following combined preparations None

QUICK REFERENCE

Drug group Drug for urinary disorders (p.112)
Overdose danger rating Medium
Dependence rating Low
Prescription needed Yes
Available as generic Yes

GENERAL INFORMATION

Tamsulosin is a selective alpha-blocker drug used to treat urinary retention as a result of benign prostatic hypertrophy, or BPH (enlarged prostate gland). The drug, as it passes through the prostate, relaxes the muscle in the wall of the urethra, thereby increasing the flow of urine.

To exclude other conditions with similar symptoms, your doctor will arrange for you to have a physical examination and a special blood test, which may be repeated at intervals during treatment.

Like other alpha-blockers, tamsulosin may lower blood pressure rapidly after the first dose is taken. For this reason, the first dose should be taken at home so that, if dizziness or weakness occur, you can lie down until they have disappeared.

INFORMATION FOR USERS

Your drug prescription is tailored for you. Do not alter dosage without checking with your doctor.

How taken/used Tablets, capsules.

Frequency and timing of doses Once daily, swallowed whole, after breakfast.

Adult dosage range 400mcg.

Onset of effect 1–2 hours.

Duration of action 24 hours.

Diet advice None.

Storage Keep in original container at room temperature out of the reach of children.

Missed dose Taken as soon as you remember. If your next dose is due within 4 hours, take a single dose now and skip the next.

Stopping the drug Do not stop taking the drug without consulting your doctor; stopping tamsulosin treatment suddenly may lead to a rise in blood pressure.

Exceeding the dose An occasional unintentional extra dose is unlikely to cause problems. Large overdoses may produce sedation, dizziness, low blood pressure and rapid pulse. Notify your doctor immediately.

POSSIBLE ADVERSE EFFECTS

Dizziness seems to be the most common adverse effect of tamsulosin, but this usually improves after the first few doses. Weakness, fainting, ejaculatory problems, headache, drowsiness, and palpitations are other common symptoms of the drug. Rarely, nausea, vomiting, diarrhoea, and constipation may also occur. If you develop a rash or itching, consult your doctor promptly.

INTERACTIONS

Antidepressants, beta blockers, calcium channel blockers, diuretics, and thymoxamine These drugs are likely to increase the blood pressure-lowering effect of tamsulosin.

SPECIAL PRECAUTIONS

Be sure to tell your doctor if:
◆ You have had low blood pressure.
◆ You have liver or kidney problems.
◆ You have heart failure.
◆ You have a history of depression.
◆ You are taking an MAOI drug.
◆ You are taking drugs for high blood pressure.
◆ You are taking other medicines.
Pregnancy Not prescribed.
Breast-feeding Not prescribed.
Infants and children Not prescribed.
Over 60 No special problems.
Driving and hazardous work Avoid such activities until you have learned how tamsulosin affects you because the drug can cause drowsiness and dizziness.
Alcohol Avoid until you know how tamsulosin affects you because alcohol can further lower blood pressure.
Surgery and general anaesthetics Tamsulosin may need to be stopped before you have any surgery. Discuss with your doctor or dentist.

PROLONGED USE

No special problems.

Temazepam

Brand names None
Used in the following combined preparations None

QUICK REFERENCE

Drug group Benzodiazepine sleeping drug (p.11)
Overdose danger rating Medium
Dependence rating High
Prescription needed Yes
Available as generic Yes

GENERAL INFORMATION

Temazepam belongs to the group of drugs known as the benzodiazepines. The actions and adverse effects of this group of drugs are described more fully under Anti-anxiety drugs (see p.13).

Temazepam is used in the short-term treatment of insomnia. Because it is short acting compared with other benzodiazepines, the drug is less likely to cause drowsiness and/or lightheadedness the following day. Temazepam is not usually effective in preventing early morning wakening.

Like other benzodiazepine drugs, temazepam can be habit-forming if taken regularly over a long period. Its effects also grow weaker with time. For these reasons, treatment with temazepam is usually only continued for a few days at a time.

INFORMATION FOR USERS

Your drug prescription is tailored for you. Do not alter dosage without checking with your doctor.
How taken/used Tablets, liquid.
Frequency and timing of doses Once daily, 30 minutes before bedtime.
Adult dosage range 10–40mg.
Onset of effect 15–40 minutes, or longer.
Duration of action 6–8 hours.
Diet advice None.
Storage Keep in original container at room temperature out of the reach of children. Protect from light.
Missed dose If you fall asleep without having taken a dose, and you wake some hours later, do not take the missed dose. If necessary, return to your normal dosing schedule the following night.

Stopping the drug If you have been taking the drug continuously for less than 2 weeks, it can be safely stopped as soon as you no longer need it. If you have been taking the drug for longer, consult your doctor, who may supervise a gradual reduction in dosage. Stopping abruptly may lead to withdrawal symptoms.

Exceeding the dose An occasional unintentional extra dose is unlikely to be a cause for concern. Large overdoses may cause unusual drowsiness. Notify your doctor.

POSSIBLE ADVERSE EFFECTS

The principal adverse effects of this drug are related to its sedative and tranquillizing properties. However, these effects, which include daytime drowsiness and headache, normally diminish after the first few days of treatment. Rarely, dizziness, unsteadiness, vivid dreams, and nightmares may occur and should be discussed with your doctor. Forgetfulness or confusion may also occur rarely and, if they do, stop taking the drug and consult your doctor.

INTERACTIONS

Sedatives All drugs that have a sedative effect on the central nervous system are likely to increase the sedative properties of temazepam. Such drugs include other anti-anxiety drugs, sleeping drugs, opioid analgesics, antidepressants, antihistamines, and antipsychotics.

SPECIAL PRECAUTIONS

Be sure to tell your doctor if:
◆ You have severe respiratory disease.
◆ You suffer from porphyria.
◆ You have liver or kidney problems.
◆ You have myasthenia gravis.
◆ You have had problems with alcohol or drug abuse.
◆ You are taking other medicines.

Pregnancy Safety in pregnancy not established. Discuss with your doctor.

Breast-feeding The drug passes into the breast milk, but at normal doses adverse effects on the baby are unlikely. Discuss with your doctor.

Infants and children Not recommended.

Over 60 Reduced dose may be necessary. Increased likelihood of adverse effects.

Driving and hazardous work Avoid such activities until you have learned how temazepam affects you because the drug can cause reduced alertness and slowed reactions.

Alcohol Avoid. Alcohol may increase the sedative effect of this drug.

PROLONGED USE

Regular use of temazepam over several weeks can lead to a reduction in its effect as the body adapts. The drug may also be habit-forming when taken for extended periods. Temazepam should not normally be used for longer than 1–2 weeks.

Tenecteplase

Brand name Metalyse
Used in the following combined preparations None

QUICK REFERENCE

Drug group Thrombolytic drug (p.40)
Overdose danger rating Medium
Dependence rating Low
Prescription needed Yes
Available as generic No

GENERAL INFORMATION

Tenecteplase is a fibrinolytic (or thrombolytic, see p.40) drug. It dissolves blood clots (thrombi) by boosting the action of the blood enzyme plasmin in breaking up the strands of fibrin that hold the clot together. It is given by intravenous injection. The sooner this is done after formation of the clot, the greater the success rate in clearing the clot from the coronary arteries in the heart, and reducing the damage to heart muscle. Tenecteplase is licensed only for treatment of heart attacks. Fibrinolytics are usually given in hospitals, where all the resources needed for this kind of urgent action are held in readiness.

After the tenecteplase has been given, aspirin and heparin are used to maintain the anticoagulant effect and to prevent further clotting. A low dose of aspirin will usually be prescribed long-term, and heparin will be given for a few days until the situation is stable.

Because tenecteplase activates the destruction of the body's fibrin (which causes clotting), the main side effect is bleeding, most often at the injection site. In addition, tenecteplase is a protein, and can therefore cause allergic reactions.

INFORMATION FOR USERS
The drug is only given under medical supervision and is not for self administration.
How taken/used Injection.
Frequency and timing of doses A single intravenous injection over 10 seconds.
Adult dosage range 30–50mg (6000–10000 units) depending on body weight.
Onset of effect The drug begins to dissolve the blood clot within minutes. Most of the clot will be gone within a few hours.
Duration of action 25–30 minutes.
Diet advice None.
Storage Not applicable. The drug is not normally kept in the home.
Missed dose Not applicable. The drug is given once, in urgent circumstances, in hospital.
Stopping the drug Not applicable.
Exceeding the dose Overdose is unlikely because dosage is carefully monitored.

POSSIBLE ADVERSE EFFECTS
Because tenecteplase is given only under close medical supervision, any of the symptoms that are listed below can be dealt with quickly. Nausea, vomiting, bleeding, palpitations, chest pain, fainting, and dizziness commonly occur. Rarely, you may experience wheezing, a rash, or itching. All adverse effects of this drug should be reported to your doctor immediately.

INTERACTIONS
Anticoagulants and drugs affecting platelet function may increase bleeding tendency.

SPECIAL PRECAUTIONS
Tenecteplase is prescribed only under close medical supervision, usually only under life-threatening circumstances.
Pregnancy Safety not established. The benefit of treatment must be weighed against the likelihood of bleeding and fetal loss.
Breast-feeding It is not known whether the drug passes into breast milk, or is harmful.

Discard breast milk for first 24 hours after treatment.
Infants and children Reduced dose necessary.
Over 60 No known problems.
Driving and hazardous work Not applicable.
Alcohol Not applicable.

PROLONGED USE
No applicable.

Terbinafine

Brand names Lamisil, Lamisil Once
Used in the following combined preparations None

QUICK REFERENCE
Drug group Antifungal drug (p.76)
Overdose danger rating Low
Dependence rating Low
Prescription needed Yes (except for some skin preparations)
Available as generic No

GENERAL INFORMATION
Terbinafine is an antifungal drug used to treat fungal infections of the skin and nails, particularly tinea (ringworm). It is also used as a cream for candida (yeast) infections.

Terbinafine has largely replaced older drugs such as griseofulvin because it is more easily absorbed and is therefore more effective.

Tinea infections are treated in 2–6 weeks, but treatment of nail infections may take up to 6 months.

Rare adverse effects of terbinafine include a sore mouth and/or throat, jaundice, a severe skin rash, bruising and/or bleeding in the mouth, and dark urine. All of these adverse effects should be reported to your doctor without delay.

INFORMATION FOR USERS
Your drug prescription is tailored for you. Do not alter dosage without checking with your doctor.
How taken/used Tablets, cream, skin solution.
Frequency and timing of doses Once daily (tablets); 1–2 x daily (cream); once only (solution).
Adult Dosage range *Tinea infections* 250mg

(tablets). *Candida infections* As directed (cream).

Onset of effect Depends on the type and severity of infection.

Duration of action 24 hours.

Diet advice None.

Storage Keep in original container at room temperature out of the reach of children. Protect from light.

Missed dose Take as soon as you remember. If your next dose is due within 4 hours, take a single dose now and skip the next.

Stopping the drug Take the full course. Even if you feel better, the original infection may still be present and may recur if treatment is stopped too soon.

Exceeding the dose An occasional unintentional extra dose is unlikely to be a cause for concern. But if you notice any unusual symptoms, or if a large overdose has been taken, notify your doctor.

POSSIBLE ADVERSE EFFECTS

Side effects of terbinafine are generally mild and transient. Nausea, indigestion, bloating, abdominal pain, diarrhoea, and headache are common. Disturbance in, or loss of, taste, dizziness, a 'pins and needles' feeling, and tiredness occur more rarely and should be discussed with your doctor. If you experience muscle or joint pain, consult your doctor promptly. A severe rash, a sore mouth or throat, bruising or bleeding in the mouth, jaundice, or dark urine are also rare, and, if they occur, stop taking the drug and contact your doctor urgently.

INTERACTIONS

Rifampicin This drug may reduce the blood level and effect of terbinafine.

Cimetidine This drug may increase blood level of terbinafine.

Oral contraceptives "Breakthrough" bleeding may occur when these are taken with terbinafine.

SPECIAL PRECAUTIONS

Be sure to tell your doctor if:
◆ You have liver or kidney problems.
◆ You have psoriasis.
◆ You are taking other medicines.

Pregnancy Safety in pregnancy not estab-

lished. Discuss with your doctor.

Breast-feeding The drug passes into the breast milk and may affect the baby adversely. Discuss with your doctor.

Infants and children Safety not established. Discuss with your doctor.

Over 60 No special problems.

Driving and hazardous work No known problems.

Alcohol No known problems.

PROLONGED USE

No special problems.

Terbutaline

Brand name Bricanyl
Used in the following combined preparations None

QUICK REFERENCE

Drug group Bronchodilator (p.23)
Overdose danger rating Low
Dependence rating Low
Prescription needed Yes
Available as generic Yes

GENERAL INFORMATION

Terbutaline is a sympathomimetic bronchodilator that dilates the small airways in the lungs. The drug is used in the treatment and prevention of the bronchospasm occurring with asthma, chronic bronchitis, and emphysema. Terbutaline is also used to delay premature labour.

Muscle tremor, especially of the hands, is common with terbutaline and usually disappears on reduction of the dose or with continued use as the body adapts to the drug. As with the other sympathomimetic drugs, it may produce nervousness and restlessness.

INFORMATION FOR USERS

Your drug prescription is tailored for you. Do not alter dosage without checking with your doctor.

How taken/used Tablets, liquid (syrup), injection, inhaler, nebules for nebulizer.

Frequency and timing of doses 3 x daily (tablets/syrup); as necessary (inhaler).

Dosage range *Adults* 7.5–15mg daily (tablets/

syrup); 0.5mg when required, up to 2mg daily (inhaler); as directed by doctor (nebules). *Children* Reduced dose according to age and weight.

Onset of effect Within a few minutes (inhaler); within 1–2 hours (tablets/syrup).

Duration of action 7–8 hours (tablets/syrup).

Diet advice None.

Storage Keep in original container at room temperature out of the reach of children. Protect from light. Do not puncture or burn aerosol containers.

Missed dose Do not take the missed dose. Take your next dose as usual.

Stopping the drug Do not stop the drug without consulting your doctor; symptoms may recur.

Exceeding the dose An occasional unintentional extra dose is unlikely to be a cause for concern. But if you notice any unusual symptoms, or if a large overdose has been taken, notify your doctor.

POSSIBLE ADVERSE EFFECTS

Possible adverse effects, including tremor, nervousness, restlessness, and nausea or vomiting, may be reduced by dosage adjustment. Anxiety also commonly occurs. Headache and sleep disturbance occur rarely; discuss with your doctor. Palpitations and headache (resulting from stimulation of the heart and narrowing of the blood vessels) and muscle cramps are also rare and, if they occur, consult your doctor promptly.

INTERACTIONS

Other sympathomimetics may add to the effects of terbutaline and vice versa, increasing the risk of adverse effects.

Monoamine oxidase inhibitors (MAOIs) Terbutaline may interact with these drugs to cause a dangerous rise in blood pressure.

Diuretics, corticosteroids, and theophylline taken with terbutaline may reduce blood levels of potassium, causing muscle weakness.

Beta blockers may reduce the beneficial effects of terbutaline.

SPECIAL PRECAUTIONS

Be sure to tell your doctor if:
◆ You have heart problems.
◆ You have high blood pressure.
◆ You have diabetes.
◆ You have an overactive thyroid.
◆ You are taking other medicines.

Pregnancy Safety in early pregnancy not established, although it is used in late pregnancy to prevent premature labour. Discuss with your doctor.

Breast-feeding The drug passes into the breast milk and may affect the baby adversely. Discuss with your doctor.

Infants and children Reduced dose necessary.

Over 60 Increased likelihood of adverse effects. Reduced dose may therefore be necessary.

Driving and hazardous work Avoid such activities until you have learned how terbutaline affects you because the drug can cause tremor of the hands.

Alcohol No special problems.

PROLONGED USE

Prolonged use may result in tolerance to the effects of terbutaline. However, failure to respond to the drug may be a result of worsening asthma, requiring prompt medical attention.

Testosterone

Brand names Andropatch, Nebido, Restandol, Striant SR, Sustanon, Testim, Testogel, Virormone
Used in the following combined preparations None

QUICK REFERENCE

Drug group Male sex hormone (p.87)
Overdose danger rating Low
Dependence rating Low
Prescription needed Yes
Available as generic Yes

GENERAL INFORMATION

Testosterone is a male sex hormone that is produced by the testes and, in small quantities, by the ovaries in women. The hormone encourages bone and muscle growth in both men and women and stimulates sexual development in men.

The drug is used to initiate puberty in male adolescents if it has been delayed due to deficiency of the natural hormone. It is also used in some cases of erectile dysfunction in men suffering from either pituitary or testicular disorders. Rarely, the drug is used to treat breast cancer.

Testosterone can interfere with growth or cause over-rapid sexual development in adolescents. High doses may cause deepening of the voice, excessive hair growth, or hair loss in women.

INFORMATION FOR USERS

Your drug prescription is tailored for you. Do not alter dosage without checking with your doctor.

How taken/used Buccal tablets, capsules, injection, implanted pellets, gel, patch.

Frequency and timing of doses 2 x daily (buccal tablets/capsules); varies according to preparation and condition being treated (injection); 5g daily, according to response, to maximum of 10g daily (gel); every 6 months (implant); once daily (patch).

Dosage range The dosage varies with the method of administration and the condition being treated.

Onset of effect 2–3 days. Full effect may take several months.

Duration of action 1–2 days (capsules and patch); 1–3 weeks (injection); approximately 6 months (implant).

Diet advice None.

Storage Keep in original container at room temperature out of the reach of children. Protect from light.

Missed dose No cause for concern, but take as soon as you remember. If your next dose (by mouth) is due within 3 hours, take a single dose now and skip the next.

Stopping the drug Do not stop taking the drug without consulting your doctor.

Exceeding the dose An occasional unintentional extra dose is unlikely to be a cause for concern. But if you notice unusual symptoms, or if a large overdose was taken, notify your doctor.

POSSIBLE ADVERSE EFFECTS

Most of the more serious adverse effects of testosterone are likely to occur only with long-term treatment, and may be helped by a reduction in dosage. Acne is a common adverse effect. Rarely, hair loss, mood changes, and water retention may occur. If jaundice occurs, stop the taking the drug and consult your doctor. Men may commonly experience abnormal erection, which should be reported to their doctor. Rarely, they may also experience breast enlargement or difficulty in passing urine, which should also be discussed with their doctor. Women may experience unusual hair growth or loss of hair, voice changes, and an enlarged clitoris; these occur rarely, but they should be discussed with their doctor.

INTERACTIONS

Anticoagulants Testosterone may increase their effect, requiring adjustment of their dosage.

Antidiabetics Testosterone enhances the effects of these drugs, requiring reduction of their dosage.

Liver enzyme inducing drugs (e.g. rifampicin and carbamazepine) These drugs may reduce the effects of testosterone.

SPECIAL PRECAUTIONS

Be sure to tell your doctor if:
◆ You have long-term liver or kidney problems.
◆ You have heart problems.
◆ You have prostate trouble.
◆ You have high blood pressure.
◆ You have epilepsy or migraine headaches.
◆ You have diabetes.
◆ You are taking other medicines.

Pregnancy Not prescribed.

Breast-feeding Not prescribed.

Infants and children Not prescribed for infants and young children. Reduced dose necessary in adolescents.

Over 60 Rarely required. Increased risk of prostate problems in elderly men. Reduced dose may therefore be necessary.

Driving and hazardous work No special problems.

Alcohol No special problems.

PROLONGED USE

Prolonged use of this drug may lead to reduced growth in adolescents.

Monitoring Regular blood tests for the effects of testosterone treatment are required.

Tetracycline/lymecycline

Brand names Economycin, Tetrachel, Tetralysal 300, Topicycline
Used in the following combined preparation Deteclo

QUICK REFERENCE

Drug group Tetracycline antibiotic (p.62)
Overdose danger rating Low
Dependence rating Low
Prescription needed Yes
Available as generic Yes

GENERAL INFORMATION

Tetracycline and lymecycline are tetracycline antibiotics, once a very widely used class of antibiotics. The development of drug-resistant bacteria has, however, reduced tetracyclines' effectiveness in many types of infection. Tetracycline and lymecycline are commonly used to treat acne and are still used for the treatment of chronic bronchitis, destructive forms of dental disease, and certain chest and genital infections due to mycoplasma organisms. They remain the treatment of choice for infections due to *chlamydia* and *rickettsia*.

Taken by mouth, these drugs can sometimes cause nausea, vomiting, and diarrhoea. Tetracyclines may discolour developing teeth if taken by children or by the mother during pregnancy. People with poor kidney function are not prescribed tetracycline drugs because they can cause further deterioration.

INFORMATION FOR USERS

Your drug prescription is tailored for you. Do not alter your dosage without checking with your doctor.

How taken/used Tablets, capsules, lotion.
Frequency and timing of doses *By mouth* 2–4 x daily, at least 1 hour before or 2 hours after meals (tetracycline); 1–2 x daily (lymecycline). Always swallow doses with water. *Skin preparations* 1–2 times daily as directed.
Adults dosage range *Infections* 1–2g daily (tetracycline); 916–1,032mg daily (lymecycline). *Acne* 1g daily (tetracycline); 408mg daily (lymecycline).
Onset of effect 4–12 hours. Improvement in acne may not be noticed for up to 4 weeks.

Duration of action Up to 6 hours.
Diet advice Milk products should be avoided for 1 hour before and 2 hours after taking the drug.
Storage Keep in original container at room temperature out of the reach of children.
Missed dose Take as soon as you remember. If your next dose is due within 2 hours, take a single dose now and skip the next.
Stopping the drug Take the full course. Even if you feel better, the original infection may still be present and may recur if treatment is stopped too soon.
Exceeding the dose An occasional unintentional extra dose is unlikely to be a cause for concern. But if you notice any unusual symptoms, or if a large overdose has been taken, notify your doctor.

POSSIBLE ADVERSE EFFECTS

Swallowing difficulties and/or oesophageal irritation may occur if the dose is taken with insufficient water. Do not take a dose prior to lying down, to prevent the drug from lodging in the oesophagus. Adverse effects from skin preparations are rare. Nausea, vomiting, or diarrhoea are common. If, rarely, you develop a light-sensitive rash, itching, jaundice, a headache, or visual disturbance, stop taking the drug and consult your doctor immediately.

INTERACTIONS

Iron may reduce the effectiveness of tetracycline/lymecycline.
Oral anticoagulants Tetracycline/lymecycline may increase the action of these drugs.
Retinoids may increase the adverse effects of tetracycline/lymecycline.
Oral contraceptives Tetracycline/lymecycline may reduce the effectiveness of oral contraceptives.
Antacids and milk These interfere with the absorption of tetracycline/lymecycline and may reduce their effectiveness. Doses should be separated by 1–2 hours.

SPECIAL PRECAUTIONS

Be sure to tell your doctor if:
◆ You have long-term liver or kidney problems.
◆ You have previously suffered an allergic reaction to a tetracycline antibiotic.

◆ You have myasthenia gravis.

◆ You have systemic lupus erythematosus.

◆ You are taking other medicines.

Pregnancy Not usually prescribed. May cause discoloured teeth and damage bones of the developing fetus. Discuss with your doctor.

Breast-feeding Not recommended. The drugs pass into the breast milk and may damage developing bones and discolour the baby's teeth. Discuss with your doctor.

Infants and children Not recommended under 12 years. Reduced dose necessary in older children. May discolour developing teeth.

Over 60 No special problems.

Driving and hazardous work No known problems.

Alcohol No known problems.

Taking your tablets To prevent irritation to the oesophagus, stand upright and take each dose with a full glass of water. Do not take immediately before going to bed.

PROLONGED USE

No problems expected.

Theophylline/aminophylline

Brand names [theophylline] Nuelin, Slo-Phyllin, Uniphyllin; [aminophylline] Amnivent, Norphyllin, Phyllocontin

Used in the following combined preparations
[theophylline] Do-Do Tablets, Franol

QUICK REFERENCE

Drug group Bronchodilator (p.23)
Overdose danger rating High
Dependence rating Low
Prescription needed No (except for injection)
Available as generic Yes

GENERAL INFORMATION

Theophylline (and aminophylline, which breaks down to theophylline in the body) is used to treat bronchospasm (constriction of the air passages). It improves breathing in patients suffering from asthma, bronchitis, and emphysema.

It is usually taken continuously for prevention, but aminophylline injections are sometimes used for acute attacks.

Slow-release formulations of the drugs produce beneficial effects lasting for up to 12 hours. These preparations may be prescribed twice daily, but they are also useful as a single dose taken at night to prevent night-time asthma and early morning wheezing.

Treatment with theophylline must be monitored closely because the effective dose is very close to the toxic dose. Some of the adverse effects, such as indigestion, nausea, headache, and agitation, can be controlled by regulating the dosage and checking blood levels of the drug.

INFORMATION FOR USERS

Follow instructions on the label. Call your doctor if symptoms worsen.

How taken/used Tablets, SR-tablets, SR-capsules, injection.

Frequency and timing of doses 3–4 x daily (tablets); every 12 or 24 hours (SR-tablets/SR-capsules). Take at the same time each day.

Dosage range Adults 375–1,000mg daily, depending on which product is used.

Onset of effect Within 30 minutes (by mouth); within 90 minutes (SR-tablets/SR-capsules).

Duration of action Up to 8 hours (by mouth); 12–24 hours (SR-tablets/SR-capsules).

Diet advice None.

Storage Keep in original container at room temperature out of the reach of children.

Missed dose Take as soon as you remember. If your next dose is due within 2 hours, take half of the dose now (short-acting preparations) or forget about the missed dose and take your next dose now (SR-preparations). Return to your normal dosing schedule thereafter.

Stopping the drug Do not stop taking the drug without consulting your doctor; stopping the drug may lead to worsening of the underlying condition.

OVERDOSE ACTION

Seek immediate medical advice in all cases. Take emergency action if chest pains, confusion, or loss of consciousness occur.

POSSIBLE ADVERSE EFFECTS

Most of the adverse effects are related to levels of the drug in the blood. The most common effects are concerned with the gastrointestinal system (and include nausea and vomiting) and the central nervous system (producing effects such as agitation and insomnia). Headaches are also common and should be discussed with your doctor. Rarely, diarrhoea and abdominal pain may occur and should also be discussed with your doctor. If you experience palpitations, stop taking the drug and consult your doctor promptly.

INTERACTIONS

General note Many drugs interact with theophylline. Some antibiotics, antidepressants, and antiepileptics increase its effects; others lower it. Taken with theophylline, high doses of Beta 2 agonists such as salbutamol increase the risk of low blood potassium levels. Discuss with your doctor.

SPECIAL PRECAUTIONS

Be sure to consult your doctor or pharmacist before taking this drug if:
◆ You have a liver problem.
◆ You have angina or an irregular heart beat.
◆ You have high blood pressure.
◆ You have epilepsy.
◆ You have hyperthyroidism.
◆ You have porphyria.
◆ You have stomach ulcers.
◆ You smoke.
◆ You are taking other medicines.
Pregnancy Safety in pregnancy not established. Discuss with your doctor.
Breast-feeding The drug passes into the breast milk and may affect the baby. Discuss with your doctor.
Infants and children Reduced dose necessary according to age and weight.
Over 60 Reduced dose may be necessary.
Driving and hazardous work No known problems.
Alcohol Avoid excess as this may alter levels of the drug and may increase gastrointestinal symptoms.
Taking your tablets Several factors such as drug interactions, certain medical conditions (heart or liver failure, for example), and smoking can affect levels of theophylline in the body. All brands release the drug differently, resulting in varying levels. For this reason, it is important that you always use the same brand.

PROLONGED USE

No problems expected.
Monitoring Periodic checks on blood levels of this drug are usually required.

Tibolone

Brand name Livial
Used in the following combined preparations None

QUICK REFERENCE

Drug group Hormone replacement therapy (p.88)
Overdose danger rating Low
Dependence rating Low
Prescription needed Yes
Available as generic No

GENERAL INFORMATION

Tibolone is a female sex hormone used to treat menopausal symptoms, such as sweating, depressed mood, and decreased sex drive, and is particularly effective in controlling hot flushes. It is usually only advised for short-term use.

The drug is taken continuously and, because it has both oestrogenic and progestogenic activity (unlike most other available types of hormone replacement therapy), the treatment does not require a cyclical course of progestogen to be taken as well.

Side effects are rare with tibolone, and the drug does not cause withdrawal bleeding in postmenopausal women. Tibolone is sometimes used in the treatment of osteoporosis when other drugs are inappropriate or ineffective.

INFORMATION FOR USERS

Your drug prescription is tailored for you. Do not alter dosage without checking with your doctor.
How taken/used Tablets.
Frequency and timing of doses Daily, preferably at the same time each day. Swallow the tablets whole – do not chew.
Adults dosage range 2.5mg daily.

Onset of effect You may notice improvement of symptoms within a few weeks, but the best results are obtained when the drug is taken for at least 3 months.

Duration of action A few days.

Diet advice None.

Storage Keep in original container at room temperature out of the reach of children. Protect from light.

Missed dose Take as soon as you remember.

Stopping the drug Do not stop the drug without consulting your doctor; symptoms may recur.

Exceeding the dose An occasional unintentional extra dose is unlikely to be a cause for concern. If several tablets are taken together, they may cause a stomach upset. Notify your doctor.

POSSIBLE ADVERSE EFFECTS

Tibolone is well tolerated, and the incidence of adverse effects is low. Vaginal bleeding is more likely to occur if less than one year has passed since you reached the menopause. For this reason, the drug is not recommended if less than 12 months have passed since your last period. Other effects include weight gain, ankle swelling, dizziness, stomach upset, facial hair growth, and acne. If headache, visual problems, vaginal bleeding, or joint or muscle pain occur, consult your doctor promptly. If you develop jaundice, stop taking the drug and consult your doctor immediately.

INTERACTIONS

Some anticonvulsants Phenytoin, phenobarbital, primidone, and carbamazepine can accelerate the metabolism of tibolone and so decrease blood levels of the drug and its effectiveness.

Rifampicin This can accelerate the metabolism of tibolone and so decrease blood levels of the drug and its effectiveness.

SPECIAL PRECAUTIONS

Be sure to tell your doctor if:
◆ You have long-term liver or kidney problems.
◆ You suffer from epilepsy.
◆ You suffer from migraine.
◆ You have diabetes.

◆ You have a tumour.
◆ You have a history of cardiovascular or cerebrovascular disease.
◆ You have a high cholesterol level.
◆ You have vaginal bleeding.
◆ You have had a period in the last 12 months.
◆ You are taking other medicines.

Pregnancy Not prescribed.

Breast-feeding Not prescribed.

Infants and children Not prescribed.

Over 60 No special problems.

Driving and hazardous work No problems expected.

Alcohol No known problems.

PROLONGED USE

HRT is usually only advised for short-term use around the menopause. Because of the increased risk of disorders such as breast cancer, thromboembolism, and stroke, it is not normally recommended for long-term use; it is only rarely recommended for the long-term treatment of osteoporosis (see General information, facing page).

Monitoring Periodic examination by your doctor is advised.

Timolol

Brand names Betim, Glau-opt, Nyogel, Timoptol
Used in the following combined preparations Cosopt, Combigan, DuoTrav, Ganfort, Moducren, Prestim, Xalacom

QUICK REFERENCE

Drug group Beta blocker (p.30) and drug for glaucoma (p.114)
Overdose danger rating High
Dependence rating Low
Prescription needed Yes
Available as generic Yes

GENERAL INFORMATION

Timolol is a beta blocker used to treat angina (pain due to narrowing of the coronary arteries). It may be given after a heart attack to prevent further damage to the heart muscle. Timolol is also used to treat hypertension (high blood pressure), but is not usually used to initiate treatment. It is also commonly given as eye drops to people with certain types of glaucoma and is occasionally given to prevent migraine.

Timolol can occasionally cause breathing difficulties, especially in people who have respiratory diseases; this is more likely to occur with the tablets, but it can also occur in people using the eye drops. As with other beta blockers, timolol may mask the body's response to low blood glucose and, for that reason, is prescribed with caution to people with diabetes.

INFORMATION FOR USERS

Your drug prescription is tailored for you. Do not alter dosage without checking with your doctor.

How taken/used Tablets, eye drops.

Frequency and timing of doses 1–3 x daily.

Adults dosage range *By mouth* 10–60mg daily (hypertension); 10–60mg daily (angina/hypertension); 10–20mg daily (after a heart attack); 10–20mg daily (migraine prevention).

Onset of effect Within 30 minutes (by mouth); 15–20 minutes (eye drops).

Duration of action Up to 24 hours.

Diet advice None.

Storage Keep in original container at room temperature out of the reach of children.

Missed dose Take as soon as you remember. If your next dose is due within 3 hours, take a single dose now and skip the next.

Stopping the drug Do not stop taking the drug without consulting your doctor; stopping the drug may lead to worsening of the underlying condition.

OVERDOSE ACTION

Seek immediate medical advice in all cases of overdose by mouth. Take emergency action if breathing difficulties, palpitations, or loss of consciousness occur.

POSSIBLE ADVERSE EFFECTS

Taken by mouth, timolol can occasionally provoke or worsen heart problems and asthma. Fainting may be a sign that the drug has slowed the heartbeat or lowered the blood pressure excessively. Eye drops cause these problems only rarely; headache or blurred vision is more likely with these. Lethargy, fatigue, headache, and eye irritation (with the eye drops) are common side effects of this drug. Cold hands or feet or blurred vision (with the eye drops) occur rarely. Dizziness, fainting, nightmares, and vivid dreams are also rare and should be discussed with your doctor. If you experience wheezing or breathlessness, stop taking the drug and seek immediate medical attention.

INTERACTIONS

Calcium channel blockers may enhance timolol's blood-pressure-lowering effects, slow the heart rate, and increase the risk of heart failure in susceptible people.

Drugs for asthma (e.g. salbutamol, salmeterol, and other beta agonists) The effects of these drugs may be reduced by timolol.

SPECIAL PRECAUTIONS

Be sure to tell your doctor if:
◆ You have heart failure.
◆ You have kidney or liver problems.
◆ You have an overactive thyroid.
  You have a lung disorder such as asthma, bronchitis, or emphysema.
◆ You have diabetes.
◆ You have myasthenia gravis.
◆ You have poor circulation.
◆ You have allergies.
◆ You are taking other medicines.

Pregnancy Safety in pregnancy not established. Discuss with your doctor.

Breast-feeding The drug passes into the breast milk, but at normal doses adverse effects on the baby are unlikely. Discuss with your doctor.

Infants and children Not usually prescribed.

Over 60 Reduced dose may be necessary.

Driving and hazardous work Avoid such activities until you have learned how timolol affects you because the tablets may cause dizziness or fatigue, and the eye drops may cause blurred vision.

Alcohol May enhance lowering of blood pressure; avoid excessive amounts.

Surgery and general anaesthetics Timolol by mouth may need to be stopped before you have a general anaesthetic. Discuss with your doctor or dentist before any surgery.

PROLONGED USE

No problems expected.

Tiotropium

Brand name Spiriva
Used in the following combined preparations None

QUICK REFERENCE

Drug group Bronchodilator (p.23)
Overdose danger rating Low
Dependence rating Low
Prescription needed Yes
Available as generic No

GENERAL INFORMATION

Tiotropium is a long-acting anticholinergic bronchodilator that relaxes the muscles surrounding the bronchioles (airways in the lung). It is used in the maintenance treatment of chronic obstructive lung disorders, such as chronic bronchitis. The drug is not suitable for acute attacks of wheezing or in the emergency treatment of asthma. Tiotropium is taken by inhalation of a powder, and it acts directly and locally on the inner surface of the lungs and not via the blood. The most common side effect is a dry mouth.

INFORMATION FOR USERS

Your drug prescription is tailored for you. Do not alter dosage without checking with your doctor.

How taken/used Powder in capsules for inhaler.
Frequency and timing of doses Once daily, at the same time each day.
Adults dosage range 18mcg daily.
Onset of effect 5–30 minutes.
Duration of action 24 hours.
Diet advice None.
Storage Keep in original container at room temperature out of the reach of children.
Missed dose Take as soon as you remember. If your next dose is due within 8 hours, take a single dose now and skip the next.
Stopping the drug Do not stop the drug without consulting your doctor; symptoms may recur.
Exceeding the dose An occasional unintentional extra dose is unlikely to be a cause for concern. But if you notice any unusual symptoms, or if a large overdose has been taken, notify your doctor.

POSSIBLE ADVERSE EFFECTS

Dry mouth, sore throat, cough, constipation, nosebleeds, thrush, and sinusitis are common adverse effects. If, rarely, a fast heart beat, palpitations, difficulty in passing urine, rash, wheezing after inhalation, eye pain, blurred vision, or visual haloes occur, seek immediate medical attention.

INTERACTIONS

Anticholinergic drugs (e.g. atropine and ipratropium) may increase the effects and toxicity of tiotropium.

SPECIAL PRECAUTIONS

Be sure to tell your doctor if:
◆ You are allergic to atropine or ipratropium.
◆ You have prostate problems.
◆ You have urinary retention.
◆ You have glaucoma.
◆ You have kidney problems.
◆ You are taking other medicines.
Pregnancy Safety not established.
Breast-feeding Safety not established.
Infants and children Not recommended under 18 years.
Over 60 No known problems.
Driving and hazardous work No known problems.
Alcohol No known problems.
Protecting your eyes. Ensure that the powder does not get into the eyes; it could trigger or worsen glaucoma. If you develop eye or vision problems, call your doctor immediately.

PROLONGED USE

No known problems.

Tolbutamide

Brand names None
Used in the following combined preparations None

QUICK REFERENCE

Drug group Antidiabetic drug (p.82)
Overdose danger rating High
Dependence rating Low
Prescription needed Yes
Available as generic Yes

GENERAL INFORMATION

Tolbutamide belongs to a group of drugs known as sulphonylureas, but is shorter acting than many in this group. It is used to treat Type 2 diabetes, and works by stimulating the cells in the pancreas to produce insulin; it will only work, therefore, if functioning cells remain. For this reason, it is not effective in juvenile diabetes, in which functioning cells are lacking. Tolbutamide may also be given to people with impaired kidney function because it is less likely to build up in the body and excessively lower blood glucose.

As with other oral antidiabetic drugs, tolbutamide may need to be replaced with insulin during serious illnesses, injury, or surgery, when diabetic control is lost. The drug is taken in conjunction with a special diabetic diet that limits the patient's carbohydrate intake.

INFORMATION FOR USERS

Your drug prescription is tailored for you. Do not alter dosage without checking with your doctor.

How taken/used Tablets.

Frequency and timing of doses Taken with meals either once daily in the morning, or 2 x daily in the morning and evening.

Adult dosage range 500mg–2g daily.

Onset of effect Within 1 hour.

Duration of action 6–10 hours.

Diet advice A low-fat, low-carbohydrate diet must be maintained for the drug to be fully effective. Follow the advice of your doctor.

Storage Keep in original container at room temperature out of the reach of children. Protect from light.

Missed dose Take as soon as you remember. If your next dose is due within 2 hours, take a single dose now and skip the next.

Stopping the drug Do not stop the drug without consulting your doctor; stopping the drug may lead to worsening of the underlying condition.

OVERDOSE ACTION

Seek immediate medical advice in all cases. If faintness, confusion, or headache occur, eat something sugary. Take emergency action if fits or loss of consciousness occur.

POSSIBLE ADVERSE EFFECTS

Serious adverse effects are rare with tolbutamide. Symptoms such as dizziness, confusion, weakness, and sweating may indicate low blood glucose levels. Rarely, headache, ringing in the ears and weight gain occur. Nausea, vomiting, and diarrhoea are also rare; consult your doctor. If jaundice, rash, or itching occur, stop taking the drug and contact your doctor immediately.

INTERACTIONS

General note A variety of drugs, including corticosteroids, oestrogens, diuretics, and rifampicin, may oppose the effect of tolbutamide and raise blood glucose levels. Others increase the risk of low blood glucose; these include sulphonamides, warfarin, chloramphenicol, aspirin and other non-steroidal anti-inflammatory drugs (NSAIDs), antidepressants, cimetidine, and some antibiotics and antifungals.

Beta blockers may mask the signs of low blood glucose.

SPECIAL PRECAUTIONS

Be sure to tell your doctor if:
◆ You have long-term liver or kidney problems.
◆ You are allergic to sulphonamides.
◆ You have thyroid problems.
◆ You have porphyria.
◆ You are taking other medicines.

Pregnancy Not prescribed. Insulin is usually substituted. May cause birth defects if taken in the first 3 months of pregnancy. Discuss with your doctor.

Breast-feeding The drug passes into the breast milk and may affect the baby. Discuss with your doctor.

Infants and children Not prescribed.

Over 60 Risk of low blood glucose. Reduced dose may therefore be necessary.

Driving and hazardous work Usually no problem. Avoid these activities if you have warning signs of low blood glucose.

Alcohol Keep consumption low. Alcohol may upset diabetic control.

Surgery and general anaesthetics Notify your doctor that you have diabetes before any surgery; insulin treatment may need to be substituted.

PROLONGED USE
No problems expected.
Monitoring Regular monitoring of urine and/or blood glucose is required.

Tolterodine

Brand name Detrusitol
Used in the following combined preparations
None

QUICK REFERENCE
Drug group Drug for urinary disorders (p.112)
Overdose danger rating Medium
Dependence rating Low
Prescription needed Yes
Available as generic No

GENERAL INFORMATION
Tolterodine is an anticholinergic and antispasmodic drug that is similar to atropine (see p.150). It is used to treat urinary frequency and incontinence in adults. Tolterodine works by reducing contraction of the bladder, allowing it to expand and hold more. It also stops spasms, and delays the desire to empty the bladder.

Tolterodine's usefulness is limited to some extent by its side effects, and dosage needs to be reduced in elderly people. Children are more susceptible than adults to the drug's anticholinergic effects. Tolterodine can also trigger glaucoma.

INFORMATION FOR USERS
Your drug prescription is tailored for you. Do not alter dosage without checking with your doctor.
How taken/used Tablets, SR-capsules.
Frequency and timing of doses 1–2 x daily.
Dosage range 4mg daily, reduced to 2mg daily, if necessary, to minimize any side effects.
Onset of effect 1 hour.
Duration of action 12 hours.
Diet advice None.
Storage Keep in original container at room temperature out of the reach of children.
Missed dose Take as soon as you remember. If your next dose is due within 2 hours, take a single dose now and skip the next.

Stopping the drug Do not stop taking the drug without consulting your doctor; symptoms may recur.
Exceeding the dose An occasional unintentional extra dose is unlikely to cause problems. Large overdoses may cause visual disturbances, urinary difficulties, hallucinations, convulsions, and breathing difficulties. Notify your doctor.

POSSIBLE ADVERSE EFFECTS
The most common side effects of tolterodine, such as dry mouth, digestive disturbance, and dry eyes, are the result of the drug's anticholinergic action. Constipation, abdominal pain, headache, blurred vision, drowsiness, nervousness, and chest pain are also some of the common side effects of this drug. However, you should discuss chest pains with your doctor. In rare cases, confusion, or urinary difficulties may occur and should be reported to your doctor promptly.

INTERACTIONS
General note All drugs that have an anticholinergic effect will have increased side effects when they are taken with tolterodine.
Domperidone and metoclopramide The effects of these drugs may be decreased by tolterodine.
Erythromycin, clarithromycin, itraconazole, ketoconazole, and miconazole These drugs may increase blood levels of tolterodine.

SPECIAL PRECAUTIONS
Be sure to tell your doctor if:
◆ You have liver or kidney problems.
◆ You have thyroid problems.
◆ You have heart problems.
◆ You have hiatus hernia.
◆ You have prostate problems or urinary retention.
◆ You have ulcerative colitis.
◆ You have glaucoma.
◆ You have myasthenia gravis.
◆ You are taking other medicines.
Pregnancy Safety in pregnancy not established. May harm the unborn baby. Discuss with your doctor.
Breast-feeding Safety not established. Discuss with your doctor.

Infants and children Not recommended. Safety not established.

Over 60 No special problems.

Driving and hazardous work Avoid such activities until you have learned how tolterodine affects you because the drug can cause drowsiness, disorientation, and blurred vision.

Alcohol Avoid. Alcohol increases the drug's sedative effects.

PROLONGED USE

No special problems. The effectiveness of tolterodine, and the continuing clinical need for taking it, are usually reviewed after 6 months.

Monitoring Periodic eye tests for glaucoma may be performed.

Tramadol

Brand names Dromadol, Larapam, Mabron, Tramake, Zamadol, Zydol

Used in the following combined preparation
Tramacet

QUICK REFERENCE

Drug group Analgesic (p.9)
Overdose danger rating High
Dependence rating Low
Prescription needed Yes
Available as generic Yes

GENERAL INFORMATION

Tramadol is a synthetic opioid analgesic drug that is used to prevent or treat moderate to severe pain. It can be used to treat acute pain such as that which follows surgery, and the chronic pain that might occur in back injuries or cancer, for example.

The painkilling effect of tramadol wears off after about 4 hours. However, a slow-release (long-acting) form of the drug can be given that will provide pain relief for up to 12 hours.

In rare cases, tramadol can be habit-forming, and dependence may occur. However, most people who take the drug for a short period of time do not become dependent and are able to stop taking it without any difficulty.

Side effects of tramadol include a dry mouth, nausea, dizziness, headaches, and occasionally, vomiting.

INFORMATION FOR USERS

Your drug prescription is tailored for you. Do not alter dosage without checking with your doctor.

How taken/used Tablets, SR-tablets, soluble tablets, capsules, SR-capsules, powder in sachets, injection.

Frequency and timing of doses Usually 2 x daily (SR-preparations) or up to 6 x daily (other preparations).

Adult dosage range Up to 400mg daily (by mouth); 600mg daily (injection).

Onset of effect 30–60 minutes (short-acting forms by mouth), at least 2 hours (SR-preparations by mouth); 15–30 minutes (injection).

Duration of action 4 hours (short-acting); 12 hours (long-acting).

Diet advice None.

Storage Keep in original container at room temperature out of the reach of children.

Missed dose Take as soon as you remember, and return to your normal schedule as soon as possible.

Stopping the drug If the reason for taking tramadol no longer exists, you may stop taking the drug and notify your doctor, who will advise you on how to stop taking it gradually. If you have been taking the drug for a long time, you may experience withdrawal effects.

OVERDOSE ACTION

Seek immediate medical advice in all cases. Take emergency action if breathing difficulties, severe drowsiness, fits, or loss of consciousness occur.

POSSIBLE ADVERSE EFFECTS

Adverse effects such as drowsiness seem to be more common with tramadol than with some other opioids. Adverse effects such as nausea, vomiting, dry mouth, tiredness, drowsiness, dizziness, and headache are common. Rarely, constipation, confusion, or hallucinations may occur and should be discussed with your doctor. If you experience convulsions, wheezing, or breathlessness, stop taking the drug and seek immediate medical attention.

INTERACTIONS

Antidepressants Tramadol may increase the risk of convulsions if taken with antidepressants and antipsychotics.

Carbamazepine This drug may reduce blood levels and effects of tramadol.

Sedatives All drugs that have a sedative effect are likely to increase the sedative effects of tramadol. Such drugs include antidepressants, antipsychotics, antihistamines, and sleeping drugs.

SPECIAL PRECAUTIONS

Be sure to tell your doctor if:
◆ You have had a head injury.
◆ You have liver or kidney problems.
◆ You have heart or circulatory problems.
◆ You have a lung disorder such as asthma or bronchitis.
◆ You have thyroid disease.
◆ You have a history of epileptic fits.
◆ You are taking other medicines.

Pregnancy Safety not established. Discuss with your doctor.

Breast-feeding The drug passes into the breast milk and may make the baby drowsy. Discuss with your doctor.

Infants and children Not recommended under 12 years.

Over 60 Reduced dose may be necessary.

Driving and hazardous work Avoid. Tramadol can cause drowsiness.

Alcohol Avoid. Alcohol increases the sedative effects of tramadol.

PROLONGED USE

Dependence may occur if tramadol is taken for long periods.

Trastuzumab

Brand name Herceptin
Used in the following combined preparations None

QUICK REFERENCE

Drug group Anticancer drug (p.96)
Overdose danger rating Low
Dependence rating Medium

Prescription needed Yes
Available as generic No

GENERAL INFORMATION

Trastuzumab belongs to a group of drugs known as monoclonal antibodies (see p.97). The drug is used in the treatment of early and advanced breast cancer. Produced synthetically, trastuzumab is similar to antibodies that occur naturally in the body to fight infection, and it attacks cancer cells in a similar way.

Around one breast cancer in five involves cancer cells that have excessive amounts of a protein called HER2 on their surface. HER2 stimulates the growth of these cancer cells, making the tumours aggressive and fast growing.

Trastuzumab blocks the HER2 protein on the cancer cells, destroying them. Therefore, in order to see whether treatment would be appropriate, it is necessary for tests to be carried out to confirm the presence of HER2.

Trastuzumab may be given on its own or in combination with other treatments. It is given by intravenous infusion, either weekly or every three weeks.

INFORMATION FOR USERS

Trastuzumab is prescribed only under close medical supervision, taking account of your present condition and medical history.

How taken/used Intravenous infusion.

Frequency and timing of doses Every 1–3 weeks.

Adult dosage range As advised by doctors, according to your bodyweight.

Onset of effect Not known.

Duration of action Up to 24 weeks.

Diet advice None.

Storage Not applicable. The drug is not normally kept in the home.

Missed dose The drug is administered in hospital under close medical supervision. If for some reason you miss your dose, contact your doctor as soon as possible.

Stopping the drug Discuss this with your doctor. Stopping the drug prematurely may lead to worsening of the underlying condition.

Exceeding the dose Overdosage is unlikely with trastuzumab because treatment is carefully monitored and supervised.

POSSIBLE ADVERSE EFFECTS

Infusion reactions are common with trastuzumab. Other common adverse effects include diarrhoea, weakness, and abdominal pain. Rarely, joint and muscle pain, breathlessness, and a cough may occur and should be discussed with your doctor. Palpitations, chest pain, swelling of the face or lips, a rash, and flu-like symptoms occur rarely and, if you experience any of these, notify your doctor immediately.

INTERACTIONS

Doxorubicin and other anticancer drugs There is a risk of heart failure when these are given with trastuzumab.

SPECIAL PRECAUTIONS

Be sure to tell your doctor if:
◆ You are allergic to trastuzumab.
◆ You have breathing difficulties.
◆ You have had heart failure, coronary artery disease, or high blood pressure.
◆ You have ever had chemotherapy with doxorubicin.
◆ You are pregnant or planning pregnancy.
◆ You are taking other medicines.
Pregnancy Rarely, trastuzumab can affect the developing baby. Discuss with your doctor before starting treatment.
Breast-feeding Not advised during treatment with trastuzumab and for six months after stopping.
Infants and children Not recommended under 18 years. Safety not established.
Over 60 No special problems.
Driving and hazardous work No known problems. However, if you experience a fever or shivering (symptoms of an infusion reaction), do not undertake such activities until these symptoms subside.
Alcohol No known problems.

PROLONGED USE

Serious problems are rare.
Monitoring Treatment is under specialist supervision; patients are usually observed for at least 6 hours after the start of treatment

and for 2 hours after subsequent treatments.

Triamterene

Brand name Dytac
Used in the following combined preparations
Dyazide (co-triamterzide), Dytide, Frusene, Kalspare, Triam-Co, TriamaxCo

QUICK REFERENCE
Drug group Potassium-sparing diuretic (p.32)
Overdose danger rating Low
Dependence rating Low
Prescription needed Yes
Available as generic Yes (in combined products)

GENERAL INFORMATION

Triamterene belongs to a group of drugs known as potassium-sparing diuretics. In combination with thiazide or loop diuretics, triamterine is given for the treatment of hypertension and oedema (fluid retention). It may be used, either on its own or, more commonly, with a thiazide diuretic such as hydrochlorothiazide (as co-triamterzide) to treat the oedema that occurs as a complication of heart failure, nephrotic syndrome, or cirrhosis of the liver.

Triamterene is fast-acting; and its effect on urine flow is apparent within two hours. For this reason, you should avoid taking the drug after about 4 pm. As with other potassium-sparing diuretics, unusually high levels of potassium may build up in the blood if the kidneys are functioning abnormally. Therefore, triamterene is prescribed with caution to people who have kidney failure.

INFORMATION FOR USERS

Your drug prescription is tailored for you. Do not alter dosage without checking with your doctor.
How taken/used Tablets, capsules.
Frequency and timing of doses 1–2 x daily after meals or on alternate days.
Adult dosage range 50–250mg daily.
Onset of effect Within 2 hours.
Duration of action 9–12 hours.
Diet advice Consume only small amounts of foods that are high in potassium, such

as bananas, tomatoes, dried fruit, and salt substitutes.

Storage Keep in original container at room temperature out of the reach of children.

Missed dose Take as soon as you remember. However, if it is late in the day, do not take the missed dose, or you may need to get up at night to pass urine. Take the next scheduled dose as usual.

Stopping the drug Do not stop the drug without consulting your doctor; symptoms may recur.

Exceeding the dose An occasional unintentional extra dose is unlikely to be a cause for concern. But if you notice any unusual symptoms, or if a large overdose has been taken, notify your doctor.

POSSIBLE ADVERSE EFFECTS

Triamterene has few adverse effects. The main problem with the drug is the possibility of potassium being retained by the body, causing muscle weakness and numbness. Triamterene may colour your urine blue but this is not a cause for concern. Digestive disturbances, headache, rash, dry mouth, or thirst are other rare adverse effects of the drug. Muscle weakness, a rash, dry mouth, or thirst are also rare, and, if any of these occur, stop taking the drug and consult your doctor promptly.

INTERACTIONS

Lithium Triamterene may increase the blood levels of lithium, leading to an increased risk of lithium toxicity.

Non-steroidal anti-inflammatory drugs (NSAIDs) may increase the risk of raised blood levels of potassium.

ACE inhibitors These drugs increase the risk of raised blood levels of potassium with triamterene.

Ciclosporin This drug may increase levels of potassium with triamterene.

SPECIAL PRECAUTIONS

Be sure to tell your doctor if:
◆ You have long-term liver or kidney problems.
◆ You have had kidney stones.
◆ You have gout.
◆ You are taking other medicines.

Pregnancy Not usually prescribed. The drug may cause a reduction in the blood supply to the developing fetus. Discuss with your doctor.

Breast-feeding The drug passes into the breast milk and may affect the baby. It could also reduce your milk supply. Discuss with your doctor.

Infants and children Not recommended.

Over 60 Increased likelihood of adverse effects. Reduced dose may therefore be necessary.

Driving and hazardous work No special problems.

Alcohol No known problems.

PROLONGED USE

Serious problems are unlikely to occur with triamterene, but levels of salts such as sodium and potassium may occasionally become abnormal during prolonged use.

Monitoring Blood tests may be performed to check on kidney function and levels of body salts.

Trimethoprim

Brand name Trimopan
Used in the following combined preparations
Fectrim, Septrin

QUICK REFERENCE

Drug group Antibacterial drug (p.66)
Overdose danger rating Low
Dependence rating Low
Prescription needed Yes
Available as generic Yes

GENERAL INFORMATION

Trimethoprim is an antibacterial drug that became popular in the 1970s for prevention and treatment of infections of the urinary and respiratory tracts. The drug has been used for many years in combination with another antibacterial drug, sulfamethoxazole, in a preparation known as co-trimoxazole (see p.203). However, trimethoprim has fewer adverse effects than co-trimoxazole and is equally effective in treating many conditions. The drug can also be given by injection to treat severe infections.

Side effects of trimethoprim are not usually troublesome, but tests to monitor blood composition are often advised when the drug is taken for prolonged periods.

INFORMATION FOR USERS

Your drug prescription is tailored for you. Do not alter dosage without checking with your doctor.

How taken/used Tablets, liquid, injection.
Frequency and timing of doses 1–2 x daily.
Adult dosage range 400mg daily (treatment); 100mg daily (prevention).
Onset of effect 1–4 hours.
Duration of action Up to 24 hours.
Diet advice None.
Storage Keep in original container at room temperature out of the reach of children. Protect from light.
Missed dose Take as soon as you remember.
Stopping the drug Take the full course. Even if you feel better, the original infection may still be present and symptoms may recur if treatment is stopped too soon.
Exceeding the dose An occasional unintentional extra dose is unlikely to be a cause for concern. But if you notice any unusual symptoms, or if a large overdose has been taken, notify your doctor.

POSSIBLE ADVERSE EFFECTS

Trimethoprim on its own rarely causes adverse effects, but additional effects may occur when it is taken in combination with sulfamethoxazole. Rarely, nausea or vomiting may occur. If a rash, itching, sore throat, fever, bruising, or bleeding occur, stop taking the drug and consult your doctor immediately.

INTERACTIONS

Cytotoxic drugs Trimethoprim increases the risk of blood problems if taken with azathioprine or mercaptopurine. Taken with methotrexate, there is an increased risk of folate deficiency.
Warfarin Trimethoprim may increase the anticoagulant effect of warfarin.
Ciclosporin Trimethoprim increases the risk of this drug causing kidney damage.
Phenytoin Taken with trimethoprim, this drug may increase the risk of folic acid deficiency, resulting in blood abnormalities.

Antimalarials containing pyrimethamine Drugs such as fansidar or maloprim may increase the risk of folic acid deficiency, resulting in blood abnormalities, if they are taken with trimethoprim.

SPECIAL PRECAUTIONS

Be sure to tell your doctor if:
◆ You have long-term liver or kidney problems.
◆ You have a blood disorder.
◆ You have porphyria.
◆ You are taking other medicines.
Pregnancy Safety in pregnancy not established. Discuss with your doctor.
Breast-feeding The drug passes into the breast milk, but at normal doses adverse effects on the baby are unlikely. Discuss with your doctor.
Infants and children Reduced dose necessary.
Over 60 Increased likelihood of adverse effects. Reduced dose may be required.
Driving and hazardous work No known problems.
Alcohol No known problems.

PROLONGED USE

Long-term use of this drug may lead to folate deficiency, which, in turn, may lead to blood abnormalities. Folate supplements may be prescribed.
Monitoring Periodic blood tests to monitor blood composition are usually advised.

Valsartan

Brand name Diovan
Used in the following combined preparation Co-Diovan

QUICK REFERENCE

Drug group Vasodilator (p.31) and antihypertensive drug (p.36)
Overdose danger rating Low
Dependence rating Low
Prescription needed Yes
Available as generic No

GENERAL INFORMATION

Valsartan belongs to the group of vasodilator drugs known as angiotensin II blockers, and is used to treat hypertension (high blood pressure). It may also be used following a myocardial infarction (heart attack) to help prevent further complications. Valsartan may be prescribed alone or in combination with other post-myocardial infarction therapies such as aspirin, beta blockers, or "statin" lipid-lowering drugs.

Valsartan works by blocking the action of angiotensin II (a powerful hormone that constricts blood vessels). This relaxes the blood vessels, thereby lowering blood pressure and easing the heart's workload.

Unlike ACE inhibitors, valsartan does not cause a persistent dry cough and may be a useful alternative for people who have to discontinue treatment with an ACE inhibitor for this reason.

INFORMATION FOR USERS

Your drug prescription is tailored for you. Do not alter dosage without checking with your doctor.

How taken/used Tablets, capsules.

Frequency and timing of doses *Hypertension* Once daily, generally in the morning. *Post-myocardial infarction* Twice daily.

Adult dosage range 20–320mg.

Onset of effect 1–2 hours; full antihypertensive effect may take 2–4 weeks.

Duration of action 24 hours for antihypertensive effect.

Diet advice None.

Storage Keep in original container at room temperature out of the reach of children.

Missed dose Take as soon as you remember, then return to your original dosing schedule. Do not make up for the missed dose.

Stopping the drug Do not stop taking the drug without consulting your doctor. Stopping the drug may lead to worsening of the underlying condition.

Exceeding the dose An occasional unintentional extra dose is unlikely to cause problems. Large overdoses may cause dizziness and fainting. Notify your doctor.

POSSIBLE ADVERSE EFFECTS

Most adverse effects of valsartan are usually mild and transient. Such effects include dizziness and hypotension (low blood pressure). Headaches are also common, but these should be reported to your doctor. If, rarely, fatigue, diarrhoea, muscle pain, joint pain, back pain, or a cough occur, consult your doctor immediately. If you develop a rash, itching, or swelling of the face or tongue, stop taking the drug and seek immediate medical attention.

INTERACTIONS

ACE inhibitors may increase potassium levels when taken with valsartan.

Diuretics taken with valsartan may alter blood potassium and sodium levels.

NSAIDs and glibenclamide may reduce the effectiveness of valsartan.

Cimetidine may increase valsartan's effect.

Potassium Salts may increase the risk of high potassium levels with valsartan.

Lithium Levels of this drug may be increased when it is combined with valsartan, leading to toxicity.

Ciclosporin may increase potassium levels when it is combined with valsartan.

SPECIAL PRECAUTIONS

Be sure to tell your doctor if:
◆ You have liver or kidney problems.
◆ You have had a recent kidney transplant.
◆ You have recently suffered from excessive sweating, diarrhoea, or dehydration.
◆ You are allergic to valsartan.
◆ You are taking other medicines.

Pregnancy Not prescribed.

Breast-feeding Not recommended. It is not known whether the drug passes into the breast milk. Discuss with your doctor.

Infants and children Not recommended.

Over 60 Increased risk of adverse effects. Reduced dose may therefore be necessary.

Driving and hazardous work Do not undertake such activities until you have learned how valsartan affects you because the drug can cause dizziness or weariness.

Alcohol Avoid. Combined with valsartan, alcohol may increase dizziness, especially at the start of treatment.

PROLONGED USE

No special problems.

Monitoring Periodic checks on blood potassium levels and kidney function may be performed.

Venlafaxine

Brand names Efexor, Efexor XL
Used in the following combined preparations None

QUICK REFERENCE

Drug group Antidepressant (p.14)
Overdose danger rating High
Dependence rating Low
Prescription needed Yes
Available as generic No

GENERAL INFORMATION

Venlafaxine is an antidepressant drug that has a chemical structure unlike any other antidepressant available. Venlafaxine combines the therapeutic properties of both the tricyclic antidepressants and selective serotonin reuptake inhibitors (SSRIs), without the anticholinergic adverse effects.

Venlafaxine is used in the treatment of depression and generalized anxiety disorder. The drug acts to elevate mood, increase physical activity, and restore interest in everyday activities.

Nausea, dizziness, drowsiness or insomnia, and restlessness are common adverse effects of venlafaxine. At high doses, the drug can elevate the blood pressure, which should be monitored during treatment.

INFORMATION FOR USERS

Your drug prescription is tailored for you. Do not alter dosage without checking with your doctor.

How taken/used Tablets, SR-capsules.
Frequency and timing of doses Twice daily (tablets); once daily (SR-capsules). The drug should be taken with food.
Dosage range 75–150mg daily for outpatients; up to 375mg daily in severely depressed patients.
Onset of effect Can appear within days, although full antidepressant effect may not be felt for 2–6 weeks. Anxiety may take longer to respond.
Duration of action About 8–12 hours (tablets); 24 hours (SR-capsules). Antidepressant effects may persist for up to 6 weeks following prolonged treatment.
Diet advice None.
Storage Keep in original container at room temperature out of the reach of children.
Missed dose Do not make up for a missed dose. Just take your next regularly scheduled dose.
Stopping the drug Do not stop the drug without consulting your doctor. Stopping abruptly can cause withdrawal symptoms.

OVERDOSE ACTION

Seek immediate medical advice in all cases. Take emergency action if fits, slow or irregular pulse, or loss of consciousness occur.

POSSIBLE ADVERSE EFFECTS

The most common adverse effects of venlafaxine are nausea, constipation, restlessness, (which can occur in the form of anxiety, nervousness, tremor, abnormal dreams, agitation, and confusion), weakness, blurred vision, drowsiness, dizziness, and sexual dysfunction. Some of these effects may wear off within 1–2 weeks of starting the drug. Rarely, hypertension (high blood pressure) occurs when the drug is taken in high doses; you should have your blood pressure monitored periodically. Palpitations are also rare and should be reported to your doctor promptly. Suicidal thoughts (or suicide attempts) may also occur in rare cases; if so, seek immediate medical attention.

INTERACTIONS

Sedatives All drugs with a sedative effect may increase those of venlafaxine.
Antihypertensive drugs Venlafaxine may reduce the effectiveness of these drugs.
Warfarin Venlafaxine may increase the effect of warfarin; dosage of warfarin may need to be reduced.
Monoamine oxidase inhibitors (MAOIs) Venlafaxine may interact with these drugs to produce a dangerous rise in blood pressure. Therefore, at least 14 days should elapse between stopping MAOIs and starting venlafaxine.

SPECIAL PRECAUTIONS

Be sure to tell your doctor if:
◆ You have had an adverse reaction to any other antidepressants.
◆ You have long-term liver or kidney problems.

◆ You have a heart problem or elevated blood pressure.

◆ You have had epileptic fits.

◆ You have had problems with alcohol or drug misuse/abuse.

◆ You have a history of mania.

◆ You are taking other medicines.

Pregnancy Safety in pregnancy not established. Discuss with your doctor.

Breast-feeding Not recommended. Discuss with your doctor.

Infants and children Not recommended under 18 years.

Over 60 Increased likelihood of adverse effects. Reduced dose may therefore be necessary.

Driving and hazardous work Avoid such activities until you have learned how venlafaxine affects you because the drug can cause dizziness, drowsiness, and blurred vision.

Alcohol Avoid. Alcohol may increase the sedative effects of this drug.

PROLONGED USE

Withdrawal symptoms (such as dizziness, electric shock sensations, anxiety, nausea, and insomnia) may occur if venlafaxine is not stopped gradually over at least 4 weeks. However, these symptoms rarely last for more than 1–2 weeks.

Monitoring The blood pressure should be measured periodically if high doses are prescribed. Anyone experiencing confusion, drowsiness, muscle cramps, or convulsions should be monitored for low sodium levels in the blood.

Verapamil

Brand names Cordilox, Securon, Univer, Verapress, Vertab, Zolvera

Used in the following combined preparations None

QUICK REFERENCE

Drug group Anti-angina drug (p.35), anti-arrhythmic drug (p.33), and antihypertensive drug (p.36)

Overdose danger rating Medium

Dependence rating Low

Prescription needed Yes

Available as generic Yes

GENERAL INFORMATION

Verapamil belongs to the group of drugs known as calcium channel blockers, which interfere with the conduction of signals in the muscles of the heart and blood vessels. Verapamil is used in the treatment of hypertension (high blood pressure), abnormal heart rhythms, and angina. It reduces the frequency of angina attacks, but it does not help to relieve the pain while an attack is in progress. Verapamil increases the ability of the body to tolerate physical exertion and, unlike some other drugs, it does not affect the breathing, and can be used safely by people with asthma.

Verapamil is also prescribed for certain types of abnormal heart rhythm. It can be administered by injection as well as in tablet form for such disorders.

Verapamil is not generally prescribed for people who have hypotension (low blood pressure), a low heart beat, or heart failure because it may worsen these conditions. The drug may also cause constipation.

INFORMATION FOR USERS

Your drug prescription is tailored for you. Do not alter dosage without checking with your doctor.

How taken/used Tablets, SR-tablets, SR-capsules, liquid, injection.

Frequency and timing of doses 2–3 x daily (tablets, liquid); 1–2 x daily (SR-tablets).

Adult dosage range 120–480mg daily.

Onset of effect 1–2 hours (tablets); 2–3 minutes (injection).

Duration of action 6–8 hours. During prolonged treatment some beneficial effects may last for up to 12 hours. SR-tablets act for 12–24 hours.

Diet advice Avoid grapefruit juice which may increase blood levels of verapamil.

Storage Keep in original container at room temperature out of the reach of children.

Missed dose Take as soon as you remember. If your next dose is due within 3 hours (tablets, liquid) or 8 hours (SR-tablets, SR-capsules), take a single dose now and skip the next.

Stopping the drug Do not stop taking the drug without consulting your doctor; symptoms may recur.

Exceeding the dose An occasional unintentional extra dose is unlikely to be a cause for concern. However, large overdoses may cause dizziness. Notify your doctor.

POSSIBLE ADVERSE EFFECTS

All adverse effects occurring with verapamil should be discussed with your doctor. The main adverse effect is constipation. Headache, nausea, vomiting, and ankle swelling also commonly occur. Flushing occurs rarely. Other rare adverse effects include dizziness, a rash, and, following long-term use, gynaecomastia (breast enlargement in men) and an increase in gum tissue; if any of these occur, stop taking the drug and consult your doctor urgently.

INTERACTIONS

Beta blockers When verapamil is taken with these drugs, there is a slight risk of abnormal heart beat and heart failure.

Carbamazepine, ciclosporin, digoxin, theophylline, sirolimus, and ivabradine The effects of these drugs may be increased by verapamil. The doses of these drug may need to be reduced or the combination avoided.

Rifampicin and barbiturates may reduce the effects of verapamil.

Clarithromycin and erythromycin may increase the effects of verapamil.

Simvastatin There is an increased risk of muscle damage if this drug is taken with verapamil.

SPECIAL PRECAUTIONS

Be sure to tell your doctor if:
◆ You have a long-term liver problem.
◆ You have heart failure.
◆ You have porphyria.
◆ You are taking other medicines.

Pregnancy Not usually prescribed. The drug may inhibit labour if it is taken during the later stages of pregnancy. Discuss with your doctor.

Breast-feeding The drug passes into the breast milk, but at normal doses adverse effects on the baby are unlikely. Discuss with your doctor.

Infants and children The drug is usually given to infants and children on specialist advice only. Reduced dose necessary.

Over 60 No special problems.

Driving and hazardous work Avoid such activities until you have learned how verapamil affects you because the drug can cause dizziness.

Alcohol Avoid. Alcohol may further reduce blood pressure, causing dizziness or other symptoms.

Surgery and general anaesthetics Tell your doctor or dentist that you are taking verapamil because the drug may need to be stopped before you have any surgery.

PROLONGED USE

No problems expected.

Warfarin

Brand name Marevan
Used in the following combined preparations None

QUICK REFERENCE

Drug group Anticoagulant drug (p.39)
Overdose danger rating High
Dependence rating Low
Prescription needed Yes
Available as generic Yes

GENERAL INFORMATION

Warfarin is an anticoagulant drug that is widely used to prevent blood clots from forming, mainly where the blood flow is slowest, particularly the leg and pelvic veins (deep-vein thromboses). Such clots can break off and travel in the bloodstream to the lungs, where they lodge and cause pulmonary embolism. The drug is also used to reduce the risk of clots in the heart in people with atrial fibrillation (irregular heart rhythm) or artificial heart valves. These clots may travel to the brain and cause a stroke. Regular monitoring is needed to ensure warfarin's proper maintenance, dosage and safety, using the INR (International Normalised Ratio) blood test. As warfarin's full beneficial effects are not felt for 2–3 days, a faster-acting drug such as heparin (see p.260) is often used initially to complement its effects in people with, or at high risk of developing, a clot.

The most serious adverse effect of treatment with warfarin is the risk of excessive bleeding. However, this usually only as a result of excessive dosage.

INFORMATION FOR USERS

Your drug prescription is tailored for you. Do not alter dosage without checking with your doctor.

How taken/used Tablets.

Frequency and timing of doses Once daily, taken at the same time each day.

Dosage range There is large variation in starting and maintenance dose, according to patient factors, but usually 10mg for 2 days (starting dose); 3–9mg daily at the same time, determined by blood tests (maintenance dose).

Onset of effect Within 24–48 hours; full effect after several days.

Duration of action 2–3 days.

Diet advice Avoid cranberry juice and major dietary changes.

Storage Keep in original container at room temperature out of the reach of children. Protect from light.

Missed dose Take as soon as you remember. Take the following dose on your original schedule.

Stopping the drug Do not stop taking the drug without consulting your doctor; stopping the drug may lead to worsening of the underlying condition.

OVERDOSE ACTION

Seek immediate medical advice in all cases. Take emergency action if severe bleeding or loss of consciousness occur.

POSSIBLE ADVERSE EFFECTS

Bleeding is the most common adverse effect. Therefore, you should stop taking the drug and contact your doctor immediately if you notice any bruising, dark stools, dark urine, or bleeding. Most of the other adverse effects caused by warfarin are rare. However, all of the following should be discussed with your doctor: nausea, vomiting, abdominal pain, diarrhoea, a rash, and hair loss. Fever and jaundice may also occur rarely and, if they do, stop taking the drug and contact your doctor urgently.

INTERACTIONS

General note A wide range of drugs, (such as aspirin and other non-steroidal anti-inflammatory drugs (NSAIDs), diuretics, chemotherapy, oral contraceptives, lipid-lowering drugs, amiodarone, barbiturates, cimetidine, steroids, and certain laxatives, antidepressants, antibiotics and herbal medicines) interact with warfarin to increase or decrease the anti-clotting effect. Consult your pharmacist before using any over-the-counter medicines, and inform your warfarin clinic of any changes to your medicines.

SPECIAL PRECAUTIONS

Be sure to tell your doctor if:
◆ You have long-term liver or kidney problems.
◆ You have high blood pressure.
◆ You have peptic ulcers.
◆ You bleed easily.
◆ You are taking other medicines.

Pregnancy Not prescribed. If the drug is given in early pregnancy, it can cause malformations in the unborn child. If it is taken near the time of delivery, it may cause the mother to bleed excessively. Discuss this with your doctor, who will prescribe alternative treatment.

Breast-feeding The drug passes into the breast milk, but at normal doses adverse effects on the baby are unlikely. Discuss with your doctor.

Infants and children Reduced dose necessary.

Over 60 No special problems.

Driving and hazardous work Use caution when undertaking such activities. Even minor bumps can cause bad bruises and excessive bleeding.

Alcohol Avoid major changes in alcohol consumption.

Surgery and general anaesthetics Warfarin may need to be stopped before surgery. Discuss with your doctor or dentist.

PROLONGED USE

No special problems.

Monitoring Regular INR blood tests are carried out. Dose is adjusted accordingly and recorded in a treatment book, which should be carried with you at all times.

Zidovudine/lamivudine

Brand names [zidovudine] Retrovir; [lamivudine] Epivir
Used in the following combined preparation Combivir

QUICK REFERENCE

Drug group Drug for HIV and immune deficiency (p.100)
Overdose danger rating Medium
Dependence rating Low
Prescription needed Yes
Available as generic No

GENERAL INFORMATION

Zidovudine and lamivudine belong to the same class of drugs – nucleoside analogues – and are used in the treatment of HIV infection. The 2 drugs can be prescribed separately or combined in one tablet, which is usually prescribed with another class of drug (either a non-nucleoside reverse transcriptase inhibitor or a protease inhibitor) to treat HIV. This combination of three drugs is more effective at treating HIV than either a single or double regime of drugs.

Although not a cure for HIV, combination retroviral therapy slows down production of the virus and, therefore, reduces the damage done to the immune system. The drugs need to be taken regularly and on a long-term basis to remain effective.

INFORMATION FOR USERS

Your drug prescription is tailored for you. Do not alter dosage without checking with your doctor.
How taken/used Tablets.
Frequency and timing of doses Every 12 hours.
Adult dosage range 1 tablet.
Onset of effect 1 hour.
Duration of action 12 hours.
Diet advice None.
Storage Keep in original container at room temperature out of the reach of children.
Missed dose Take as soon as you remember. If your next dose is due within 2 hours, take a single dose now and skip the next. It is very important not to miss doses on a regular basis as this can lead to the development of drug-resistant HIV.

Stopping the drug Do not stop taking the drug without consulting your doctor.
Exceeding the dose An occasional unintentional extra dose is unlikely to cause problems. But if you notice any unusual symptoms, or if a large overdose has been taken, notify your doctor.

POSSIBLE ADVERSE EFFECTS

The most common adverse effect of zidovudine and lamivudine are nausea, vomiting, and diarrhoea. Sometimes, following prolonged use of the drugs, you may develop anaemia. Fatigue also commonly occurs. In rare cases, you may experience discoloration of the skin and anaemia. Severe abdominal pain is also rare, and, if it occurs, seek immediate medical attention.

INTERACTIONS

General note A wide range of drugs may interact with zidovudine and lamivudine causing either an increase in adverse effects or a reduction in the effect of the antiretroviral drugs. Check with your doctor or pharmacist before taking any new drugs, including those from the dentist and supermarket, and herbal medicines.

SPECIAL PRECAUTIONS

Be sure to tell your doctor if:
◆ You have liver or kidney problems.
◆ You have other infections, such as hepatitis B or C.
◆ You are taking other medicines.
Pregnancy Safety in pregnancy not established. If you are pregnant or planning pregnancy, discuss with your doctor.
Breast-feeding Safety in breast-feeding not established. Breast-feeding is not recommended by HIV-positive mothers as the virus may be passed to the baby.
Infants and children Reduced dose necessary.
Over 60 Increased likelihood of adverse effects. Reduced dose may therefore be necessary.
Driving and hazardous work No special problems.
Alcohol No known problems.

PROLONGED USE

Increased risk of serious blood disorders, such as anaemia, with long-term use.

Monitoring Regular blood checks will be carried out in order to monitor the effects of the drugs on the virus and to look for signs of anaemia.

Zopiclone

Brand names Zileze, Zimovane, Zimovane LS
Used in the following combined preparations None

QUICK REFERENCE

Drug group Sleeping drug (p.11)
Overdose danger rating Medium
Dependence rating Medium
Prescription needed Yes
Available as generic Yes

GENERAL INFORMATION

Zopiclone is a hypnotic (sleeping drug) that is used for the short-term treatment of insomnia. Sleep problems can take the form of difficulty in falling asleep, frequent night-time awakenings, and/or early morning awakenings. Hypnotic drugs are given only when other, non-drug, measures – for example, avoidance of caffeine – have proved to be ineffective. Unlike the benzodiazepines, zopiclone possesses no anti-anxiety properties. Therefore, it may be suitable for instances of insomnia that are not accompanied by anxiety – for example, international travel or change in shift work routine.

Hypnotics are intended for occasional use only. Dependence can develop after as little as one week of continuous use.

INFORMATION FOR USERS

Your drug prescription is tailored for you. Do not alter dosage without checking with your doctor.
How taken/used Tablets.
Frequency and timing of doses Once daily at bedtime when required.
Dosage range 3.75–7.5mg.
Onset of effect Within 30 minutes.
Duration of action 4–6 hours.
Diet advice None.
Storage Keep in original container at room temperature out of the reach of children. Protect from light.

Missed dose If you fall asleep without having taken a dose and wake some hours later, do not take the missed dose.
Stopping the drug If you have been taking the drug continuously for less than 1 week, it can be safely stopped as soon as you feel you no longer need it. However, if you have been taking the drug for longer, consult your doctor.
Exceeding the dose An occasional, unintentional extra dose is unlikely to cause problems. Large overdoses may cause prolonged sleep, drowsiness, lethargy, and poor muscle coordination and reflexes. Notify your doctor immediately.

POSSIBLE ADVERSE EFFECTS

The most common adverse effects of zopiclone are headache, daytime drowsiness (which normally diminishes after the first few days of treatment), and a bitter or metallic taste in the mouth. If headaches and daytime drowsiness persist, you should discuss them with your doctor. Persistent morning drowsiness or impaired coordination are signs of excessive dose. Dizziness, weakness, nausea, vomiting, and diarrhoea are rare. Amnesia, confusion, and a rash are also rare and, if they occur, stop taking the drug and seek immediate medical attention.

INTERACTIONS

Sedatives All drugs, including alcohol, that have a sedative effect on the central nervous system are likely to increase the sedative effects of zopiclone. Such drugs include other sleeping and anti-anxiety drugs, antihistamines, antidepressants, opioid analgesics, and antipsychotics.
Erythromycin, clarithromycin, and ketoconazole These drugs may increase the levels and effect of zopiclone, leading to adverse effects.

SPECIAL PRECAUTIONS

Be sure to tell your doctor if:
◆ You have or have had any problems with alcohol or drug misuse/abuse.
◆ You have myasthenia gravis.
◆ You have severe respiratory disease.
◆ You have liver or kidney problems.
◆ You are taking other medicines.

Pregnancy Not recommended.

Breast-feeding Not recommended.

Infants and children Not recommended.

Over 60 Increased likelihood of adverse effects. Reduced dose may therefore be necessary.

Driving and hazardous work Avoid such activities until you have learned how zopiclone affects you because the drug can cause drowsiness, reduced alertness, and slowed reactions.

Alcohol Avoid. Alcohol increases the sedative effects of this drug.

PROLONGED USE

Intended for occasional use only. Continuous use of zopiclone, or any other sleeping drug, for as little as one or two weeks may cause dependence.

PART 3

DRUG FINDER AND INDEX

This part of the book consists of a combined
drug finder and index, which helps you to
find information on specific brand-name
drugs and generic substances, as well as
directing you to further information about
them throughout the book.

DRUG FINDER AND INDEX

This section contains the names of approximately 2,500 individual drug products and substances. It provides a quick and easy reference for readers interested in finding out about a specific drug or medication, as well as directing the reader to information about them throughout the book. There is no need for you to know what group a drug belongs to, whether an item is a brand name or a generic name, or whether it is a prescription or an over-the-counter drug; all types of drug and the major drug groups are listed.

WHAT IT CONTAINS

The drugs are listed alphabetically and include all major generic drugs and many less widely used substances. A broad range of brand names, as well as many vitamins and minerals, are also included. This comprehensive selection reflects the wide diversity of products available for the treatment and prevention of disease. Inclusion of a drug or product does not imply BMA endorsement, nor does the exclusion of a particular drug or product indicate BMA disapproval.

HOW THE REFERENCES WORK

References are to the pages in Part 2, containing the drug profiles of each principal generic drug, and to the section in Part 1 that describes the relevant drug group, as appropriate. Some entries for generic drugs that do not have a full profile contain a brief description here.

A

abacavir an antiretroviral for HIV/AIDS 100

abciximab an antiplatelet drug 39

Abelcet a brand name for amphotericin 143 (an antifungal 76)

Abidec a brand-name multivitamin 90

Abilify a brand name for aripiprazole (an antipsychotic 15)

acamprosate 130 (an alcohol abuse deterrent used in addition to counselling)

acarbose an oral antidiabetic 82

Accolate a brand name for zafirlukast (a leukotriene receptor antagonist for asthma 24 and bronchospasm 23)

Accupro a brand name for quinapril (an ACE inhibitor 31)

Accuretic a brand name for quinapril (an ACE inhibitor 31) with hydrochlorothiazide 261 (a diuretic 32)

acebutolol a beta blocker 30

aceclofenac a non-steroidal anti-inflammatory 50

acemetacin a non-steroidal anti-inflammatory 50

acenocoumarol an anticoagulant 39 previously known as nicoumalone

Acepril a brand name for captopril 169 (an ACE inhibitor 31)

acetaminophen see paracetamol 340

acetazolamide a carbonic anhydrase inhibitor diuretic 32 and drug for glaucoma 114

acetomenaphthone a vitamin K substance used in multivitamin preparations 90

acetylcholine a neurotransmitter that stimulates parasympathetic nervous system 9 and miotic for glaucoma 114 and to constrict the pupil 116

acetylcysteine a mucolytic 27 (also used for paracetamol 340 overdose)

Acezide a brand name for captopril 169 (an ACE inhibitor 31) with hydrochlorothiazide 261 (a thiazide diuretic 32)

aciclovir 131, an antiviral 69

acipimox a lipid-lowering drug 37

acitretin a drug for psoriasis 124

Aclasta a brand name for zoledronic acid (a drug for bone disorders 56 in cancer 96)

Acne, drugs used to treat 123

Acnecide a brand name for benzoyl peroxide 156 (a drug for acne 123)

Acnisal a brand name for salicylic acid (a drug for acne 123)

Acoflam a brand name for diclofenac 210 (a non-steroidal anti-inflammatory 50)

Acomplia a brand name for rimonabant 373 (an appetite suppressant 19 and adjunct for treatment of obesity)

acrivastine an antihistamine 58

Actifed Dry Coughs a brand name for dextromethorphan (a cough suppressant 27) with pseudoephedrine (a decongestant 26) and triprolidine (an antihistamine 58)

Actifed Chesty Coughs a brand name for guaifenesin (an expectorant 27) with pseudoephedrine (a decongestant 26) and triprolidine (an antihistamine 58)

Actilyse a brand name for alteplase (a thrombolytic 40)

Actinac a brand-name acne preparation 123 containing chloramphenicol 177, hydrocortisone 263, allantoin, butoxyethyl nicotinate, and sulphur

actinomycin D another name for dactinomycin (an anticancer drug 96)

Actiq a brand name for fentanyl (an opioid analgesic 9)

activated charcoal a substance used in the emergency treatment of poisoning

Actonel a brand name for risedronate 374 (a drug for bone disorders 56)

Actos a brand name for poiglitazone (an oral antidiabetic 82)

Acular a brand name for ketorolac (a non-steroidal anti-inflammatory 50)

Acupan a brand name for nefopam (a non-opioid analgesic 9)

ACWY Vax a brand-name vaccine 70 to protect against meningococcal infections

Adalat a brand name for nifedipine 328 (a calcium-channel blocker anti-angina drug 35 and antihypertensive 36)

Adalat Retard a brand name for nifedipine 328 (a calcium-channel blocker, anti-angina drug 35, and antihypertensive 36)

adapalene a retinoid for acne 123

adalimumab a disease-modifying antirheumatic drug 51

Adartrel a brand name for ropinirole (a drug for parkinsonism 18)

Adcal D3 a brand name for calcium carbonate (a mineral 93) with vitamin D (a vitamin 90)

adefovir an antiviral 69 for chronic hepatitis B

Adcortyl a brand name for triamcinolone (a corticosteroid 80)

Adenocor a brand name for adenosine (an anti-arrhythmic 33)

adenosine an anti-arrhythmic 33

Adipine MR a brand name for nifedipine 328 (a calcium channel blocker 35)

Adizem-SR a brand name for diltiazem 215 (a calcium channel blocker 35)

Adizem-XL a brand name for diltiazem 215 (a calcium channel blocker 35)

adrenaline see epinephrine 231, a bronchodilator 23 and drug for glaucoma 114 and cardiac resuscitation and anaphylaxis 512)

AeroBec a brand name for beclometasone 153 (a corticosteroid 80)

Aerodiol a brand-name preparation for menopausal symptoms 88 containing estradiol 235

Aerrane a brand name for isoflurane (a general anaesthetic 486)

Afrazine a brand name for oxymetazoline (a topical decongestant 26)

Agalsidase alfa and beta drugs for metabolic disorders

Agenerase a brand name for amprenavir (an antiretroviral for HIV/AIDS 100)

Aggrastat a brand name for tirofiban (an antiplatelet drug 39 used to prevent heart attacks)

Airomir a brand name for salbutamol 379 (a bronchodilator 23)

Aknemin a brand name for minocycline 315 (a tetracycline antibiotic 62)

Aknemycin Plus a brand-name product containing tretinoin (a drug for acne 123) and erythromycin 233 (an antibiotic 62)

albendazole an anthelmintic 78

aclometasone a topical corticosteroid 120

Aldactide a brand name for co-flumactone (spironolactone 390 with hydroflumethiazide, both diuretics 32)

Aldactone a brand name for spironolactone 390 (a potassium-sparing diuretic 32)

Aldara a brand name for imiquimod (a drug to treat genital and perianal warts)

aldesleukin an anticancer drug 96

Aldomet a brand name for methyldopa (an antihypertensive 36)

alemtuzumab a monoclonal antibody anticancer drug 96

alendronic acid 132 (a drug for bone disorders 56)

alfacalcidol vitamin D (a vitamin 90)

alfentanil an anaesthetic 9

alfuzosin an alpha blocker for prostate disorders 112

alginates 133 substances extracted from brown seaweed used to protect the stomach and oesophagus from acid reflux (antacids 42)

alimemazine an antihistamine 58 and antipruritic 118 previously known as trimeprazine

Alka-Seltzer Original a brand-name analgesic 9 and antacid 42 containing aspirin 146, sodium bicarbonate, and citric acid

Alkeran a brand name for melphalan (an anticancer drug 96)

allantoin a mild antibacterial 66

Allegron a brand name for nortriptyline (a tricyclic antidepressant 14)

Aller-Eze a brand name for azelastine (a topical antihistamine 58)

allopurinol 134 (a drug for gout 53)

Almogran a brand name for almotriptan (a drug for migraine 20)

almotriptan a drug for migraine 20

Alomide a brand name for lodoxamide (an anti-allergy drug 58)

Alopecia (see Drugs for hair loss 127)

Aloxi a brand name for palonosetron (an anti-emetic 21)

Alphaderm a brand name for hydrocortisone 263 (a corticosteroid 80) with urea (an emollient)

Alphagan a brand name for brimonidine (a drug for glaucoma 114)

alpha tocopheryl acetate vitamin E (a vitamin 90)

Alphosyl HC a brand-name drug for eczema 125 and psoriasis 124 containing coal tar and allantoin (a mild antibacterial 66) and hydrocortisone 263 (a corticosteroid 80)

alprazolam a benzodiazepine anti-anxiety drug 13

alprostadil a prostaglandin used for erectile dysfunction 87, 109

Altacite Plus a brand name for hydrotalcite (an antacid 42) with dimeticone (an antifoaming agent 42)

alteplase a thrombolytic 40

Alu-Cap a brand name for aluminium hydroxide 135 (an antacid 42)

Aludrox a brand name for aluminium hydroxide 135, magnesium carbonate, and magnesium hydroxide 296 (all antacids 42)

aluminium acetate an astringent used for inflammation of the skin or outer ear canal 120; also used in rectal preparations 47

aluminium chloride an antiperspirant

aluminium hydroxide 135 (an antacid 42)

Alupent a brand name for orciprenaline (a bronchodilator 23)

Alvedon a brand name for paracetamol 340 (a non-opioid analgesic 9)

alverine an antispasmodic for irritable bowel syndrome 45

amantadine an antiviral 69 and drug used for parkinsonism 18

Amaryl a brand name for glimepiride (an oral antidiabetic 82)

AmBisome a brand name for amphotericin 143 (an antifungal 76)

amethocaine see tetracaine, a local anaesthetic 9

Ametop a brand name for tetracaine (a local anaesthetic 9)

amfebutamone see bupropion 166 (an adjunct to smoking cessation with counselling)

Amias a brand name for candesartan 168 (an angiotensin II blocker (a vasodilator 31 and antihypertensive 36)

amikacin an aminoglycoside antibiotic 62

Amikin a brand name for amikacin (an aminoglycoside antibiotic 62)

Amil-Co a brand name for co-amilozide (amiloride 136 with hydrochlorothiazide 261, both diuretics 32)

Amilamont a brand name for amiloride 136 (a potassium-sparing diuretic 32)

amiloride 136 (a potassium-sparing diuretic 32)

Amilospare a brand name for amiloride 136 (a potassium-sparing diuretic 32)

aminobenzoic acid an ingredient of sunscreen preparations 127

aminoglycosides antibiotics 62

aminophylline a bronchodilator 23 related to theophylline 405

amiodarone 137, an anti-arrhythmic 33

amisulpride 138, an antipsychotic 15

amitriptyline 139, a tricyclic antidepressant 14

Amix a brand name for amoxicillin 142 (a penicillin antibiotic 62)

amlodipine 141, a calcium channel blocker 35

Amlostin a brand name for amlodipine 141 (a calcium channel blocker 35)

Ammonaps a brand name for sodium phenylbutyrate (a drug for metabolic disorders)

ammonium chloride a drug that increases urine acidity 112 and speeds excretion of poisons, and is an expectorant 27

Amnivent a brand name for aminophylline 405 (a bronchodilator 23)

amobarbital a barbiturate sleeping drug 11

Amoram a brand name for amoxicillin 142 (a penicillin antibiotic 62)

amorolfine an antifungal 76

amoxicillin 142, a penicillin antibiotic 62

Amoxil a brand name for amoxicillin 142 (a penicillin antibiotic 62)

Amphocil a brand name for amphotericin 143 (an antifungal 76)

amphotericin 143, an antifungal 76

ampicillin a penicillin antibiotic 62

amprenavir an antiretroviral 69 for HIV/AIDS 100

amsacrine an anticancer drug 96

Amsidine a brand name for amsacrine (an anticancer drug 96)

Amytal a brand name for amobarbital (a barbiturate sleeping drug 11)

Anabact a brand name for metronidazole 313 (an antibacterial 66)

anabolic steroids 88 male sex hormones 87

Anadin Original a brand-name analgesic 9 containing aspirin 146 and caffeine

Anadin Extra a brand-name analgesic 9 containing aspirin 146, paracetamol 340, and caffeine

Anadin Paracetamol a brand name for paracetamol 340 (an analgesic 9)

Anadin Ultra a brand name for ibuprofen 265 (a non-steroidal anti-inflammatory 50)

Anaesthetics, local 11 (drugs used as anaelgesics 9, in antipruritics 118, in labour 110, and in rectal and anal disorders 47)

Anafranil, Anafranil SR brand names for clomipramine 192 (a tricyclic antidepressant 14)

anagrelide a drug for platelet disorders 39

Ana-Guard a brand name for epinephrine 231 (a drug for anaphylaxis 512)

Ana-Kit a brand name for epinephrine 231 (a drug for anaphylaxis 512

anakinra a disease-modifying antirheumatic drug 51

Analgesics 9

Anapen a brand name for epinephrine 231 (for anaphylactic shock 512)

anastrozole 144, an anticancer drug 96

Anbesol a brand-name topical liquid for mouth ulcers and teething pain, containing lidocaine (a local anaesthetic 9), cetylpyridinium, and chlorocresol (both topical antiseptics 120)

Ancotil a brand name for flucytosine (an antifungal 76)

Andrews Plus a brand-name preparation for headache with gastric upset 42 containing paracetamol 340, citric acid, sodium and potassium bicarbonate, sodium carbonate and vitamin C (a vitamin 90)

Androcur a brand name for cyproterone acetate (a synthetic sex hormone 87 for male sexual disorders)

Andropatch a brand name for testosterone 402 (a male sex hormone 87)

Anectine a brand name for suxamethonium (a muscle relaxant 54)

Anexate a brand name for flumazenil (an antidote for benzodiazepine overdose)

Angettes 75 a brand-name antiplatelet drug 39 containing aspirin 146

Angilol a brand name for propranolol 359 (a beta blocker 30)

Angitak a brand name for isosorbide dinitrate 275 (an anti-angina drug 35)

Angitil SR, Angitil XL brand names for diltiazem 215 (a calcium channel blocker 35)

Anhydrol Forte a brand name for aluminium chloride (an antiperspirant)

anistreplase a thrombolytic 40

Anodesyn a brand-name preparation for haemorrhoids 47 containing allantoin (a mild antibacterial 66), lidocaine (a local anaesthetic 9), and ephedrine 230

Antabuse a brand name for disulfiram 217 (an alcohol abuse deterrent)

antacids 42

antazoline an antihistamine 58

Antepsin a brand name for sucralfate 392 (an ulcer-healing drug 43)

anthelmintic drugs 78

Anthisan a brand name for mepyramine (a topical antihistamine 58)

anti-angina drugs 35

anti-anxiety drugs 13

antibacterial drugs 66

antibiotics 62

anticoagulants drugs that affect blood clotting 38

anticancer drugs 96

anticonvulsant drugs 16

antidepressant drugs 14

antidiarrhoeal drugs 44

anti-D immunoglobulin 72 a drug used to prevent sensitization to Rhesus antigen

anti-emetics 21

antifungal drugs 76

antihaemophilic fraction a blood protein used to promote blood clotting in haemophilia 39

antihistamines 58 (also used as anti-emetics 21 and antipruritics 118)

antihypertensive drugs 36

anti-infective skin preparations 120

anti-inflammatory drugs, non-steroidal 50

antimanic drugs 16

antimalarial drugs 75

antiplatelet drugs drugs that affect blood clotting 38

antiprotozoal drugs 73

antipruritics 118

antipsychotic drugs 15

antiretroviral drugs drugs for HIV/AIDS 100

antirheumatic drugs 51

antituberculous drugs 67

anti-ulcer drugs 43

antiviral drugs 69

Antizol a brand name for fomepizole (an antidote for ethylene glycol and methanol poisoning)

Anturan a brand name for sulphinpyrazone (a drug for gout 53)

Anusol a brand-name preparation for haemorrhoids 47 containing zinc oxide, bismuth and Peru balsam

Apidra a brand name for insulin glulisine 269 (a drug for diabetes 82)

apomorphine 145, a drug used to treat Parkinson's disease 18 and erectile dysfunction 87, 109

apraclonidine a drug for glaucoma 114

aprepitant an anti-emetic 21

Apresoline a brand name for hydralazine (an antihypertensive 36)

Aprinox a brand name for bendroflumethiazide 154 (a thiazide diuretic 32)

aprotinin an antifibrinolytic drug used to promote blood clotting 39

Aprovel a brand name for irbesartan 273 an angiotensin II blocker (a vasodilator 31 and antihypertensive 36)

Aptivus a brand name for tipranavir (an antiretroviral for HIV/AIDS 100)

AquaBan a brand name for caffeine with ammonium chloride as a mild diuretic 32

Aquadrate a brand name for urea (an emollient)

Aramine a brand name for metaraminol (a drug for low blood pressure)

Aranesp a brand name for darbepoetin alfa (a drug for anaemia)

Arava a brand name for leflunomide (a disease-modifying antirheumatic drug 51)

Arcoxia a brand name for etoricoxib (an analgesic 9 and non-steroidal anti-inflammatory 50)

Aredia a brand name for pamidronate (a drug for bone disorders 56)

argipressin synthetic vasopressin (a drug for diabetes insipidus 86)

Aricept a brand name for donepezil 219 (a drug for Alzheimer's disease)

Aridil a brand name for amiloride 136 with furosemide 251 (both diuretics 32)

Arimidex a brand name for anastrozole 144 (a drug for breast cancer 96)

aripiprazole an antipsychotic 15

Arixtra a brand name for fondaparinux (an anticoagulant 39)

Aromasin a brand name for exemestane (a drug for breast cancer 96)

Arpicolin a brand name for procyclidine 355 (a drug for parkinsonism 18)

Artelac SDU a brand name for hypromellose (artificial tears 116)

artemether an antimalarial 75

artesunate an antimalarial 75

Arthrocin a brand name for naproxen 325 (a non-steroidal anti-inflammatory 50 and drug for gout 53)

Arthrofen a brand name for ibuprofen 265 (an analgesic 9 and non-steroidal anti-inflammatory 50)

Arthrotec a brand-name antirheumatic drug 51 containing diclofenac 210 with misoprostol 319

Arthroxen a brand name for naproxen 325 (a non-steroidal anti-inflammatory 50 and drug for gout 53)

articaine a local anaesthetic 9

artificial tear preparations drugs affecting the pupil 116

Arythmol a brand name for propafenone (an anti-arrhythmic 33)

Asacol a brand name for mesalazine 305 (a drug for ulcerative colitis 46)

Asasantin a brand name for aspirin 146 with dipyridamole 216 (an antiplatelet drug 39)

Ascabiol a brand name for topical benzyl benzoate (an antiparasitic 122)

ascorbic acid vitamin C (a vitamin 90)

Aserbine a brand-name product for wound cleaning

Asilone a brand name for aluminium hydroxide 135 and magnesium oxide (both antacids 42) with simeticone (an antifoaming agent 42)

Asmanex a brand name for mometasone 320 (a topical corticosteroid 120)

asparaginase a drug for leukaemia 96

Aspav a brand-name analgesic 9 containing aspirin 146 and papaveretum

aspirin/aspirin dispersible 146, a non-opioid analgesic 9 and antiplatelet drug 39

Aspro Clear a brand name for soluble aspirin 146 (a non-opioid analgesic 9)

AS Saliva Orthana a brand name for artificial saliva

Asthma, drugs for 24

AT 10 a brand name for dihydrotachysterol (vitamin D, a vitamin 90)

Atarax a brand name for hydroxyzine (an antihistamine 58 and an anti-anxiety drug 13)

atazanavir an antiretroviral for HIV/AIDS 100

Atenix a brand name for atenolol 147 (a beta blocker 30)

atenolol 147, a beta blocker 30

Ativan a brand name for lorazepam 209 (a benzodiazepine, an anti-anxiety drug 13 and sleeping drug 11)

Atomoxetine a drug for attention deficit hyperactivity disorder 19

atorvastatin 148, a lipid-lowering drug 37

atosiban a drug used to stop premature labour 110

atovaquone an antiprotozoal 73 and antimalarial 75

atracurium a drug used to relax the muscles in general anaesthesia

atropine 150, an anticholinergic for irritable bowel syndrome 45 and a mydriatic 116

Atrovent a brand name for ipratropium bromide 272 (a bronchodilator 23)

Audax a brand-name analgesic ear preparation 117 containing choline salicylate and glycerol

Augmentin a brand name for amoxicillin 142 (a penicillin antibiotic 62) with clavulanic acid (a substance that increases the effectiveness of amoxicillin)

auranofin a disease-modifying antirheumatic drug 51

Aureocort a brand name for chlortetracycline (a tetracycline antibiotic 62) with triamcinolone (a corticosteroid 80)

aurothiomalate a disease-modifying antirheumatic drug 51

Avandamet a brand name for rosiglitazone 377 (an oral antidiabetic 82) with metformin 306 (an oral antidiabetic 82)

Avandia a brand name for rosiglitazone 377 (an oral antidiabetic 82)

Avastin a brand name for bevacizumab (an anticancer drug 96)

Avaxim a brand-name vaccine 70 to protect against viral hepatitis A

Avelox a brand name for moxifloxacin (an antibiotic 62)

Avloclor a brand name for chloroquine 178 (an antimalarial 75 and disease-modifying antirheumatic drug 51)

Avodart a brand name for dutasteride (a male sex hormone 87 for benign prostatic hypertrophy 112)

Avomine a brand name for promethazine 358 (an antihistamine 58 and anti-emetic 21)

Avonex a brand name for interferon beta 271 (a drug for multiple sclerosis)

Axid a brand name for nizatidine (an anti-ulcer drug 43)

Axsain a brand name for capsaicin (a rubefacient)

Azactam a brand name for aztreonam (an antibiotic 62)

Azamune a brand name for azathioprine 151 (a disease-modifying antirheumatic drug 51 and immunosuppressant 99)

azathioprine 151, a disease-modifying antirheumatic drug 51 and immunosuppressant 99

azelaic acid an antibacterial 66, a drug for acne 123

azelastine an antihistamine 58

azidothymidine zidovudine 422 (an antiretroviral for HIV/AIDS 100)

Azilect a brand name for rasagiline (a drug for parkinsonism 18)

azithromycin an antibiotic 62

Azopt a brand name for brinzolamide (a carbonic anhydrase inhibitor drug used for glaucoma 114)

AZT zidovudine 422 (an antiretroviral for HIV/AIDS 100)

aztreonam an antibiotic 62

B

bacitracin an antibiotic 62

baclofen 152, a muscle relaxant 54

Baclospas a brand of baclofen 152 (a muscle relaxant 54)

Bactroban a brand name for mupirocin (an antibacterial 66 for skin infections 120)

balsalazide a drug for ulcerative colitis 46

Bambec a brand name for bambuterol (a sympathomimetic bronchodilator 23)

bambuterol a sympathomimetic bronchodilator 23

Baraclude a brand name for entecavir (an antiviral 69 for hepatitis B)

Baratol a brand name for indoramin (an alpha blocker antihypertensive 36 and drug for urinary disorders 112)

basiliximab an immunosuppressant 99

Baxan a brand name for cefadroxil (a cephalosporin antibiotic 62)

Bazuka a brand-name preparation for verrucas containing salicylic acid (a keratolytic 123) and lactic acid

becaplermin a drug for healing skin ulcers

Beclazone a brand name for beclometasone 153 (a corticosteroid 80)

Becloforte a brand name for beclometasone 153 (a corticosteroid 80)

beclometasone 153, a corticosteroid 80

Becodisks a brand of beclometasone 153 (a corticosteroid 80)

Beconase a brand name for beclometasone 153 (a corticosteroid 80)

Becotide a brand name for beclometasone 153 (a corticosteroid 80)

Bedol a brand-name preparation for menopausal symptoms 88 containing estradiol 235

Bedranol a brand name for propranolol 359 (a beta blocker 30)

Beechams Powders a brand name for aspirin 146 (a non-opioid analgesic 9) and caffeine

Beechams Powders Capsules a brand name for paracetamol 340 (a non-opioid analgesic 9) with phenylephrine (a de-congestant 95) and caffeine (a stimulant 19)

Begrivac a brand name for vaccine 70 to protect against influenza

belladonna an antispasmodic anticholinergic for irritable bowel syndrome 45

bemiparin a type of heparin 260 (an anticoagulant 39)

bendroflumethiazide 154, a thiazide diuretic 32 previously known as bendrofluazide

Benerva a brand name for thiamine (vitamin B_1, a vitamin 90)

benign prostatic hyperplasia (BPH) (see male sex hormones 87)

benperidol an antipsychotic 15

Benquil a brand name for benperidol (an antipsychotic 15)

benserazide a drug used to enhance the effect of levodopa 284 (a drug for parkinsonism 18)

Bonefos a brand name for sodium clodronate (a drug for high blood calcium in cancer patients 96)

Bonjela a brand name for choline salicylate (a drug similar to aspirin 146) and cetalkonium chloride used for cold sores, mouth ulcers, and teething pain

Bonjela Teething gel a brand-name preparation containing lidocaine (a local anaesthetic 9) and cetalkonium (an antiseptic 120)

Bonviva a brand name for ibandronic acid (a drug for bone disorders 56)

Bortezomib an anticancer drug 96

bosentan a drug for pulmonary arterial hypertension

Botox a brand name for botulinum toxin 161 (a muscle relaxant 54)

botulinum toxin 161, a muscle relaxant 54

BPH (benign prostatic hyperplasia) (see male sex hormones 87)

Bradosol a brand name for benzalkonium chloride (an antiseptic 120) lozenges

Brasivol a brand-name abrasive paste for acne 123

bretylium tosilate an anti-arrhythmic 33

Brevibloc a brand name for esmolol (a beta blocker 30)

Brevinor a brand-name oral contraceptive 105 containing ethinylestradiol 238 and norethisterone 331

Brevoxyl a brand name for benzoyl peroxide (a drug for acne 123)

Brexidol a brand name for piroxicam 349 (a non-steroidal anti-inflammatory 50)

Bricanyl a brand name for terbutaline 401 (a bronchodilator 23 and drug used in premature labour 110)

brimonidine a drug for glaucoma 114

brinzolamide a drug for glaucoma 114

BritLofex a brand name for lofexidine (a drug to treat opioid withdrawal symptoms)

Broflex a brand name for trihexyphenidyl (a drug for parkinsonism 18)

Brolene a brand name for propamidine isethionate (an antibacterial 66) for eye infections

bromocriptine 162, a pituitary agent 85 and drug for parkinsonism 18

brompheniramine an antihistamine 58

Bronchodilators 23

Brufen, Brufen Retard brand names for ibuprofen 265 (a non-steroidal anti-inflammatory 50)

Buccastem a brand name for prochlorperazine 354 (an anti-emetic 21)

buclizine an antihistamine 58 and anti-emetic 21 used for motion sickness

Budenofalk a brand name for budesonide 163 (a corticosteroid 80)

budesonide 163, a corticosteroid 80

bulk-forming agents laxatives 45

bumetanide 165, a loop diuretic 32

bupivacaine a long-lasting local anaesthetic 9 used in labour 110

buprenorphine an opioid analgesic 9

bupropion 166, an antidepressant 14 used as an aid to smoking cessation in addition to counselling

Burinex a brand name for bumetanide 165 (a loop diuretic 32)

Burinex-A a brand name for bumetanide 165 (a loop diuretic 32) with amiloride 136 (a potassium-sparing diuretic 32)

Burinex-K a brand name for bumetanide 165 (a loop diuretic 32) with potassium

BurnEze a brand name for benzocaine (a local anaesthetic 9)

Buscopan a brand name for hyoscine butylbromide 264 (an antispasmodic for irritable bowel syndrome 45)

buserelin a drug for menstrual disorders 104 and prostate cancer 96

Buspar a brand name for buspirone (an anti-anxiety drug 13)

buspirone a non-benzodiazepine anti-anxiety drug 13

busulfan an alkylating agent for certain leukaemias 96

butobarbital a barbiturate sleeping drug 11

butoxyethyl nicotinate a vasodilator 31

BuTrans a brand name for buprenorphine (an opioid analgesic 9)

butylcyanoacrylate a tissue and skin adhesive for closing wounds

C

Cabaser a brand name for cabergoline (a drug for parkinsonism 18)

cabergoline a drug for parkinsonism 18 and endocrine disorders 85

Cacit a brand name for calcium carbonate (a mineral 93)

Caelyx a brand name for doxorubicin 224 (a cytotoxic anticancer drug 96)

Cafergot a brand name for ergotamine 232 (a drug for migraine 20) with caffeine (a stimulant 19)

caffeine a stimulant 19 in coffee, tea, and cola drinks, added to some analgesics 9

calamine a substance containing zinc carbonate (an antipruritic 118) used to soothe irritated skin

Calceos a brand name for colecalciferol (vitamin D, a vitamin 90) and calcium carbonate (a mineral 93)

Calcicard CR a brand of diltiazem 215 (a calcium channel blocker anti-angina drug 35 and antihypertensive 36)

calciferol vitamin D (a vitamin 90)

Calcijex a brand name for calcitriol (vitamin D 90)

Calciparine a brand of heparin 260 (an anticoagulant 39)

calcipotriol 167 a drug for psoriasis 124

calcitonin a drug for bone disorders 56

calcitonin (salmon) a drug for bone disorders 56 previously known as salcatonin

calcitriol vitamin D (a vitamin 90)

calcium a mineral 93

calcium acetate calcium (a mineral 93)

calcium carbonate a calcium salt (a mineral 93) used as an antacid 42

calcium chloride calcium (a mineral 93)

calcium folinate folinic acid salt used to reduce side effects of methotrexate 308

calcium gluconate calcium (a mineral 93)

Calcium resonium a drug to lower the amount of potassium in the blood

Calcort a brand name for deflazacort (a corticosteroid 80)

Calgel a brand-name teething gel containing lidocaine (a local anaesthetic 9) and cetylpyridinium (an antibacterial 66)

Calmurid HC a brand-name substance for eczema 125 containing hydrocortisone 263, lactic acid, and urea (an emollient)

Calpol a brand name for paracetamol 340 (a non-opioid analgesic 9)

Cam a brand name for ephedrine 230, a bronchodilator 23 and decongestant 26

Camcolit a brand name for lithium 290 (a drug for mania 15)

camphor a topical antipruritic 118

Campral EC a brand name for acamprosate 130 (an alcohol abuse deterrent)

Campto a brand name for irinotecan (an anticancer drug 96)

Cancidas a brand name for caspofungin (an antifungal 76)

candesartan 168, an angiotensin II blocker (a vasodilator 31 and antihypertensive 36)

Canesten a brand name for clotrimazole 195 (an antifungal 76)

Canesten HC a brand name for clotrimazole 195 (an antifungal 76) with hydrocortisone 263 (a corticosteroid 80)

Canesten Oral a brand name for fluconazole 246 (an antifungal 76)

Capasal a brand-name coal tar shampoo for dandruff 126 and psoriasis 124

Capastat a brand name for capreomycin sulphate (an antituberculous drug 67)

capecitabine an antimetabolite anticancer drug 96

Capoten a brand name for captopril 169 (an ACE inhibitor 31)

Capozide a brand name for captopril 169 (an ACE inhibitor 31) with hydrochlorothiazide 261 (a thiazide diuretic 32)

capreomycin an antituberculous drug 67

Caprin a brand name for aspirin 146 (a non-opioid analgesic 9 and antiplatelet drug 39)

capsaicin a rubefacient

Capsal a brand-name preparation for dry and scaly scalp conditions 126 containing coal tar with salicylic acid

captopril 169, an ACE inhibitor 31

Carace a brand name for lisinopril 289 (an ACE inhibitor 31)

Carace Plus a brand-name preparation containing lisinopril 289 and hydrochlorothiazide 261 (a product for high blood pressure 36)

Caralpha a brand name for lisinopril 289 (an ACE inhibitor 31)

Carbagen SR a brand name for carbamazepine 170 (an anticonvulsant 16)

Carbalax a brand name for sodium acid phosphate (a laxative 45) and sodium bicarbonate (an antacid 42)

carbamazepine 170 (an anticonvulsant 16 and antipsychotic 15)

carbaryl 172, an antiparasitic 122 for head lice

carbetocin a drug to control bleeding after childbirth

carbidopa a substance that enhances the therapeutic effect of levodopa 284 (a drug for parkinsonism 18)

carbimazole 172 (an antithyroid drug 84)

carbocisteine a mucolytic 95

Carbo-Dome a brand name for coal tar (a substance for psoriasis 124)

carboplatin an anticancer drug 96

carboprost a drug to control bleeding after childbirth 110

Cardene a brand name for nicardipine (a calcium channel blocker 35)

Cardicor a brand name for bisoprolol 160 (a beta blocker 30)

Cardilate MR a brand name for nifedipine 328 (a calcium channel blocker 35)

Cardura a brand name for doxazosin 223 (an antihypertensive 36, also used for prostate disorders 112)

Carisoma a brand name for carisoprodol (a muscle relaxant 54 related to meprobamate)

carisoprodol a muscle relaxant 54 related to meprobamate

carmustine an alkylating agent for Hodgkin's disease and solid tumours 96

carnitine an amino acid used as a nutritional supplement

Carnitor a brand name for carnitine (an amino acid used as a nutritional supplement)

carteolol a beta blocker 30 for glaucoma 114

carvedilol a beta blocker 30

Carylderm a brand name for carbaryl 172 (an antiparasitic 122 for head lice)

cascara a stimulant laxative 45

Casodex a brand name for bicalutamide (an anticancer drug 96)

caspofungin an antifungal 76

castor oil a stimulant laxative 45

Catapres a brand name for clonidine (an antihypertensive 36 and drug for migraine 20)

Caverject a brand name for alprostadil (a prostaglandin used for erectile dysfunction 87, 109)

Ceanel Concentrate a brand-name shampoo for dandruff 126 and psoriasis 124

Cedocard a brand name for isosorbide dinitrate 275 (a nitrate vasodilator 31 and anti-angina drug 35)

cefaclor a cephalosporin antibiotic 62

cefadroxil a cephalosporin antibiotic 62

cefalexin 174 (a cephalosporin antibiotic 62)

cefixime a cephalosporin antibiotic 62

cefotaxime a cephalosporin antibiotic 62

cefpodoxime a cephalosporin antibiotic 62

cefradine a cephalosporin antibiotic 62

ceftazidime a cephalosporin antibiotic 62

ceftriaxone a cephalosporin antibiotic 62

cefuroxime a cephalosporin antibiotic 62

Celance a brand name for pergolide (a drug for parkinsonism 18)

Celebrex a brand name for celecoxib 175 (a non-steroidal anti-inflammatory 50)

celecoxib 175, a non-steroidal anti-inflammatory 50

Celectol a brand name for celiprolol (a beta blocker 30)

Celevac a brand name for methylcellulose 309 (a laxative 45 and antidiarrhoeal 44)

celiprolol a beta blocker 30

CellCept a brand name for mycophenolate mofetil (an immunosuppressant 99)

Celluvisc a brand name for carmellose (artificial tears 116)

Centyl K a brand name for bendroflumethiazide (a thiazide diuretic 32) with potassium

cephalosporins antibiotics 62

Ceporex a brand name for cefalexin 174 (a cephalosporin antibiotic 62)

Ceprotin a brand name for protein C concentrate (a blood product to promote blood clotting 39)

Cerazette a brand name for oral contraceptive 105 containing desogestrel 206 (a female sex hormone 88)

Cerezyme a brand name for imiglucerase (enzyme for replacement therapy)

Cerumol a brand-name preparation for ear wax removal 117

cetirizine 176, an antihistamine 58

cetrimide an antiseptic 120

cetrorelix a drug for infertility 109

Cetrotide a brand name for cetrorelix (a drug for infertility 109)

cetuximab an anticancer drug 96

cetylpyridium an antiseptic 120

Chemydur a brand name for isosorbide mononitrate 275 (a nitrate vasodilator 31 anti-angina drug 35)

Chloractil a brand name for chlorpromazine 180 (a phenothiazine antipsychotic 15 and anti-emetic 21)

chloral hydrate a sleeping drug 11

chlorambucil an anticancer drug 96 used for chronic lymphocytic leukaemia and lymphatic and ovarian cancers, and as an immunosuppressant 99 for rheumatoid arthritis 51

chloramphenicol 177, an antibiotic 62

chlordiazepoxide a benzodiazepine anti-anxiety drug 13

chlorhexidine an antiseptic 120

Chloromycetin a brand name for chloramphenicol 177 (an antibiotic 62)

chloroquine 178, an antimalarial 75 and disease-modifying antirheumatic drug 51

chloroxylenol an antiseptic 120

chlorphenamine 179, an antihistamine 58 previously known as chlorpheniramine

chlorpromazine 180, a phenothiazine antipsychotic 15 and anti-emetic 21

chlorpropamide a drug for diabetes 82

chlortalidone a thiazide diuretic 32

choline salicylate a drug similar to aspirin 146 used in pain-relieving mouth gels 9 and ear drops 117

Choragon a brand name for chorionic gonadotrophin (a drug for infertility 109)

choriogonadotropin alfa a drug for infertility 109

chorionic gonadotrophin a drug for infertility 109

chromium a mineral 93

Cialis a brand name for tadalafil (a drug for erectile dysfunction 109)

Cicatrin a brand name for bacitracin (an antibacterial 66) with neomycin (an antibiotic 62)

ciclosporin 182, an immunosuppressant 99

cidofovir an antiviral 69 used for cytomegalovirus infection in HIV/AIDS 100

Cidomycin a brand name for gentamicin 253 (an aminoglycoside antibiotic 62)

cilastatin an enzyme inhibitor used to make imipenem (an antibiotic 62) more effective

cilazapril an ACE inhibitor 31

Cilest a brand-name oral contraceptive 105 containing ethinylestradiol 238 and norgestimate

cilostazol a vasodilator 31

Ciloxan a brand name for ciprofloxacin 185 (a quinolone antibacterial 66)

cimetidine 183, an anti-ulcer drug 43

Cinaziere a brand name of cinnarizine 184 (an antihistamine 58 and anti-emetic 21)

cinchocaine a local anaesthetic 9

cinnarizine 184 (an antihistamine 58 anti-emetic 21)

Cipralex a brand name for escitalopram (an antidepressant 14)

Cipramil a brand name for citalopram 187 (an antidepressant 14)

ciprofibrate a lipid-lowering drug 37

ciprofloxacin 185, a quinolone antibacterial 66, 67

Ciproxin a brand name for ciprofloxacin 185 (an antibacterial 66)

cisatracurium a drug used to relax the muscles in general anaesthesia

cisplatin 186, an anticancer drug 96

citalopram 187, an antidepressant 14

Citanest a brand name for prilocaine (a local anaesthetic 9)

Citramag a brand name for magnesium citrate (an osmotic laxative 45)

cladribine an anticancer drug 96

Claforan a brand name for cefotaxime (a cephalosporin antibiotic 62)

Clarelux a brand name for clobetasol (a topical corticosteroid 120)

clarithromycin 189, a macrolide antibiotic 62

Clarityn a brand name for loratadine 294 (an antihistamine 58)

Clarosip a brand name for clarithromycin 189 (a macrolide antibiotic 62)

clavulanic acid a substance given with amoxicillin 142 (a penicillin antibiotic 62) to make it more effective

clemastine an antihistamine 58

Clenil Modulite a brand name for beclometasone (a corticosteroid 80)

Clexane a brand name for enoxaparin (a low-molecular-weight heparin 260, an anticoagulant 39)

Climagest a brand-name preparation for menopausal symptoms 88 containing estradiol 235 and norethisterone 331

Climanor a brand name for medroxyprogesterone 299 (a female sex hormone 88)

Climaval a brand-name preparation for menopausal symptoms 88 containing estradiol 235

Climesse a brand-name preparation for menopausal symptoms 88 containing estradiol 235 and norethisterone 331

clindamycin a lincosamide antibiotic 62

Clinitar a brand name for coal tar (a substance used for psoriasis 124 and dandruff 126)

Clinorette a brand-name preparation containing estradiol 235 with norethisterone 331 (both female sex hormones 88)

Clinoril a brand name for sulindac (a non-steroidal anti-inflammatory 50)

clioquinol an antibacterial 66 and antifungal 76 for outer ear infections 117

Clivarine a brand name for reviparin (a type of heparin 260 an anticoagulant 39)

clobazam a benzodiazepine anti-anxiety drug 13 and anticonvulsant 16

clobetasol 190, a topical corticosteroid 120

clobetasone a topical corticosteroid 120

clodronate a drug for bone disorders 56 in cancer 96

clofarabine an anticancer drug 96

clofazimine a drug for leprosy 66

clomethiazole a non-benzodiazepine, non-barbiturate sleeping drug 11

Clomid a brand name for clomifene 191 (a drug for infertility 109)

clomifene 191, a drug for infertility 109

clomipramine 192, a tricyclic antidepressant 14

clonazepam 193, a benzodiazepine anticonvulsant 16

clonidine an antihypertensive 36 and drug for migraine 20

clopamide a thiazide diuretic 32

clopidogrel 194, an antiplatelet drug 39

Clopixol a brand name for zuclopenthixol (an antipsychotic 15)

cloral betaine a sleeping drug 11

Clotam a brand name for tolfenamic acid (a drug for migraine 20)

clotrimazole 195, an antifungal 76

clozapine 196, an antipsychotic 15

Clozaril a brand name for clozapine 196 (an antipsychotic 15)

coal tar a substance for psoriasis 124 and eczema 125

co-amilofruse a generic product containing amiloride 136 with furosemide 251 (both diuretics 32)

co-amilozide a generic product containing amiloride 136 with hydrochlorothiazide 261 (both diuretics 32)

co-amoxiclav a generic product containing amoxicillin 142 (a penicillin antibiotic 62) with clavulanic acid (a substance that increases the effectiveness of amoxicillin)

CoAprovel a brand name for irbesartan (an antihypertensive 36) with hydrochlorothiazide (a thiazide diuretic 32)

Cobalin-H a brand name for hydroxocobalamin (a vitamin 90)

co-beneldopa a generic product containing levodopa 284 (a drug for parkinsonism 18) with benserazide (a drug that enhances the effect of levodopa)

cocaine a local anaesthetic 9

co-careldopa a generic product containing levodopa 284 (a drug for parkinsonism 18) with carbidopa (a drug that enhances the effect of levodopa)

co-codamol a generic product containing codeine 197 with paracetamol 340 (both analgesics 9)

co-codaprin a generic product containing aspirin 146 with codeine 197 (both analgesics 9)

co-cyprindiol a generic product containing cyproterone (an anti-androgen 87) with ethinylestradiol (an oestrogen 88)

Codafen Continus a brand name for codeine 197 (an opioid analgesic 9) and ibuprofen 265 (a non-steroidal anti-inflammatory 50)

Codalax a brand name for co-danthramer (a stimulant laxative 45)

co-danthramer a generic product containing dantron with poloxamer (both stimulant laxatives 45)

co-danthrusate a generic product containing dantron with docusate (both stimulant laxatives 45)

codeine 197 (an opioid analgesic 9, cough suppressant 27, and antidiarrhoeal 44)

Codipar a brand name for codeine 197 with paracetamol 340 (both analgesics 9)

Codis 500 a brand name for aspirin 146 with codeine 197 (both analgesics 9)

co-dydramol a generic product containing paracetamol 340 with dihydrocodeine 214 (both analgesics 9)

co-fluampicil a generic product containing flucloxacillin 245 with ampicillin (both penicillin antibiotics 62)

co-flumactone a generic product containing hydroflumethiazide with spironolactone (both diuretics 32)

Cogentin a brand name for benztropine (an anticholinergic for parkinsonism 18)

Colazide a brand name for balsalazide (a drug for ulcerative colitis 46)

colchicine 198, a drug for gout 53

cold cream an antipruritic 118

Cold cures 28

colecalciferol vitamin D (a vitamin 90)

Colestid a brand name for colestipol (a lipid-lowering drug 37)

colestipol a lipid-lowering drug 37

colestyramine 200, a lipid-lowering drug 37

Colifoam a brand name for hydrocortisone 263 (a corticosteroid 80)

colistimethate the injection form of colistin (an antibiotic 62)

colistin an antibiotic 62

collodion a substance that dries to form a sticky film, protecting broken skin 120

Colofac a brand name for mebeverine 298 (an antispasmodic for irritable bowel syndrome 45)

Colomycin a brand name for colistin (an antibiotic 62)

Colpermin a brand name for peppermint oil (a substance for indigestion 42 and spasm of the bowel 44)

co-magaldrox a generic product containing aluminium hydroxide 135 with magnesium hydroxide 296 (both antacids 42)

Combigan a brand-name preparation for glaucoma 114 containing brimonidine with timolol 407 (a beta blocker 30)

Combivent a brand-name inhaler containing salbutamol 379 and ipratropium bromide 272 (both bronchodilators 23)

Combivir a brand-name preparation containing zidovudine/lamivudine 422 (antiretrovirals used for HIV/AIDS 100)

co-methiamol a generic product containing paracetamol 340 and methionine (an antidote to paracetamol poisoning)

competact a brand-name preparation containing metformin 306 and pioglitazone (both oral antidiabetics 82)

Compound W a brand-name keratolytic 123 for warts, containing salicylic acid

Comtess a brand name for entacapone (a drug for parkinsonism 18)

Concavit a brand-name multivitamin 90

Concerta XL a brand name for methylphenidate (a drug for attention-deficit hyperactivity disorder 19)

Condyline a brand name for podophyllotoxin (a drug for genital warts)

conjugated oestrogens 201 (a female sex hormone 88)

Conotrane a brand name for benzalkonium chloride (an antiseptic 120) with dimeticone (a base for skin preparations 120)

Contac Non Drowsy 12 Hour Relief a brand name for pseudoephedrine (a decongestant 26)

contraception, postcoital 109 (oral contraceptives 105)

contraceptives, oral (see oral contraceptives 105)

Convulex a brand name for sodium valproate 387 (an anticonvulsant 16)

Copaxone a brand name for glatiramer (a drug for multiple sclerosis)

Copegus a brand name for ribavirin (an antiviral 69)

co-phenotrope 202 a generic antidiarrhoeal 44 containing diphenoxylate with atropine 150

copper a mineral 93

co-prenozide a generic product containing oxprenolol (a beta blocker 30) with cyclopenthiazide (a thiazide diuretic 32)

co-proxamol a generic product containing paracetamol 340 with dextropropoxyphene (an opioid analgesic 9)

Coracten a brand name for nifedipine 328 (an anti-angina drug 35 and antihypertensive 36)

Cordarone X a brand name for amiodarone 137 (an anti-arrhythmic 33)

Cordilox a brand name for verapamil 419 (an anti-angina drug 35 and anti-arrhythmic 33)

Corgard a brand name for nadolol (a beta blocker 30)

Corlan a brand name for hydrocortisone 263 (a corticosteroid 80)

Coro-Nitro a brand name for glyceryl trinitrate 257 (an anti-angina drug 35)

Corsodyl a brand-name mouthwash and oral gel containing chlorhexidine (an antiseptic 120)

Corticosteroids 80

Corticosteroids for rheumatic disorders 53

Corticosteroids, topical 120

corticotropin a pituitary hormone 85

cortisol a former name for hydrocortisone 263

cortisone a corticosteroid 80

Cosalgesic a brand name for co-proxamol (an opioid analgesic 9)

co-simalcite a generic product containing hydrotalcite (an antacid 42) with dimeticone (an antifoaming agent 42)

Cosmegen Lyovac a brand name for dactinomycin (a cytotoxic anticancer drug 96)

CosmoFer a brand name for iron dextran (a mineral 93)

Cosopt a brand-name preparation containing dorzolamide 220 and timolol 407 (drugs for glaucoma 114)

co-tenidone a generic product containing atenolol 147 (a beta blocker 30) with chlortalidone (a thiazide diuretic 32)

co-triamterzide a generic product containing hydrochlorothiazide 261 with triamterene 414 (both diuretics 32)

co-trimoxazole 203 a generic product containing trimethoprim 415 with sulfamethoxazole (an antibacterial 66 and antiprotozoal 73)

Coughs, drugs to treat 27

Covermark a brand name for a masking cream for skin disfigurement

Coversyl a brand name for perindopril 342 (an ACE inhibitor 31)

cox-2 inhibitors non-steroidal anti-inflammatory drugs 50

Cozaar a brand name for losartan 295 (an antihypertensive 36)

Cozaar-Comp a brand-name preparation containing losartan 295 and hydrochlorothiazide 261 (a thiazide diuretic 32)

Cream of Magnesia a brand name for magnesium hydroxide 296 (an antacid 42 and laxative 45)

Creon a brand name for pancreatin (a preparation of pancreatic enzymes 49)

Crestor a brand name for rosuvastatin 378 (a lipid-lowering drug 37)

Crinone a brand name for progesterone (a female sex hormone 88)

crisantaspase an anticancer drug 96

Crixivan a brand name for indinavir (antiretroviral for HIV/AIDS 100)

Crohn's disease (see drugs for inflammatory bowel disease 46)

Cromogen a brand name for sodium cromoglicate 386 (an anti-allergy drug 58)

cromoglicate 386, an anti-allergy drug 58

crotamiton an antipruritic 118 and antiparasitic 122 for scabies

Crystacide a brand name for hydrogen peroxide cream (an antiseptic 120)

Crystapen a brand name for penicillin G (a penicillin antibiotic 62)

Cubicin a brand name for daptomycin (an antibiotic 62)

Cuplex a brand-name wart preparation containing copper acetate, lactic acid, and salicylic acid

Cuprofen a brand name for ibuprofen 265 (a non-steroidal anti-inflammatory 50)

Curatoderm a brand name for tacalcitol (a drug for psoriasis 124)

Curosurf a brand name for poractant alfa (a drug to mature the lungs of premature babies)

Cutivate a brand name for fluticasone 250 (a corticosteroid 80)

cyanocobalamin vitamin B_{12} (a vitamin 90)

Cyclimorph a brand name for morphine 322 (an opioid analgesic 9) with cyclizine (an anti-emetic 21)

cyclizine an antihistamine 58 used as an anti-emetic 21

Cyclogest a brand name for progesterone (a female sex hormone 88)

cyclopenthiazide a thiazide diuretic 32

cyclopentolate an anticholinergic mydriatic 116

cyclophosphamide 204, an anticancer drug 96

Cyclo-Progynova a brand name for estradiol 235 with levonorgestrel 286 (both female sex hormones 88)

cycloserine an antibiotic 62 for tuberculosis 67

Cyklokapron a brand name for tranexamic acid (an antifibrinolytic used to promote blood clotting 39)

Cymalon a brand-name preparation for cystitis 112 containing sodium bicarbonate, citric acid, sodium citrate, and sodium carbonate

Cymbalta a brand name for duloxetine (an antidepressant 14 and drug for diabetic neuropathy)

Cymevene a brand name for ganciclovir (an antiviral 69)

cyproheptadine an antihistamine 58 and drug for migraine 20

Cyprostat a brand name for cyproterone acetate, a synthetic sex hormone used for acne 123 and cancer of the prostate 96

cyproterone acetate a synthetic sex hormone used for acne 123, cancer of the prostate 96, and male sexual disorders 87

Cystagon a brand name for mercaptamine (a drug used for a metabolic disorder)

Cysticide a brand name for praziquantel (an anthelmintic 78)

Cystopurin a brand name for potassium citrate (used for cystitis 112)

Cystrin a brand name for oxybutynin 339 (a drug for urinary disorders 112)

cytarabine a drug for leukaemia 96

cytokines anticancer drugs 96

Cytotec a brand name for misoprostol 319 (an anti-ulcer drug 43)

cytotoxic drugs anticancer drugs 96

D

dacarbazine a drug for malignant melanoma and cancer of soft tissues 96

daclizumab an immunosuppressant 99

dactinomycin a cytotoxic antibiotic for cancer 96

Daktacort a brand name for hydrocortisone 263 (a corticosteroid 80) with miconazole 314 (an antifungal 76)

Daktarin a brand name for miconazole 314 (an antifungal 76)

Dalacin C a brand name for clindamycin (a lincosamide antibiotic 62)

dalfopristin an antibiotic 62

Dalivit a brand-name multivitamin 90

Dalmane a brand name for flurazepam (a benzodiazepine sleeping drug 11)

dalteparin a type of heparin 260 (an anticoagulant 39)

danaparoid an anticoagulant 39

danazol a drug for menstrual disorders 104

Dandrazol a brand name for ketoconazole 277 (an antifungal 76)

dandruff, drugs for 126

Danol a brand name for danazol (a drug for menstrual disorders 104)

Dantrium a brand name for dantrolene (a muscle relaxant 54)

dantrolene a muscle relaxant 54

dantron a stimulant laxative 45

Daonil a brand name for glibenclamide 255 (an oral antidiabetic 82)

dapsone an antibacterial 66 and antiprotozoal 73

daptomycin a lipopeptide antibiotic 62

Daraprim a brand name for pyrimethamine 362 (an antimalarial 75)

darbepoetin alfa a drug used to treat anaemia

daunorubicin a cytotoxic antibiotic (an anticancer drug 96)

DaunoXome a brand name for daunorubicin (an anticancer drug 96)

Day Nurse a brand-name preparation containing paracetamol 340 (a non-opioid analgesic 9), pseudoephedrine (a decongestant 26) and pholcodine (a cough suppressant 27)

DDAVP a brand name for desmopressin 205 (a pituitary hormone 85)

DDI see didanosine

Deca-Durabolin a brand name for nandrolone (an anabolic steroid 88)

De-capeptyl SR a brand name for triptorelin (an anticancer drug 96)

Decongestants 26

DEET another name for diethyltoluamide (a mosquito repellent)

Deep Relief a brand-name preparation containing ibuprofen 265 (a non-steroidal anti-inflammatory 50) with levomenthol

deferiprone a drug used to remove excess iron from the blood in thalassaemia

deflazacort a corticosteroid 80

Deltacortril Enteric a brand name for prednisolone 352 (a corticosteroid 80)

Deltastab a brand name for prednisolone 352 (a corticosteroid 80)

demeclocycline a tetracycline antibiotic 62

Dementia, drugs for 19

Demser a brand name for metirosine (a drug for phaeochromocytoma – an adrenal gland tumour 96)

De-Nol a brand name for bismuth (a substance for gastric and duodenal ulcers 43)

Dentomycin a brand name for minocycline 315 (a tetracycline antibiotic 62)

Denzapine a brand name for clozapine (an antipsychotic 15)

Depakote a brand name for valproic acid (a drug for mania 15)

Depixol a brand name for flupentixol 248 (an antipsychotic 15 and antidepressant 14)

Depo-Medrone a brand name for methylprednisolone (a corticosteroid 80)

Deponit a brand name for glyceryl trinitrate 257 (an anti-angina drug 35)

Depo-Provera a brand name for medroxyprogesterone 299 (a female sex hormone 88)

Dequacaine a brand name for benzocaine (a local anaesthetic 9) with dequalinium (an antibacterial 66)

Dequadin a brand name for dequalinium (an antibacterial 66)

dequalinium an antibacterial 66 used for mouth infections

Derbac-M a brand-name shampoo containing malathion 297 (an anti-parasitic 122)

Dermabond a brand name for octylcyanoacrylate (a skin adhesive)

Dermacolor a brand name for a masking cream for skin disfigurement

Dermacort a brand-name preparation for hydrocortisone cream 263

Dermidex Cream a brand-name topical preparation for skin irritation 120 containing chlorobutanol, lignocaine, cetrimide, and alcloxa

Dermovate a brand name for clobetasol 190 (a topical corticosteroid 120)

Dermovate-NN a brand name for nystatin 332 (an antifungal 76) with clobetasol 190 (a topical corticosteroid 120) and neomycin (an aminoglycoside antibiotic 62)

Deseril a brand name for methysergide (a drug to prevent migraine 20)

Desferal a brand name for desferrioxamine (an antidote for iron overdose)

desferrioxamine an antidote for iron overdose

desflurane a general anaesthetic

desloratadine 294, an antihistamine 58

desmopressin 205, a pituitary hormone 85 used for diabetes insipidus 86

desogestrel 206, a female sex hormone 88 and oral contraceptive 105

Destolit a brand name for ursodeoxycholic acid (a drug for gallstones 48)

Deteclo a brand name for tetracycline 404 with chlortetracycline and demeclocycline (all tetracycline antibiotics 62)

Detrunorm a brand name for propiverine (drug for urinary frequency 112)

Detrusitol a brand name for tolterodine 411 (an anticholinergic and antispasmodic for urinary disorders 112)

Dettol a brand-name liquid skin antiseptic 120 containing chloroxylenol

dexamethasone 208, a corticosteroid 80

dexamfetamine an amfetamine (a drug for narcolepsy and hyperactivity in children 19)

Dexa-Rhinaspray Duo a brand name for dexamethasone 208 (a corticosteroid 80) with tramazoline (a nasal decongestant 26)

Dexedrine a brand name for dexamfetamine (a drug for narcolepsy and hyperactivity in children 19)

dexibuprofen a non-steroidal anti-inflammatory 50

dexketoprofen a non-steroidal anti-inflammatory 50

dextromethorphan a cough suppressant 27

dextropropoxyphene a constituent of co-proxamol (an opioid analgesic 9)

DF 50 a brand name for dihydrocodeine 214 (an opioid analgesic 9)

DHC Continus a brand name for dihydrocodeine 214 (an opioid analgesic 9)

diabetes, drugs used in 82

diabetes insipidus, drugs for (see drugs for pituitary disorders 85)

DIAGLYK a brand name for gliclazide 256 (an oral antidiabetic 82)

Dialar a brand of diazepam 209 (a benzodiazepine anti-anxiety drug 13, muscle relaxant 54, and anticonvulsant 16)

Diamicron a brand name for gliclazide 256 (an oral antidiabetic 82)

diamorphine an opioid analgesic 9

Diamox a brand name for acetazolamide (a carbonic anhydrase inhibitor diuretic 32 and drug for glaucoma 114)

Dianette a brand name for cyproterone acetate (a synthetic sex hormone used for acne 123) with ethinylestradiol 238 (a female sex hormone 88)

Diazemuls a brand name for diazepam 209
(a benzodiazepine anti-anxiety drug 13, muscle
relaxant 54, and anticonvulsant 16)

diazepam 209, a benzodiazepine anti-anxiety drug
13, muscle relaxant 54, and anticonvulsant 16

diazoxide an antihypertensive 36 also used for
hypoglycaemia 82

Dibenyline a brand name for phenoxybenzamine
(a drug for phaeochromocytoma 96)

dibromopropamidine an antibacterial agent 66

diclofenac 210, a non-steroidal anti-inflammatory
50

Dicloflex a brand name for diclofenac 210 (a non-
steroidal anti-inflammatory 50)

Diclomax Retard a brand name for diclofenac 210
(a non-steroidal anti-inflammatory 50)

dicobalt edetate an antidote for cyanide
poisoning

Diconal a brand name for dipipanone (an opioid
analgesic 9) with cyclizine (an anti-emetic 21)

dicycloverine 211, a drug for irritable bowel
syndrome 45 previously known as
chlorpheniramine

Dicynene a brand name for etamsylate
(an antifibrinolytic used to promote blood
clotting 39)

didanosine an antiretroviral for HIV/AIDS 100

Didronel a brand name for etidronate 239 (a drug
for bone disorders 56)

Didronel PMO a brand name for etidronate 239
(a drug for bone disorders 56) and calcium
carbonate

diethylamine salicylate a rubefacient

diethylcarbamazine an anthelmintic drug 78

diethylstilbestrol a female sex hormone 88
previously known as stilboestrol

diethyltoluamide (DEET) a mosquito repellent

Differin a brand name for adapalene (a retinoid for
acne 123)

Difflam a brand name for benzydamine
(an analgesic 9)

Diflucan a brand name for fluconazole 246
(an antifungal 76)

diflucortolone a topical corticosteroid 120

diflunisal a non-steroidal anti-inflammatory 50

Diftavax a brand-name vaccine 70 to protect
against diphtheria/tetanus

Digibind an antidote for overdose of digoxin 213

Digitalis drugs 29

digitoxin a digitalis drug 29

digoxin 213, a digitalis drug 29

dihydrocodeine 214, an opioid analgesic 9

dihydrotachysterol vitamin D (a vitamin 90)

Dilcardia SR a brand name for diltiazem 215
(a calcium channel blocker 35)

diloxanide furoate an antiprotozoal 73 for amoebic
dysentery

diltiazem 215, a calcium channel blocker 35 and
antihypertensive 36

Dilzem a brand name for diltiazem 215
(an antihypertensive 36 and calcium channel
blocker 35)

dimercaprol an antidote for heavy metal poisoning

dimethyl sulfoxide a drug to treat bladder
inflammation

dimeticone a silicone-based substance used in
barrier creams 120 and as an antifoaming agent
42

Dimetriose a brand name for gestrinone (a drug for
menstrual disorders 104)

dinoprostone a prostaglandin used to terminate
pregnancy 110

Diocalm a brand-name antidiarrhoeal 44
containing attapulgite and morphine 322

Diocalm Ultra a brand name for loperamide 292
(an antidiarrhoeal 44)

Dioctyl a brand name for docusate (a stimulant
laxative 45)

Dioderm a brand name for hydrocortisone 263
(a corticosteroid 80)

Dioralyte a brand name for rehydration salts
containing sodium bicarbonate, glucose,
potassium chloride, and sodium chloride

Diovan a brand name for valsartan 416
(an antihypertensive 36)

Dipentum a brand name for olsalazine (a drug for
ulcerative colitis 46)

diphenhydramine an antihistamine 58, anti-emetic
21, and antipruritic 118

diphenoxylate an opioid antidiarrhoeal 44

dipipanone an opioid analgesic 9

dipivefrine a sympathomimetic for glaucoma 114

Diprobase a brand-name emollient preparation

Diprosalic a brand-name skin preparation
containing betamethasone 158 (a corticosteroid
80) and salicylic acid (a keratolytic 123)

Diprosone a brand name for betamethasone 158
(a corticosteroid 80)

dipyridamole 216, an antiplatelet drug 39

Dirythmin SA a brand name for disopyramide
(an anti-arrhythmic 33)

Disipal a brand name for orphenadrine 337 (a drug
for parkinsonism 18)

disopyramide an anti-arrhythmic 33

Disprin a brand name for soluble aspirin 146
(a non-opioid analgesic 9)

Disprin Extra a brand-name soluble analgesic 9
containing aspirin 146 and paracetamol 340

Disprol a brand name for paracetamol 340 (a non-
opioid analgesic 9)

Dutasteride a male sex hormone 87 for benign prostatic hyperplasia 112

Dyazide a brand name for hydrochlorothiazide 261 with triamterene 414 (both diuretics 32)

dydrogesterone 226, a female sex hormone 88

Dymotil a brand-name product containing atropine 150 and diphenoxylate (an opioid antidiarrhoeal 44)

Dynastat a brand name for parecoxib (an analgesic 9 and non-steroidal anti-inflammatory 50)

Dyspamet a brand name for cimetidine 183 (an anti-ulcer drug 43)

Dysport a brand name for botulinum toxin 161 (used as a muscle relaxant 54)

Dytac a brand name for triamterene 414 (a potassium-sparing diuretic 32)

Dytide a brand name for benzthiazide with triamterene 414 (both diuretics 32)

E

EarCalm a brand-name preparation for treatment of superficial ear infections 117 containing acetic acid

ear disorders, drugs for 117

Earex a brand-name preparation for ear wax removal 117

Ebixa a brand name for memantidine, used to treat Alzheimer's disease 18

Ebufac a brand name for ibuprofen 265 (a non-steroidal anti-inflammatory 50)

Eccoxolac a brand name for etodolac (a non-steroidal anti-inflammatory 50)

Econacort a brand name for econazole (an antifungal 76) with hydrocortisone 263 (a corticosteroid 80)

econazole an antifungal 76

Ecostatin a brand name for econazole (an antifungal 76)

eczema, treatments for 125

Edronax a brand name for reboxetine (an antidepressant 14)

edrophonium a drug for diagnosis of myasthenia gravis 55

efalizumab a drug for severe psoriasis 124

efavirenz 227, an antiretroviral for HIV/AIDS 100

Efcortelan a brand name for hydrocortisone 263 (a corticosteroid 80)

Efcortesol a brand name for hydrocortisone 263 (a corticosteroid 80)

Efexor a brand name for venlafaxine 418 (an antidepressant 14)

Effercitrate a brand name for potassium citrate used for cystitis

eflornithine a drug for treatment of facial hair in women

eformoterol see formoterol (a sympathomimetic bronchodilator 23)

Efudix a brand name for fluorouracil (an anticancer drug 96)

Elantan a brand name for isosorbide mononitrate 275 (a nitrate vasodilator 31 and anti-angina drug 35)

Eldepryl a brand name for selegiline (a drug for parkinsonism 18)

Eldisine a brand name for vindesine (an anticancer drug 96)

Electrolade a brand-name oral rehydration salts with potassium, sodium chloride, sodium bicarbonate, and glucose

eletriptan a drug for migraine 20

Elidel cream a brand name for pimecrolimus (an anti-inflammatory used for eczema 125)

Elleste Duet a brand-name preparation for menopausal symptoms 88 containing estradiol 235 and norethisterone 331

Elleste Solo a brand name for estradiol 235 (an oestrogen 88 for menopausal symptoms)

Elocon a brand name for mometasone 320 (a topical corticosteroid 120)

Eloxatin a brand name for oxaliplatin (an anticancer drug 96)

Eltroxin a brand name for levothyroxine 288 (a thyroid hormone 84)

Eludril a brand-name antiseptic preparation containing chlorhexidine with chlorobutanol

Elyzol a brand name for metronidazole 313 (an antibacterial 66 and antiprotozoal 73)

Emadine a brand name for emedastine (an antihistamine 58)

Emcor a brand name for bisoprolol 160 (a beta blocker 30)

emedastine an antihistamine 58

Emend a brand name for aprepitant (an anti-emetic 21)

Emeside a brand name for ethosuximide (an anticonvulsant 16)

Emflex a brand name for acemetacin (a non-steroidal anti-inflammatory 50)

Emla a brand-name local anaesthetic 9 containing lignocaine and prilocaine

emtricitabine an antiretroviral for HIV/AIDS 100

Emtriva a brand name for emtricitabine (an antiretroviral for HIV/AIDS 100)

enalapril 228, an ACE inhibitor vasodilator 31 and antihypertensive 36

Enbrel a brand name for etanercept (an immunosuppressant 99 and disease-modifying antirheumatic drug 51)

enbucrilate a tissue and skin adhesive for closing wounds

En-De-Kay a brand name for fluoride (a mineral 93)

Endoxana a brand name for cyclophosphamide 204 (an anticancer drug 96)

Enfuvirtide an antiretroviral for HIV/AIDS 100

Engerix B a brand-name vaccine 70 to protect against viral hepatitis B

ENO's a brand-name antacid 42 containing sodium bicarbonate, sodium carbonate, and citric acid

enoxaparin a type of heparin 260 (an anticoagulant 39)

enoximone a drug for heart failure 97

entacapone a drug for parkinsonism 18

entecavir an antiviral 69 for hepatitis B

Entocort a brand name for budesonide 163 (a corticosteroid 80)

Entonox a brand name for a mixture of nitrous oxide and oxygen used as an analgesic 9

Epanutin a brand name for phenytoin 347 (an anticonvulsant 16)

ephedrine 230, a bronchodilator 23 and decongestant 26

Ephynal a brand name for vitamin E (a vitamin 90)

Epiglu a brand name for ethylcyanoacrylate (a tissue and skin adhesive)

Epilim a brand name for sodium valproate 387 (an anticonvulsant 16)

epinastine an antihistamine 58

epinephrine 231, a bronchodilator 23 and drug for glaucoma 114. Also known as adrenaline.

EpiPen a brand name for epinephrine 231 (an anti-allergy drug 58)

epirubicin a cytotoxic anticancer drug 96

Epivir a brand name for lamivudine 422 an antiretroviral for HIV/AIDS 100

eplerenone a drug for heart failure following a heart attack 97

epoetin a kidney hormone 80 (used for anaemia due to kidney failure). Also known as erythropoietin 234.

epoprostenol a prostaglandin used for its vasodilator effects 31

Eprex a brand name for erythropoietin 234 (a kidney hormone 80 used for anaemia due to kidney failure)

eprosartan an angiotensin II blocker (a vasodilator 31 and antihypertensive 36)

eptifibatide an antiplatelet drug 39 for prevention of heart attacks

Equanox a brand name for a mixture of nitrous oxide and oxygen used as an analgesic 9

Equasym a brand name for methylphenidate (a drug used for attention deficit hyperactivity disorder 19)

Erbitux a brand name for cetuximab (an anticancer drug 96)

ergocalciferol vitamin D (a vitamin 90)

ergometrine a uterine stimulant 110

ergotamine 232, a drug for migraine 20

erlotinib an anticancer drug 96

ertapenem an antibiotic 62

Erwinase a brand name for crisantaspase (an anticancer drug 96)

Erymax a brand name for erythromycin 233 (an antibiotic 62)

Erythrocin a brand name for erythromycin 233 (an antibiotic 62)

erythromycin 233, an antibiotic 62

Erythroped a brand name for erythromycin 233 (an antibiotic 62)

erythropoietin 234, a kidney hormone 80 (used for anaemia due to kidney failure). Also known as epoetin.

escitalopram 187, an antidepressant 14

Eskamel a brand name for resorcinol (a drug for acne 123) with sulphur (a topical antibacterial 66 and antifungal 76)

esmolol a beta blocker 30

esomeprazole an anti-ulcer drug 43

Estracombi a brand-name preparation to treat menopausal symptoms 88 containing estradiol 235 and norethisterone 331

Estracyt a brand name for estramustine (an anticancer drug 96)

Estraderm a brand name for estradiol 235 (an oestrogen 88)

estradiol 235, an oestrogen 88

estramustine an alkylating agent for cancer of the prostate 96

Estring a brand-name vaginal ring for menopausal symptoms 88 containing estradiol 235

estriol an oestrogen 88

estrone an oestrogen 88

estropipate an oestrogen 88

etamsylate an antifibrinolytic used to promote blood clotting 39

etanercept an immunosuppressant 99 and disease-modifying antirheumatic drug 51

ethambutol 237, an antituberculous drug 67

ethinylestradiol 238, a female sex hormone 88 and oral contraceptive 105

Ethmozine a brand name for moracizine (an anti-arrhythmic 33)

ethosuximide an anticonvulsant 16

etidronate 239, a drug for bone disorders 56

etodolac a non-steroidal anti-inflammatory 50

etomidate a drug for induction of general anaesthesia

etonorgestrel a progestogen 88

Etopophos a brand name for etoposide (an anticancer drug 96)

etoposide a drug for cancers of the lung, lymphatic system, and testes 96

etoricoxib an analgesic 9 and non-steroidal anti-inflammatory 50

etynodiol a progestogen, a female sex hormone 88

Eucardic a brand name for carvedilol (an antihypertensive 36)

Eudemine a brand name for diazoxide (used to treat hypoglycaemia 82 and as an antihypertensive 36)

Euglucon a brand name for glibenclamide 255 (an oral antidiabetic 82)

Eumovate a brand name for clobetasone (a topical corticosteroid 120)

Eurax a brand name for crotamiton (an antipruritic 118)

Eurax-Hydrocortisone a brand name for hydrocortisone 263 (a corticosteroid 80) with crotamiton (an antipruritic 118)

Evista a brand name for raloxifene 367 (an anti-oestrogen sex hormone antagonist 88 for osteoporosis 56)

Evorel a brand name for estradiol 235 (an oestrogen 88)

Evra a brand-name contraceptive patch containing ethinylestradiol 238 with norelgestromin (both female sex hormones 88)

Exelderm a brand name for sulconazole (an antifungal 76)

Exelon a brand name for rivastigmine 376 (a drug for Alzheimer's disease)

exemestane an anti-breast cancer drug 96

Ex-Lax a brand name for senna (a stimulant laxative 45)

Exocin a brand name for ofloxacin (an antibiotic 62)

Exorex a brand name for coal tar lotion (for psoriasis 124 and eczema 125)

Exterol brand-name ear drops for wax removal 117 containing urea (an emollient) and hydrogen peroxide (an antiseptic 120)

Exubera a brand name for inhaled insulin 269 (a drug for diabetes 82)

ezetimibe 240, a lipid-lowering drug 37

Ezetrol a brand name for ezetimibe 240 (a lipid-lowering drug 37)

F

factor VIIa a blood extract to promote blood clotting 39

factor VIII a blood extract to promote blood clotting 39

factor IX a blood extract to promote blood clotting 39

factor XIII a blood extract to promote blood clotting 39

famciclovir an antiviral 69

famotidine an anti-ulcer drug 43

Famvir a brand name for famciclovir (an antiviral 69)

Fansidar a brand-name antimalarial 75 containing pyrimethamine 362 and sulfadoxine

Fareston a brand name for toremifene (an anticancer drug 96)

Farlutal a brand name for medroxyprogesterone 299 (a female sex hormone 88)

Fasigyn a brand name for tinidazole (an antibacterial 66)

Faslodex a brand name for fluvestrant (an anti-breast cancer drug 96)

Faverin a brand name for fluvoxamine (an antidepressant 14)

Fectrim a brand name for co-trimoxazole 203 (an antibacterial 66 and antiprotozoal 73)

Fefol a brand name for folic acid (a vitamin 90) with iron (a mineral 93)

felbinac a non-steroidal anti-inflammatory 50

Feldene a brand name for piroxicam 349 (a non-steroidal anti-inflammatory 50 and drug for gout 53)

felodipine 242, a calcium channel blocker 35

felypressin a vasoconstrictor 97 used in dentistry

female sex hormones 88

Femapak a brand-name preparation for menopausal symptoms 88 containing estradiol 235 and dydrogesterone 226

Femara a brand name for letrozole (an anticancer drug 96)

Fematrix a brand name for estradiol 235 (an oestrogen 88)

Feminax a brand-name analgesic 9 for dysmenorrhoea containing paracetamol 340, codeine 197, hyoscine 264, and caffeine

Femodene a brand-name oral contraceptive 105 containing ethinylestradiol 238 and gestodene

Femodette a brand-name oral contraceptive 105 containing gestodene and ethinylestradiol 238

Femoston a brand-name preparation for menopausal symptoms 88 containing estradiol 235 and dydrogesterone 226

FemSeven a brand name for estradiol 235 (an oestrogen 88)

FemSeven Conti a brand name for estradiol with levonorgestrel for hormone replacement therapy 88

Femulen a brand-name oral contraceptive 105 containing etynodiol diacetate

Fenbid a brand name for ibuprofen 265 (a non-steroidal anti-inflammatory 50)

fenbufen a non-steroidal anti-inflammatory 50

fenofibrate a lipid-lowering drug 37

fenoprofen a non-steroidal anti-inflammatory 50

Fenopron a brand name for fenoprofen (a non-steroidal anti-inflammatory 50)

fenoterol a sympathomimetic bronchodilator 23

Fenox a brand name for phenylephrine (a decongestant 26)

fentanyl an opioid analgesic 9 used in general anaesthesia and labour 110

Fentazin a brand name for perphenazine (an antipsychotic 15 and anti-emetic 21)

Feospan a brand name for iron (a mineral 93)

Feprapax a brand name for lofepramine (a tricyclic antidepressant 14)

ferric ammonium citrate iron (a mineral 93)

Ferriprox a brand name for deferiprone (used to treat iron overload)

Ferrograd a brand name for iron (a mineral 93)

Ferrograd C a brand name for iron (a mineral 93) with vitamin C (a vitamin 90)

Ferrograd Folic a brand name for folic acid (a vitamin 90) with iron (a mineral 93)

ferrous fumarate iron (a mineral 93)

ferrous gluconate iron (a mineral 93)

ferrous glycine sulphate iron (a mineral 93)

ferrous sulphate iron (a mineral 93)

Fersaday a brand name for iron (a mineral 93)

Fersamal a brand name for iron (a mineral 93)

fexofenadine an antihistamine 58

Fibrogammin P a brand name for factor XIII (a blood extract to promote blood clotting 39)

Fibro-vein a brand name for sodium tetradecyl sulphate (a drug for varicose veins)

Filair a brand name for beclometasone 153 (a corticosteroid 80)

filgrastim 243, a blood growth stimulant

finasteride 244, a male sex hormone 87 for benign prostatic hypertrophy 112

Flagyl a brand name for metronidazole 313 (an antibacterial 66 and antiprotozoal 73)

Flamazine a brand name for silver sulfadiazine (a topical antibacterial 66)

flavoxate a urinary antispasmodic 112

Flebogamma a brand name for human immunoglobulin 72 (a preparation injected to prevent infectious diseases 70)

flecainide an anti-arrhythmic 33

Flexin Continus a brand name for indometacin (a non-steroidal anti-inflammatory 50)

Flixonase a brand name for fluticasone 250 (a corticosteroid 80)

Flixotide a brand name for fluticasone 250 (a corticosteroid 80)

Flolan a brand name for epoprostenol (an anticoagulant 39 and vasodilator 31)

Flomaxtra XL a brand name for tamsulosin 397, an alpha blocker for prostate disorders 112

Florinef a brand name for fludrocortisone (a corticosteroid 80)

Floxapen a brand name for flucloxacillin 245 (a penicillin antibiotic 62)

Fluanxol a brand name for flupentixol 248 (an antipsychotic 15 used in the treatment of depression 14)

Fluarix a brand-name vaccine 70 to protect against influenza

flucloxacillin 245, a penicillin antibiotic 62

fluconazole 246, an antifungal 76

flucytosine an antifungal 76

Fludara a brand name for fludarabine (an anticancer drug 96)

fludarabine an anticancer drug 96

fludrocortisone a corticosteroid 80

fludroxycortide a topical corticosteroid 120 previously known as flurandrenolone

flumazenil an antidote for benzodiazepine overdose

flumetasone a corticosteroid 80

flunisolide a corticosteroid 80

flunitrazepam a benzodiazepine sleeping drug 11

fluocinolone a topical corticosteroid 120

fluocinonide a topical corticosteroid 120

fluocortolone a topical corticosteroid 120

Fluor-a-day a brand name for fluoride (a mineral 93)

fluorescein a drug used to stain the eye before examination

fluoride a mineral 93

Fluorigard a brand name for fluoride (a mineral 93)

fluorometholone a corticosteroid 80 for eye disorders

fluorouracil an anticancer drug 96

fluoxetine 247, an antidepressant 14

flupentixol 248, an antipsychotic 15 used in depression 14

fluphenazine an antipsychotic 15 used in depression 14

flurandrenolone see fludroxycortide, a topical corticosteroid 120

flurazepam a benzodiazepine sleeping drug 11

flurbiprofen a non-steroidal anti-inflammatory 50

flutamide 249, an anticancer drug 96

fluticasone 250, a corticosteroid 80

fluvastatin a lipid-lowering drug 37

DRUG FINDER AND INDEX

fluvoxamine an antidepressant 14

FML a brand name for fluorometholone (a corticosteroid 80)

folate sodium folic acid (a vitamin 90)

folic acid a vitamin 90

folinic acid a vitamin 90

follicle-stimulating hormone (FSH) a natural hormone for infertility 109

follitropin alfa a drug for infertility 109

follitropin beta a drug for infertility 109

fomepizole an antidote for ethylene glycol and methanol poisoning

fondaparinux an anticoagulant 39

Foradil a brand name for formoterol (a bronchodilator 23)

Forceval a brand-name multivitamin preparation 90

formoterol formerly known as eformoterol (a sympathomimetic bronchodilator 23)

Forsteo a brand name for teriparatide (a drug for bone disorders 56)

Fortral a brand name for pentazocine (an opioid analgesic 9)

Fortum a brand name for ceftazidime (a cephalosporin antibiotic 62)

Fosamax a brand name for alendronic acid 132 (a drug for bone disorders 56)

fosamprenavir an antiretroviral for HIV/AIDS 100

Fosavance a brand name for alendronic acid (a drug for bone disorders 56) with colecalciferol (vitamin D, a vitamin 90)

Foscan a brand name for temoprofin (an anticancer drug 96)

foscarnet an antiviral 69

Foscavir a brand name for foscarnet (an antiviral 69)

fosphenytoin 347, an anticonvulsant 16

fosinopril an ACE inhibitor 31

Fragmin a brand name for dalteparin (a low-molecular-weight heparin 260 used as an anticoagulant 39)

framycetin a topical aminoglycoside antibiotic 62 for ear, eye, and skin infections

frangula a mild stimulant laxative 45

Frisium a brand name for clobazam (a benzodiazepine anti-anxiety drug 13)

Froben a brand name for flurbiprofen (a non-steroidal anti-inflammatory 50)

Froop a brand name for furosemide 251 (a loop diuretic 32)

Frovatriptan a drug for migraine 20

Fru-Co a brand name for amiloride 136 with furosemide 251 (both diuretics 32)

Frumil a brand name for amiloride 136 with furosemide 251 (both diuretics 32)

Frusene a brand name for furosemide 251 with triamterene 414 (both diuretics 32)

FSH follicle-stimulating hormone a natural hormone for infertility 109

FuciBET a brand name for betamethasone 158 (a corticosteroid 80) with fusidic acid (an antibiotic 62)

Fucidin a brand name for fusidic acid (an antibiotic 62)

Fucidin H a brand name for fusidic acid (an antibiotic 62) and hydrocortisone 263 (a corticosteroid 80)

Fucithalmic a brand name for fusidic acid (an antibiotic 62)

Full Marks a brand name for phenothrin (a topical antiparasitic 122)

Fungilin a brand name for amphotericin 143 (an antifungal 76)

Fungizone a brand name for amphotericin 143 (an antifungal 76)

Furadantin a brand name for nitrofurantoin (an antibacterial 66)

furosemide 251, a loop diuretic 32 previously known as frusemide

fusidic acid an antibiotic 62

Fuzeon a brand name for enfuviritide (an antiretroviral for HIV/AIDS 100)

Fybogel a brand name for ispaghula (a bulk-forming agent used as a laxative 45 and antidiarrhoeal 44)

G

gabapentin 252 an anticonvulsant 16

Gabitril a brand name for tiagabine (an anticonvulsant 16)

galantamine a drug for dementia 19

Galcodine a brand name for codeine 197 (a cough suppressant 27)

Galenamox a brand name for amoxicillin 142 (a penicillin antibiotic 62)

Galenphol a brand name for pholcodine (a cough suppressant 27)

Galfer a brand name for iron (a mineral 93)

Galfer FA a brand name for folic acid (a vitamin 90) with iron (a mineral 93)

gallamine a drug used to relax the muscles in general anaesthesia

Galpseud a brand name for pseudoephedrine (a sympathomimetic decongestant 26)

gallstones, drug treatment for 48

Gamanil a brand name for lofepramine 291 (a tricyclic antidepressant 14)

gamma globulin an immunoglobulin 72

447

gamolenic acid an extract of evening primrose

ganciclovir an antiviral 69

Ganfort a brand-name preparation containing bimatoprost (a drug for glaucoma 114) with timolol (a beta blocker 30)

ganirelix a drug for treatment of infertility 109

Gastrobid Continus a brand name for metoclopramide 310 (a gastrointestinal motility regulator and anti-emetic 21)

Gastrocote a brand-name antacid 42 containing aluminium hydroxide 135, sodium bicarbonate, magnesium trisilicate, and alginic acid

Gavilast a brand name for ranitidine 369 (an anti-ulcer drug 43)

Gaviscon Advance a brand-name antacid 42 containing potassium bicarbonate with alginate

Gaviscon Extra Strength a brand-name antacid 42 containing aluminium hydroxide 135, sodium bicarbonate, magnesium trisilicate, and alginic acid

GelTears a brand of artificial tears 116

gemcitabine an anticancer drug 96

gemeprost a drug used in labour 110

gemfibrozil a lipid-lowering drug 37

Gemzar a brand name for gemcitabine (an anticancer drug 96)

Genotropin a brand name for somatropin (a synthetic pituitary hormone 85)

gentamicin 253, an aminoglycoside antibiotic 62

gentian mixture acid and alkaline, an appetite stimulant 19

Genticin a brand name for gentamicin 253 (an aminoglycoside antibiotic 62)

Gentisone HC a brand name for gentamicin 253 (an aminoglycoside antibiotic 62) with hydrocortisone 263 (a corticosteroid 80)

Germolene a brand-name preparation containing phenol with chlorhexidine (both antiseptics 120)

gestodene a progestogen 88 and oral contraceptive 105

Gestone a brand name for progesterone (a female sex hormone 88)

gestrinone a drug for menstrual disorders 104

Glandosane a brand name for artificial saliva

glatiramer a drug for treatment of multiple sclerosis

glaucoma, drugs for 114

glibenclamide 255, an oral antidiabetic 82

Glibenese a brand name for glipizide (an oral antidiabetic 82)

gliclazide 256, an oral antidiabetic 82

glimepiride an oral antidiabetic 82

glipizide an oral antidiabetic 82

gliquidone an oral antidiabetic 82

Glivec a brand name for imatinib (an anticancer drug 96)

GlucaGen a brand name for glucagon (a drug for hypoglycaemia 82)

glucagon a pancreatic hormone for hypoglycaemia 82

Glucobay a brand name for acarbose (an oral antidiabetic 82)

Glucophage a brand name for metformin 306 (an oral antidiabetic 82)

Glurenorm a brand name for gliquidone (an oral antidiabetic 82)

glutaraldehyde a topical preparation for treating warts

Glutarol a brand name for glutaraldehyde (a topical wart preparation)

glycerol a drug used to reduce pressure inside the eye in glaucoma 114, and an ingredient in cough mixtures 27, skin preparations 120, laxative suppositories 45, and ear-wax softening drops 117

glyceryl trinitrate 257, an anti-angina drug 35

glycopyrronium bromide an anticholinergic used in general anaesthesia

Glypressin a brand name for terlipressin (a drug similar to vasopressin, a pituitary hormone 85, used to stop bleeding)

Glytrin a brand name for glyceryl trinitrate 257 (an anti-angina drug 35)

gold a metal used medically as a disease-modifying anitrheumatic drug 52

Golden Eye a brand name for propamidine isethionate (an antibacterial 66)

gonadorelin a drug for infertility 109

gonadotrophin chorionic a drug for infertility 109

Gopten a brand name for trandolapril (an antihypertensive 36)

goserelin 258 a female sex hormone 88 and anticancer drug 96, also used for menstrual disorders 104 and infertility 109

gout, drug for 53

gramicidin an aminoglycoside antibiotic 62 for eye, ear, and skin infections

Graneodin a brand name for gramicidin with neomycin (both aminoglycoside antibiotics 62)

granisetron an anti-emetic 21

Granocyte a brand name for lenograstim (a blood growth stimulant)

griseofulvin an antifungal 76

growth-factor inhibitors anticancer drugs 96

growth hormone somatropin (a pituitary hormone 85)

GTN 300-mcg a brand name for glyceryl trinitrate 257 (an anti-angina drug 35)

guaifenesin an expectorant 27

guanethidine an antihypertensive 36

Gyno-Daktarin a brand name for miconazole 314 (an antifungal 76)

Gyno-Pevaryl a brand name for econazole (an antifungal 76)

H

Haelan a brand name for fludroxycortide (a topical corticosteroid 120)

haem arginate a drug to treat porphyria

hair loss, drugs for 127

Halciderm Topical a brand name for halcinonide (a topical corticosteroid 120)

halcinonide a topical corticosteroid 120

Haldol a brand name for haloperidol 259 (a butyrophenone antipsychotic 15)

Half Inderal a brand name for propranolol 359 (a beta blocker 30)

halibut liver oil a natural fish oil rich in vitamin A and vitamin D (both vitamins 90)

haloperidol 259, a butyrophenone antipsychotic 15

halothane a gas used to induce general anaesthesia

Halycitrol a brand name for vitamin A with vitamin D (both vitamins 90)

hamamelis an astringent in rectal preparations 47

Hansen's disease, drug treatment for 67

Harmogen a brand name for estropipate (a drug for hormone replacement therapy 88)

Hay-Crom a brand name for sodium cromoglicate 386 (an anti-allergy drug 58)

Hayfever and Allergy Relief/Hayfever Relief brand names for cetirizine 176 (an antihistamine 58)

HBvaxPRO a brand-name vaccine 70 to protect against viral hepatitis B

HCG human chorionic gonadotrophin (a drug for infertility 109)

Hedex a brand name for paracetamol 340 (a non-opioid analgesic 9)

Hedex Extra a brand name for paracetamol 340 (a non-opioid analgesic 9) with caffeine

HeliClear a brand-name product containing lansoprazole 282 (an anti-ulcer drug 43), amoxicillin 142, and clarithromycin 189 (both antibiotics 62)

Hemabate a brand name for carboprost (a drug to control bleeding after childbirth 110)

Heminevrin a brand name for clomethiazole (a non-benzodiazepine, non-barbiturate sleeping drug 11)

heparin 260, an anticoagulant 39

heparinoid a drug applied topically to reduce inflammation of the skin 120

Hepatyrix a brand-name vaccine 70 to protect against viral hepatitis A/typhoid

Hepsera a brand name for adefovir (an antiviral 69 for chronic hepatitis B)

Herceptin brand name for trastuzumab 413 (an anticancer drug 96)

Herpid a brand name for idoxuridine (an antiviral 69)

hexachlorophene an antiseptic 120

hexamine another name for methenamine, a drug for urinary tract infections 112

hexetidine an antiseptic 120

Hexopal a brand name for inositol nicotinate (a vasodilator 31)

Hibisol a brand name for chlorhexidine (an antiseptic 120)

Hibitane a brand name for chlorhexidine (an antiseptic 120)

Hioxyl a brand name for hydrogen peroxide (an antiseptic 120)

Hiprex a brand name for hexamine/methenamine (a drug for urinary tract infections 112)

Hirudoid a brand name for heparinoid (a topical anti-inflammatory 120)

Histalix a brand-name cough preparation 27 containing diphenhydramine (an antihistamine 58), ammonium chloride, and menthol

Histoacryl a brand name for enbucrilate (a tissue adhesive)

HIV and AIDS, drugs for 100

homatropine a mydriatic 116

hormone replacement therapy (HRT), effects of (see female sex hormones 88)

hormone therapies (see anticancer drugs 96)

Hormonin a brand name for estradiol 235 (a female sex hormone 88)

Humalog a brand name for insulin lispro 269 (a drug for diabetes 82)

Human Actrapid a brand name for insulin 269 (a drug for diabetes 82)

Human Insulatard a brand name for insulin 269 (a drug for diabetes 82)

human menopausal gonadotrophins also known as menotrophin, a drug for infertility 109

Human Mixtard a brand name for insulin 269 (a drug for diabetes 82)

Human Velosulin a brand name for insulin 269 (a drug for diabetes 82)

Humatrope a brand name for somatropin, a pituitary hormone 85 (a synthetic pituitary hormone 85)

Humira a brand name for adalimumab (a disease-modifying antirheumatic drug 51)

Humulin preparations a brand name for insulin 269 (a drug for diabetes 82)

Hyalase a brand name for hyaluronidase (helps injections to penetrate tissues)

hyaluronidase helps injections penetrate tissues

Hycamtin a brand name for topotecan (an anticancer drug 96)

hydralazine an antihypertensive 36

Hydrea a brand name for hydroxycarbamide (an anticancer drug 96)

hydrochlorothiazide 261, a thiazide diuretic 32

hydrocortisone 263, a corticosteroid 80 and antipruritic 118

Hydrocortistab a brand name for hydrocortisone 263 (a corticosteroid 80)

Hydrocortone a brand name for hydrocortisone 263 (a corticosteroid 80)

hydroflumethiazide a thiazide diuretic 32

hydrogen peroxide an antiseptic mouthwash 120

hydromorphone an opioid analgesic 9

hydrotalcite an antacid 42

hydroxocobalamin vitamin B_{12} (a vitamin 90)

hydroxycarbamide a drug for chronic myeloid leukaemia 96 previously known as hydroxyurea

hydroxychloroquine an antimalarial 75 and disease-modifying antirheumatic drug 51

hydroxyurea see hydroxycarbamide, a drug for leukaemia 96

hydroxyzine an antihistamine 58 and anti-anxiety drug 13

Hygroton a brand name for chlortalidone (a thiazide diuretic 32)

hyoscine 264, a drug for irritable bowel syndrome 45, affecting the pupil 116, and to prevent motion sickness 21

hyperthyroidism (see drugs for thyroid disorders 84)

Hypnovel a brand name for midazolam (a benzodiazepine 11 used as premedication)

hypothyroidism (see drugs for thyroid disorders 84)

Hypovase a brand name for prazosin (an alpha blocker 36 antihypertensive 36 and drug for prostate disorders 112)

hypromellose a substance in artificial tear preparations 116

Hypurin a brand name for insulin 269 (a drug for diabetes 82)

Hytrin a brand name for terazosin (an alpha blocker 31 antihypertensive 36 and drug for prostate disorders 112)

I

ibandronic acid a drug for bone disorders 56

Ibugel a brand name for ibuprofen 265 (a non-steroidal anti-inflammatory 50)

Ibuleve a brand name for gel for muscular pain relief containing ibuprofen 265 (a non-steroidal anti-inflammatory 50)

ibuprofen 265, a non-opioid analgesic 9 and non-steroidal anti-inflammatory 50

Ibuspray a brand name for ibuprofen 265 (a non-steroidal anti-inflammatory 50)

ichthammol a substance in skin preparations for eczema 125

idarubicin a cytotoxic antibiotic (an anticancer drug 96)

idoxuridine an antiviral 69

ifosfamide an anticancer drug 96

Ikorel a brand name for nicorandil 326 (an anti-angina drug 35)

Ilube a brand name for acetylcysteine (a mucolytic 27) with hypromellose (a substance in artificial tear preparations 116)

imatinib an anticancer drug 96

Imdur a brand name for isosorbide mononitrate 275 (a nitrate vasodilator 31 and anti-angina drug 35)

imidapril an ACE inhibitor 31

imiglucerase an enzyme used in replacement therapy

Imigran a brand name for sumatriptan 395 (a drug for migraine 20)

imipenem an antibiotic 62

imipramine 266, a tricyclic antidepressant 14 and drug for urinary disorders 112

imiquimod a drug to treat genital warts

Immukin a brand name for interferon gamma 271 (an antiviral 69)

immunoglobulins 72 preparations injected to prevent infectious diseases (see vaccines and immunization 70)

Immunoprin a brand name for azathioprine 151 (a disease-modifying antirheumatic drug 51 and immunosuppressant 99)

immunosuppressant drugs 99

Imodium a brand name for loperamide 292 (an antidiarrhoeal 44)

Implanon a brand name for etonorgestrel (a progestogen 88)

impotence, drugs for (see drugs for infertility 109)

Imunovir a brand name for inosine pranobex (an antiviral 69)

Imuran a brand name for azathioprine 151 (a disease-modifying antirheumatic drug 51 and immunosuppressant 99)

indapamide 267 a thiazide-like diuretic 32

Inderal a brand name for propranolol 359 (a beta blocker 30)

Inderal-LA a brand name for propranolol 359 (a beta blocker 30)

Indermil a brand name for enbucrilate (a tissue adhesive)

indinavir an antiretroviral for HIV/AIDS 100

Indivina a brand-name preparation for menopausal symptoms 88 containing estradiol 235 with medroxyprogesterone 299

Indocid PDA a brand name for indometacin (a non-steroidal anti-inflammatory 50 and drug for gout 53)

Indolar a brand name for indometacin, a non-steroidal anti-inflammatory 50 and drug for gout 53

indometacin a non-steroidal anti-inflammatory 50 and drug for gout 53

indoramin an antihypertensive 36 and drug for urinary disorders 112

Inegy a brand-name preparation containing simvastatin 385 with ezetimibe 240 (both lipid-lowering drugs 37)

Infacol a brand name for dimeticone (an antifoaming agent 42)

infertility, drugs for 109

inflammatory bowel disease, drugs for 46

infliximab 268, a drug for inflammatory bowel disease 46 and disease-modifying antirheumatic drug 51

Influvac Sub-unit a brand-name influenza vaccine 70

Innohep a brand name for tinzaparin (a low-molecular-weight heparin 260 used as an anticoagulant 39)

Innovace a brand name for enalapril 228 (a vasodilator 31 and antihypertensive 36)

Innozide a brand name for enalapril 228 (a vasodilator 31 and antihypertensive 36)

inosine pranobex an antiviral 69

inositol a drug related to nicotinic acid

Inspra a brand name for eplerenone (a drug for heart failure following a heart attack 97)

Insulatard a brand name for insulin 269 (a drug for diabetes 82)

insulin 269, a drug for diabetes 82

insulin aspart a type of insulin 269 (a drug for diabetes 82)

insulin detemir a type of insulin 269 (a drug for diabetes 82)

insulin glargine a type of insulin 269 (a drug for diabetes 82)

insulin glulisine a type of insulin 269 (a drug for diabetes 82)

insulin isphane a type of insulin 269 (a drug for diabetes 82)

insulin lispro a type of insulin 269 (a drug for diabetes 82)

Insuman a brand name for insulin (human) 269 (a drug for diabetes 82)

Intal a brand name for sodium cromoglicate 386 (an anti-allergy drug 58)

Integrilin a brand name for eptifibatide (an antiplatelet drug 39 for prevention of heart attacks 95)

interferon 271, an antiviral 69 and anticancer drug 96

Intralgin a brand-name topical gel for muscle strains and sprains

Intron-A a brand name for interferon 271 (an antiviral 69 and anticancer drug 96)

Invanz a brand name for ertapenem (an antibiotic 62)

Invirase a brand name for saquinavir (an antiretroviral for HIV/AIDS 100)

Invivac a brand name for influenza vaccine 70

iodine a mineral 93

Iopidine a brand name for apraclonidine (a drug for glaucoma 114)

ipecacuanha a drug used to induce vomiting in drug overdose and poisoning, also used as an expectorant 27

Ipocol a brand name for mesalazine 305 (a drug for ulcerative colitis 46)

ipratropium bromide 272, a bronchodilator 23

irbesartan 273, an angiotensin II blocker (a vasodilator 31 and antihypertensive 36)

irinotecan an anticancer drug 96

iron a mineral 93

irritable bowel syndrome, drugs for 45

Isib a brand name for isosorbide mononitrate 275 (a nitrate vasodilator 31 and anti-angina drug 35)

Ismelin a brand name for guanethidine (an antihypertensive 36 also used to treat glaucoma 114)

Ismo a brand name for isosorbide mononitrate 275 (a nitrate vasodilator 31 and anti-angina drug 35)

isocarboxazid an MAOI antidepressant 14

isoflurane a volatile liquid inhaled as a general anaesthetic

Isogel a brand name for ispaghula (a laxative 45 and antidiarrhoeal 44)

Isoket a brand name for isosorbide dinitrate 275 (a nitrate vasodilator 31 and anti-angina drug 35)

isometheptene mucate a drug for migraine 20

isoniazid 274, an antituberculous drug 67

isophane insulin a type of insulin 269 (a drug for diabetes 82)

isoprenaline a bronchodilator 23

Isopto Alkaline a brand name for hypromellose (a substance in artificial tear preparations 116)

Isopto Atropine a brand name for atropine 150 (an anticholinergic mydriatic 116) with hypromellose (a substance in artificial tear preparations 116)

Isopto Frin brand-name eye drops containing phenylephrine (a decongestant 26) and hypromellose (a substance in artificial tear preparations 116)

Isopto Plain brand-name eye drops containing phenylephrine (a decongestant 26) and hypromellose (a substance in artificial tear preparations 116)

isosorbide dinitrate 275, a nitrate vasodilator 31 and anti-angina drug 35

isosorbide mononitrate 275, a nitrate vasodilator 31 and anti-angina drug 35

Isotard a brand name for isosorbide mononitrate 275 (a nitrate vasodilator 31 and anti-angina drug 35)

Isodur a brand name for isosorbide mononitrate 275 (a nitrate vasodilator 31 and anti-angina drug 35)

isotretinoin 276, a drug for acne 123

Isotrex a brand name for isotretinoin 276 (a drug for acne 123)

Isotrexin a brand name for isotretinoin 276 with erythromycin 233 (a drug for acne 123)

ispaghula a bulk-forming agent for constipation 45 and diarrhoea 44

isradipine a calcium channel blocker 35

Istin a brand name for amlodipine 141 (a calcium channel blocker 35 and antihypertensive 36)

itraconazole an antifungal 76

ivabradine an anti-angina drug 35

ivermectin an anthelmintic 78

J

Joy-rides a brand name for hyoscine hydrobromide 264 (used to prevent motion sickness 21)

K

Kaletra a brand name for lopinavir 293 with ritonavir (both antiretrovirals for HIV/AIDS 100)

Kalspare a brand name for triamterene 414 with chlortalidone (both diuretics 32)

Kalten a brand name for amiloride 136 with hydrochlorothiazide 261 (both diuretics 32) and atenolol 147 (a beta blocker 30)

Kamillosan an ointment 120 containing chamomile used for treating nappy rash, sore nipples, and chapped skin

kaolin an absorbent used as an antidiarrhoeal 44

Kapake a brand name for codeine 197 (an opioid analgesic 9) and paracetamol 340 (a non-opioid analgesic 9)

Karvol a brand name for menthol (a decongestant 26 inhalant)

Kay-Cee-L a brand name for potassium supplement (a mineral 93)

Kefadim a brand name for ceftazidime (a cephalosporin antibiotic 62)

Keflex a brand name for cefalexin 174 (a cephalosporin antibiotic 62)

Keftid a brand name for cefaclor (a cephalosporin antibiotic 62)

Kemadrin a brand name for procyclidine 355 (a drug for parkinsonism 18)

Kemicetine a brand name for chloramphenicol 177 (an antibiotic 62)

Kenalog a brand name for triamcinolone (a corticosteroid 80)

Kentera a brand name for oxybutynin 339 (a drug for urinary disorders 112)

Keppra a brand name for levetiracetam (an anticonvulsant 16)

Keral a brand name for dexketoprofen (a non-steroidal anti-inflammatory 50)

ketamine a drug used to induce general anaesthesia

Ketek a brand name for telithromycin (an antibiotic 62)

Ketocid a brand name for ketoprofen 279 (a non-steroidal anti-inflammatory 50)

ketoconazole 277, an antifungal 76

ketoprofen 279, a non-steroidal anti-inflammatory 50

ketorolac a non-steroidal anti-inflammatory 50 used as an analgesic 9

ketotifen an antihistamine 58 similar to sodium cromoglicate 386 used to treat allergies and asthma 24

Ketovail a brand name for ketoprofen 279 (a non-steroidal anti-inflammatory 50)

Ketovite a brand-name vitamin supplement 90

Kineret a brand name for anakinra (a disease-modifying antirheumatic drug 51)

Kivexa a brand name for abacavir with lamivudine 422 (both antiretrovirals for HIV/AIDS 100)

Klaricid a brand name for clarithromycin 189 (an antibiotic 62)

Klean-prep a brand-name osmotic laxative 45

Kliofem a brand-name product for menopausal symptoms 88 containing estradiol 235 and norethisterone 331

Kliovance a brand-name product for menopausal symptoms 88 containing estradiol 235 and norethisterone 331

Kloref a brand-name potassium (a mineral 93) supplement

Kolanticon a brand name for aluminium hydroxide 135 and magnesium oxide (both antacids 42) with dicycloverine 211 (an anticholinergic antispasmodic 44) and simeticone (an antifoaming agent 42)

Konakion a brand name for phytomenadione (vitamin K, a vitamin 90)

Kwells/Kwells Adult a brand name for hyoscine hydrobromide 264 used to prevent motion sickness 21

Kytril a brand name for granisetron (an anti-emetic 21)

L

labetalol a beta blocker 30

labour, drugs used in 110

lacidipine a calcium channel blocker 35

Lacri-Lube a brand-name eye ointment for dry eyes 116

lactic acid an ingredient in wart preparations, emollients, and pessaries

Lactugal a brand name for lactulose 280 (an osmotic laxative 45)

lactulose 280, an osmotic laxative 45

Ladropen a brand name for flucloxacillin 245 (a penicillin antibiotic 62)

Lamictal a brand name for lamotrigine 281 (an anticonvulsant 16)

Lamisil, Lamisil Once brand names for terbinafine 400 (an antifungal 76)

lamivudine 422, an antiretroviral for HIV/AIDS 100 and hepatitis B

lamotrigine 281, an anticonvulsant 16

Lanoxin a brand name for digoxin 213 (a digitalis drug 29)

lanreotide an anticancer drug 96, also used for endocrine disorders 85

lansoprazole 282, an anti-ulcer drug 43

Lantus a brand name for insulin glargine (a type of insulin 269 a drug for diabetes 82)

Lanvis a brand name for tioguanine (an anticancer drug 96)

Larafen a brand name for ketoprofen 279 (a non-steroidal anti-inflammatory 50)

Larapam a brand name for tramadol 412 (an opioid analgesic 9)

Largactil a brand name for chlorpromazine 180 (a phenothiazine antipsychotic 15 and anti-emetic 21)

Lariam a brand name for mefloquine 302 (an antimalarial 75)

Lasikal a brand name for furosemide 251 (a loop diuretic 32) with potassium (a mineral 93)

Lasilactone a brand name for furosemide 251 with spironolactone 390 (both diuretics 32)

Lasix a brand name for furosemide 251 (a loop diuretic 32)

Lasonil a brand name for heparinoid (a topical anti-inflammatory 120)

Lasoride a brand name for amiloride 136 (a potassium-sparing diuretic 32) with furosemide 251 (a loop diuretic 32 and antihypertensive 36)

Lassar's Paste a preparation for psoriasis 124 containing zinc oxide, salicylic acid and starch

latanoprost 283 a drug for glaucoma 114

laxatives 45

Laxoberal a brand name for sodium picosulfate (a stimulant laxative 45)

Ledclair a brand name for sodium calcium edetate (an antidote for poisoning with lead and heavy metals)

Lederfen a brand name for fenbufen (a non-steroidal anti-inflammatory 50)

Lederfolin a brand name for calcium folinate (used to reduce side effects of methotrexate 308)

Ledermycin a brand name for demeclocycline (a tetracycline antibiotic 62)

leflunomide a disease-modifying antirheumatic drug 51

Lemsip Max a brand name for paracetamol 340 (a non-opioid analgesic 9) with phenylephrine (a decongestant 26) and caffeine

lenograstim a blood growth stimulant

lepirudin an anticoagulant 39

lercanidipine a calcium channel blocker 35

Lescol a brand name for fluvastatin (a lipid-lowering drug 37)

letrozole an anticancer drug 96

leucovorin a vitamin 90 (also called calcium folinate or folinic acid)

Leukeran a brand name for chlorambucil (an anticancer drug 96)

leukotriene antagonists antihistamines 58

leuprorelin a drug for menstrual disorders 104 and prostate cancer 96

levamisole an anthelmintic 78

Levemir a brand name for insulin 269 (a drug for diabetes 82)

levetiracetam an anticonvulsant 16

Levitra a brand name for vardenafil (a drug for erectile dysfunction 109)

levobunolol a beta blocker 30 and drug for glaucoma 114

levobupivacaine a local anaesthetic 9

levocetirizine 176, an antihistamine 58

levodopa 284, a drug for parkinsonism 18

levofloxacin 285, an antibacterial 66

levomenthol an alcohol from mint oils used as an inhalation and topical antipruritic 118

levomepromazine an antipsychotic 15 previously known as methotrimeprazine

Levonelle 1500 a brand name for levonorgestrel 286 (a female sex hormone 88 and oral contraceptive 105)

Levonelle One Step a brand name for levonorgestrel 286 (a female sex hormone 88 and oral contraceptive 105)

levonorgestrel 286, a female sex hormone 88 and oral contraceptive 105

levothyroxine 288, a thyroid hormone 84 previously known as thyroxine

Librium a brand name for chlordiazepoxide (a benzodiazepine anti-anxiety drug 13)

lidocaine a local anaesthetic 9, anti-arrhythmic 33, and antipruritic 118 previously known as lignocaine

lignocaine see lidocaine

Li-liquid a brand name for lithium 290 (a drug for mania 15)

linezolid an antibiotic 62

lincosamides antibiotics 62

Lioresal a brand name for baclofen 152 (a muscle relaxant 54)

liothyronine a thyroid hormone 84

Lipantil a brand name for fenofibrate (a lipid-lowering drug 37)

Lipid-lowering drugs 37

Lipitor a brand name for atorvastatin 148 (a lipid-lowering drug 37)

Lipostat a brand name for pravastatin 351 (a cholesterol lowering agent 37)

liquid paraffin a lubricating agent used as a laxative 45 and in artificial tear preparations 116

Liquifilm Tears brand-name eye drops containing polyvinyl acetate (artificial tears 116)

liquorice a substance for peptic ulcers 43

Lisicostad a brand-name preparation containing lisinopril 289 (an ACE inhibitor 31) and hydrochlorothiazide 261 (a thiazide diuretic 32)

lisinopril 289, an ACE inhibitor 31

Liskonum a brand name for lithium 290 (a drug for mania 15)

lisuride a drug for parkinsonism 18

lithium 290, a drug for mania 15

Lithonate a brand name for lithium 290 (a drug for mania 15)

Livial a brand name for tibolone 406 (a female sex hormone 88)

Loceryl a brand name for amorolfine (an antifungal 76)

Locoid a brand name for hydrocortisone 263 (a corticosteroid 80)

Locorten-Vioform a brand name for clioquinol (an anti-infective skin preparation 120) with flumetasone (a corticosteroid 80)

Lodine a brand name for etodolac (a non-steroidal anti-inflammatory 50)

lodoxamide an anti-allergy drug 58

Loestrin 20, Loestrin 30 brand-name oral contraceptives 105 containing ethinylestradiol 238 and norethisterone 331

lofepramine 291, tricyclic antidepressant 14

lofexidine a drug to treat opioid withdrawal symptoms 24

Logynon a brand-name oral contraceptive 105 containing ethinylestradiol 238 and levonorgestrel 286

Lomont a brand name for lofepramine 291 (a tricyclic antidepressant 14)

Lomotil a brand-name antidiarrhoeal 44 containing atropine 150 and diphenoxylate

lomustine an alkylating agent for Hodgkin's disease 96

Loniten a brand name for minoxidil 316 (an antihypertensive 36)

loop diuretics diuretics 32

loperamide 292, an antidiarrhoeal 44

Lopid a brand name for gemfibrozil (a lipid-lowering drug 37)

lopinavir 293 an antiretroviral used for HIV/AIDS 100

loprazolam a benzodiazepine sleeping drug 11

Lopresor a brand name for metoprolol 312 (a cardioselective beta blocker 30)

loratadine 294 an antihistamine 58

lorazepam 209, a benzodiazepine anti-anxiety drug 13 and sleeping drug 11

lormetazepam a benzodiazepine sleeping drug 11

Loron a brand name for sodium clodronate (a drug for bone disorders 56 in some types of cancer 96)

losartan 295, an angiotensin II blocker (a vasodilator 31 and antihypertensive 36)

Losec a brand name for omeprazole 334 (an anti-ulcer drug 43)

Lotriderm a brand-name product containing betamethasone 158 (a corticosteroid 80) and clotrimazole 195 (an antifungal 76)

low molecular weight heparins heparin 260

Luborant a brand name for artificial saliva

Lugol's solution an iodine (a mineral 93) solution for an overactive thyroid gland 84

lumefantrine an antimalarial 75

Lumigan a brand name for bimatoprost (a drug for glaucoma 114)

Lumiracoxib a non-steroidal anti-inflammatory 50

Lustral a brand name for sertraline 382 (an antidepressant 14)

luteinizing hormone (LH) an infertility drug 109

lutropin alfa a drug for infertility 109

Lyclear a brand name for permethrin 343 (a topical antiparasitic 122)

Lyflex a brand of baclofen 152 (a muscle relaxant 54)

lymecycline 404 a tetracycline antibiotic 62

Lyrinel XL a brand name for oxybutynin 339 (a drug for urinary disorders 112)

Lyrica a brand name for pregabalin (an anticonvulsant 16) also used for neuropathic pain

Lysovir a brand name for amantadine (an antiviral 69 for influenza and parkinsonism 18)

M

Maalox a brand-name antacid 42 containing aluminium hydroxide 135 and magnesium hydroxide 296

Maalox Plus a brand-name antacid 42 containing aluminium hydroxide 135, magnesium hydroxide 296, and simeticone (an antifoaming agent 42)

MabCampath a brand name for alemtuzumab (an anticancer drug 96)

Mabron a brand name for tramadol 412 (an opioid analgesic 9)

MabThera a brand name for rituximab (an anticancer drug 96)

Macrobid a brand name for nitrofurantoin (an antibacterial 66)

Macrodantin a brand name for nitrofurantoin (an antibacterial 66)

macrolides antibiotics 62

Macugen a brand name for pegaptanib (a drug for age-related macular degeneration)

Madopar a brand name for levodopa 284 (a drug for parkinsonism 18) with benserazide (a drug to enhance the effect of levodopa)

Magnapen a brand name for ampicillin with flucloxacillin 245 (both penicillin antibiotics 62)

magnesium a mineral 93

magnesium alginate an antifoaming agent 42

magnesium aspartate a magnesium (a mineral 93) supplement

magnesium carbonate an antacid 42

magnesium citrate an osmotic laxative 45

magnesium glycerol phosphate a magnesium supplement (a mineral 93)

magnesium hydroxide 296, an antacid 42 and laxative 45

magnesium oxide an antacid 42

magnesium sulphate an osmotic laxative 45

magnesium trisilicate an antacid 42

Malarivon a brand-name antimalarial 75 containing chloroquine 178

Malarone a brand-name antimalarial 75 containing proguanil 356 with atovaquone

malathion 297, an antiparasitic 122 for head lice and scabies

male sex hormones 87

Manerix a brand name for moclobemide (a reversible MAOI antidepressant 14)

Manevac a brand name for ispaghula (a bulk-forming agent 42) with senna (a stimulant laxative 45)

mannitol an osmotic diuretic 32

Marcain a brand name for bupivacaine (a local anaesthetic 9 used in labour 110)

Marevan a brand name for warfarin 420 (an anticoagulant 39)

Marvelon a brand-name oral contraceptive 105 containing ethinylestradiol 238 and desogestrel 206 (both female sex hormones 88)

Maxalt a brand name for rizatriptan (a drug for migraine 20)

Maxepa a brand name for concentrated fish oils (used to reduce fats in the blood 37)

Maxidex a brand name for dexamethasone 208 (a corticosteroid 80) with hypromellose (a substance in artificial tear preparations 116)

Maxitrol a brand name for dexamethasone 208 (a corticosteroid 80) with hypromellose (a substance used in artificial tear preparations 116), and neomycin and polymyxin B (both antibiotics 62)

Maxolon a brand name for metoclopramide 310 (a gastrointestinal motility regulator and anti-emetic 21)

Maxtrex a brand name for methotrexate 308 an antimetabolite anticancer drug 96

MCT Oil used to treat cystic fibrosis

mebendazole an anthelmintic 78

mebeverine 298, an antispasmodic for irritable bowel syndrome 45

mecysteine a mucolytic for coughs 27

Medijel a brand name for a pain-relieving mouth gel containing lidocaine (a local anaesthetic 9) and aminacrine (an antiseptic 120)

Medinol a brand name for paracetamol 340 (a non-opioid analgesic 9)

Medised a brand name for paracetamol 340 (a non-opioid analgesic 9) with diphenhydramine (an antihistamine 58)

Medrone a brand name for methylprednisolone (a corticosteroid 80)

medroxyprogesterone 299, a female sex hormone 88 and anticancer drug 96

mefenamic acid 300, a non-steroidal anti-inflammatory 50

mefloquine 302, an antimalarial 75

Megace a brand name for megestrol (a female sex hormone 88 and anticancer drug 96)

megestrol a female sex hormone 88 and anticancer drug 96

melatonin a hormone 80

meloxicam 303, a non-steroidal anti-inflammatory 50 and non-opioid analgesic 9

melphalan an alkylating agent for multiple myeloma 96

memantidine an NMDA receptor antagonist used to treat Alzheimer's disease 18

menadiol vitamin K (a vitamin 90)

Meningitis, drugs for 66

Menitorix a brand-name vaccine 70 to protect against haemophilus influenzae/Neisseria meningitidis

menopause (see female sex hormones 88)

menotrophin a drug for infertility 109. Also known as human menopausal gonadotrophins

menstrual cycle (see drugs used to treat menstrual disorders 104)

menstrual disorders, drugs used to treat 104

menthol an alcohol from mint oils used as an inhalation and topical antipruritic 118

mepacrine an antiprotozoal 73 for giardiasis

mepivacaine a local anaesthetic 9

Mepradec a brand name for omeprazole 334 (an anti-ulcer drug 43)

meprobamate an anti-anxiety drug 13

meptazinol an opioid analgesic 9

Meptid a brand name for meptazinol (an opioid analgesic 9)

Merbentyl a brand name for dicycloverine 211 (a drug for irritable bowel syndrome 45)

mercaptamine a drug used for metabolic disorders

mercaptopurine 304, anticancer drug 96

Mercilon a brand-name oral contraceptive 105 containing ethinylestradiol 238 and desogestrel 206 (a female sex hormone 88)

Merocaine Lozenges a brand-name preparation for sore throat and minor mouth infections, containing benzocaine (a local anaesthetic 9) and cetylpyridinium (a topical antiseptic 120)

Merocets a brand-name preparation for sore throat and minor mouth infections, containing cetylpyridinium (a topical antiseptic 120)

Meronem a brand name for meropenem (an antibiotic 62)

meropenem an antibiotic 62

mesalazine 305, a drug used to treat ulcerative colitis 46

mesna a drug used to protect the urinary tract from damage caused by some anticancer drugs 96

mesterolone a male sex hormone 87

Mestinon a brand name for pyridostigmine 361 (a drug for myasthenia gravis 55)

mestranol an oestrogen 88 and oral contraceptive 105

Metalyse a brand name for tenecteplase 399 (a drug that affects blood clotting 38)

Metanium a brand-name barrier ointment 120 containing titanium dioxide, titanium peroxide and titanium salicylate

metaraminol a drug used to treat hypotension (low blood pressure)

Metenix-5 a brand name for metolazone (a thiazide-like diuretic 32)

metformin 306, a drug for diabetes 82

methadone 307, an opioid used as an analgesic 9 and to ease heroin withdrawal

Methadose a brand name for methadone 307 (an opioid used as an analgesic 9 and to ease heroin withdrawal)

Metharose a brand name for methadone 307 (an opioid used as an analgesic 9 and to ease heroin withdrawal)

methenamine a drug for urinary tract infections 112

methionine an antidote for paracetamol 340 poisoning

methocarbamol a muscle relaxant 54

methotrexate 308 (an antimetabolite anticancer drug 96 and disease-modifying antirheumatic drug 51)

methotrimeprazine see levomepromazine (an antipsychotic 15)

methylcellulose 309, a laxative 45, antidiarrhoeal 44, and artificial tear preparation 116

methyldopa an antihypertensive 36

methylphenidate a drug used to treat hyperactivity in children 19

methylprednisolone a corticosteroid 80

methyl salicylate a topical analgesic 9 for muscle and joint pain

methysergide a drug to prevent migraine 20

metipranolol a beta blocker 30 used to treat glaucoma 114

metirosine a drug for phaeochromocytoma (tumour of the adrenal glands 96)

metoclopramide 310, a gastrointestinal motility regulator and anti-emetic 21

metolazone a thiazide-like diuretic 32

Metopirone a brand name for metyrapone (a diuretic 32)

metoprolol 312, a beta blocker 30

Metosyn a brand name for fluocinonide (a topical corticosteroid 120)

Metrogel a brand name for topical metronidazole 313 (an antibacterial 66)

Metrolyl a brand name for metronidazole 313 (an antibacterial 66 and antiprotozoal 73)

metronidazole 313, an antibacterial 66 and antiprotozoal 73

Metrotop a brand name for topical metronidazole 313 (an antibacterial 66)

metyrapone a diuretic 32 to reduce fluid retention in Cushing's syndrome (an adrenal disorder 80)

mexiletine an anti-arrhythmic 33

Mexitil a brand name for mexiletine (an anti-arrhythmic 33)

Miacalcit a brand name for calcitonin (salmon) (a drug for bone disorders 56)

mianserin an antidepressant 14

Micardis a brand name for telmisartan (an angiotensin II blocker vasodilator 31 and antihypertensive 36)

Micardis Plus a brand-name antihypertensive 36 containing telmisartan (an angiotensin II blocker vasodilator 31) with hydrochlorothiazide 261 (a thiazide diuretic 32)

miconazole 314, an antifungal 76

Microgynon 30 a brand-name oral contraceptive 105 containing ethinylestradiol 238 and levonorgestrel 286

Micronor a brand-name oral contraceptive 105 containing norethisterone 331

Microval a brand-name oral contraceptive 105 containing levonorgestrel 286

midazolam a benzodiazepine 11 used as premedication

Midrid a brand-name drug for migraine 20 containing paracetamol 340 and isometheptene mucate

Mifegyne a brand name for mifepristone (a drug used during labour 110)

mifepristone a drug used during labour 110

Migraine, drugs used for 20

MigraMax a brand-name drug for migraine 20 containing aspirin (a non-opioid analgesic 9) with metoclopramide 310 (a gastrointestinal motility regulator and anti-emetic 21)

Migraleve a brand-name drug for migraine 20 containing codeine 197, paracetamol 340, and buclizine

Migril a brand-name drug for migraine 20 containing ergotamine 232, caffeine, and cyclizine

Mildison a brand name for hydrocortisone 263 (a corticosteroid 80)

Milk of Magnesia a brand name for magnesium hydroxide 296 (an antacid 42 and laxative 45)

Milpar a brand-name laxative 45 containing magnesium hydroxide 296 and liquid paraffin

milrinone a vasodilator 31 and drug for heart failure

minerals 93

Minijet Adrenaline a brand name for epinephrine 231 (a drug for anaphylaxis 512)

Minims Atropine a brand name for atropine 150 (a mydriatic 116)

Minims Chloramphenicol a brand name for chloramphenicol 177 (an antibiotic 62)

Minims Cyclopentolate a brand name for cyclopentolate (an anticholinergic mydriatic 116)

Minims Dexamethasone a brand name for dexamethasone (a corticosteroid 80)

Minims Gentamicin a brand name for gentamicin 253 (an aminoglycoside antibiotic 62)

Minims Phenylephrine a brand name for phenylephrine (a decongestant 26)

Minims Pilocarpine a brand name for pilocarpine 348 (a miotic for glaucoma 114 and to constrict pupil 116)

Minims Prednisolone a brand name for prednisolone 352 (a corticosteroid 80)

Minitran a brand name for glyceryl trinitrate 257 (an anti-angina drug 35)

Minocin a brand name for minocycline 315 (a tetracycline antibiotic 62)

minocycline 315, a tetracycline antibiotic 62

Minodiab a brand name for glipizide (an oral antidiabetic 82)

minoxidil 316, an antihypertensive 36 and treatment for male pattern baldness 127

Mintec a brand name for peppermint oil (a substance for irritable bowel syndrome 45)

Mintezol a brand name for tiabendazole (an anthelmintic 78)

Minulet a brand-name oral contraceptive 105 containing ethinylestradiol 238 and gestodene

Mirapexin a brand name for pramipexole (a drug for parkinsonism 18)

Mirena an intrauterine contraceptive device 105 containing levonorgestrel 286 (a female sex hormone 88)

mirtazapine 318, an antidepressant 14

misoprostol 319, an anti-ulcer drug 43

mitobronitol an anticancer drug 96

mitomycin a cytotoxic antibiotic for breast, stomach, and bladder cancer 96

mitoxantrone an anticancer drug 96 previously known as mitozantrone

mivacurium a drug used to relax muscles during general anaesthesia

Mixtard preparations brand names for insulin 269 (a drug for diabetes 82)

mizolastine an antihistamine 58

Mizollen a brand name for mizolastine (an antihistamine 58)

MMR II a brand-name vaccine 70 to protect against mumps/measles/rubella

Mobic a brand name for meloxicam 303 (a non-steroidal anti-inflammatory 50 and non-opioid analgesic 9)

Mobiflex a brand name for tenoxicam (a non-steroidal anti-inflammatory 50)

moclobemide a reversible MAOI antidepressant 14

modafinil a drug for narcolepsy 19

Modalim a brand name for ciprofibrate (a lipid-lowering drug 37)

Modecate a brand name for fluphenazine (an antipsychotic 15)

Modisal a brand name for isosorbide mononitrate 275 (a nitrate vasodilator 31 and anti-angina drug 35)

Moditen a brand name for fluphenazine (an antipsychotic 15)

Modrasone a brand name for alclometasone (a topical corticosteroid 120)

Modrenal a brand name for trilostane (an adrenal antagonist used for Cushing's syndrome (an adrenal disorder 80) and for breast cancer 96)

Moducren a brand-name antihypertensive 36 containing amiloride 136, hydrochlorothiazide 261, and timolol 407

Moduret-25 a brand name for amiloride 136 with hydrochlorothiazide 261 (both diuretics 32)

Moduretic a brand name for amiloride 136 with hydrochlorothiazide 261 (both diuretics 32)

moexipril an ACE inhibitor 31

Mogadon a brand name for nitrazepam 329 (a benzodiazepine sleeping drug 11)

Molipaxin a brand name for trazodone (an antidepressant 14)

molybdenum a mineral 93 required in minute amounts in the diet, poisonous if ingested in large quantities

mometasone 320, a topical corticosteroid 120

Monigen XL a brand name for isosorbide mononitrate 275 (an anti-angina drug 35)

Momomil a brand name for isosorbide mononitrate 275 (a nitrate vasodilator 31 and anti-angina drug 35)

monoclonal antibodies anticancer drugs 96

Monoparin, Monoparin CA brand names for heparin 260 (an anticoagulant 39)

Monosorb XL a brand name for isosorbide mononitrate 275 (an anti-angina drug 35)

Monphytol a brand-name antifungal 76 for athlete's foot

montelukast 321 (a leukotriene antagonist for asthma 24 and bronchospasm 23)

moracizine an anti-arrhythmic agent 33

Morphgesic SR a brand name for morphine 322 (an opioid analgesic 9)

morphine 322, an opioid analgesic 9

Morvesin XL a brand-name product containing tamsulosin 397 (an alpha blocker for prostate disorders 112)

Motens a brand name for lacidipine (a calcium channel blocker 35)

Motifene a brand name for diclofenac 210 (a non-steroidal anti-inflammatory 50)

Motilium a brand name for domperidone 218 (an anti-emetic 21)

Movelat a brand-name topical anti-inflammatory 120 containing mucopolysaccharide and salicylic acid

Movicol a brand-name osmotic laxative 45

moxifloxacin an antibiotic 62

moxisylyte a drug used to reduce pupil size after examination 116 and as a vasodilator 31 to improve blood supply to the limbs. Previously known as thymoxamine

moxonidine 323, a centrally acting antihypertensive 36

MST Continus a brand name for morphine 322 (an opioid analgesic 9)

Mucodyne a brand name for carbocisteine (a mucolytic decongestant 26)

Mucogel a brand-name antacid 42 containing aluminium hydroxide 135 and magnesium hydroxide 296

Multiparin a brand name for heparin 260 (an anticoagulant 39)

mupirocin an antibacterial 66 for skin infections 120

Murine Eye Drops a brand-name preparation containing naphazoline (a topical sympathomimetic 79)

muscle relaxants 54

MXL a brand name for morphine sulphate 322 (an opioid analgesic 9)

myasthenia gravis, drugs used for 55

Mycil a brand name for tolnaftate (an antifungal 76)

Mycobutin a brand name for rifabutin (an antituberculous drug 67)

mycophenolate mofetil an immunosuppressant drug 99

Mycota a brand name for undecanoate acid (an antifungal 76)

Mydriacyl a brand name for tropicamide (a mydriatic 116)

Mydrilate a brand name for cyclopentolate (an anticholinergic mydriatic 116)

Myelobromol a brand name for mitobronitol (an anticancer drug 96)

Myforic a brand name for mycophenolic acid (an immunosuppressant 99)

Myleran a brand name for busulphan (an alkylating anticancer drug 96)

Myocrisin a brand name for sodium aurothiomalate (a disease-modifying antirheumatic drug 51)

Myotonine a brand name for bethanechol (a parasympathomimetic for urinary retention 112)

Mysoline a brand name for primidone (an anticonvulsant 16)

N

nabilone an anti-emetic 21 derived from marijuana for nausea and vomiting induced by anticancer drugs 96

nabumetone a non-steroidal anti-inflammatory 50

nadolol a beta blocker 30

nafarelin a drug for menstrual disorders 104

naftidrofuryl 324, a vasodilator 31

Nalcrom a brand name for sodium cromoglicate 386 (an anti-allergy drug 58)

nalidixic acid an antibacterial 66

Nalorex a brand name for naltrexone (a drug for opioid withdrawal 24)

naloxone an antidote for opioid poisoning

naltrexone a drug for opioid withdrawal 24

nandrolone an anabolic steroid 88

naphazoline a topical sympathomimetic 79

Napratec a brand-name antirheumatic drug containing naproxen 325 (a non-steroidal anti-inflammatory 50 and drug for gout 53) and misoprostol 319 (an anti-ulcer drug 43)

Naprosyn a brand name for naproxen 325 (a non-steroidal anti-inflammatory 50 and drug for gout 53)

naproxen 325, a non-steroidal anti-inflammatory 50 and drug for gout 53

Naramig a brand name for naratriptan (drug for migraine 20)

naratriptan drug for migraine 20

Nardil a brand name for phenelzine (an MAOI antidepressant 14)

Naropin a brand name for ropivacaine (a local anaesthetic 9)

Nasacort a brand name for triamcinolone (a corticosteroid 80)

Naseptin a brand name for chlorhexidine (an antiseptic 120) with neomycin (an aminoglycoside antibiotic 62)

Nasonex a brand name for mometasone 320

(a topical corticosteroid 120)

nateglinide a drug for diabetes 82

Natrilix a brand name for indapamide 267 (a thiazide-like diuretic 32)

Navelbine a brand name for vinorelbine (anticancer drug 96)

Navidrex a brand name for cyclopenthiazide (a thiazide diuretic 32)

Navispare a brand name for cyclopenthiazide with amiloride 136 (both diuretics 32)

Navoban a brand name for tropisetron (an anti-emetic 21)

Nebido a brand name for testosterone 402 (a male sex hormone 87)

Nebilet a brand name for nebivolol (a beta blocker 30 antihypertensive 36)

nebivolol a beta blocker 30 (an antihypertensive 36)

nedocromil a drug similar to sodium cromoglicate 386 used to prevent asthma attacks 24

nefopam a non-opioid analgesic 9

Negaban a brand name for temocillin (an antibiotic 62)

nelfinavir an antiretroviral for HIV/AIDS 100

Neoclarityn a brand name for desloratadine 294 (an anithistamine 58)

Neo-Cortef a brand name for hydrocortisone 263 (a corticosteroid 80) and neomycin an aminoglycoside antibiotic 62

Neo-Mercazole a brand name for carbimazole 172 (an antithyroid drug 84)

neomycin an aminoglycoside antibiotic 62 used in ear drops 117

Neo-NaClex a brand name for bendroflumethiazide 154 (a thiazide diuretic 32)

Neo-NaClex-K a brand name for bendroflumethiazide 154 (a thiazide diuretic 32) with potassium

Neoral a brand name for ciclosporin 182 (an immunosuppressant 99)

NeoRecormon a brand name for erythropoietin 234 (a kidney hormone 80)

Neosporin a brand name for gramicidin with neomycin and polymyxin B (all antibiotics 62)

neostigmine a drug for myasthenia gravis 55

Neotigason a brand name for acitretin (a drug for psoriasis 124)

Nerisone a brand name for diflucortolone (a topical corticosteroid 120)

Nervous system stimulants 19

Netillin a brand name for netilmicin (an aminoglycoside antibiotic 62)

netilmicin an aminoglycoside antibiotic 62

Neulactil a brand name for pericyazine

(an antipsychotic 15)

Neulasta a brand name for pegfilgrastim (a blood growth stimulant)

Neupogen a brand name for filgrastim 243 (a blood growth stimulant)

Neupro a brand name for rotigotine (a drug for parkinsonism 18)

Neurontin a brand name for gabapentin 252 (an anticonvulsant 16) also used for neuropathic pain

nevirapine an antiretroviral for HIV/AIDS 100

Nexium a brand name for esomeprazole (an anti-ulcer drug 43)

niacin a vitamin 90

niacinamide a former name for niacin (a vitamin 90)

nicardipine a calcium channel blocker 35

niclosamide an anthelmintic 78 for tapeworm infestation

nicorandil 326, an anti-angina drug 35

Nicorette a brand of nicotine 327 (used for relief of smoking withdrawal symptoms)

nicotinamide a B vitamin (vitamins 90)

nicotine 327, a nervous system stimulant 19 and an insecticide

Nicotinell a brand name for nicotine 327 (used for relief of smoking withdrawal symptoms)

nicotinic acid a vasodilator 31, lipid-lowering drug 37, and vitamin 90

nicotinyl alcohol tartrate niacin (a vitamin 90)

nicoumalone see acenocoumarol, an anticoagulant 39

nifedipine 328, a calcium channel blocker 35

Nifedipress MR a brand name for nifedipine 328 (a calcium channel blocker 35)

Niferex a brand name for iron (a mineral 93)

Night Nurse a brand-name preparation for the relief of cold symptoms containing paracetamol 340 (a non-opioid analgesic 9) with promethazine 358 (an antihistamine 58 and anti-emetic 21) and dextromethorphan (a cough suppressant 27)

nimodipine a calcium channel blocker 35

Nimotop a brand name for nimodipine (a calcium channel blocker 35)

Nindaxa a brand name for indapamide 267 (a thiazide-like diuretic 32)

Nipent a brand name for pentostatin (an anticancer drug 96)

NiQuitin CQ a brand name for nicotine 327 (used for relief of smoking withdrawal symptoms)

nisoldipine a calcium channel blocker 35

nitrazepam 329, a benzodiazepine sleeping drug 11

Nitrocine a brand name for glyceryl trinitrate 257

(an anti-angina drug 35)

Nitro-Dur a brand name for glyceryl trinitrate 257 (an anti-angina drug 35)

nitrofurantoin an antibacterial 66

Nitrolingual a brand name for glyceryl trinitrate 257 (an anti-angina drug 35)

Nitronal a brand name for glyceryl trinitrate 257 (an anti-angina drug 35)

nitroprusside antihypertensive 36

nitrous oxide anaesthetic gas

Nivaquine a brand name for chloroquine 178 (an antimalarial 75 and disease-modifying antirheumatic drug 51)

Nivemycin a brand name for neomycin (an aminoglycoside antibiotic 62)

nizatidine an anti-ulcer drug 43

Nizoral a brand name for ketoconazole 277 (an antifungal 76)

Nocutil a brand name for desmopressin 205 (a pituitary hormone 85 used for diabetes insipidus 86)

Nolvadex-D a brand name for tamoxifen 396 (an anticancer drug 96)

nonacog alfa a synthetic form of factor IX to promote blood clotting 39

Non-Drowsy Sudafed a brand name for phenylephrine (a decongestant 26)

nonoxinol '9' a spermicidal agent

non-steroidal anti-inflammatory drugs 50

Nootropil a brand name for piracetam (an anticonvulsant 16)

noradrenaline see norepinephrine

Norditropin a brand name for somatropin (a synthetic pituitary hormone 85)

norepinephrine a drug similar to epinephrine 231 used to raise the blood pressure during shock. Previously known as noradrenaline

norethisterone 331, a female sex hormone 88 and oral contraceptive 105

norfloxacin an antibacterial 66

Norgalax a brand name for docusate (a stimulant laxative 45)

norgestimate an oral contraceptive 105

Norgeston a brand-name oral contraceptive 105 containing levonorgestrel 286

norgestrel a progestogen 88

Noriday a brand-name oral contraceptive 105 containing norethisterone 331

Norimin a brand-name oral contraceptive 105 containing ethinylestradiol 238 and norethisterone 331

Norimode a brand name for loperamide 292 (an antidiarrhoeal 44)

Norinyl-1 a brand-name oral contraceptive 105 containing norethisterone 331 and mestranol

Noristerat a brand-name injectable contraceptive 105 containing norethisterone 331 (a female sex hormone 88)

Noritate a brand name for metronidazole 313 (an antibacterial 66 and antiprotozoal 73)

Normacol Plus a brand name for frangula with sterculia (both laxatives 45)

Normax a brand name for dantron and docusate (both laxatives 45)

Normosang a brand name for haem arginate (a drug to treat porphyria)

Norphyllin SR a brand name for aminophylline 405 (a bronchodilator 23)

Norprolac a brand name for quinagolide (a drug for infertility 109 and to treat hyperprolactinaemia 85)

nortriptyline a tricyclic antidepressant 14

Norvir a brand name for ritonavir 293 (an antiretroviral for HIV/AIDS 100)

Novofem a brand-name preparation containing estradiol 235 with norethisterone 331 (both female sex hormones 88)

Novolizer a brand name for budesonide 163 (a corticosteroid 80)

NovoMix a brand name for insulin 269 (a drug for diabetes 82)

NovoNorm a brand name for repaglinide 370 an oral antidiabetic 82

NovoRapid a brand name for insulin 269 (a drug for diabetes 82)

NovoSeven a brand of factor VIIa (a blood extract to promote blood clotting 39)

Nozinan a brand name for methotrimeprazine (an antipsychotic 15)

Nuelin a brand name for theophylline 405 (a bronchodilator 23)

Nurofen a brand name for ibuprofen 265 (a non-opioid analgesic 9 and non-steroidal anti-inflammatory 50)

Nurofen Plus a brand name for ibuprofen 265 (a non-steroidal anti-inflammatory 50) with codeine 197 (an opioid analgesic 9)

Nu-Seals Aspirin a brand name for aspirin 146 (a non-opioid analgesic 9 and antiplatelet drug 39)

Nutraplus a brand name for urea (an emollient)

Nutrizym GR a brand name for pancreatin (a preparation of pancreatic enzymes 49)

Nuvelle a brand-name preparation for menopausal symptoms 88 containing estradiol 235 and levonorgestrel 286 (both female sex hormones 88)

Nylax a brand-name stimulant laxative 45

Nyogel a brand name for timolol (a beta blocker 30 and drug for glaucoma 114)

Nystaform a brand name for nystatin 332 (an antifungal 76) with chlorhexidine (an antiseptic 120)

Nystaform-HC a brand name for hydrocortisone 263 (a corticosteroid 80) with nystatin 332 (an antifungal 76) and chlorhexidine (an antiseptic 120)

Nystan a brand name for nystatin 332 (an antifungal 76)

nystatin 332, an antifungal 76

Nytol a brand-name preparation for sleep disturbance containing diphenhydramine (an antihistamine 58)

O

Oasis a brand-name preparation for cystitis containing sodium citrate and sucrose

Occlusal a brand name for salicylic acid (a wart remover)

Octim a brand name for desmopressin 205 (a pituitary hormone 85 used for diabetes insipidus 86)

octocog alfa synthetic form of factor VIII (a blood extract to promote blood clotting 39)

octreotide a synthetic pituitary hormone 85 used to relieve symptoms of cancer of the pancreas 96

Ocufen a brand name for flurbiprofen (a non-steroidal anti-inflammatory 50)

Oestrogel a brand name for estradiol 235 (an oestrogen 88)

oestrogen a female sex hormone 88

ofloxacin an antibacterial 66

Oftaquix a brand-name topical preparation of levofloxacin 285 (an antibacterial 66)

Oilatum Emollient a brand-name bath additive containing liquid paraffin for dry skin conditions 120

Oilatum Gel a brand name for a shower gel containing liquid paraffin for dry skin conditions 120

olanzapine 333, an antipsychotic 15

Olbetam a brand name for acipimox (a lipid-lowering drug 37)

Olmesartan an angiotensin II blocker (a vasodilator 31 and antihypertensive 36)

Olmetec a brand name for olmesartan (an angiotensin II blocker vasodilator 31 and antihypertensive 36)

olopatadine an anithistamine 58

Opatanol a brand name for olopatadine (an antihistamine 58)

olsalazine a drug for ulcerative colitis 46

Omacor a brand name for omega 3 acid ethyl esters (a lipid-lowering drug 37)

omalizumab a drug for asthma 24

omega-3-acid ethyl esters lipid-lowering drugs 37

omega-3-marine triglycerides lipid-lowering drugs 37

omeprazole 334, an anti-ulcer drug 43

Omnic MR a brand name for tamsulosin 397, an alpha blocker for prostate disorders 112

Oncovin a brand name for vincristine (an anticancer drug 96)

ondansetron 335, an anti-emetic 21

One-Alpha a brand name for alfacalcidol (a vitamin 90)

Opilon a brand name for moxisylyte (a vasodilator 31)

opium morphine 322 (an opioid analgesic 9)

Opticrom a brand name for sodium cromoglicate 386 (an anti-allergy drug 58)

Optil a brand name for diltiazem (a calcium channel blocker 35)

Optrex Allergy a brand name for sodium cromoglicate 386 (an anti-allergy drug 58)

Optrex Infected Eyes a brand-name preparation containing chloramphenicol 177 (an antibiotic 62)

Optrex Sore Eyes a brand-name preparation containing witch hazel (an astringent)

Optrex Red Eyes a brand-name preparation containing naphazoline (a topical sympathomimetic)

Orabase a brand-name ointment containing carmellose to protect the skin or mouth from damage

oral contraceptives 105

Oraldene a brand-name antiseptic mouthwash containing hexetidine

Oramorph a brand name for morphine 322 (an opioid analgesic 9)

Orap a brand name for pimozide (an antipsychotic 15)

Orbifen a brand name for ibuprofen 265 (a non-steroidal anti-inflammatory 50)

orciprenaline a sympathomimetic used as a bronchodilator 23

Orelox a brand name for cefpodoxime (a cephalosporin antibiotic 62)

Orgaran a brand name for danaparoid (an anticoagulant 39)

Orlept a brand name for sodium valproate 387 (an anticonvulsant 16)

orlistat 336 an anti-obesity drug

Orovite a brand-name multivitamin 90

orphenadrine 337, an anticholinergic muscle relaxant 54 and drug for parkinsonism 18

Ortho-Creme a brand name for nonoxinol '9' a spermicidal agent

Orthoforms a brand name for nonoxinol '9' a spermicidal agent

Ortho-Gynest a brand name for estriol (an oestrogen 88)

Orudis a brand name for ketoprofen 279 (a non-steroidal anti-inflammatory 50)

Oruvail a brand name for ketoprofen 279 (a non-steroidal anti-inflammatory 50)

oseltamivir 338, an antiviral 69 to protect against influenza

osmotic diuretics diuretics 32

osmotic laxatives laxatives 45

osteoporosis (see drugs for bone disorders 56)

osteomalacia and rickets (see drugs for bone disorders 56)

Otex a brand-name preparation for removal of ear wax containing urea (an emollient) and hydrogen peroxide (an antiseptic 120)

Otomize a brand name for dexamethasone 208 (a corticosteroid 80) and neomycin (an aminoglycoside antibiotic 62)

Otosporin a brand name for hydrocortisone 263 (a corticosteroid 80) with neomycin and polymyxin B (both antibiotics 62)

Otrivine a brand name for xylometazoline (a decongestant 26)

Otrivine-Antistin a brand name for antazoline (an antihistamine 58) with xylometazoline (a decongestant 26)

Ovestin a brand name for estriol (an oestrogen 88)

Ovex a brand name for mebendazole (an anthelmintic 78)

Ovranette a brand-name oral contraceptive 105 containing ethinylestradiol 238 and levonorgestrel 286

Ovysmen a brand-name oral contraceptive 105 containing ethinylestradiol 238 and norethisterone 331

oxaliplatin an anticancer drug 96

oxazepam a benzodiazepine anti-anxiety drug 13

oxcarbazepine an anticonvulsant 16

oxerutins a drug used to treat peripheral vascular disease 31

Oxis a brand name for formoterol (a bronchodilator 23)

oxpentifylline see pentoxifylline, a vasodilator 31 used to improve blood flow to the limbs in peripheral vascular disease

oxprenolol a beta blocker 30

oxybenzone a sunscreen 127

oxybuprocaine a local anaesthetic 9

oxybutynin 339, an anticholinergic and antispasmodic for urinary disorders 112

OxyContin a brand name for oxycodone (an opioid analgesic 9)

oxycodone an opioid analgesic 9

oxymetazoline a topical decongestant 26 also used for ear disorders 117

Oxymycin a brand name for oxytetracycline (a tetracycline antibiotic 62)

OxyNorm a brand name for oxycodone (an opioid analgesic 9)

oxytetracycline a tetracycline antibiotic 62

oxytocin a uterine stimulant 110

P

paclitaxel an anticancer drug 96

Paldesic a brand name for paracetamol 340 (a non-opioid analgesic 9)

palivizumab an antiviral 69

Palladone a brand name for hydromorphone (an opioid analgesic 9)

palonosetron an anti-emetic 21

Paludrine a brand name for proguanil 356 (an antimalarial 75)

Pamergan P100 a brand name for pethidine (an opioid analgesic 9) with promethazine 358 (an antihistamine 58 and anti-emetic 21)

pamidronate a drug for bone disorders 56

Panadeine a brand name for paracetamol 340 (a non-opioid analgesic 9) with codeine 197

Panadol a brand name for paracetamol 340 (a non-opioid analgesic 9)

Panadol Extra a brand name for paracetamol 340 (a non-opioid analgesic 9) with caffeine

Panadol NightPain a brand name for paracetamol 340 (a non-opioid analgesic 9) with diphenhydramine (an antihistamine 58)

Panadol Ultra a brand name for paracetamol 340 with codeine 197 (both analgesics 9)

Pancrease a brand name for pancreatin (a preparation of pancreatic enzymes 49)

pancreatic disorders, drug treatment for 49

pancreatin a preparation of pancreatic enzymes 49

Pancrex a brand name for pancreatin (a preparation of pancreatic enzymes 49)

pancuronium a muscle relaxant 54 used during general anaesthesia

Panoxyl a brand name for benzoyl peroxide 156 (a drug for acne 123)

panthenol pantothenic acid (a vitamin 90)

pantoprazole an ulcer healing drug 43

pantothenic acid a vitamin 90

papaveretum an opioid analgesic 9 containing morphine 322, codeine 197, and papaverine (a muscle relaxant 54)

Papaveretum and Hyoscine Injection a preparation containing papaveretum (an opioid analgesic 9) and hyoscine (an anticholinergic) used in general anaesthesia

papaverine a muscle relaxant 54

Papulex a brand name for nicotinamide (a drug for acne 123)

paracetamol 340, a non-opioid analgesic 9

Paracodol a brand-name analgesic 9 containing codeine 197 and paracetamol 340

Paradote a brand-name analgesic 9 containing paracetamol 340 and methionine (an antidote for paracetamol poisoning)

paraldehyde an anticonvulsant 16 used for status epilepticus

Paramax a brand-name drug for migraine 20 containing paracetamol 340 and metoclopramide 310 (a gastrointestinal motility regulator and anti-emetic 21)

Paramol a brand name for paracetamol 340 with dihydrocodeine 214 (both analgesics 9)

Paraplatin a brand name for carboplatin (an anticancer drug 96)

parecoxib an analgesic 9 and non-steroidal anti-inflammatory 50

Pariet a brand name for rabeprazole 366 (an anti-ulcer drug 43)

Parkinsonism, drugs for 18

Parlodel a brand name for bromocriptine 162 (a pituitary agent 85 and drug for parkinsonism 18)

paromomycin an antiprotozoal 73

Paroven a brand name for oxerutin (a drug used to treat peripheral vascular disease 31)

paroxetine 341, an antidepressant 14

Parvolex a brand name for acetylcysteine (a mucolytic 27) and antidote for paracetamol 340 poisoning

patch testing see treatments for eczema 125

Pavacol-D a brand name for pholcodine (a cough suppressant 27)

pegaptanib a drug for age-related macular degeneration

Pegasys a brand name for peginterferon alfa (an antiviral 69 for hepatitis C)

pegfilgrastim a blood growth stimulant

peginterferon alfa an antiviral 69 for hepatitis C

pemetrexed an anticancer drug 96

Penbritin a brand name for ampicillin (a penicillin antibiotic 62)

penciclovir an antiviral 69

penicillamine a disease-modifying antirheumatic drug 51

penicillins antibiotics 62

penicillin G see benzylpenicillin (a penicillin antibiotic 62)

Plaquenil a brand name for hydroxychloroquine (an antimalarial 75 and disease-modifying antirheumatic drug 51)

Platinex a brand name for cisplatin 186, an anticancer drug 96

Plavix a brand name for clopidogrel 194 (an antiplatelet drug 39)

Plendil a brand name for felodipine 242 (a calcium channel blocker 35)

Pletal a brand name for cilostazol (a vasodilator 31)

Pneumovax a brand-name pneumococcal vaccine 70

podophyllin a topical treatment for genital warts

podophyllotoxin a topical treatment for genital warts

podophyllum a topical treatment for warts

poloxamer a stimulant laxative 45

Polyfax a brand name for bacitracin with polymyxin B (both antibiotics 62)

polymyxin B an antibiotic 62

polystyrene sulphonate a drug to remove excess potassium from the blood

Polytar a brand name for coal tar (a substance used for eczema 125, psoriasis 124, and dandruff 126)

polyvinyl alcohol an ingredient of artificial tear preparations 116

Ponstan a brand name for mefenamic acid 300 (a non-steroidal anti-inflammatory 50)

Poractant alfa a drug to mature the lungs of premature babies

porfimer an anticancer drug 96

Pork Insulatard a brand name for insulin 269 (a drug for diabetes 82)

Pork Mixtard a brand name for insulin 269 (a drug for diabetes 82)

Posaconazole an antifungal 76

Posalfilin a brand name for podophyllum with salicylic acid (both drugs for warts)

postcoital contraception 109 (oral contraceptives 105)

potassium a mineral 93

potassium bicarbonate an antacid 42

potassium chloride potassium (a mineral 93)

potassium citrate a drug for cystitis that reduces the acidity of urine 112

potassium clavulanate a preparation of clavulanic acid (a substance given with amoxicillin 142 to make it more effective)

potassium hydroxyquinolone sulphate an agent with antibacterial 66, antifungal 76, and deodorant properties, used for skin infections 120 and acne 123

potassium iodide a drug used for overactive thyroid before surgery 84

potassium permanganate an antiseptic 120

potassium-sparing diuretics diuretics 32

povidone-iodine an antiseptic 117

pralidoxime mesylate an antidote for organophosphorus poisoning

pramipexole a drug for parkinsonism 18

pramocaine a local anaesthetic 9

pravastatin 351, a cholesterol lowering agent 37

Praxilene a brand name for naftidrofuryl 324 (a vasodilator 31)

praziquantel an anthelmintic 78 for tapeworms

prazosin an antihypertensive 36 also used to relieve urinary obstruction 112

Predenema a brand name for prednisolone 352 (a corticosteroid 80)

Predfoam a brand name for prednisolone 352 (a corticosteroid 80)

prednisolone 352 (a corticosteroid 80)

Predsol a brand name for prednisolone 352 (a corticosteroid 80)

Predsol-N a brand name for prednisolone 352 (a corticosteroid 80) with neomycin (an aminoglycoside antibiotic 62)

pregabalin an anticonvulsant 16 and drug for treatment of neuropathic pain

Pregaday a brand name for folic acid (a vitamin 90) with iron (a mineral 93)

Pregnyl a brand name for chorionic gonadotrophin (a drug for infertility 109)

Premarin a brand name for conjugated oestrogens 201 (a female sex hormone 88)

Premique a brand-name preparation for menopausal symptoms 88 containing conjugated oestrogens 201 with medroxyprogesterone 299

Prempak-C a brand-name drug for menopausal symptoms 88 containing conjugated oestrogens 201 and norgestrel

Prepadine a brand name for dosulepin 221 (a tricyclic antidepressant 14)

Prescal a brand name for isradipine (a calcium channel blocker 35)

Preservex a brand name for aceclofenac (a non-steroidal anti-inflammatory 50)

Prestim a brand name for bendroflumethiazide 154 (a thiazide diuretic 32) with timolol 407 (a beta blocker 30)

Priadel a brand name for lithium 290 (a drug for mania 15)

prilocaine a local anaesthetic 9

Primacine a brand name for erythromycin 233 (an antibiotic 62)

primaquine an antimalarial 75 and antiprotozoal 73

Primaxin a brand name for imipenem (an antibiotic 62) with cilastatin (used to make imipenem more effective)

primidone an anticonvulsant 16

Primolut N a brand name for norethisterone 331 (a female sex hormone 88)

Prioderm a brand name for malathion 297 (a topical antiparasitic 122)

Pripsen a brand name for piperazine (an anthelmintic 78) with senna (a stimulant laxative 45)

Pro-Banthine a brand name for propantheline (an anticholinergic antispasmodic for irritable bowel syndrome 45 and urinary incontinence 112)

probenecid a uricosuric for gout 53

procainamide an anti-arrhythmic 33

procaine a local anaesthetic 9

procaine benzylpenicillin a penicillin antibiotic 62

procarbazine a drug for lymphatic cancers and small-cell cancer of the lung 96

prochlorperazine 354, a phenothiazine anti-emetic 21 and antipsychotic 15

Procoralan a brand name for ivabradine (an anti-angina drug 35)

Proctofoam HC a brand name for hydrocortisone 263 (a corticosteroid 80) with pramocaine (a local anaesthetic 9)

Proctosedyl a brand name for hydrocortisone 263 (a corticosteroid 80) with cinchocaine (a local anaesthetic 9)

procyclidine 355 an anticholinergic drug for parkinsonism 18

Pro-Epanutin a brand name for fosphenytoin 347 (an anticonvulsant 16)

Proflex a brand name for ibuprofen 265 (a non-steroidal anti-inflammatory 50)

progesterone a female sex hormone 88

Prograf a brand name for tacrolimus (an immunosuppressant 99)

proguanil 356, an antimalarial 75

Progynova a brand name for estradiol 235 (an oestrogen 88)

Progynova TS a brand name for estradiol 235 (an oestrogen 88)

promazine 357, a phenothiazine antipsychotic 15

promethazine 358, an antihistamine 58 and anti-emetic 21

Propaderm a brand name for beclometasone 153 (a corticosteroid 80)

propafenone an anti-arrhythmic 33

Propain a brand-name analgesic 9 containing codeine 197, diphenhydramine, paracetamol 340, and caffeine

propamidine isetionate an antibacterial 66 for eye infections

propantheline an anticholinergic anti-spasmodic for irritable bowel syndrome 45 and urinary incontinence 112

Propine a brand name for dipivefrine (a sympathomimetic for glaucoma 114)

propiverine drug for urinary frequency 112

Pro-Plus a brand name for caffeine (a stimulant 19)

propofol an anaesthetic agent 9

propranolol 359, a beta blocker 30 and anti-anxiety drug 13

propylthiouracil 360, an antithyroid drug 84

Proscar a brand name for finasteride 244 (a drug for benign prostatic hypertrophy 112)

Prostap SR a brand name for leuprorelin (a drug for menstrual disorders 104)

protamine an antidote for heparin 260

Protelos a brand name for strontium (a drug for bone disorders 56)

Prothiaden a brand name for dosulepin 221 (a tricyclic antidepressant 14)

protirelin test of thyroid function 84

Protium a brand name for pantoprazole (an ulcer healing drug 43)

Protopic a brand name for tacrolimus (an immunosuppressant 99)

Provera a brand name for medroxyprogesterone 299 (a female sex hormone 88)

Provigil a brand name for modafinil (a drug for narcolepsy 19)

Pro-Viron a brand name for mesterolone (a male sex hormone 87)

proxymetacaine a local anaesthetic 9

Prozac a brand name for fluoxetine 247 (an antidepressant 14)

Proziere a brand name for prochlorperazine 354 (a phenothiazine anti-emetic 21)

pseudoephedrine a sympathomimetic decongestant 26

psoriasis, drugs for 124

Psorin a brand-name drug for psoriasis 124 containing dithranol, coal tar, and salicylic acid

Pulmicort a brand name for budesonide 163 (a corticosteroid 80)

Pulmozyme a brand name for dornase alfa (a drug for cystic fibrosis 27)

pupil, drugs affecting the 116

Puri-Nethol a brand name for mercaptopurine 304 (an anticancer drug 96)

PUVA (see drugs for psoriasis 124)

Pylorid a brand name for ranitidine bismuth citrate (an anti-ulcer drug 43)

Pyralvex an brand-name preparation for mouth ulcers containing salicylic acid

pyrazinamide an antituberculous drug 67

pyridostigmine 361, a drug for myasthenia gravis 55

pyridoxine a vitamin 90

pyrimethamine 362, an antimalarial 75

pyrithione zinc an antimicrobial for dandruff 126

Q

Quellada M a brand name for malathion 297 (an antiparasitic 122)

Questran a brand name for colestyramine 200 (a lipid-lowering drug 37)

quetiapine 364, an antipsychotic 15

quinagolide a drug for hyperprolactinaemia 85

quinapril an ACE inhibitor 31

quinidine an anti-arrhythmic drug 33

Quinil a brand name for quinapril (an ACE inhibitor 31)

quinine 365, an antimalarial 75

Quinoderm a brand-name preparation for acne 123 containing benzoyl peroxide 156 and potassium hydroxyquinoline sulphate (an agent for skin infections 120)

Quinoped a brand-name antifungal 76 containing benzoyl peroxide 156 and potassium hydroxyquinoline sulphate (an agent for skin infections 120)

quinolones antibiotics 62

quinupristin an antibiotic 62

Qvar a brand name for beclomethasone (a corticosteroid 80)

R

rabeprazole 366, an anti-ulcer drug 43

Radian B a brand-name topical preparation for muscle aches and sprains

raloxifene 367, an anti-oestrogen sex hormone antagonist 88 used for osteoporosis 56

raltitrexed an anticancer drug 96

ramipril 368, an ACE inhibitor 31

Ranitic a brand name for ranitidine 369 (an anti-ulcer drug 43)

ranitidine 369, an anti-ulcer drug 43

ranitidine bismuth citrate an anti-ulcer drug 43

Ranitil a brand name for ranitidine 369 (an anti-ulcer drug 43)

Rantec a brand name for ranitidine 369 (an anti-ulcer drug 43)

Ranzac a brand name for ranitidine 369 (an anti-ulcer drug 43)

Rapamune a brand name for sirolimus (an immunosuppressant 99)

Rapilysin a brand name for reteplase (a thrombolytic 40)

Rapitil a brand name for nedocromilan (an anti-allergy drug 58)

Rasagiline a drug for parkinsonism 18

rasburicase a drug used to reduce high uric acid blood levels

Rebetol a brand name for ribavirin (an antiviral 69)

reboxetine antidepressant 14

rectal and anal disorders, drugs for 47

Rectogesic a rectal preparation 47 containing glyceryl trinitrate 257 (an anti-angina drug 35)

Redoxon a brand name for vitamin C (a vitamin 90)

Reductil a brand name for sibutramine 383 (an appetite suppressant and nervous system stimulant 19)

Refludan a brand name for lepirudin (an anticoagulant 39)

Refolinon a brand name for calcium folinate (used to reduce toxicity of methotrexate 308)

Regaine a brand name for minoxidil 316 (for treatment of male pattern baldness 127)

Regranex a brand name for becaplermin, a drug for healing skin ulcers

Regulan a brand name for ispaghula (a bulk-forming agent used as a laxative 45)

Regulose a brand of lactulose 280 (an osmotic laxative 45)

Relaxit a brand-name lubricant laxative 45

Relenza a brand name for zanamivir, an antiviral 69

Relifex a brand name for nabumetone (a non-steroidal anti-inflammatory 50)

Relpax a brand name for eletriptan (a drug for migraine 20)

Remedeine a brand name for paracetamol 340 (a non-opioid analgesic 9) with dihydrocodeine 214 (an opioid analgesic 9)

Remicade a brand of infliximab 268 (a drug for Crohn's disease 46 and disease-modifying antirheumatic drug 51)

remifentanil a drug used in anaesthesia

Remegel a brand-name antacid 42 containing calcium carbonate

Reminyl a brand name for galantamine (a drug for dementia 19)

Remnos a brand name for nitrazepam 329 (a benzodiazepine sleeping drug 11)

Rennie a brand name for calcium carbonate with magnesium carbonate (both antacids 42)

Rennie Deflatine a brand-name antacid 42 containing calcium carbonate with magnesium carbonate and simeticone (an antifoaming agent)

Rennie Duo a brand-name antacid 42 containing calcium carbonate with magnesium carbonate and alginate (an antifoaming agent)

ReoPro a brand name for abciximab (an anti-platelet drug 39 to prevent heart attacks)

repaglinide 370, an oral antidiabetic 82

Requip a brand name for ropinirole (a drug for parkinsonism 18)

Resolve a brand-name analgesic 9 and antacid 42
with paracetamol 340, sodium bicarbonate,
potassium bicarbonate, sodium carbonate, citric
acid, and vitamin C (a vitamin 90)

Resonium A a brand name for polystyrene
sulphonate (a drug to remove excess potassium
from the blood)

resorcinol a keratolytic mainly for acne 123

Restandol a brand name for testosterone 402
(a male sex hormone 87)

reteplase a thrombolytic 40

Retin-A a brand name for tretinoin (a drug for
acne 123)

retinoic acid vitamin A (a vitamin 90)

retinoids vitamin A (a vitamin 90) derivatives
(drugs for psoriasis 124)

retinol vitamin A (a vitamin 90)

Retinova a brand name for tretinoin (a drug for
acne 123)

Retrovir a brand name for zidovudine 422
(an antiretroviral for HIV/AIDS 100)

Revatio a brand name for sildenafil 384 (a drug for
pulmonary hypertension)

Revaxis a brand-name vaccine 70 to protect aganst
diphtheria/tetanus/poliomyelitis

reviparin a type of heparin 260 an anticoagulant
39

Reyataz a brand name for atazanavir
(an antiretroviral for HIV/AIDS 100)

Rheumacin LA a brand name for indometacin
(a non-steroidal anti-inflammatory 50 and drug
for gout 53)

Rheumatic disorders, corticosteroids for 53

Rhinocort a brand name for budesonide 163
(a corticosteroid 80)

Rhinolast a brand name for azelastine
(an antihistamine 58)

Rhumalgan a brand name for diclofenac 210
(a non-steroidal anti-inflammatory 50)

Riamet a brand name for artemether with
lumefantrine (both antimalarials 75)

ribavirin an antiviral 69 used for certain lung
infections in infants and children

riboflavin a vitamin 90

Ridaura a brand name for auranofin (a disease-
modifying antirheumatic drug 51)

Rideril a brand name for thioridazine
(a phenothiazine antipsychotic 15)

rifabutin an antituberculous drug 67

Rifadin a brand name for rifampicin 371
(an antituberculous drug 67)

rifampicin 371, an antituberculous drug 67

Rifater a brand name for isoniazid 274 with
rifampicin 371 and pyrazinamide (all
antituberculous drugs 67)

Rifinah a brand name for isoniazid 274 with
rifampicin 371 (both antituberculous drugs 67)

Rilutek a brand name for riluzole (glutamate
inhibitor used to help patients with sclerosis)

riluzole a glutamate inhibitor used to help patients
with sclerosis

Rimactane a brand name for rifampicin 371
(an antituberculous drug 67)

Rimactazid a brand name for isoniazid 274 with
rifampicin 371 (both antituberculous drugs 67)

Rimapam a brand name for diazepam 209
(a benzodiazepine anti-anxiety drug 13, muscle
relaxant 54, and anticonvulsant 16)

rimexolone a corticosteroid 80

rimonabant 373, an appetite suppressant

Rimoxallin a brand name for amoxicillin 142
(a penicillin antibiotic 62)

Rimso-50 a brand name for dimethyl sulfoxide
(a drug for urinary infection 112)

Rinatec a brand name for ipratropium bromide
272 (a bronchodilator 23)

Rinstead pastilles a brand-name preparation for
mouth ulcers and denture sores containing
cetylpyridinium (a topical antiseptic 120) and
menthol

risedronate 374, a drug for bone disorders 56

Risperdal a brand name for risperidone 375
(an antipsychotic 15)

risperidone 375, an antipsychotic 15

Ritalin a brand name for methylphenidate (a drug
for attention-deficit hyperactivity disorder 19)

ritodrine a uterine muscle relaxant 111

ritonavir 293 an antiretroviral for HIV/AIDS 100

rituximab an anticancer drug 96

rivastigmine 376, a drug for Alzheimer's disease

Rivotril a brand name for clonazepam 193
(a benzodiazepine anticonvulsant 16)

rizatriptan a drug for migraine 20

Roaccutane a brand name for isotretinoin 276
(a drug for acne 123)

Robaxin a brand name for methocarbamol
(a muscle relaxant 54)

Robinul a brand name for glycopyrronium
bromide (an anticholinergic used in general
anaesthesia)

Robinul-Neostigmine a brand name for neostigmine
(a drug for myasthenia gravis 55)

Robitussin Chesty Cough a brand name for
guaifenesin (an expectorant 27)

Robitussin Dry Cough a brand name for
dextromethorphan (a cough suppressant 27)

Rocaltrol a brand name for calcitriol (a vitamin
90)

Rocephin a brand name for ceftriaxone
(an antibiotic 62)

rocuronium a drug to relax the muscles during general anaesthesia

Roferon-A a brand name for interferon 271 (an antiviral 69 and anticancer drug 96)

Rohypnol a brand name for flunitrazepam (a benzodiazepine sleeping drug 11)

Rommix a brand name for erythromycin 233 (an antibiotic 62)

ropinirole a drug for parkinsonism 18

ropivacaine a local anaesthetic 9

rosiglitazone 377, an oral antidiabetic 82

rosuvastatin 378, a lipid-lowering drug 37

Rotarix a brand-name vaccine 70 to protect against gastroenteritis caused by rotavirus infection

rotigotine a drug for parkinsonism 18

Rowachol a brand-name preparation of essential oils for gallstones 48

Rowatinex a brand-name preparation to dissolve kidney stones 53 and to treat kidney infections

Rozex a brand name for metronidazole 313 (an antibacterial 66)

Rusyde a brand name for furosemide 251 (a loop diuretic 32)

Rynacrom a brand name for sodium cromoglicate 386 (an anti-allergy drug 58)

Rynacrom Compound a brand name for sodium cromoglicate 386 (an anti-allergy drug 58) with xylometazoline (a decongestant 26)

Rythmodan a brand name for disopyramide (an anti-arrhythmic 33)

S

Sabril a brand name for vigabatrin (an anticonvulsant 16)

Saizen a brand name for somatropin (a synthetic pituitary hormone 85)

Salactol a brand-name wart preparation containing salicylic acid, lactic acid, and collodion 120

Salagen a brand name for pilocarpine 348 (a miotic for glaucoma 114 and to constrict the pupil 116)

Salamol a brand name for salbutamol 379 (a bronchodilator 23)

Salatac a brand-name wart preparation containing salicylic acid, lactic acid, and collodion 120

Salazopyrin a brand name for sulfasalazine 393 (a drug for inflammatory bowel disease 46 and disease-modifying antirheumatic drug 51)

salbutamol 379, a bronchodilator 23 and drug used in labour 110

salcatonin see calcitonin (salmon), a drug used for bone disorders 56

salicylic acid a keratolytic for acne 123, dandruff 126, psoriasis 124, and warts

Saliveze a brand name for artificial saliva

Salivix a brand name for artificial saliva

salmeterol 381, a bronchodilator 23

Salofalk a brand name for mesalazine 305 (a drug for ulcerative colitis 46)

Sanatogen preparations brand-name multivitamin preparations 90

Sandimmun a brand name for ciclosporin 182 (an immunosuppressant 99)

Sandocal a brand name for calcium (a mineral 93)

Sando-K a brand name for potassium (a mineral 93)

Sandostatin a brand name for octreotide (a synthetic pituitary hormone 85 used to relieve symptoms of cancer of the pancreas 96)

Sandrena a brand-name preparation for menopausal symptoms 88 containing estradiol 235

Sanomigran a brand name for pizotifen 350 (a drug for migraine 20)

saquinavir an antiretroviral for HIV/AIDS 100

Savlon a brand name for chlorhexidine with cetrimide (both skin antiseptics 120)

Scheriproct a brand name for prednisolone 352 (a corticosteroid 80) with cinchocaine (a local anaesthetic 9)

Scopoderm TTS a brand-name anti-emetic 21 containing hyoscine 264

Sea-Legs a brand name for meclozine (an antihistamine 58 used to prevent motion sickness 90)

Sebomin MR a brand name for minocycline (an antibiotic 62)

secobarbital a barbiturate sleeping drug 11

Seconal Sodium a brand name for secobarbital (a barbiturate sleeping drug 11)

Sectral a brand name for acebutolol (a beta blocker 30)

Securon SR a brand name for verapamil 419 (an anti-arrhythmic 33 and anti-angina drug 35)

selegiline a drug for severe parkinsonism 18

selenium a mineral 93

selenium sulphide a substance for skin inflammation 120 and dandruff 126

Selsun a brand-name dandruff shampoo 126 containing selenium sulphide

Semi-Daonil a brand name for glibenclamide 255 (an oral antidiabetic 82)

senna a stimulant laxative 45

Senokot a brand name for senna (a stimulant laxative 45)

Septanest a brand name for articaine (a local anaesthetic 9) with epinephrine 231

Solpadeine Plus a brand-name analgesic 9 containing codeine 197, paracetamol 340, and caffeine

Solpaflex a brand-name analgesic 9 containing ibuprofen 265 (a non-steroidal anti-inflammatory 50) with codeine 197

Soltamox a brand name for tamoxifen 396, an anti-oestrogen anticancer drug 96

Solu-Cortef a brand name for hydrocortisone 263 (a corticosteroid 80)

Solu-Medrone a brand name for methylprednisolone (a corticosteroid 80)

Solvazinc a brand name for zinc (a mineral 93)

somatropin a synthetic pituitary hormone 85

Somatuline a brand name for lanreotide (an anticancer drug 96 and drug for endocrine disorders 85)

Sominex a brand-name sleeping drug 11 containing promethazine 358

Somnite a brand name for nitrazepam 329 (a benzodiazepine sleeping drug 11)

Sonata a brand name for zaleplon (a sleeping drug 11)

Soneryl a brand name for butobarbital (a barbiturate sleeping drug 11)

Soothelip a brand-name cold-sore cream containing aciclovir 131 (an antiviral 69)

sorafenib an anticancer drug 96

sorbitol a sweetening agent used in diabetic foods, and included in skin creams as a moisturizer 120

Sotacor a brand name for sotalol 389 (a beta blocker 30)

sotalol 389, a beta blocker 30

Spasmonal a brand name for alverine citrate (an antispasmodic for irritable bowel syndrome 45)

Spectraban a brand name for aminobenzoic acid with padimate-O (both sunscreens 127)

Spiriva a brand name for tiotropium 409 (a bronchodilator 23)

spironolactone 390, a potassium-sparing diuretic 32

Sporanox a brand name for itraconazole (an antifungal 76)

Sprilon a brand-name skin preparation 120 containing dimeticone and zinc oxide

Stalevo a brand-name product containing levodopa 284 with carbidopa (a drug that enhances the effect of levodopa) and entacapone (drugs for parkinsonism 18)

Staril a brand name for fosinopril (an ACE inhibitor 31)

Starlix a brand name for netaglenide (an oral antidiabetic 82)

stavudine an antiretroviral used to treat HIV/AIDS 100

Stelazine a brand name for trifluoperazine (a phenothiazine antipsychotic 15 and anti-emetic 21)

Stemetil a brand name for prochlorperazine 354 (a phenothiazine anti-emetic 21 and antipsychotic 15)

sterculia a bulk-forming agent used as an antidiarrhoeal 44 and laxative 45

Ster-Zac a brand name for triclosan (an antimicrobial 118)

Stesolid a brand name for diazepam 209 (a benzodiazepine anti-anxiety drug 13, muscle relaxant 54, and anticonvulsant 16)

Stiemycin a brand name for erythromycin 233 (an antibiotic 62)

stilboestrol see diethylstilbestrol (a female sex hormone 88)

Stilnoct a brand name for zolpidem (a sleeping drug 11)

stimulant (contact) laxatives laxatives 45

St John's Wort a herbal antidepressant 14 that interacts with many other drugs

Strattera a brand name for atomoxetine (a drug for attention-deficit hyperactivity disorder 19)

Strefen a brand-name preparation for sore throats containing flurbiprofen (a non-steroidal anti-inflammatory 50)

Strepsils a brand-name preparation for mouth and throat infections containing amylmetacresol and dichlorobenzyl alcohol (both antiseptics 120)

Streptase a brand name for streptokinase 391 (a thrombolytic 40)

streptokinase 391, a thrombolytic 40

streptomycin an antituberculous drug 67 and aminoglycoside antibiotic 62

Striant SR a brand name for testosterone 402 (a male sex hormone 87)

Stronazon MR a brand name for tamsulosin 397, an alpha blocker for prostate disorders 112

strontium ranelate a drug for bone disorders 56

Stugeron a brand name for cinnarizine 184 (an antihistamine 58 anti-emetic 21)

Sublimaze a brand name for fentanyl (an opioid analgesic 9)

Subutex a brand name for buprenorphine (an opioid analgesic 9)

sucralfate 392, an ulcer-healing drug 43

Sudafed a brand name for pseudoephedrine (a decongestant 26)

Sudafed-Congestion Cold and Flu a brand name for paracetamol 340 (a non-opioid analgesic 9) and pseudoephedrine (a decongestant 26)

Sudocrem a brand-name skin preparation 120 containing benzyl benzoate and zinc oxide

sulconazole an antifungal 76

Suleo-M a brand name for malathion 297 (a topical antiparasitic 120)

sulfacetamide a sulphonamide antibacterial 66

sulfadiazine a sulphonamide antibacterial 66

sulfadoxine a drug used with pyrimethamine 362 for malaria 75

sulfamethoxazole a sulphonamide antibacterial 66 combined with trimethoprim 415 in co-trimoxazole 203

sulfasalazine 393, a drug for inflammatory bowel disease 46 and disease-modifying antirheumatic drug 51

sulfinpyrazone a drug for gout 53

sulindac a non-steroidal anti-inflammatory 50

sulphur a topical antibacterial 66 and anti-fungal 76 for acne 123 and dandruff 126

sulpiride 138 an antipsychotic 15

Sulpitil a brand name for sulpiride 138 (an antipsychotic 15)

Sulpor a brand name for sulpiride 138 (an antipsychotic 15)

sumatriptan 395, a drug for migraine 20

sunscreens 127

Supralip a brand name for a fenofibrate (a lipid-lowering drug 37)

Suprane a brand name for desflurane (a general anaesthetic)

Suprax a brand name for cefixime (a cephalosporin antibiotic 62)

Suprecur a brand name for buserelin (a drug for menstrual disorders 104 and prostate cancer 96)

Suprefact a brand name for buserelin (a drug for menstrual disorders 104 and prostate cancer 96)

Surgam a brand name for tiaprofenic acid (a non-steroidal anti-inflammatory 50)

Surmontil a brand name for trimipramine (a tricyclic antidepressant 14)

Suscard a brand name for glyceryl trinitrate 257 (an anti-angina drug 35)

Sustac a brand name for glyceryl trinitrate 257 (an anti-angina drug 35)

Sustanon a brand name for testosterone 402 (a male sex hormone 87)

Sustiva a brand name for efavirenz 227 (an antiretroviral for HIV/AIDS 100)

suxamethonium a muscle relaxant used during general anaesthesia

Symbicort a brand name for formoterol (a bronchodilator 23) with budesonide (a corticosteroid 80)

Symmetrel a brand name for amantadine (an antiviral 69 and drug for parkinsonism 18)

Synacthen a brand name for tetracosactide (a drug used to assess adrenal gland function 85)

Synagis a brand name for palivizumab, an antiviral 69

Synalar a brand name for fluocinolone (a topical corticosteroid 120)

Synalar C a brand name for fluocinolone (a topical corticosteroid 120) with clioquinol (an antiseptic 120)

Synalar N a brand name for fluocinolone (a topical corticosteroid 120) with neomycin (an aminoglycoside antibiotic 62)

Synarel a brand name for nafarelin (a drug for menstrual disorders 104)

Syndol a brand name for codeine 197 and paracetamol 340 (both analgesics 9), with caffeine (a stimulant 19) and doxylamine (an antihistamine 58)

Synercid a brand name preparation of quinupristin and dalfopristin (both antibiotics 62)

Synflex a brand name for naproxen 325 (a non-steroidal anti-inflammatory 50 and drug for gout 53)

Synphase a brand-name oral contraceptive 105 containing ethinylestradiol 238 and norethisterone 331

Syntaris a brand name for flunisolide (a corticosteroid 80)

Syntocinon a brand name for oxytocin (a uterine stimulant 110)

Syntometrine a brand name for ergometrine with oxytocin (both uterine stimulants 110)

Syprol a brand name for propranolol 359 (a beta blocker 30)

Syscor MR a brand name for nisoldipine (a calcium channel blocker 35)

Sytron a brand name for sodium feredetate (iron, a mineral 93)

T

Tabphyn MR a brand name for tamsulosin 397, an alpha blocker for prostate disorders 112

tacalcitol a drug for psoriasis 124

tacrolimus an immunosuppressant 99

tadalafil a drug for erectile dysfunction 109

Tagamet a brand name for cimetidine 183 (an anti-ulcer drug 43)

Tambocor a brand name for flecainide (an anti-arrhythmic 33)

Tamiflu a brand name for oseltamivir 338 (an antiviral 69 to protect against influenza)

tamoxifen 396, an anticancer drug 96

tamsulosin 397, an alpha blocker for prostate disorders 112

Tanatril a brand name for imidapril (an ACE inhibitor 31)

Tarceva a brand name for erlotinib (an anticancer drug 96)

Targocid a brand name for teicoplanin (an antibiotic 62)

Targretin a brand name for bexarotene (an anticancer drug 96)

Tarivid a brand name for ofloxacin (an antibiotic 62)

Tarka a brand-name preparation containing trandolapril (an ACE inhibitor 31) with verapamil 419 (an anti-arrhythmic 33 and anti-angina drug 35)

Tasmar a brand name for tolcapone (a drug for parkinsonism 18)

Tavanic a brand name for levofloxacin 285 (an antibacterial 66)

Tavegil a brand name for clemastine (an antihistamine 58)

Taxol a brand name for paclitaxel (an anticancer drug 96)

Taxotere a brand name for docetaxel (an anticancer drug 96)

tazarotene a retinoid (vitamin A 90) for psoriasis 124

tazobactam an antibiotic 62

Tazocin a brand name for piperacillin (an antibiotic 62) with tazobactam (a substance that increases the effectiveness of piperacillin)

TCP a brand-name antiseptic 120 containing phenol, chlorinated and halogenated phenols, sodium salicylate, and glycerol

tear preparations, artificial drugs affecting the pupil 116

Tears Naturale a brand-name artificial tear preparation 116 containing hypromellose

tegafur an anticancer drug 96

Tegretol a brand name for carbamazepine 170 (an anticonvulsant 16)

teicoplanin an antibiotic 62

Telfast a brand name for fexofenadine (an antihistamine 58)

telithromycin an antibiotic 62

telmisartan a vasodilator 31 and antihypertensive drug 36

Telzir a brand name for fosamprenavir (an antiretroviral for HIV/AIDS 100)

temazepam 398, a benzodiazepine sleeping drug 11

Temgesic a brand name for buprenorphine (an opioid analgesic 9)

temocillin an antibiotic 62

Temodal a brand name for temozolomide (anticancer drug 96)

temozolomide anticancer drug 96

tenecteplase 399, a thrombolytic 40

Tenif a brand name for atenolol 147 (a beta blocker 30) with nifedipine 328 (an anti-angina drug 35 and antihypertensive 36)

tenofovir an antiretroviral used for HIV/AIDS 100

Tenoret-50 a brand name for atenolol 147 (a beta blocker 30) with chlortalidone (a thiazide diuretic 32)

Tenoretic a brand name for atenolol 147 (a beta blocker 30) with chlortalidone (a thiazide diuretic 32)

Tenormin a brand name for atenolol 147 (a beta blocker 30)

tenoxicam a non-steroidal anti-inflammatory 50

Tensipine MR a brand name for nifedipine 328 (a calcium channel blocker 35)

Tensium a brand name for diazepam 209 (a benzodiazepine anti-anxiety drug 13 and muscle relaxant 54)

Teoptic a brand name for carteolol (a beta blocker 30 used for glaucoma 114)

terazosin a sympatholytic antihypertensive 36, also used for prostate disorders 112

terbinafine 400 an antifungal 76

terbutaline 401, a sympathomimetic bronchodilator 23 and uterine muscle relaxant 111

terfenadine an antihistamine 58

teriparatide a drug for bone disorders 56

terlipressin a drug similar to vasopressin (a pituitary hormone 85) used to stop bleeding

Tertroxin a brand name for liothyronine (a thyroid hormone 84)

Testim a brand name for testosterone 402 (a male sex hormone 87)

Testogel a brand name for testosterone 402 (a male sex hormone 87)

testosterone 402, a male sex hormone 87

tetrabenazine a drug for tremor

tetracaine a local anaesthetic 9 previously known as amethocaine

tetracosactide a drug similar to corticotropin, used to assess adrenal gland function 85

tetracycline 404 an antibiotic 62 and antimalarial 75

tetracyclines antibiotics 62

Tetralysal-300 a brand name for lymecycline 404 (a tetracycline antibiotic 62)

T-Gel a brand name for coal tar (an agent for dandruff 126 and psoriasis 124)

thalidomide a drug for leprosy 66 and some types of cancer 96

theophylline/aminophylline 405, a bronchodilator 23

Tropium a brand name for chlordiazepoxide (a benzodiazepine anti-anxiety drug 13)

trospium an anticholinergic drug for urinary disorders 112

Trosyl a brand name for tioconazole (an antifungal 76)

Trusopt a brand name for dorzolamide 220 (a drug for glaucoma 114)

Truvada a brand name for tenofovir with emtricitabine (both antiretrovirals for HIV/AIDS 100)

trypanosomiasis see antiprotozoal drugs 73

tryptophan an antidepressant 14

Tuinal a brand name for amobarbital with secobarbital (both barbiturate sleeping drugs 11)

Twinrix a brand-name vaccine 70 to protect against hepatitis A/hepatitis B

Tygacil a brand name for tigecycline (an antibiotic 62)

Tylex a brand-name analgesic 9 containing codeine 197 and paracetamol 340

Tyrozets a brand name for benzocaine (a local anaesthetic 9) with tyrothricin (an antibiotic 62)

U

Ubretid a brand name for distigmine (a parasympathomimetic for urinary retention 112 and myasthenia gravis 55)

Ucerax a brand name for hydroxyzine (an antihistamine 58 and anti-anxiety drug 13)

Uftoral a brand name for tegafur (an anticancer drug 96) with uracil (to prolong the drug's effects)

ulcerative colitis see drugs for inflammatory bowel disease 46

Ultiva a brand name for remifentanil (a drug used in anaesthesia)

Ultralanum Plain a brand name for fluocortolone (a topical corticosteroid 120)

Ultraproct a brand name for fluocortolone (a topical corticosteroid 120) with cinchocaine (a local anaesthetic 9)

undecenoic acid an antifungal 76 to treat athlete's foot

Unguentum M a brand-name preparation for dry skin conditions 120

Uniflu a brand name for codeine 197 (an opioid analgesic 9 and cough suppressant 27) with diphenhydramine (an antihistamine 58), paracetamol 340 (a non-opioid analgesic 9), phenylephrine (a decongestant 26), and caffeine (a stimulant 19)

Uniphyllin Continus a brand name for theophylline 405 (a bronchodilator 23)

Uniroid HC a brand name for hydrocortisone 263 (a corticosteroid 80) with cinchocaine (a local anaesthetic 9)

Univer a brand name for verapamil 419 (an anti-arrhythmic 33 and anti-angina drug 35)

urea a topical treatment to moisturize dry skin 120 and soften ear wax 117

Urdox a brand name for ursodeoxycholic acid (a drug for gallstones 48)

Uriben a brand name for nalidixic acid (an antibacterial 66)

urinary disorders, drugs used for 112

Urispas-199 a brand name for flavoxate (a urinary antispasmodic 112)

urofollitropin a drug for pituitary disorders 85

Uromitexan a brand name for mesna (used to protect the urinary tract from damage caused by some anticancer drugs 96)

ursodeoxycholic acid a drug for gallstones 48

Ursofalk a brand name for ursodeoxycholic acid (a drug for gallstones 48)

Uterine muscle relaxants 111

Utinor a brand name for norfloxacin (an antibiotic 62)

Utovlan a brand name for norethisterone 331 (a female sex hormone 88)

Uvistat a brand name for a sunscreen preparation 127

V

vaccines and immunization 70

Vagifem a brand name for estradiol 235 (a female sex hormone 88)

Vaginyl a brand name for metronidazole 313 (an antibacterial 66 and antiprotozoal 73)

valaciclovir an antiviral 69

Valclair a brand name for diazepam 209 (a benzodiazepine anti-anxiety drug 13, muscle relaxant 54 and anticonvulsant 16)

Valcyte a brand name for valganciclovir (an antiviral 69)

Valderma Cream a brand-name preparation for minor skin troubles, containing potassium hydroxyquinoline sulphate (an antibacterial 66 and antifungal 76), and chlorocresol (a topical antiseptic 120)

valganciclovir an antiviral 69 used for cytomegalovirus infection in HIV/AIDS 100

Vallergan a brand name for trimeprazine (an antihistamine 58)

Virazole a brand name for ribavirin (an antiviral 69)

Viread a brand name for tenofovir (an antiretroviral for HIV/AIDS 100)

Viridal Duo a brand name for alprostadil (a prostaglandin for erectile dysfunction 87, 109)

Virormone a brand name for testosterone 402 (a male sex hormone 87)

Visclair a brand name for mecysteine (a mucolytic for coughs 27)

Viscotears a brand of artificial tears 116

Viskaldix a brand name for pindolol (a beta blocker 30) and clopamide (a thiazide diuretic 32)

Visken a brand name for pindolol (a beta blocker 30)

Vistabel a brand name for botulinum toxin 161 (a muscle relaxant 54)

Vista-Methasone a brand name for betamethasone 158 (a corticosteroid 80)

Vistide a brand name for cidofovir (an antiviral 69 used for cytomegalovirus infections in HIV/AIDS 100)

vitamin A a vitamin 90

vitamin B Complex vitamins 90

vitamin B₁ another name for thiamine (a vitamin 90)

vitamin B₂ another name for riboflavin (a vitamin 90)

vitamin B₆ another name for pyridoxine (a vitamin 90)

vitamin B₁₂ another name for hydroxocobalamin (a vitamin 90)

vitamin C another name for ascorbic acid (a vitamin 90)

vitamin D a vitamin 90

vitamin D analogues drugs for psoriasis 124

vitamin E a vitamin 90

vitamin K a vitamin 90

vitamins 90

Vivacor a brand name for bisoprolol 160 (a beta blocker 30)

Vivotif a brand-name vaccine 70 to protect against typhoid fever

Volmax a brand name for salbutamol 379 (a bronchodilator 23 also used in uncomplicated premature labour 110)

Volraman a brand name for diclofenac 210 (a non-steroidal anti-inflammatory 50)

Volsaid Retard a brand name for diclofenac 210 (a non-steroidal anti-inflammatory 50)

Voltarol a brand name for diclofenac 210 (a non-steroidal anti-inflammatory 50)

voriconazole an antifungal 76

W

warfarin 420, an anticoagulant 39

Warticon a brand name for podophyllotoxin (a drug for genital warts)

WaspEze a brand-name aerosol preparation for insect bites and stings containing benzocaine (a local anaesthetic 9) and mepyramine (an antihistamine 58)

Waxsol a brand name for docusate (an ear wax softener 117)

Welldorm Elixir a brand name for cloral hydrate (non-benzodiazepine, non-barbiturate sleeping drug 11)

Welldorm Tablets a brand name for cloral betaine (non-benzodiazepine, non-barbiturate sleeping drug 11)

Wellvone a brand name for atovaquone (an antiprotozoal 73 and antimalarial 75)

what to do if you miss a pill see oral contraceptives 105

Windeze a brand-name preparation for flatulance and abdominal distension containing simethicone (an antifoaming agent)

WinRho SDF a brand-name immunoglobulin 72 used to prevent sensitization to Rhesus antigen

witch hazel an astringent used in topical 120 and rectal preparations 47

Woodward's Gripe Water a brand-name preparation for wind pain in infants, containing sodium bicarbonate (an antacid 42) and dill seed oil

X

Xagrid a brand name for anagrelide

Xalacom a brand name for latanoprost 283 with timolol 407 (both drugs for glaucoma 114)

Xalatan a brand name for latanoprost 283 (a drug for glaucoma 114)

Xanax a brand name for alprazolam (a benzodiazepine anti-anxiety drug 13)

Xatral XL a brand name for alfuzosin (a drug for prostate disorders 87)

Xeloda a brand name for capecitabine (an anticancer drug 96)

Xenical a brand name for orlistat 336 (an anti-obesity drug)

Xigris a brand name for drotrecogin alfa (a drug that affects blood clotting 38)

xipamide a thiazide-like diuretic 32

Xolair a brand name for omalizumab a drug for severe asthma 24

Xylocaine a brand name for lidocaine (a local anaesthetic 9)

xylometazoline a decongestant 26

Xyloproct a brand-name anal preparation 47 containing hydrocortisone 263, aluminium acetate, lidocaine, and zinc oxide

Xyzal a brand name for levocetirizine 176 (an antihistamine 58)

Y

Yasmin a brand-name oral contraceptive 105 containing ethinylestradiol 238 with drospirenone (a progestogen 88)

Yentreve a brand name for duloxetine (a drug for stress incontinence 112)

Yutopar a brand name for ritodrine (a uterine muscle relaxant 111)

Z

Zaditen a brand name for ketotifen (a drug used to prevent asthma 24)

zafirlukast a leukotriene antagonist for asthma 24 and bronchospasm 23

zaleplon a sleeping drug 11

Zamadol a brand name for tramadol 412 (an opioid analgesic 9)

Zanaflex a brand name for tizanidine

zanamivir an antiviral 69

Zanidip a brand name for lercanidipine (a calcium channel blocker 35)

Zanprol a brand name for omeprazole (an anti-ulcer drug 43)

Zantac a brand name for ranitidine 369 (an anti-ulcer drug 43)

Zaponex a brand name for clozapine 196 (an antipsychotic 15)

Zarontin a brand name for ethosuximide (an anticonvulsant 16)

Zeffix a brand name for lamivudine 422 (an antiretroviral 100 for hepatitis B)

Zenapax a brand name for daclizumab (an immunosuppressant 99)

Zerit a brand name for stavudine (an antiretroviral for HIV/AIDS 100)

Zestoretic a brand name for lisinopril 289 (an ACE inhibitor 31) and hydrochlorothiazide 261 (a diuretic 32)

Zestril a brand name for lisinopril 289 (an ACE inhibitor 31)

Ziagen a brand name for abacavir (an antiretroviral for HIV/AIDS 100)

Zibor a brand name for bemiparin (a type of heparin 260, an anticoagulant 39)

Zidoval a brand name for topical metronidazole 313 (an antibacterial 66 and antiprotozoal 73)

zidovudine (AZT) 422, an antiretroviral for HIV/AIDS 100

Zileze a brand name for zopiclone 423 (a sleeping drug 11)

Zimbacol XL a brand name for bezafibrate 159 (a lipid-lowering drug 37)

Zimovane, Zimovane LS brand names for zopiclone 423 (a sleeping drug 11)

Zinacef a brand name for cefuroxime (a cephalosporin antibiotic 62)

zinc a mineral 93

zinc acetate a drug used in Wilson's disease (a metabolic disorder)

zinc oxide a soothing agent 120

zinc pyrithione an antimicrobial with antibacterial 66 and antifungal 76 properties used for dandruff 126

zinc sulphate zinc (a mineral 93)

Zineryt a brand-name acne preparation 123 containing erythromycin 233 (an antibiotic 62) and zinc (a mineral 93)

Zinnat a brand name for cefuroxime (a cephalosporin antibiotic 62)

Zirtek a brand name for cetirizine 176 (an antihistamine 58)

Zispin a brand name for mirtazapine 318 (an antidepressant 14)

Zita a brand name for cimetidine 183 (an anti-ulcer drug 43)

Zithromax a brand name for azithromycin (an antibiotic 62)

Zocor a brand name for simvastatin 385 (a lipid-lowering drug 37)

Zocor Heart-Pro a brand name for simvastatin 385 (a lipid-lowering drug 37)

Zofran a brand name for ondansetron 335 (an anti-emetic 21)

Zoladex a brand name for goserelin 258 (a female sex hormone 88 and anticancer drug 96)

zoledronic acid a drug for bone disorders 56 in cancer 96

Zoleptil a brand name for zotepine (an antipsychotic 15)

zolmitriptan drug for migraine 20

zolpidem a sleeping drug 11

Zolvera a brand name for verapamil 419 (an anti-angina drug 35 and anti-arrhythmic 33)

Zomacton a brand name for somatropin (a synthetic pituitary hormone 85)

Zometa a brand name for zoledronic acid (a drug for bone disorders 56)

Zomig a brand name for zolmitriptan (a drug for migraine 20)

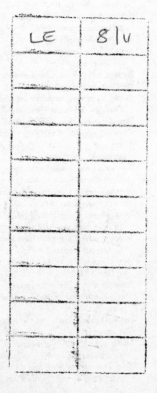